Current Progress in Sarcoma Research

Current Progress in Sarcoma Research

Edited by Natalie Kasey

hayle medical

New York

Hayle Medical,
750 Third Avenue, 9th Floor,
New York, NY 10017, USA

Visit us on the World Wide Web at:
www.haylemedical.com

ISBN: 978-1-63241-843-2

Cataloging-in-Publication Data

Current progress in sarcoma research / edited by Natalie Kasey.
p. cm.
Includes bibliographical references and index.
ISBN 978-1-63241-843-2
1. Sarcoma. 2. Sarcoma--Research. 3. Cancer. 4. Tumors. I. Kasey, Natalie.
RC262 .C87 2020
616.994--dc23

Table of Contents

Preface

Every book is a source of knowledge and this one is no exception. The idea that led to the conceptualization of this book was the fact that the world is advancing rapidly; which makes it crucial to document the progress in every field. I am aware that a lot of data is already available, yet, there is a lot more to learn. Hence, I accepted the responsibility of editing this book and contributing my knowledge to the community.

Sarcoma is a cancer which originates in the transformed cells of mesenchymal origin. All malignant tumors consisting of the cartilage, cancellous bone, muscle, fat, hematopoietic or vascular tissues are sarcomas. Askin's tumor, malignant hemangioendothelioma, osteosarcoma, chondrosarcoma, malignant schwannoma, etc. are certain types of sarcomas. Surgery is commonly used in the treatment of sarcoma. Limb-sparing surgery is performed in extremity tumor cases. Along with surgery, chemotherapy and radiation therapy can also be used. Sarcomas in humans are quite rare, though it can affect people of all ages. Oncology is an upcoming field of science that has undergone rapid development over the past few decades. This book aims to shed light on some of the unexplored aspects of sarcoma and the recent researches in this condition. For all readers who are interested in sarcoma diagnosis and management, the case studies included in this book will serve as an excellent guide to develop a comprehensive understanding.

While editing this book, I had multiple visions for it. Then I finally narrowed down to make every chapter a sole standing text explaining a particular topic, so that they can be used independently. However, the umbrella subject sinews them into a common theme. This makes the book a unique platform of knowledge.

I would like to give the major credit of this book to the experts from every corner of the world, who took the time to share their expertise with us. Also, I owe the completion of this book to the never-ending support of my family, who supported me throughout the project.

Editor

1

Mesenchymal stromal cells of osteosarcoma patients do not show evidence of neoplastic changes during long-term culture

Emilie P Buddingh[1], S Eriaty N Ruslan[1], Christianne M A Reijnders[2], Karoly Szuhai[3], Marieke L Kuijjer[2], Helene Roelofs[4], Pancras C W Hogendoorn[2], R Maarten Egeler[1], Anne-Marie Cleton-Jansen[2†] and Arjan C Lankester[1*†]

Abstract

Background: In vitro expanded mesenchymal stromal cells (MSCs) are increasingly used as experimental cellular therapy. However, there have been concerns regarding the safety of their use, particularly with regard to possible oncogenic transformation. MSCs are the hypothesized precursor cells of high-grade osteosarcoma, a tumor with often complex karyotypes occurring mainly in adolescents and young adults.

Methods: To determine if MSCs from osteosarcoma patients could be predisposed to malignant transformation we cultured MSCs of nine osteosarcoma patients and five healthy donors for an average of 649 days (range 601–679 days). Also, we compared MSCs derived from osteosarcoma patients at diagnosis and from healthy donors using genome wide gene expression profiling.

Results: Upon increasing passage, increasing frequencies of binucleate cells were detected, but no increase in proliferation suggestive of malignant transformation occurred in MSCs from either patients or donors. Hematopoietic cell specific Lyn substrate 1 (*HLCS1*) was differentially expressed (fold change 0.25, *P* value 0.0005) between MSCs of osteosarcoma patients (n = 14) and healthy donors (n = 9).

Conclusions: This study shows that although *HCLS1* expression was downregulated in MSCs of osteosarcoma patients and binucleate cells were present in both patient and donor derived MSCs, there was no evidence of neoplastic changes to occur during long-term culture.

Background

Mesenchymal stromal cells (MSCs) are increasingly used as experimental cellular therapy in a wide range of conditions, such as graft-versus-host disease in the context of allogeneic bone marrow transplantation, auto-immune diseases and for regenerative purposes in for example myocardial injury or cartilage defects [1–6]. However, since MSCs have to be expanded in vitro to achieve sufficient numbers, there have been concerns regarding the safety of their use, particularly with regard to possible oncogenic transformation [7]. Cultured murine MSCs readily transform and form sarcoma-like tumors in vivo [8–12]. Similarly, MSCs derived from rhesus macaques become polyploid and subsequently aneuploid during long-term culture [13]. In contrast, human MSCs appear resistant to spontaneous in vitro transformation [14]. Studies reporting that human MSCs undergo malignant transformation in vitro have been retracted because of cross-contamination issues [15–20]. Despite the apparent difference between human and murine MSCs in their propensity to spontaneously transform in vitro, concerns remain. MSCs are hypothesized to be the precursor cells of high-grade osteosarcoma (OS) and a patient transplanted with bone marrow (containing hematopoietic

*Correspondence: a.lankester@lumc.nl
†Anne-Marie Cleton-Jansen and Arjan C Lankester contributed equally to this work
[1] Department of Pediatrics, J6-S, Leiden University Medical Center, PO Box 9600, 2300 RC Leiden, The Netherlands

stem cells and MSCs) from a sibling was diagnosed with OS originating from donor stem cells 17 years later [21]. This case demonstrates that donor-derived (pre-) cancerous MSCs can survive in a host and cause disease many years later. Another cause for concern is the observation that cultured MSCs can acquire chromosomal aberrations, although these do not seem to confer a selective growth advantage in vitro [22, 23].

High-grade osteosarcoma is a malignant primary bone tumor which often occurs at a relatively young age [24]. OS tumor cells are characterized by aneuploid karyotypes and gross chromosomal instability [25]. Such highly complex chromosomal rearrangements can occur as a result of a single catastrophic event, termed chromothripsis [26, 27]. However, this probably has to occur in a susceptible background, either as a genetic predisposition or acquired as a de novo event. In a murine model failed cytokinesis can lead to tetraploidy and subsequent tumorigenesis only in a p53 deficient host [28]. We previously showed loss of CDKN2A/p16 protein expression in tetraploid tumorigenic murine MSCs [9]. We hypothesized that normal MSCs from OS patients could be predisposed to malignant transformation, and performed long term in vitro culture and genome wide expression profiling of early passage MSCs from OS patients and healthy donors. Here we show that OS patient-derived MSCs do not transform in vitro, confirming previous reports in healthy individuals that spontaneous transformation of human MSCs in vitro is an extremely unlikely event.

Methods

Patients

Characteristics of OS patients and healthy stem cell donors can be found in Table 1. Bone marrow cells of OS patients were harvested under general anesthesia prior to start of the chemotherapeutic treatment. The site of MSC harvest (iliac crest) was different from the location of the primary tumor (metaphyseal ends of the long bones) in all cases. Healthy donors were either identical sibling donors for patients with malignant or benign disease requiring hematopoietic stem cell transplantation; or haploidentical donors for either hematopoietical stem

Table 1 Characteristics of osteosarcoma patients (OS) and healthy donors (HD) and overview of experiments

Culture	OS (UI)/HD	Sex	Age (years)	Histology	Location of the primary tumor	Included in experiment		
						Microarray	qPCR	Long-term culture
001OS	OS (352)	M	12	Osteoblastic	Distal femur	Y	Y	Y
002OS	OS (340)	F	13	Osteoblastic	Distal femur	Y	Y	Y
003OS	OS (376)	F	13	Telangiectatic	Distal femur	Y	Y	Y
004OS	OS (377)	F	14	Sclerosing	Proximal tibia	Y	Y	Y
005OS	OS (348)	F	15	Telangiectatic	Distal tibia	N	N	Y
006OS	OS (349)	M	8	Osteoblastic	Distal femur	Y	Y	Y
007OS	OS (350)	F	15	Osteoblastic	Distal femur	N	N	Y
008OS	OS (378)	F	9	Osteoblastic	Proximal humerus	Y	Y	Y
009OS	OS (382)	M	15	Chondroblastic	Proximal humerus	Y	Y	Y
010OS	OS (388)	M	14	Osteoblastic	Proximal humerus	N	Y	N
011OS	OS (391)	F	14	Osteoblastic	Proximal tibia	N	Y	N
012OS	OS (394)	F	5	Osteoblastic	Distal femur	N	Y	N
013OS	OS (393)	F	14	Osteoblastic	Distal femur	N	Y	N
014OS	OS (395)	M	10	Sclerosing	Distal femur	N	Y	N
015OS	OS (396)	M	13	Osteoblastic	Distal femur	N	Y	N
016OS	OS (402)	F	15	Sclerosing	Proximal tibia	N	Y	N
HB	HD (HB)	M	15			Y	Y	Y
HD3	HD (HD3)	F	27			Y	Y	Y
HD5	HD (HD5)	M	50			Y	Y	Y
MH	HD (MH)	M	15			Y	Y	Y
TD1	HD (TD1)	F	11			Y	Y	Y
TD2	HD (TD2)	F	43			N	Y	N
TD3	HD (TD3)	F	43			N	Y	N
TD4	HD (TD4)	F	25			N	Y	N
TD5	HD (TD5)	M	5			N	Y	N

UI unique identifier.

cell transplantation or the therapeutic infusion of MSCs for steroid-resistant graft-versus-host disease. Written informed consent was obtained from all patients and donors prior to bone marrow harvesting. The study was approved by the Institutional Review Board on Medical Ethics [LUMC Medical Ethics Committee (CME), P06.152].

Mesenchymal stromal cell cultures

Bone marrow derived mononuclear cells were obtained from 5 to 15 mL of heparinized bone marrow aspirate by density gradient centrifugation on Ficoll. Cells were plated on non-coated 75 cm^2 polystyrene flasks at a cell density of 160,000/cm^2 in complete culture medium (LG-DMEM; Invitrogen, Paisley, UK) supplemented with penicillin/streptomycin (Invitrogen) and 10% fetal bovine serum (FBS; HyClone, Verviers, Belgium). We used a characterized and defined FBS batch preselected for its potential to support MSC expansion and continued to use this specific batch throughout the culture period. MSCs were plastic adherent and had spindle shaped morphology. Chondrogenic, adipogenic and osteoblastic differentiation were performed as described earlier [29]. Medium was refreshed twice a week and cells were replated when reaching 80–90% confluence at a density of 4,000/cm^2. The first nine OS patient and first five healthy donor MSC samples that were obtained were cultured long-term, the subsequent samples were used for confirmatory mRNA expression analysis (Table 1). Morphology of the cells was recorded and population doublings per passage (PD) were calculated using the log ratio of the harvesting cell count (N) to the starting (baseline) count (X0), divided by the log of 2 ($PD = [\log(N/X0)]/\log 2$).

Flow cytometry

Expression of the cell surface markers CD73, CD90 and CD105 and absence of hematopoietic markers on MSCs was determined using flow cytometry, according to the statement by the International Society for Cellular Therapy [30]. Cells were detached using Trypsin/EDTA and washed in PBS/0.05% bovine serum albumin. Antibodies used were (FITC) conjugated anti-CD86-fluorescein isothiocyanate (FITC) (cat. no. 555657), anti-HLA-DR-FITC (cat. no. 347400), anti-CD31-phycoerythrin (PE) (cat no 555446), anti-CD34-PE (cat no 348057), anti-CD73-PE (cat no 550257), anti-CD90-PE (cat no 555596), anti-CD3-peridinin chlorophyll protein(PerCP)-Cy5.5 (cat no 332771), anti-CD45-PerCPCy5.5 (cat no 332784), all from BD (San Diego, CA, USA) and anti-CD105-PE (cat no SN6), from Ancell (Bayport, MN, USA). Flow cytometry was performed on a FACScalibur, and analyzed using Cellquest software (both Becton–Dickinson). Mean fluorescence intensity (MFI) ratio was calculated by determining the MFI of the specific staining relative to the MFI of the appropriate isotype control staining.

Analysis of binucleate cells

MSCs were grown on coverslips. Coverslips were washed with PBS and fixed in 4% PFA. Coverslips were incubated for 10 min in 1 μg/mL acridine orange (Sigma-Aldrich, Zwijndrecht, the Netherlands) to stain cytoplasm and 1 μg/mL wheat-germ agglutinin with an Alexa Fluor® 594 conjugate (Invitrogen) in PBS to stain cell membranes. Following washes in PBS, coverslips were mounted using Vectashield with DAPI (Vector laboratories, Burlingame, CA, USA) to stain nuclei. Images were acquired using a COHU 4910 series monochrome CCD camera (COHU, San Diego, CA, USA) attached to a DM fluorescence microscope (Leica, Wetzlar, Germany) and analyzed using ImageJ software with the Cell Counter plug-in (National Institute of Mental Health, Bethesda, MD, USA).

RNA isolation

RNA was isolated from frozen cell pellets of at least 1*10e6 undifferentiated MSCs at passage 2–5 using TRIzol reagent (Invitrogen). Cells were lysed in TRIzol, followed by phase separation in chloroform, precipitation using 2-propanolol and washing in 75% ethanol. RNA clean-up was performed using the QIAGEN Rneasy mini kit (Venlo, the Netherlands) with on-column DNAse treatment. RNA quality and concentration were measured using an Agilent 2100 Bioanalyzer (Santa Clara, CA, USA) and Nanodrop ND-1000 (Thermo Fisher Scientific, Waltham, MA, USA), respectively.

cDNA synthesis, cRNA amplification, and Illumina Human v2.0 Expression BeadChip hybridization

Gene expression profiling was performed using Human-6 v2 Expression BeadChips (San Diego, CA, USA) containing >48,000 transcript probes. Synthesis of cDNA, cRNA amplification, and hybridization of cRNA onto the Illumina Human v2.0 Expression BeadChips were performed as described previously [31, 32].

qPCR

cDNA synthesis for qPCR was performed as described earlier [32]. qPCR was performed using the iQ™ SYBR® Green Supermix (Bio-Rad, Hercules, CA, USA) according to the manufacture's instructions, reverse transcriptase negative (RT−) and H_2O controls were taken along for each sample. For normalization, three genes with stable expression in the microarray experiments were chosen (*CPSF6*, *GPR108* and *CAPNS1*). Data were normalized by geometric mean expression levels of the three reference genes using geNorm (http://medgen.ugent.be/jvdesomp/genorm/). Primer sequences can be found in Additional file 1: Table S1. A standard curve was taken along for each primer set and used for quantification, PCR efficiencies ranged from 93 to 104%.

Karyotyping

Six early passage samples (three derived from OS patients, three derived from healthy donors) were subjected to a multicolor FISH based karyotyping test (COBRA-FISH) as described earlier [33]. From each sample at least 20 metaphase cells were recorded and analyzed.

Statistical analysis

Microarray data were normalized using the Cubic Spline normalization method with the Illumina BeadStudio Gene Expression Module. Microarray data are available at GEO using the accession no. GSE42572. Statistical analysis of microarray was performed using Significance Analysis for Microarrays, using a false discovery rate of 20% (SAM, http://www-stat.stanford.edu/~tibs/SAM/) [34]. Univariate statistical analyses were performed using GraphPad Prism software (version 5.01, La Jolla, CA, USA). Two-sided *P* values lower than 0.05 were determined to be significant.

Results

MSCs of OS patients and healthy donors do not differ in expression of cell surface markers or differentiation capacity

We tested the MSC cultures from OS patients and healthy donors for phenotypic markers and functionality. Samples from 16/16 patients and 9/9 controls were able to differentiate into chondrogenic (Additional file 2: Figure S1A), adipogenic (Additional file 2: Figures S1B and C) and osteoblastic lineages (Additional file 2: Figures S1D and E). Also, all MSC cultures expressed CD73, CD90 and CD105 and lacked expression of hematopoietic markers (Additional file 2: Figure S1F). Level of expression of CD73, CD90 and CD105 as determined by MFI-ratios (specific staining/isotype control) did not differ between MSC cultures derived from OS patients and healthy donors. Early passage samples from three OS patient derived MSCs and three healthy donor derived MSCs were karyotyped; no structural or numerical aberrations were observed in the analyzed samples (Additional file 3: Figure S2): MSC001: 46,XY (26 metaphases), MSC003: 46,XX (27 metaphases), MSC008:46,XX (22 metaphases), MSC-HB: 46,XY (21 metaphases), MSC-MH: 46,XY (20 metaphases), MSC-TD: 46,XX (21 metaphases). Late passage cells could not be karyotypically analyzed due to the low numbers of dividing cells.

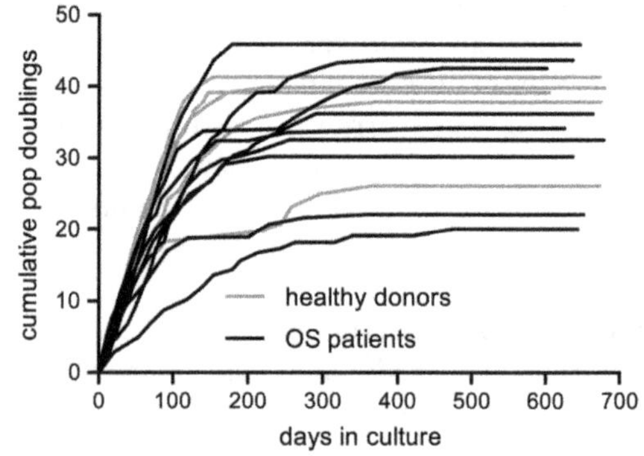

Figure 1 Cumulative population doublings of cultured MSCs from nine osteosarcoma (OS) patients and five healthy donors. All samples were grown in duplicate, averages of each duplicate are shown.

Long-term in vitro culture of MSCs results in increased binucleation but not in malignant transformation

MSCs of nine OS patients and five healthy donors were long term cultured (average number of days in culture 649, range 601–679 days). From each individual sample, duplicate cultures were established. There were no significant differences between growth rate, cumulative population doublings (median cumulative population doublings OS patients 34 vs. healthy donors 39; *P* value Mann–Whitney U test 0.70), passage number at termination of culture (mean passage number OS patients 21 vs. healthy donors 23; *P* value Mann–Whitney U test 0.74) or time to growth arrest (median days to growth arrest OS patients 441 days vs. healthy donors 222 days; *P* value Mann–Whitney U test 0.15) between MSCs of OS patients and healthy donors. The cumulative population doublings are shown in Figure 1 (averages of the duplicate cultures are shown per sample). All cultures exhibited rapid exponential growth in the first few passages. Later, proliferation slowed down and eventually stopped, characteristic of cultured cells in crisis. At termination of the cultures, viable cells were present in all samples. Cultures were terminated at the end of the growth curves. At this point, in none of the cultures there was evidence of cells escaping the crisis by an increase in proliferation and corresponding morphological changes indicative for spontaneous in vitro malignant transformation.

Morphology of the cells was inspected with every passage. Low passage cells were spindle-shaped, higher passage cells were larger. Upon increasing passage number, increasing frequencies of binucleate cells were noted using phase contrast microscopy. To quantify binucleation, cells were grown on coverslips and cytoplasm, cell membranes and nuclei were stained. Mono- and binucleate cells were counted (Figure 2a–d). There was no difference in percentage of binucleate cells between MSCs derived from OS patients and healthy donors (Figure 2e).

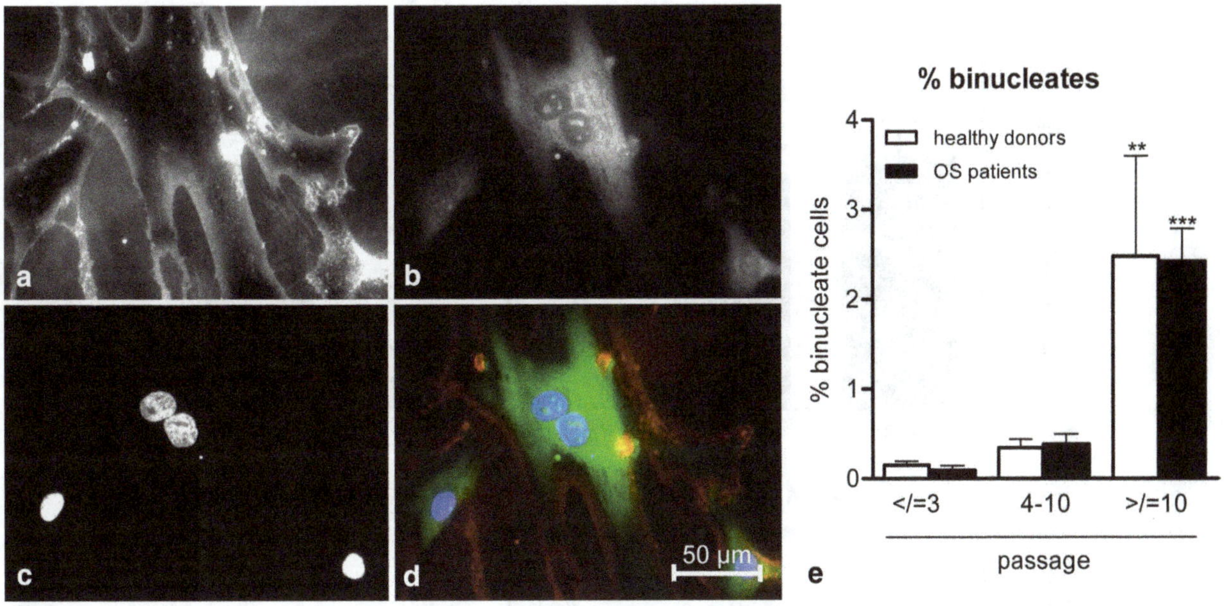

Figure 2 Increased binucleation upon increasing passage number. To facilitate cell staining and counting of nuclei, cells were grown on glass coverslips and stained using wheat-germ agglutinin (**a** cell membranes), acridine orange (**b** cytoplasm) and DAPI (**c** nuclei), shown in ×100 magnification. **d** Overlay with cell membrane in *red*, cytoplasm in *green* and nuclei in *blue*. A representative example of a high passage binucleate cell is shown. Note also the presence of a micronucleus (*panel* **c**). **e** Upon increasing passage number, more binucleate cells were noted, but no differences were seen between healthy donor-derived and osteosarcoma (OS) patient-derived MSCs (Kruskal–Wallis test *P* value <0.0001, Dunn's post-test compared to early passage cells; P value **<0.01; ***<0.001.

HCLS1 mRNA expression is downregulated in OS patient derived MSCs

Using microarray gene expression analysis, five genes were found to be differentially expressed between early passage healthy donor derived MSCs (n = 5) and OS patient derived MSCs (n = 7), with a false discovery rate of 20%. Expression of *HCLS1, ADM, EEF1A1, LOC644739* (or *WASF4*) and *LOC441155* was lower in patient derived MSCs as compared to healthy donor derived MSCs. To perform simultaneous technical and biological validation of the microarray results, the original low passage MSC samples were recultured and the original series expanded to now include four additional healthy donor derived MSCs (total of n = 9) and seven additional OS patient derived MSCs (total of n = 14). Four of the differentially expressed genes were validated using qPCR: hematopoietic cell specific Lyn substrate 1 (*HCLS1*), adrenomedullin (*ADM*), eukaryotic translation elongation factor 1 alpha 1 (*EEF1A1*) and *LOC644739* (or WAS protein family, member 4; *WASF4*). *LOC441155* is a pseudogene for which we did not succeed in designing a sufficiently specific and efficient primer pair. In this second, newly cultured and expanded series, expression of *HCLS1* was significantly lower in OS patient derived MSCs as compared to healthy donor derived MSCs (Figure 3, fold change 0.25, *P* value 0.0005). The other genes were not differentially expressed in this series, perhaps because this was a newly expanded batch of cells. We tried to determine if the observed difference in *HCLS1* expression was also true at the protein level. Although HCLS1 protein could be clearly detected in the positive control cell line Jurkat, we were unable to reproducibly detect HCLS1 in MSCs. For five OS patients we had mRNA available from both bone-marrow derived MSCs and the primary tumor. In these samples, expression of *HCLS1* was higher in tumor tissue as compared to MSCs, but there was no correlation between level of expression of *HCLS1* in low passage MSCs and in the corresponding tumor tissue.

Discussion

In recent years, MSCs have gained increasing interest as a therapeutic modality for immune modulatory and regenerative purposes [1–4]. In order to achieve sufficient numbers of cells for therapeutic utility, MSCs need to be expanded in vitro prior to infusion. Since long-term culture of non-human MSCs can result in oncogenic transformation and the occurrence of sarcomas in the receiving hosts, there is ongoing debate regarding the safety of using cultured MSCs in clinical studies [35]. In the present study, we compared human MSCs derived from OS patients at diagnosis and from healthy donors

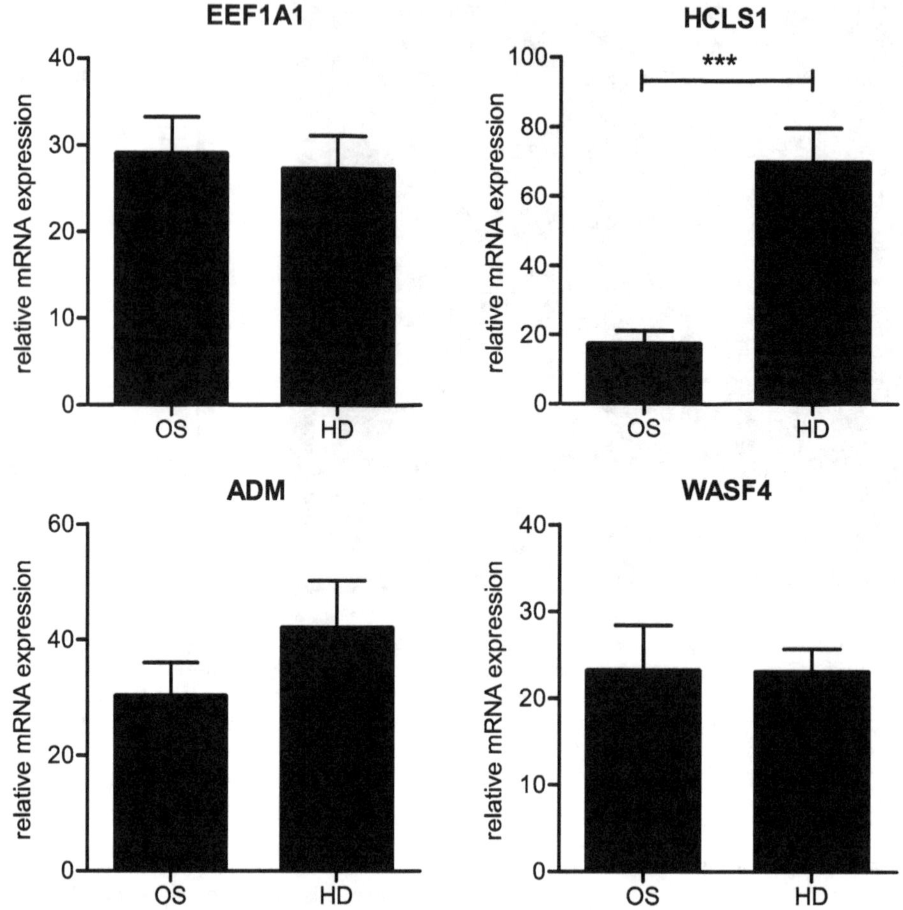

Figure 3 *HCLS1* gene expression is lower in MSCs from osteosarcoma patients as compared to healthy donors. Expression of *HCLS1* as determined by qPCR in bone-marrow derived MSCs no later than passage 5 is lower in MSCs derived from newly diagnosed osteosarcoma patients (OS; n = 14) than in MSCs derived from healthy donors (HD; n = 9). ****P* value Mann–Whitney-U test = 0.0005. Expression levels for *EEF1A1*, *ADM* and *WASF4* were not significantly different.

to answer two questions. First, do human MSCs transform to a malignant phenotype when cultured in vitro, as has been shown for murine MSCs? Second, are MSCs derived from OS patients more likely to transform than healthy donor derived MSCs?

MSCs from patients and controls exhibited similar growth patterns during long-term in vitro culture. During this time, all cultures reached a plateau in proliferation characteristic of cells in crisis. In contrast to what we have previously observed in murine MSCs [9], we never observed escape of this crisis by a rapidly dividing cell population with changed morphology, even after almost 2 years of continuous culture. There were no phenotypical or functional differences between OS patient derived and healthy donor derived MSCs and early passage karyotypes were normal in both groups. Differentiation capacity and expression of specific cell surface markers was similar.

During prolonged culture, progressive shortening of telomeres occurs [36]. This can cause anaphase chromatin bridges, resulting in failed cytokinesis and consequently in binucleate cells [37]. In the context of loss of expression or function of tumor suppressor proteins and corresponding cell cycle checkpoints, tetraploidy and ultimately aneuploidy will occur [28]. Upon increasing passage, increasing frequencies of binucleate cells were noted; both in patient derived MSCs and healthy donor derived MSCs (Figure 2). However, since we did not observe an increase in proliferation in these cells despite the presence of increasingly high frequencies of binucleate cells, cell cycle checkpoints were probably functionally intact, both in MSCs derived from OS patients and from healthy donors.

In addition to the functional read-out of long-term culture, we also performed gene expression analysis on early passage cells. Expression of *HCLS1* was downregulated in MSCs from OS patients as compared to MSCs of healthy donors. *HCLS1* is primarily known for its role in the signaling cascade that follows B cell receptor activation. It is highly expressed in B-cell derived malignancies and is associated with a poor outcome [38, 39]. Further studies are needed to determine if *HCLS1* might have a tumor suppressor function and if its loss of expression in OS patients derived MSCs has any relationship to in vivo tumorigenesis. Although we show no functional difference between healthy donor and OS patient derived MSCs, we do not advocate the use of MSCs from known cancer patients for clinical purposes. The relevance of the differential expression of *HCLS1* remains unknown and there might be other undetected (pre-) malignant alterations.

Both on a transcriptional and on a functional level, OS patient and healthy donor derived MSCs were very similar. There are several possible explanations for the observed similarities between OS patient derived and donor derived MSCs. First, we obtained MSCs from the iliac crest, while all tumors in our series were located at the metaphyseal ends of the long bones. OS occurs at a time and place of active growth and perhaps this pro-proliferative microenvironment (with high expression of growth factors) is an essential prerequisite for oncogenic transformation of MSCs. Second, (pre-) oncogenic alterations may be present in only one or a few local mesenchymal tumor precursor cells and not in MSCs at a distant site such as the iliac crest. This could be due to somatic mosaicism, similar to what has been shown for the enchondromatosis syndromes Ollier disease and Maffucci syndrome [40]. Third, according to the 'multiple hit hypothesis', there may not have been sufficient 'hits' for in vitro transformation to occur, even if relevant predisposing alterations are present. Ionizing radiation is a well-known risk factor for developing osteosarcoma and low-dose radiation facilitates oncogenic transformation in telomerase-transduced immortalized MSCs [41, 42]. Perhaps one or two additional 'hits' (for example loss of cell cycle checkpoint control or radiation-induced DNA damage) would be enough for oncogenic transformation to occur.

Fourth, pre-malignant alterations may have been present in only a few cells, which would not lead to large enough differences in gene expression to be picked up by genome wide expression analysis. Novel techniques to study genetic alterations at a single cell level might be able to pick up these rare events [43, 44]. Finally, although there is compelling evidence to suggest MSCs are the precursor cells for human OS, this has not yet been unequivocally proven.

Conclusions

During long-term in vitro culture of human OS patient and healthy donor derived MSCs, there was no evidence for neoplastic changes to occur. We could not confirm our hypothesis that MSCs of OS patients might have a higher propensity to oncogenic transformation than healthy donor derived MSCs. In contrast to what has been reported for other species, under the tested conditions, human MSCs do not easily transform. Although we cannot exclude the occurrence of low frequencies of cells with genomic alterations, we did not see a selective growth advantage of aberrant cells nor did we observe karyotypic abnormalities in low passage cells. This data supports the currently held view that administration of low passage cultured healthy donor derived human MSCs for therapeutic purposes is unlikely to result in sarcomas in the host.

Additional files

Additional file 1: Table S1. Primer sequences used for qPCR experiments.

Additional file 2: Figure S1. Differentiation capacity and expression of membranous markers of MSCs. Representative examples are shown (40× magnification). A, chondrogenic differentiation was performed using cell pellet cultures and assessed using toluidine blue staining. Adipogenic differentiation was assessed using phase contrast microscopy (B) and Oil-red-O staining (C). Osteogenic differentiation was assessed using phase contrast microscopy (D) and Alizarin red staining (E). F, all samples expressed CD73, CD90 and CD105 (bold histograms) as determined by flow cytometry (isotype controle staining shown for comparison).

Additional file 3: Figure S2. Representative example of karyotypic analysis of early passage MSCs (OS patient derived MSC003OS; 46,XX).

Abbreviations

ADM: adrenomedullin; EEF1A1: eukaryotic translation elongation factor 1 alpha 1; FBS: fetal bovine serum; FITC: fluorescein isothiocyanate; HCLS1: hematopoietic cell specific lyn substrate 1; MFI: mean fluorescence intensity; MSC: mesenchymal stromal cell; OS: osteosarcoma; PD: population doublings; PE: phycoerythrin; PerCP: peridinin chlorophyll protein; WASF4: WAS protein family member 4.

Authors' contributions

EB participated in design of the study, harvested and cultured bone marrow derived MSCs and performed and analyzed flow cytometry, differentiation assays, binucleate cell assays and qPCR, and drafted the manuscript. SR cultured bone marrow derived MSCs and performed and analyzed flow cytometry, differentiation assays, binucleate cell assays and qPCR. CR cultured bone marrow derived MSCs and performed and analyzed flow cytometry and differentiation assays. KS performed and analyzed karyotypic analyses. MK performed and analyzed genome wide profiling studies. HR harvested, cultured and analyzed BM derived MSCs. PH and RE participated in design of the study and helped to draft the manuscript. AC and AL conceived of the study, participated in the design and coordination and helped to draft the manuscript. All authors read and approved the final manuscript.

Author details

Department of Pediatrics, J6-S, Leiden University Medical Center, PO Box 9600, 2300 RC Leiden, The Netherlands. [2] Department of Pathology, Leiden University Medical Center, Leiden, The Netherlands. [3] Department of Molecular Cell Biology, Leiden University Medical Center, Leiden, The Netherlands. [4] Department of Immunohematology and Blood Transfusion, Leiden University Medical Center, Leiden, The Netherlands.

Acknowledgements
The authors like to thank Ronald Duim for technical assistance, Marco Schilham for critical review, and Maarten Morsink for help in analysis of microarray data. Also, the authors would like to thank the medical and nursing staff of the departments of pediatrics and clinical oncology for help in obtaining informed consent. This work was financially supported by EuroBoNet, a European Commission granted Network of Excellence for studying the pathology and genetics of bone tumors (Grant Number LSHC-CT-2006-018814) and by the Netherlands Organization for Health Research and Development (ZonMw, Grant Number 92003-399 to EB).

Competing interests
The authors declare that they have no competing interests.

References
1. Le Blanc K, Frassoni F, Ball L, Locatelli F, Roelofs H, Lewis I et al (2008) Mesenchymal stem cells for treatment of steroid-resistant, severe, acute graft-versus-host disease: a phase II study. Lancet 371:1579–1586
2. Uccelli A, Prockop DJ (2010) Why should mesenchymal stem cells (MSCs) cure autoimmune diseases? Curr Opin Immunol 22:768–774
3. Orlic D, Kajstura J, Chimenti S, Jakoniuk I, Anderson SM, Li B et al (2001) Bone marrow cells regenerate infarcted myocardium. Nature 410:701–705
4. Cipriani P, Carubbi F, Liakouli V, Marrelli A, Perricone C, Perricone R et al (2013) Stem cells in autoimmune diseases: implications for pathogenesis and future trends in therapy. Autoimmun Rev 12(7):709–716
5. Ball LM, Bernardo ME, Roelofs H, Lankester A, Cometa A, Egeler RM et al (2007) Cotransplantation of ex vivo-expanded mesenchymal stem cells accelerates lymphocyte recovery and may reduce the risk of graft failure in haploidentical hematopoietic stem-cell transplantation. Blood 110:2764–2767
6. Wakitani S, Imoto K, Yamamoto T, Saito M, Murata N, Yoneda M (2002) Human autologous culture expanded bone marrow mesenchymal cell transplantation for repair of cartilage defects in osteoarthritic knees. Osteoarthritis Cartilage 10:199–206
7. Ross AL, Leder DE, Weiss J, Izakovic J, Grichnik JM (2011) Genomic instability in cultured stem cells: associated risks and underlying mechanisms. Regen Med 6:653–662
8. Miura M, Miura Y, Padilla-Nash HM, Molinolo AA, Fu BJ, Patel V et al (2006) Accumulated chromosomal instability in murine bone marrow mesenchymal stem cells leads to malignant transformation. Stem Cells 24:1095–1103
9. Mohseny AB, Szuhai K, Romeo S, Buddingh EP, Briaire-de Bruijn I, de Jong D et al (2009) Osteosarcoma originates from mesenchymal stem cells in consequence of aneuploidization and genomic loss of Cdkn2. J Pathol 219:294–305
10. Tolar J, Nauta AJ, Osborn MJ, Mortari AP, McElmurry RT, Bell S et al (2007) Sarcoma derived from cultured mesenchymal stem cells. Stem Cells 25:371–379
11. Jeong JO, Han JW, Kim JM, Cho HJ, Park C, Lee N et al (2011) Malignant tumor formation after transplantation of short-term cultured bone marrow mesenchymal stem cells in experimental myocardial infarction and diabetic neuropathy. Circ Res 108:1340–1347
12. Josse C, Schoemans R, Niessen NA, Delgaudine M, Hellin AC, Herens C et al (2010) Systematic chromosomal aberrations found in murine bone marrow-derived mesenchymal stem cells. Stem Cells Dev 19:1167–1173
13. Izadpanah R, Kaushal D, Kriedt C, Tsien F, Patel B, Dufour J et al (2008) Long-term in vitro expansion alters the biology of adult mesenchymal stem cells. Cancer Res 68:4229–4238
14. Bernardo ME, Zaffaroni N, Novara F, Cometa AM, Avanzini MA, Moretta A et al (2007) Human bone marrow-derived mesenchymal stem cells do not undergo transformation after long-term In vitro culture and do not exhibit telomere maintenance mechanisms. Cancer Res 67:9142–9149
15. Rubio D, Garcia-Castro J, Martin MC, de la Fuente R, Cigudosa JC, Lloyd AC et al (2005) Spontaneous human adult stem cell transformation. Cancer Res 65:3035–3039
16. Rubio D, Garcia S, De la Cueva T, Paz MF, Lloyd AC, Bernad A et al (2008) Human mesenchymal stem cell transformation is associated with a mesenchymal-epithelial transition. Exp Cell Res 314:691–698
17. Rubio D, Garcia S, Paz MF, De la CT, Lopez-Fernandez LA, Lloyd AC et al (2008) Molecular characterization of spontaneous mesenchymal stem cell transformation. PLoS One 3:e1398
18. Rosland GV, Svendsen A, Torsvik A, Sobala E, McCormack E, Immervoll H et al (2009) Long-term cultures of bone marrow-derived human mesenchymal stem cells frequently undergo spontaneous malignant transformation. Cancer Res 69:5331–5339
19. Torsvik A, Rosland GV, Svendsen A, Molven A, Immervoll H, McCormack E et al (2010) Spontaneous malignant transformation of human mesenchymal stem cells reflects cross-contamination: putting the research field on track-letter. Cancer Res 70:6393–6396
20. de la Fuente R, Bernad A, Garcia-Castro J, Martin MC, Cigudosa JC (2010) Retraction: spontaneous human adult stem cell transformation. Cancer Res 70:6682
21. Berger M, Muraro M, Fagioli F, Ferrari S (2008) Osteosarcoma derived from donor stem cells carrying the Norrie's disease gene. N Engl J Med 359:2502–2504
22. Ben-David U, Mayshar Y, Benvenisty N (2011) Large-scale analysis reveals acquisition of lineage-specific chromosomal aberrations in human adult stem cells. Cell Stem Cell 9:97–102
23. Tarte K, Gaillard J, Lataillade JJ, Fouillard L, Becker M, Mossafa H et al (2010) Clinical-grade production of human mesenchymal stromal cells: occurrence of aneuploidy without transformation. Blood 115:1549–1553
24. Fletcher CDM, Bridge JA, Hogendoorn PCW, Mertens F (2013) WHO classification of tumours of soft tissue and bone. International Agency for Research on Cancer, Lyon
25. Szuhai K, Cleton-Jansen AM, Hogendoorn PC, Bovee JV (2012) Molecular pathology and its diagnostic use in bone tumors. Cancer Genet 205:193–204
26. Stephens PJ, Greenman CD, Fu B, Yang F, Bignell GR, Mudie LJ et al (2011) Massive genomic rearrangement acquired in a single catastrophic event during cancer development. Cell 144:27–40
27. Holland AJ, Cleveland DW (2012) Chromoanagenesis and cancer: mechanisms and consequences of localized, complex chromosomal rearrangements. Nat Med 18:1630–1638
28. Fujiwara T, Bandi M, Nitta M, Ivanova EV, Bronson RT, Pellman D (2005) Cytokinesis failure generating tetraploids promotes tumorigenesis in p53-null cells. Nature 437:1043–1047
29. Bernardo ME, Emons JAM, Karperien M, Nauta AJ, Willemze R, Roelofs H et al (2007) Human mesenchymal stem cells derived from bone marrow display a better chondrogenic differentiation compared with other sources. Connect Tissue Res 48:132–140
30. Dominici M, Le Blanc K, Mueller I, Slaper-Cortenbach I, Marini FC, Krause DS et al (2006) Minimal criteria for defining multipotent mesenchymal stromal cells. The International Society for Cellular Therapy position statement. Cytotherapy 8:315–317
31. Hallor KH, Staaf J, Bovee JVMG, Hogendoorn PCW, Cleton-Jansen AM, Knuutila S et al (2009) Genomic profiling of chondrosarcoma: chromosomal patterns in central and peripheral tumors. Clin Cancer Res 15:2685–2694
32. Buddingh EP, Kuijjer ML, Duim RA, Burger H, Agelopoulos K, Myklebost O et al (2011) Tumor-infiltrating macrophages are associated with metastasis suppression in high-grade osteosarcoma: a rationale for treatment with macrophage activating agents. Clin Cancer Res 17:2110–2119
33. Szuhai K, Tanke HJ (2006) COBRA: combined binary ratio labeling of nucleicacid probes for multi-color fluorescence in situ hybridization karyotyping. Nat Protoc 1:264–275
34. Tusher VG, Tibshirani R, Chu G (2001) Significance analysis of microarrays applied to the ionizing radiation response. Proc Natl Acad Sci USA 98:5116–5121
35. Prockop DJ, Keating A (2012) Relearning the lessons of genomic stability of human cells during expansion in culture: implications for clinical research. Stem Cells 30:1051–1052
36. Kim J, Kang JW, Park JH, Choi Y, Choi KS, Park KD et al (2009) Biological characterization of long-term cultured human mesenchymal stem cells. Arch Pharm Res 32:117–126

37. Pampalona J, Frias C, Genesca A, Tusell L (2012) Progressive telomere dysfunction causes cytokinesis failure and leads to the accumulation of polyploid cells. PLoS Genet 8:e1002679
38. Scielzo C, Ghia P, Conti A, Bachi A, Guida G, Geuna M et al (2005) HS1 protein is differentially expressed in chronic lymphocytic leukemia patient subsets with good or poor prognoses. J Clin Invest 115:1644–1650
39. Frezzato F, Gattazzo C, Martini V, Trimarco V, Teramo A, Carraro S et al (2012) HS1, a Lyn kinase substrate, is abnormally expressed in B-chronic lymphocytic leukemia and correlates with response to fludarabine-based regimen. PLoS One 7:e39902
40. Pansuriya TC, van ER, d'Adamo P, van Ruler MA, Kuijjer ML, Oosting J et al (2011) Somatic mosaic IDH1 and IDH2 mutations are associated with enchondroma and spindle cell hemangioma in Ollier disease and Maffucci syndrome. Nat Genet 43:1256–1261
41. Christensen R, Alsner J, Brandt SF, Dagnaes-Hansen F, Kolvraa S, Serakinci N (2008) Transformation of human mesenchymal stem cells in radiation carcinogenesis: long-term effect of ionizing radiation. Regen Med 3:849–861
42. Ottaviani G, Jaffe N (2009) The etiology of osteosarcoma. Cancer Treat Res 152:15–32
43. Navin N, Kendall J, Troge J, Andrews P, Rodgers L, McIndoo J et al (2011) Tumour evolution inferred by single-cell sequencing. Nature 472:90–94
44. Zamani EM, Dimitriadou E, Mateiu L, Melotte C, Van der Aa N, Kumar P et al (2015) Concurrent whole-genome haplotyping and copy-number profiling of single cells. Am J Hum Genet 96(6):894–912

2

Radiotherapy in the management of gist: state of the art and new potential scenarios

L. Gatto[1], M. Nannini[1], M. Saponara[1], V. Di Scioscio[2], G. Beltramo[3], G. P. Frezza[4], G. Ercolani[5], A. D. Pinna[5], A. Astolfi[6], M. Urbini[6], G. Brandi[1,6], G. Biasco[1,6] and M. A. Pantaleo[1,6*]

Abstract

Background: Gastrointestinal stromal tumor (GIST) is the most common mesenchymal neoplasm of the gastrointestinal tract. The main treatment for localized gastrointestinal stromal tumors is surgical resection. Unresectable or advanced GIST are poorly responsive to conventional cytotoxic chemotherapy but the introduction of tyrosine kinase inhibitors (TKIs) marked a revolutionary step in the treatment of these patients, radically improving prognosis and clinical benefit. Historically GIST has been considered radiation-resistant, and the role of radiotherapy in the management of patients with GIST is currently restricted to symptomatic palliation in current treatment guidelines.

Case presentation: Here we report two patients affected by metastatic GIST, treated with radiotherapy and radiosurgery in combination with TKIs, achieving an unexpected objective response in the first case and a significant clinical benefit associated with a local tumor control of several months in the second case.

Conclusions: These and other successful experiences that are progressively accumulating, open up new scenarios of use of radiation therapy in various settings of treatment. GIST is not universally radioresistant and radiotherapy, especially if combined with molecularly targeted therapy, can improve the outcomes for patients diagnosed with GIST.

Keywords: Radiotherapy, GIST, Treatment

Background

Gastrointestinal stromal tumors (GISTs) are the most common mesenchymal tumors of the gastrointestinal tract. Previously classified as leiomyomas, leiomyosarcomas, leiomyoblastomas or schwannomas, they are now recognized as a distinct entity, arising from the interstitial cells of Cajal or their precursors, specialized pacemaker playing a critical role in the coordination of normal motility within the gastrointestinal tract.

GIST molecular pathophysiology is a mutation-driven process, in most cases (85–90%) a gain-of-function KIT gene mutations, which lead to constitutive activation of KIT kinase activity and to uncontrolled cell proliferation. A notably smaller proportion (5–8%) is associated with analogous mutations in platelet-derived growth factor receptor α (PDGFRα) and <10% contain no identified receptor tyrosine-kinase mutations, referred as KIT/PDGFRA wild-type GISTs [1–4].

The advent of the tyrosine kinase inhibitors has dramatically revolutionized the therapeutic approach to gastrointestinal stromal tumor and improved the outcome of these patients, becoming the standard systemic therapies for locally advanced/metastatic GIST [5, 6].

Most patients obtain good, durable responses to treatment; nevertheless, almost the great majority of patients in a metastatic setting develop resistance, leading to failure of tyrosine-kinase inhibitors and bringing the clinicians to consider an increasingly wide spectrum of loco-regional treatment options.

The decisions are based on the specific clinical history of each patient and have the aim of maximizing the

*Correspondence: maria.pantaleo@unibo.it
[1] Department of Specialized, Experimental, and Diagnostic Medicine, S. Orsola-Malpighi Hospital, University of Bologna, Bologna, Italy

duration of each therapeutic method and, ultimately, the overall sequential treatment strategy.

Historically GIST has been considered radiation-resistant, and radiotherapy is recommended only for palliative purpose of bone metastases in current treatment guidelines [7].

However, some experiences accumulated in recent times, including ours, suggest that GIST metastases are moderately radiosensitive, and frequently stabilize for several months with radiotherapy.

Radiotherapy appears to be a well-tolerated treatment that should be considered in the management of metastatic GIST not only with palliative purposes but, in our opinion, even in other settings of treatment.

In this article, we report the strategy of integration between radiotherapy and medical treatment, focusing on new potential scenarios not explored yet, that may enlarge the treatment opportunities for these patients.

Cases presentation

Case 1

In October 2008 a 62 years old male underwent urgency total gastrectomy due to a massive hematemesis. Histological examination revealed a CD 117 positive, DOG 1 positive gastric GIST with high risk of recurrence according to Miettinen classification (6 cm of diameter, 15 mitoses per 50 high power field). No tumor rupture was observed.

In January 2010, a CT scan documented the appearance of multiple liver metastases, thus the patient was enrolled in CAMN107G2301 trial and a first line therapy with imatinib mesylate at a daily dose of 400 mg was started. The treatment was pursued regularly, with good tolerance and stability of disease until July 2011, when a mild increase in size of hepatic lesions led to stop the trial and an imatinib dose escalation to 800 mg/day was started.

In May 2012 a new solid paracaval lesion with thrombosis of the inferior vena cava was identified (diameter 27 × 45 mm), and therapy was switched to a second line treatment with oral sunitinib at the dose of 37.5 mg/day.

A CT scan after 5 months of sunitinib treatment showed progression in the size of the paracaval lesion (diameter 130 × 110 mm) with compression of the vena cava and coeliac trunk, therefore we discontinued sunitinib and prescribed regorafenib 160 mg/day (21 days on, 7 days off). The mass became quickly symptomatic with local pain and hiccup. A surgical consultation excluded reintervention because of the site of disease, inseparable from the great vessels, and because of the sequelae of previous surgery.

In view of the symptoms development, of the rapid increase in size of the mass (about 8 cm in few months) and in absence of surgical options, in November 2012 we administered external radiotherapy combined with regorafenib at a dose of 160 mg/day.

A dose of 35 Gray was administered in 14 sessions, with good subjective tolerance by the patient and without complications, obtaining an objective response, with decrease in size of the paracaval mass from 130 to 80 mm and clinical benefit on pain (Fig. 1).

Despite a regorafenib dose reduction for toxicity (120 mg/day—21 days on, 7 days off schedule) the patient has maintained a stable disease, both in the liver and in the radio-treated mass, for over three years, until now.

Case 2

In January 2012, a 44 years-old male diagnosed with gastric GIST with multiple liver metastases and previously treated with imatinib and sunitinib was referred to our institution.

Clinically the patient complained a number of symptoms related to compression of the tumor, mainly nausea, vomiting and abdominal pain.

Because of the clinical picture, the young age and the lack, at that time, of approved third-line therapies, we decided for a debulking surgery.

In March 2012 a partial gastrectomy and right hepatectomy were performed, histology confirming the diagnosis of GIST with a high mitotic index (mitoses 30/50 high power field). The surgical approach was no radical, with residual hepatic disease, thus, after post-operative recovery, a medical treatment with imatinib 400 mg/day was resumed, subsequently increased to 800 mg/day for increase in size of liver metastases.

In October 2013 a CT scan documented the appearance of a new lesion below the diaphragm in the right pararenal (diameter 34 mm) associated with significant pain, poorly responsive to opioids.

Considering the exclusively focal progression of disease and the symptoms development we decided for local radiosurgery: a cyberknife treatment was performed (at first 4500 cGy delivered in 5 sessions; after 60 days repeated a second dose of 4000 cGy fractionated in 4 sessions), well-tolerated, burdened only by nausea which required a discontinuation of imatinib during sessions. Radiological assessment after cyberknife showed disease stabilization without shrinkage of tumor size, but with a decrease in hypervascularity of the mass, and the patient referred an early improvement in pain (Fig. 2). Few months later the patient developed a critical left supraclavicular mass (diameter 46 × 37 mm), progressively increasing and displacing the trachea, causing worsening pain, hacking cough and dysphagia. In this phase we decided for a combination strategy, integrating medical treatment with sunitinib rechallange with a cyberknife

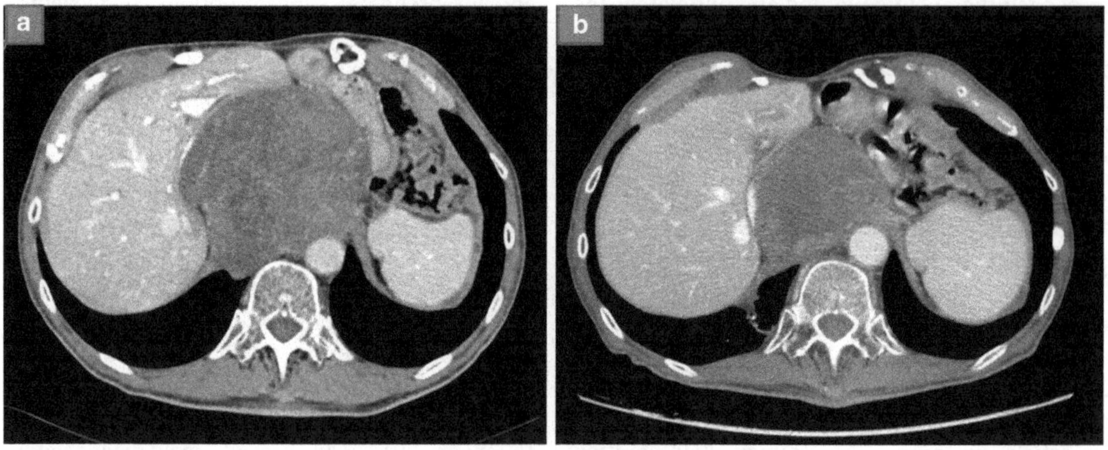

Fig. 1 **a** CT scan documenting a voluminous GIST metastasis compressing the vena cava (diameter 130 × 110 mm). **b** CT scan performed 4 months after radiotherapy showing significant tumor shrinkage

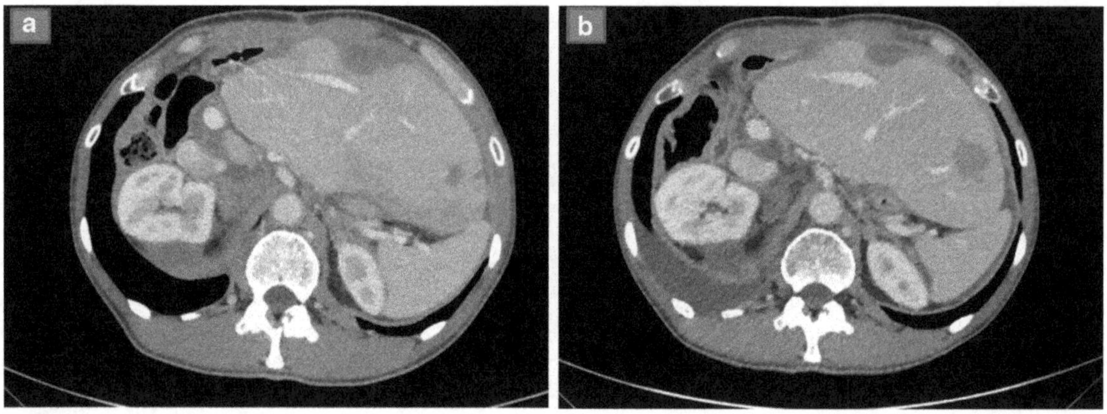

Fig. 2 **a** CT scan documenting right pararenal hypervascular metastatsis (diameter 34 mm). **b** CT scan performed after cyberknife. The lesion, substantially stable in size, became completely hypodense

treatment of the supraclavicular mass (total dosage of 32 Gy in 5 sessions). Also in this case, in addition to a dimensional stabilization of the lesion, the patient obtained a substantial clinical benefit.

Unfortunately, in the following months, our patient exhibited a rapid disease progression, whilst maintaining a dimensional stability of the radiosurgical-treated masses (for about 5 months) and a prolonged symptoms control.

Discussion

Although the role of radiation therapy is well established for the treatment of soft tissue sarcomas, GIST has been historically considered radioresistant [8, 9], and the use of this method has been discouraged mainly because of the elective abdominal pattern of spread, which require too large fields of irradiation, often resulting in unacceptable bowel toxicity.

Based on these considerations, currently the use of radiation therapy in GIST is rarely considered and is recommended only for the palliative treatment of bone metastases [7].

However, to date some publications suggest the efficacy of radiation therapy in the management of GIST [10–12].

Herein we report two very peculiar cases suggesting a possible successful use of radiotherapy as an integrated approach in GIST management, to obtain a long lasting disease stabilization, and, in selected cases, even objective responses.

In the first case we combined radiotherapy with regorafenib for the treatment of a voluminous, progressively increasing and symptomatic paracaval lesion, obtaining not only a symptoms control but also a significant tumor shrinkage for three years.

The second case, instead, is the first published experience, to our knowledge, of cyberknife treatment in GIST. Cyberknife is a device that combines a robotic arm with a linear accelerator, has been developed for stereotactic radiotherapy and may provide an adequate dose to the tumor while decreasing the dose to the surrounding normal tissue. Cyberknife was administered in both a pararenal and a supraclavicular mass, at different times, and resulted in a well-tolerated treatment which provided local control of the masses and rapid improvement of the symptoms.

Currently the standard of care for resectable GIST is surgery, followed by adjuvant imatinib for high risk recurrence. Inoperable or metastatic tumors are treated primarily with imatinib, which should be pursued indefinitely until the development of progression that occurs, generally, after a median time of 24 months [13].

For patients who progress to imatinib, sunitinib is an effective treatment option and currently represent the only proven second-line therapy for advanced GISTs [14]. However, due to the development of resistance to both of these two drugs in the majority of patients, the need for third-line therapy arose. Based on the phase III placebo-controlled GRID trial, regorafenib, an oral multi-targeted inhibitor with activity against multiple kinases including KIT, RET, RAF1, BRAF, PDGFR, FGFR and angiogenesis (VEGFR), has shown an increase of median PFS (4–8 vs 0–9 months in regorafenib group, $p < 0.0001$)and is now established as the third-line therapy of metastatic GISTs [15].

In recent years the development of three lines of therapy has improved a lot the prognosis and survival of patients with GIST, making more and more evident the need not only of further lines of therapy, but, above all, the necessity of multidisciplinary approaches in order to maximize the clinical benefit and the duration of treatment with each single agent. In this context we invite to consider much more the role of radiation therapy in GIST, which could prove to be invaluable, as it has been for the radiofrequency ablation of liver metastases, now definitively imposed as a successful option in providing effective local tumor control, especially if combined with TKIs therapy [16, 17].

There are several scenarios in which radiation therapy may provide a potential benefit:

I. radiotherapy of metastases for palliation of local symptoms with low toxicities, a possibility already widely explored
II. radiotherapy of focally progressing lesions, with the aim of overcoming emergent resistant clones, not only with a palliative intent but also cytoreductive, in combination with systemic therapy which continue acting on the sensitive clones
III. in the peri-operative setting, combined with imatinib, especially for GIST at high risk of local recurrence, where surgery is often demolitive, such as rectal and esophageal GIST
IV. definitive radiotherapy alternative to surgery in localized GIST in elderly patients with comorbidities or in case of unresectable tumors

In the largest published series, Joensuu et al. presented a phase II prospective study of 25 patients affected by liver, soft-tissue, intra-abdominal and bone GIST metastases, treated with external beam radiotherapy, at a cumulative dose of approximately 40 Gy, whilst maintaining systemic therapy during irradiation (11 patients continued to receive imatinib, 4 sunitinib, 2 nilotinib, 1 regorafenib and 1 a combination of sorafenib and everolimus). Two patients achieved partial remission, 20 patients had a durable stabilization of the target lesion, with a median duration of stabilization of 16 months, and only 3 progressed (9).

Obviously it is difficult to determine if the systemic therapy is a confounding factor in assessing the response to a local treatment and if it can increase sensitivity to radiotherapy. Realistically the efficacy achieved could result rather from the combined effects of radiotherapy and tyrosine kinase inhibitors, and might be less with radiation alone.

Some studies suggest that imatinib can increase the radiosensitivity in cell lines, specifically human glioma and anaplastic thyroid cancer cell lines. In particular, imatinib can reduce the levels of cellular RAD51, an essential component of the homologous DNA repair pathway implicated as a determinant of cellular radiosensitivity, leading to increased radiosensitivity in vitro and in vivo without undue toxicity toward normal cells and tissues [18, 19].

Ciresa et al. described a successful use of neo-adjuvant radiotherapy in a case of rectal GIST extending to the anal canal, who received imatinib 400 mg/day and concomitant radiotherapy (total dose 50.4 Gy in fractions of 1.8 Gy daily) obtaining a partial clinical response 3 weeks after the end of combination treatment. The patient then underwent a sphincter-saving surgical procedure, with a complete pathological response at the histological examination [20].

Although there are no prospective data that produce this evidence, radiotherapy may be considered, associated with TKI and preferably in the context of clinical studies, in the treatment of GIST and in particular of those in the rectal, esophageal and duodenal site, to evaluate the effectiveness of this approach in both the down-staging and the prevention of local recurrence as well as for the epithelial counterpart, even though it is well known the histology is completely different.

Regarding the cyberknife, it is an image-guided frameless robotic technology for whole-body radiosurgery, used for classic single-fraction radiosurgery and for hypofractionated treatments, which treat tumors with supreme accuracy, essentially "painting" the mass with radiation and sparing surrounding healthy tissue.

Unlike some radiosurgery systems, which can only treat primary or secondary brain neoplasms, the cyberknife may be applicated to extracranial use and has been tested in a broad range of tumors, including prostate, lung, spine, liver, pancreas, and kidney. However, to our knowledge, no experience has so far been published regarding the application of the cyberknife in GIST.

This radiosurgery strategy has emerged as an additional tool in oncology armamentarium, extremely attractive for the high tumor control, the low toxicity and the repeatability of the treatments for recurrent metastases [21, 22].

Optimal management of patients diagnosed with GIST is multidisciplinary, should be performed only at specialized oncological center, and requires strong cooperation among different expertises, including oncology, surgery, ultrasound, radiology, radiotherapy, radiosurgery and interventional radiology.

It is not excluded that in the very near future, not only radiation but also other approaches such as arterial embolization, cyber-knife and HIFU ablation (high intensity focused ultrasound) can carve out a role in the treatment of this tumor, increasingly articulate and complex.

Conclusions

To date, the evidence regarding the use of radiation therapy in GIST is limited to small case series, therefore, the impression emerging from these experiences is that this approach is effective not only in a strictly palliative field, but may also provide objective responses and long-term disease control in selected patients, without any significant toxicity or impact on quality of life.

We decided to report these two cases because, in our view, are very interesting in several aspects: the unexpected significant objective response obtained with the combination of regorafenib and radiotherapy in the first case, and the experience with the technique of cyberknife in the second case, which we hope could find an increasingly wide range of use in the immediate future.

We can certainly conclude that radiation therapy, unjustifiably underutilized until now, should be considered a viable option in the treatment of locally advanced\ metastatic GISTs. Nevertheless further studies are needed to standardize its correct role in the different settings of treatment, but also the effective dosage and the irradiation techniques.

Abbreviations

CT: computed tomography; GIST: gastrointestinal stromal tumor; PDGFRα: platelet-derived growth factor receptor α; TKIs: tyrosine kinase inhibitors.

Authors' contributions

GL collected data and wrote the manuscript. MN and MS contributed in collecting data. DSV, BeGi and FGP provided radiological data. EG and PAD provided surgical informations. AA and UM performed molecular analysis. BrGi, BG and PMA reviewed the manuscript and gave final approval. All authors read and approved the final manuscript.

Author details

[1] Department of Specialized, Experimental, and Diagnostic Medicine, S. Orsola-Malpighi Hospital, University of Bologna, Bologna, Italy. [2] Department of Radiology, S. Orsola Malpighi Hospital, Bologna University, Bologna, Italy. [3] Centro Diagnostico Italiano, Reparto Cyberknife, Milan, Italy. [4] Radiation Oncology Unit, Bellaria Hospital, Bologna, Italy. [5] Department of General and Emergency Surgery and Organ Transplantation, S. Orsola-Malpighi Hospital, University of Bologna, Bologna, Italy. [6] Interdepartmental Centre of Cancer Research "G. Prodi", University of Bologna, Bologna, Italy.

Acknowledgements

Not applicable.

Competing interests

The authors declare that they have no competing financial interests.

References

1. Miettinen M, Lasota J. Gastrointestinal stromal tumors—definition, clinical, histological, immunohistochemical, and molecular genetic features and differential diagnosis. Virchows Arch. 2001;438(1):1–12.
2. Hirota S, Isozaki K, Moriyama Y, Hashimoto K, Nishida T, Ishiguro S, et al. Gain-of-function mutations of c-kit in human gastrointestinal stromal tumors. Science. 1998;279(5350):577–80.
3. Heinrich MC, Corless CL, Duensing A, McGreevey L, Chen CJ, Joseph N, et al. PDGFRA activating mutations in gastrointestinal stromal tumors. Science. 2003;299:708–10.
4. Nannini M, Astolfi A, Urbini M, Indio V, Santini D, Heinrich MC, et al. Integrated genomic study of quadruple-WT GIST (KIT/PDGFRA/SDH/RAS pathway wild-type GIST). BMC Cancer. 2014;20(14):685.
5. Dematteo RP, Heinrich MC, El-Rifai WM, Demetri G. Clinical management of gastrointestinal stromal tumors: before and after STI-571. Hum Pathol. 2002;33:466–77.
6. Biasco G, Velo D, Angriman I. Gastrointestinal stromal tumors: report of an audit and review of the literature. Eur J Cancer Prev. 2009;18(2):106–16.
7. ESMO/European Sarcoma Network Working Group. Gastrointestinal stromal tumors: ESMO Clinical Practice Guidelines for diagnosis, treatment and follow-up. Ann Oncol 2014;25(Suppl 3):iii21–6
8. Crosby JA, Catton CN, Davis A, Couture J, O'Sullivan B, Kandel R, Swallow CJ. Malignant gastrointestinal stromal tumors of the small intestine: a review of 50 cases from a prospective database. Ann Surg Oncol. 2001;8(1):50–9.

9. Pierie JP, Choudry U, Muzikansky A, Yeap BY, Souba WW, Ott MJ. The effect of surgery and grade on outcome of gastrointestinal stromal tumors. Arch Surg. 2001;136(4):383–9.
10. Joensuu H, Eriksson M, Collan J, Balk MH, Leyvraz S, Montemurro M. Radiotherapy for GIST progressing during or after tyrosine kinase inhibitor therapy: a prospective study. Radiother Oncol. 2015;116(2):233–8.
11. Cuaron JJ, Goodman KA, Lee N, Wu AJ. External beam radiation therapy for locally advanced and metastatic gastrointestinal stromal tumors. Radiat Oncol. 2013;23(8):274.
12. Lolli C, Pantaleo MA, Nannini M, Saponara M, Pallotti MC, Scioscio VD, et al. Successful radiotherapy for local control of progressively increasing metastasis of gastrointestinal stromal tumor. Rare Tumors. 2011;3(4):e49.
13. Maleddu A, Pantaleo MA, Nannini M, Di Battista M, Saponara M, Lolli C, Biasco G. Mechanisms of secondary resistance to tyrosine kinase inhibitors in gastrointestinal stromal tumours (Review). Oncol Rep. 2009;21(6):1359–66.
14. Demetri GD, van Oosterom AT, Garrett CR, Blackstein ME, Shah MH, Verweij J, et al. Efficacy and safety of sunitinib in patients with advanced gastrointestinal stromal tumor after failure of imatinib: a randomised controlled trial. Lancet. 2006;368:1329–38.
15. Demetri GD, Reichardt P, Kang YK, Blay JY, Rutkowski P, Gelderblom H, et al. Efficacy and safety of regorafenib for advanced gastrointestinal stromal tumours after failure of imatinib and sunitinib: an international, multicentre, prospective, randomised, placebo-controlled phase 3 trial (GRID). Lancet. 2013;381(9863):295–302.
16. Chunchuan F, Nianzhou L, Qingsong D, Yunhua T, Kuansheng M, Ping B. Successful treatment of gastrointestinal stromal tumor with multiple liver metastases with radiofrequency ablation and imatinib: a case report. Oncol Lett. 2015;10(2):875–8.
17. Jung JH, Won HJ, Shin YM, Kim PN. Safety and efficacy of radiofrequency ablation for hepatic metastases from gastrointestinal stromal tumor. J Vasc Interv Radiol. 2015;26(12):1797–802.
18. Podtcheko A, Ohtsuru A, Namba H, Saenko V, Starenki D, Palona I, et al. Inhibition of ABL tyrosine kinase potentiates radiation-induced terminal growth arrest in anaplastic thyroid cancer cells. Radiat Res. 2006;165(1):35–42.
19. Choudhury A, Zhao H, Jalali F, Al Rashid S, Ran J, Supiot S, et al. Targeting homologous recombination using imatinib results in enhanced tumor cell chemosensitivity and radiosensitivity. Mol Cancer Ther. 2009;8(1):203–13.
20. Ciresa M, D'Angelillo RA, Ramella S, Cellini F, Gaudino D, Stimato G, et al. Molecularly targeted therapy and radiotherapy in the management of localized gastrointestinal stromal tumor (GIST) of the rectum: a case report. Tumori. 2009;95:236–9.
21. Wowra B, Muacevic A, Tonn JC. CyberKnife radiosurgery for brain metastases. Prog Neurol Surg. 2012;25:201–9.
22. Kato H, Yoshida H, Taniguch H, Nomura R, Sato K, Suzuki I, Nakata R. Cyberknife treatment for advanced or terminal stage hepatocellular carcinoma. World J Gastroenterol. 2015;21(46):13101–12.

Metastatic mesenteric dedifferentiated leiomyosarcoma

Mercy Varghese[1,7*], Oyvind Bruland[1,2], Anne Marit Wiedswang[3], Ingvild Lobmaier[4], Bård Røsok[5], Robert S. Benjamin[6] and Kirsten Sundby Hall[1]

Abstract

Background: Abdominal leiomyosarcoma arising from the mesentery is a rare malignancy. It is an aggressive entity with an overall 5 year survival rate between 20 and 30 %. Surgical resection is the cornerstone of primary treatment and may be curative for localized disease. However, patients often develop intra-abdominal relapse and/or metastatic disease. If surgical resection is not feasible, palliative chemotherapy is the treatment of choice. However, there are no clear guidelines regarding chemotherapy; neither in the adjuvant nor advanced setting.

Case presentation: We present a 40 year-old woman, with a mesenteric leiomyosarcoma, who underwent radical tumor resection and did not receive adjuvant oncological therapy. Three months postoperatively, she developed metastatic disease to the lungs and liver. After multidisciplinary assessment she received an unconventional histological-subtype-tailored chemotherapy comprising 3–4 regimens. Initially, there was a decrease both in number and size of metastases. Ultimately, an almost complete radiological response was seen. Subsequent surgical resection and radiofrequency ablation of residual metastatic foci in the liver and lung brought her into complete clinical remission. She is presently tumor free, 36 months following diagnosis of metastatic disease.

Conclusions: To our knowledge, this is the first report of a patient with metastatic mesenteric leiomyosarcoma who is in complete clinical and radiological long-term remission following very aggressive multimodal treatment; including intense poly-drug chemotherapy and without any demonstrable long-term side effects. Given the rarity of mesenteric leiomyosarcoma and lack of guidelines regarding oncological therapy, we suggest that multimodal therapy including aggressive chemotherapy, guided by a multidisciplinary team, is essential to achieve an optimal outcome.

Keywords: Leiomyosarcoma, Mesenteric, Abdominal, Histological-subtype, Chemotherapy, Metastases, Multimodal

Background

Leiomyosarcoma (LMS) represents between 10 and 20 % of all newly diagnosed soft tissue sarcomas [1]. It is classified based on anatomical site of origin, a factor that is important for outcome and prognosis [2]. Abdominal LMS is highly aggressive with an overall 5 year survival rate between 20 and 30 % [3]. Although histologically similar, the different anatomic variants of abdominal LMS have varying clinical behaviour and differ in prognosis [4]. Surgical resection is the cornerstone of curative treatment for localized disease if adequate margins are obtained [1, 5]. However, this is often not possible due to anatomical restrictions and large tumor size at diagnosis. Moreover, LMS tends to metastasize, most commonly to the lungs and liver. Unfortunately, there are no clear guidelines regarding the role of oncological treatment; neither in the primary nor metastatic setting [5]. In fact, almost all patients with metastatic disease are considered incurable and, thus, offered only palliative treatment.

Here, we present a patient with an abdominal LMS, specifically a mesenteric LMS. This is a rare malignancy,

*Correspondence: Mercy.verghese@gmail.com
[7] Department of Surgery, Nordland Hospital, 8092 Bodoe, Norway
Full list of author information is available at the end of the article

with only a few cases reported in the literature [6–9]. The LMS was surgically resected with an R0 margin and no adjuvant oncological therapy was given. Unfortunately, the patient developed metastatic disease both to the liver and lungs. Histological evaluation of metastases revealed a highly malignant, pleomorphic sarcoma that resembled her primary tumor, but was not morphologically identical. It was categorized as dedifferentiated LMS [3, 10]. An aggressive multimodal therapeutic strategy was chosen, including staggered intensive chemotherapy tailored to the histological-subtype of the metastasis [11]. Presently, she is in complete clinical remission about 36 months following diagnosis of metastatic disease and without any demonstrable long-term side effects from chemotherapy.

Case report

Our patient is a 40 year old woman who had no significant medical history except for an appendectomy when she was 20 years-old. She presented with a two-month history of left sided abdominal pain accompanied by abdominal discomfort and distention. Additionally, she suffered from nausea and vomiting without any changes in stool pattern.

On physical examination, a large palpable mass was detected in the left quadrant. This mass was very tender upon palpation, but there were no signs of peritonitis. Blood tests revealed increased acute phase proteins and reduced haemoglobin but were otherwise unremarkable. Computerized tomography (CT) of the abdomen revealed an intraperitoneal tumor in the left quadrant measuring 8 × 7 cm axially and 7 cm craniocaudally (Fig. 1a). The tumor was closely related to the descending colon and small intestine and revealed heterogenous contrast enhancement with necrotic areas (Fig. 1b). There was no pelvic or retroperitoneal adenopathy, though some ascites was seen in the pelvis minor. A sarcoma was suspected and the patient was referred to the Section for Sarcoma at The Norwegian Radium Hospital.

About two weeks later, the patient was operated via a midline laparotomy. The tumor, which was partly adherent to the sigmoid mesocolon, was removed en bloc together with 15 cm of small intestine and colon. An antiperistaltic side-to-side-anastomosis was established at the splenic flexure as well as a small intestinal anastomosis about 120 cm proximal to the ileocaecal valve. No intraperitoneal metastases were seen, but tumor perforation to the peritoneal cavity and resulting bloody ascites was documented perioperatively. Despite this high risk for tumor relapse, no adjuvant therapy was given to the patient in line with guidelines regarding adjuvant therapy for abdominal LMS [5].

Histopathological investigations revealed that the resected tumor measured 11 × 9 × 7 cm, was well circumscribed and without infiltration of the small or large intestine. However, the tumor diffusely invaded the serosal surface. More than 50 % of the tumor showed necrosis macroscopically. Histologically, the tumor consisted of pleomorphic, spindle cells with eosinophilic cytoplasm and focally cigar shaped nuclei resembling a high grade, pleomorphic leiomyosarcoma. Up to 14 mitoses per 10

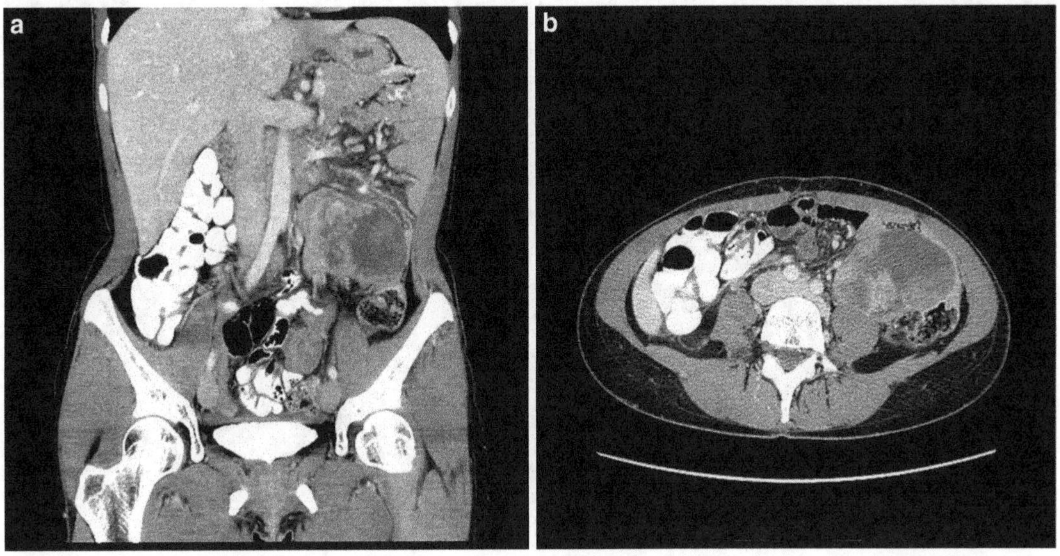

Fig. 1 CT of the primary LMS. CT of the abdomen and pelvis showing an intraperitoneal tumor in the left quadrant measuring 8 × 7 × 7 cm (**a** coronal section). The tumor is located in the mesentery and is in close relation to both the small bowel and the sigmoid colon (**b** axial section). The low-density region within the tumor indicates necrosis

high power fields (1734 mm^2) were found (French malignancy grade 3) (Fig. 2a, b). No invasion of blood vessels was seen. Immunohistochemical examination showed distinct, focal positivity for caldesmon, SMA and desmin, supporting the diagnosis of LMS (Fig. 2 c–e).

About three months after the operation, the patient experienced intermittent abdominal pain. No local tumor recurrence was seen on the CT of the abdomen, but multiple contrast enhancing lesions, typical for metastases, were seen in the liver, the largest measuring close to 3 cm (Fig. 3a). Chest CT revealed multiple round, well-circumscribed lesions in both lungs consistent with metastases (Fig. 3b). Biopsy of a liver lesion confirmed metastatic disease and showed only large, pleomorphic cells (Fig. 3a insert) consistent with a highly malignant pleomorphic sarcoma. After multidisciplinary assessment, we decided to treat the patient with 6 cycles of doxorubicin (50 mg/m^2, for the first treatment and 75 mg/m^2 for the other cycles) and ifosfamide (5 g/m^2) with granulocyte colony-stimulating factor (G-CSF) given at 3 weeks interval. The patient showed a radiological response, exhibiting partial remission with a reduction in size and number of liver and lung metastases (Fig. 4). No new metastases were seen. Moreover, her side effects of treatment were surprisingly modest. Hence, to further enhance the chemotherapeutic effect, we added 5 cycles of weekly doxorubicin monotherapy (20 mg) and 6 cycles with gemcitabine 675 mg/m^2 days 1 and 8 with docetaxel 75 mg/m^2 on day 8 and G-CSF on day 9 (every three weeks). This induced a further reduction in the number and size of metastases in the liver and lungs. Due to side effects with water retention and muscle pain we switched to 3 cycles of high dose ifosfamide 12 g/m^2. Subsequent radiological assessment confirmed an almost complete radiological response to this intense schedule of chemotherapies (Fig. 4).

After a multidisciplinary discussion, we considered the remaining visible lesions in the lungs and liver to be resectable. Therefore, the patient underwent combined left hepatectomy in combination with radiofrequency ablation of metastatic foci in the right liver lobe, followed by a thoracoscopic wedge resection of metastasis in the right lung. The rationale of removing metastases was to decrease tumor burden, as this has been shown to prolong disease-free survival and probably also overall survival, similar to what is seen in patients who undergo resection of metastases limited to the lungs [12]. This combination of surgery and/or radiofrequency ablation of residual lesions was performed to improve chances of long-term clinical remission, as there was no evidence of tumor outside the liver and lungs. An immediate postoperative MRI of the abdomen showed three

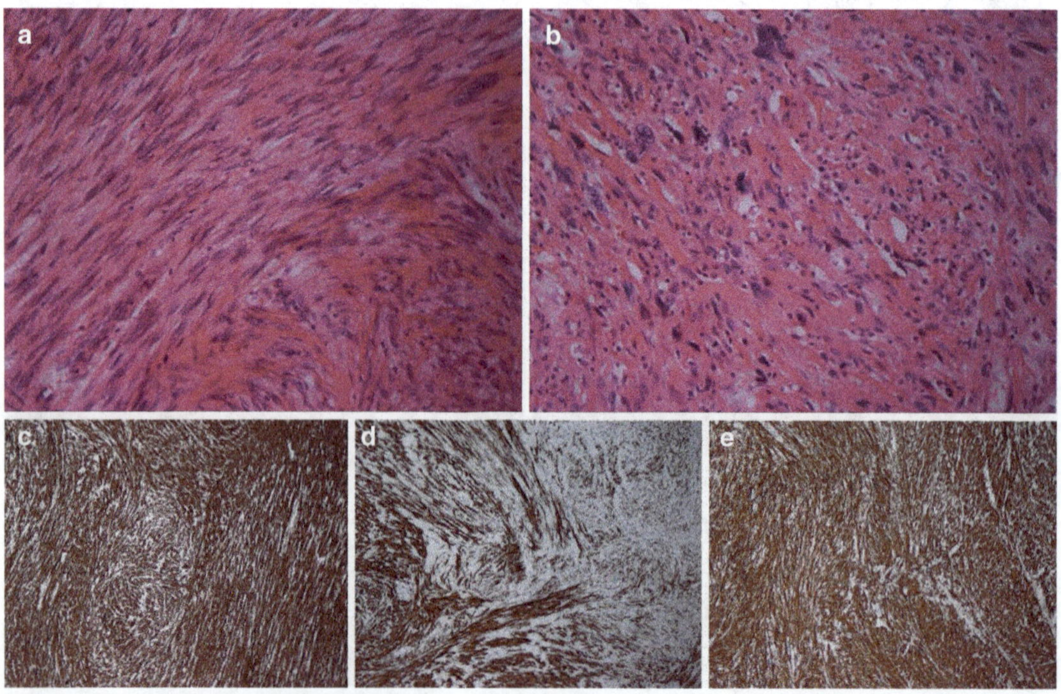

Fig. 2 Histopathology of tumor. Histopathological analysis of primary tumor revealed pleomorphic, spindle cells (**a**) and pleomorphic cells (**b**) with eosinophilic cytoplasm consistent with a high grade, pleomorphic leiomyosarcoma. Immunohistochemical examination showed distinct, focal positivity for SMA (**c**), desmin (**d**) and H-caldesmon (**e**), markers that are characteristic for LMS

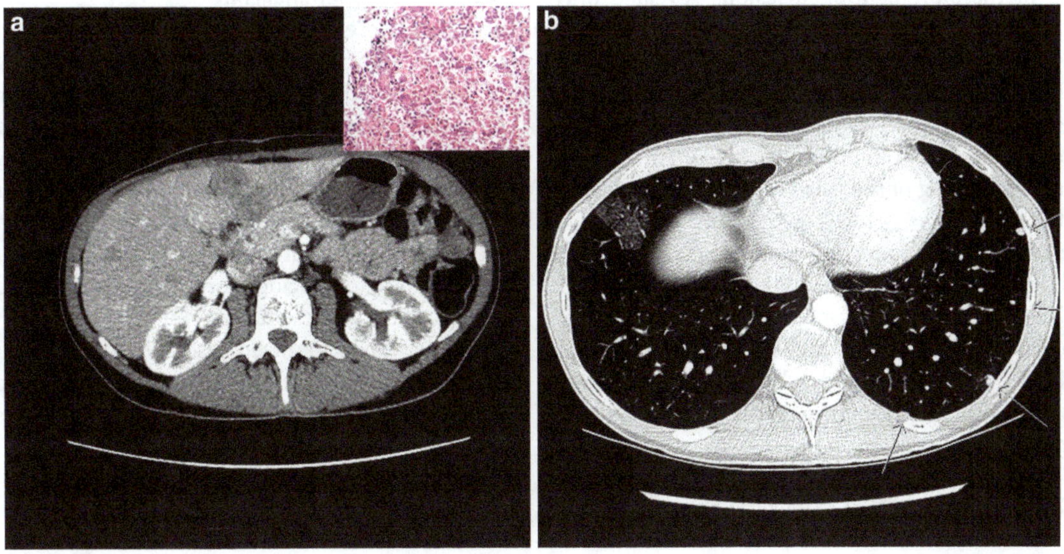

Fig. 3 CT of metastatic disease. Axial CT of the abdomen and thorax. Multiple contrast-enhancing lesions in the liver with irregular borders typical for metastases (**a**). Histopathological analysis of a liver metastasis revealed only large, pleomorphic cells (**a** inset) consistent with a highly malignant dedifferentiated pleomorphic sarcoma. CT of thorax showing multiple round, well-circumscribed lung lesions consistent with metastases. The ground-glass opacity around the lesions may be caused by hemorrhage (**b**)

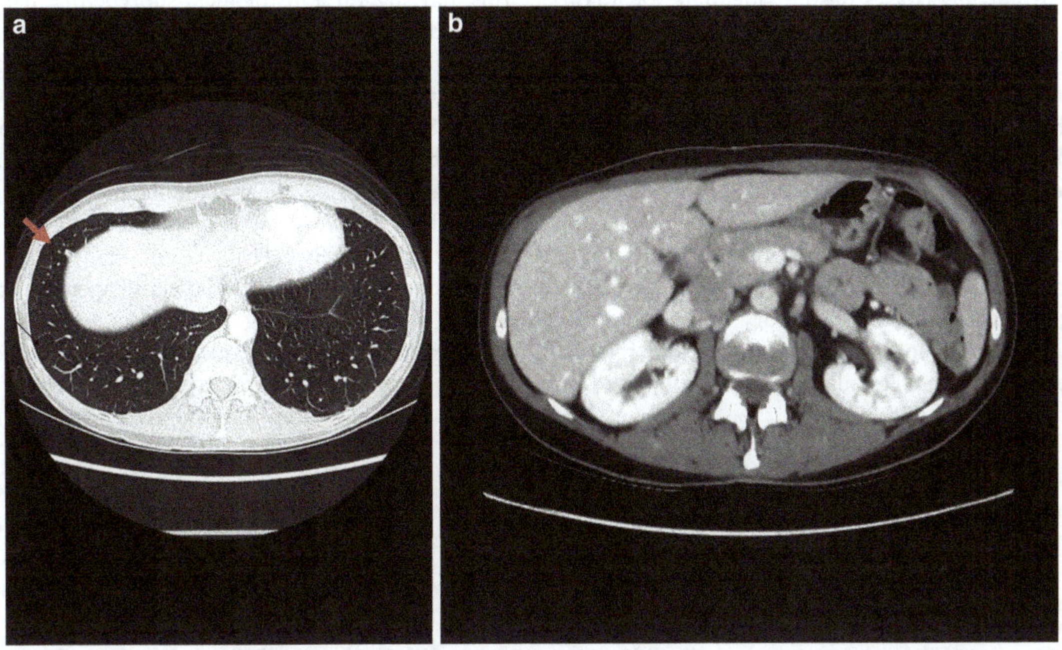

Fig. 4 CT showing radiological response. Axial CT of the thorax and abdomen showing almost complete radiological response after histological subtype-specific chemotherapy. A small metastatic lesion measuring 5 × 6 mm (**a**, arrow) and no other visible metastatic foci in the lungs or the liver (**b**) are seen after chemotherapy

residual lesions in the liver which were not visible on the perioperative ultrasound and suspicious subcutaneous lesions near the midline laparotomy scar. A repeat laparotomy was then performed in which the abdominal scar was removed in combination with ultrasound/MRI-image fusion guided re-ablation of the liver. Histological evaluation of the aforementioned lesions revealed only fibrotic changes with no viable tumor cells. Postoperatively, the patient received 2 cycles of weekly doxorubicin 20 mg due to a strong desire from the patient. Post operative CT of the abdomen and thorax revealed only postoperative changes in the liver and lungs. A complete outline and scheduling of the various chemotherapies are displayed in Fig. 5.

Five months after surgery for metastatic disease, the patient developed abdominal pain and constipation. CT of the abdomen and thorax revealed only postoperative changes. Moreover, upper and lower endoscopy was unremarkable. A contrast study showed no pathology, only stenosis of the small intestine, which was dilatated, and the patient showed symptomatic relief after laxative therapy. The patient is presently in clinical remission, 36 months following diagnosis of metastatic disease.

Discussion

Abdominal LMS

Mesenteric LMS was first described in 1963 [13] and is most likely derived from the smooth muscle cells of blood vessels in the mesentery [3]. It is an aggressive disease and approximately half of all patients will develop distant metastases despite adequate local control [14]. The overall 5 year survival rate is only 20–30 % [3], partly because mesenteric LMS often remains undetected until late in the course of disease development, due to the large available space of the abdominal cavity. As in the case of our patient, abdominal distension and discomfort are common presenting symptoms [1]. Additionally, altered bowel movements and weight loss are also seen. Blood tests are non-specific but may reveal anaemia [1] and elevated acute phase proteins. Radiological assessment is mandatory for preoperative evaluation of tumor location, dimensions and relation to adjacent structures. Definitive diagnosis is based on histopathology.

Treatment of abdominal LMS

Localized disease

Surgery is the cornerstone of treatment and is the only therapeutic modality proven to provide cure [5]. However, complete resection is often difficult due to large tumor size at presentation and recent studies have shown that resection margins may be the only significant predictor of local recurrence [4, 15]. Moreover, complete primary surgical resection is critical for achieving the best overall outcome [16]. Other factors include tumor depth, histological grade, and metastasis at presentation [15, 17]. The role of adjuvant chemotherapy in localized disease is not established and therefore is not standard treatment [5]. It can be proposed to high-risk patients, after multidisciplinary assessment or within clinical trials. In keeping with current guidelines, our patient did not receive adjuvant treatment.

Metastatic disease

Chemotherapy

When our patient developed metastatic disease, a core needle biopsy of a liver metastasis was obtained. Though the biopsy material was limited, a highly malignant tumor, displaying only large pleomorphic cells similar to the cells focally present in the primary tumor, was seen. This may suggest a histological-subtype that had evolved into a dedifferentiated phenotype compared to the primary tumor. This was the reason for choosing to add ifosfamide, rather than dacarbazine, to the initial regimen [18]. Such biological heterogeneity is documented between primary and metastatic disease in a number of malignancies [19]. Patients with pleomorphic or dedifferentiated LMS have a particularly poor prognosis, with a metastatic rate of 89 % [10].

The choice of chemotherapeutic agents depend on several factors including histological-subtype, age, comorbidity and expected tolerance of side effects. Our present knowledge regarding chemotherapy of LMS is mainly based on non-randomized phase II studies or

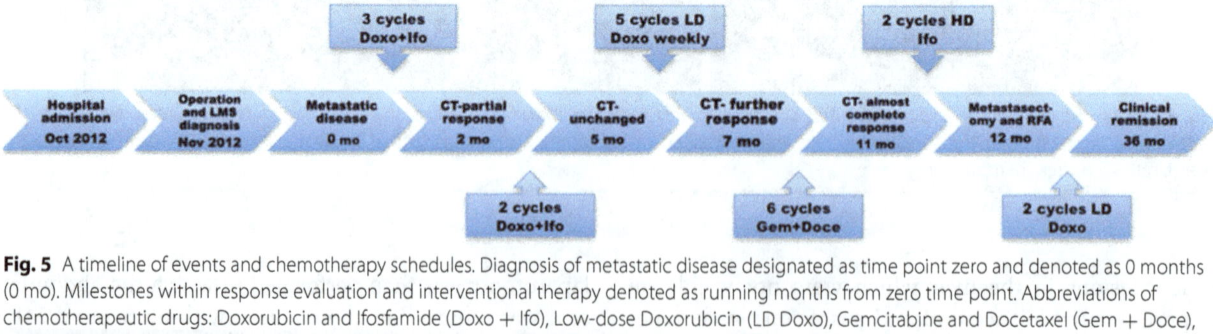

Fig. 5 A timeline of events and chemotherapy schedules. Diagnosis of metastatic disease designated as time point zero and denoted as 0 months (0 mo). Milestones within response evaluation and interventional therapy denoted as running months from zero time point. Abbreviations of chemotherapeutic drugs: Doxorubicin and Ifosfamide (Doxo + Ifo), Low-dose Doxorubicin (LD Doxo), Gemcitabine and Docetaxel (Gem + Doce), High-dose Ifosfamide (HD Ifo)

retrospective case series [11]. Furthermore, the rarity and heterogeneity of soft tissue sarcomas, as well as the high variability of patient characteristics, chemotherapeutic regimens, histological and molecular subtypes (early trials might even have included GIST patients), the variable follow-up and differing definitions of end points all preclude the available evidence of chemotherapeutic effectiveness.

Despite the paucity of randomized trials, anthracyclines, either as a single-or-multi-agent chemotherapy, are the first-line of treatment for abdominal LMS [5], according to the ESMO-guidelines. Moreover, depending on the histological-subtype, doxorubicin and dacarbazine (for a purely LMS) [20] or doxorubicin and ifosfamide (for malignancies with a pleomorphic cellular component) [21] have been advocated. Second-line chemotherapeutic agents recommended include (1) standard ifosfamide or high-dose ifosfamide (around 14 g/m^2) [22], (2) a combination of gemcitabine and docetaxel [23] (which showed improved progression free survival and overall survival than gemcitabine alone) [24], (3) a combination of dacarbazine and gemcitabine [25] and (4) trabectedin [26]. The rationale for giving the patient such intense and sequential chemotherapy has previously been shown to be successful [27] in achieving a maximal radiological and clinical response. It has also been reported to improve long-term survival [28]. We chose not to use trabectedin and pazopanib as there is not much experience with these drugs in a curative treatment setting.

For advanced metastatic disease, surgery or radiofrequency ablation is usually not the treatment of choice, but may be considered in selected cases where the number of metastatic foci are few and amenable to intervention. Given the remarkable response of our patient to chemotherapy, we decided to remove remaining lesions in the lung and liver using surgical resection and radiofrequency ablation with the hope of achieving long-term, complete clinical remission [29]. The rational for such an approach is that the smallest lesions, including micrometastases, may have been completely eradicated by the chemotherapy. Hence, removing the larger metastases, which may still contain foci of viable sarcoma cells, eliminates the nidus for subsequent relapse. While the degree of response to preoperative chemotherapy has not been demonstrated to influence post-resection survival, largely due to small sample size, the progression of disease prior to resection is a known adverse prognostic factor [30]. The presence of disease outside the chest has been considered a contraindication to resection of pulmonary metastases. More recently, however, it has been shown that resection of pulmonary and extrapulmonary metastases results in disease-free survival and overall survival, similar to that seen in patients who undergo resection of metastases limited to the lungs [12].

Conclusions

To our knowledge, this is the first report of a patient with metastatic mesenteric LMS who developed complete clinical and radiological remission without any demonstrable long-term side effects from chemotherapy, after receiving multimodal therapy including an unconventional histological-subtype-tailored chemotherapy comprising 3–4 regimens, surgical resection and radiofrequency ablation of metastatic foci. Given the rarity of mesenteric leiomyosarcoma and lack of guidelines regarding oncological therapy, we suggest that multimodal therapy including aggressive histological-subtype tailored chemotherapy can result in complete remission under the guidance of a multidisciplinary team.

Authors' contributions

Study Concept and Study Design: RB, KSH, OB. Data Acquisition: KSH, MV, IL, AMW. Quality control of data: KSH, OB. Data analysis and interpretation: KSH, OB, MV. Manuscript preparation: MV. Manuscript editing: RB, KSH, OB. Manuscript review: All authors. All authors read and approved the final manuscript.

Author details

[1] Department of Oncology, Oslo University Hospital, The Norwegian Radium Hospital, Ullernchausseen 70, 0379 Oslo, Norway. [2] Institute for Clinical Medicine, Faculty of Medicine, University of Oslo, Box 1171, Blindern, 0450 Oslo, Norway. [3] Department of Radiology, Oslo University Hospital, The Norwegian Radium Hospital, Ullernchausseen 70, 0379 Oslo, Norway. [4] Department of Pathology, Oslo University Hospital, The Norwegian Radium Hospital, Ullernchausseen 70, 0379 Oslo, Norway. [5] Gastrointestinal and pediatric surgery, Section for Hepatopancreatobiliary Surgery, Oslo University Hospital Rikshospitalet, Sognsvannsveien 20, 0424 Oslo, Norway. [6] Department of Sarcoma Medical Oncology, The University of Texas M. D. Anderson Cancer Center, Texas, Houston 77030, USA. [7] Department of Surgery, Nordland Hospital, 8092 Bodoe, Norway.

Acknowledgements

We would like to acknowledge gastrointestinal surgeons T. Hølmebakk and S. Stoldt and thoracic surgeon L. Jørgensen.

Competing interests

The authors declare that they have no competing interests.

References

1. Serrano C, George S. Leiomyosarcoma. Hematol Oncol Clin North Am. 2013;27(5):957–74.
2. Fiore M, Colombo C, Locati P, Berselli M, Radaelli S, Morosi C, Casali PG, Gronchi A. Surgical technique, morbidity, and outcome of primary retroperitoneal sarcoma involving inferior vena cava. Ann Surg Oncol. 2012;19(2):511–8.
3. Hashimoto H, Tsuneyoshi M, Enjoji M. Malignant smooth muscle tumors of the retroperitoneum and mesentery: a clinicopathologic analysis of 44 cases. J Surg Oncol. 1985;28(3):177–86.
4. Bathan AJ, Constantinidou A, Pollack SM, Jones RL. Diagnosis, prognosis, and management of leiomyosarcoma: recognition of anatomic variants. Curr Opin Oncol. 2013;25(4):384–9.

5. ESMO. Soft tissue and visceral sarcomas: ESMO Clinical Practice Guidelines for diagnosis, treatment and follow-up. Ann Oncol. 2014;25(3):iii102–12.
6. Kim KJ, Lee WS, Chang SE, Choi JH, Sung KJ, Moon KC, Koh JK. Metastatic cutaneous leiomyosarcoma from primary neoplasm of the mesentery. Int J Dermatol. 2001;40(8):527–9.
7. Koczkowska M, Lipska BS, Grzeszewska J, Limon J, Biernat W, Jassem J. Primary leiomyosarcoma of the mesentery in two sisters: clinical and molecular characteristics. Pol J Pathol. 2013;64(1):59–63.
8. Natarajan A, Rudresh HK, D'Souza RE, Lahoti NG. Primary leiomyosarcoma of jejunal mesentery: a rare case. Trop Gastroenterol. 2000;21(1):30–2.
9. Simonovich CJ, Hardman JM, Navin JJ, Jacobs J, Fergusson N. An unusual abdominal tumor–leiomyosarcoma of the mesentery: a case report. Hawaii Med J. 2006;65(1):18–20.
10. Nicolas MM, Tamboli P, Gomez JA, Czerniak BA. Pleomorphic and dedifferentiated leiomyosarcoma: clinicopathologic and immunohistochemical study of 41 cases. Hum Pathol. 2010;41(5):663–71.
11. Eriksson M. Histology-driven chemotherapy of soft-tissue sarcoma. Ann Oncol. 2010;21(Suppl 7):vii270–6.
12. Blackmon SH, Shah N, Roth JA, Correa AM, Vaporciyan AA, Rice DC, Hofstetter W, Walsh GL, Benjamin R, Pollock R, et al. Resection of pulmonary and extrapulmonary sarcomatous metastases is associated with long-term survival. Ann Thorac Surg. 2009;88(3):877–84.
13. Yannopoulous K, Stout AP. Primary solid tumors of the mesentery. Cancer. 1963;16:914–27.
14. Penel N, Italiano A, Isambert N, Bompas E, Bousquet G, Duffaud F. Factors affecting the outcome of patients with metastatic leiomyosarcoma treated with doxorubicin-containing chemotherapy. Ann Oncol. 2010;21(6):1361–5.
15. Abraham JA, Weaver MJ, Hornick JL, Zurakowski D, Ready JE. Outcomes and prognostic factors for a consecutive case series of 115 patients with somatic leiomyosarcoma. J Bone Joint Surg Am. 2012;94(8):736–44.
16. Nagarsheth NP, Nicastri DG, Kashani M, Fried K. Complete surgical resection of a 40-cm leiomyosarcoma of the large bowel mesentery. J Surg Educ. 2007;64(3):162–4.
17. Italiano A, Lagarde P, Brulard C, Terrier P, Lae M, Marques B, Ranchere-Vince D, Michels JJ, Trassard M, Cioffi A, et al. Genetic profiling identifies two classes of soft-tissue leiomyosarcomas with distinct clinical characteristics. Clin Cancer Res. 2013;19(5):1190–6.
18. Judson I, Verweij J, Gelderblom H, Hartmann JT, Schoffski P, Blay JY, Kerst JM, Sufliarsky J, Whelan J, Hohenberger P, et al. Doxorubicin alone versus intensified doxorubicin plus ifosfamide for first-line treatment of advanced or metastatic soft-tissue sarcoma: a randomised controlled phase 3 trial. Lancet Oncol. 2014;15(4):415–23.
19. Fidler IJ. The pathogenesis of cancer metastasis: the 'seed and soil' hypothesis revisited. Nat Rev Cancer. 2003;3(6):453–8.
20. Lorigan P, Verweij J, Papai Z, Rodenhuis S, Le CA, Leahy MG, Radford JA, Van Glabbeke MM, Kirkpatrick A, Hogendoorn PC, et al. Phase III trial of two investigational schedules of ifosfamide compared with standard-dose doxorubicin in advanced or metastatic soft tissue sarcoma: a European Organisation for Research and Treatment of Cancer Soft Tissue and Bone Sarcoma Group Study. J Clin Oncol. 2007;25(21):3144–50.
21. Nascimento AF, Raut CP. Diagnosis and management of pleomorphic sarcomas (so-called "MFH") in adults. J Surg Oncol. 2008;97(4):330–9.
22. Le CA, Antoine E, Spielmann M, Le CT, Brain E, Toussaint C, Janin N, Kayitalire L, Fontaine F, Genin J, et al. High-dose ifosfamide: circumvention of resistance to standard-dose ifosfamide in advanced soft tissue sarcomas. J Clin Oncol. 1995;13(7):1600–8.
23. Hensley ML, Maki R, Venkatraman E, Geller G, Lovegren M, Aghajanian C, Sabbatini P, Tong W, Barakat R, Spriggs DR. Gemcitabine and docetaxel in patients with unresectable leiomyosarcoma: results of a phase II trial. J Clin Oncol. 2002;20(12):2824–31.
24. Maki RG, Wathen JK, Patel SR, Priebat DA, Okuno SH, Samuels B, Fanucchi M, Harmon DC, Schuetze SM, Reinke D, et al. Randomized phase II study of gemcitabine and docetaxel compared with gemcitabine alone in patients with metastatic soft tissue sarcomas: results of sarcoma alliance for research through collaboration study 002 [corrected]. J Clin Oncol. 2007;25(19):2755–63.
25. Garcia-Del-Muro X, Lopez-Pousa A, Maurel J, Martin J, Martinez-Trufero J, Casado A, Gomez-Espana A, Fra J, Cruz J, Poveda A, et al. Randomized phase II study comparing gemcitabine plus dacarbazine versus dacarbazine alone in patients with previously treated soft tissue sarcoma: a Spanish Group for Research on Sarcomas study. J Clin Oncol. 2011;29(18):2528–33.
26. Grosso F, Jones RL, Demetri GD, Judson IR, Blay JY, Le CA, Sanfilippo R, Casieri P, Collini P, Dileo P, et al. Efficacy of trabectedin (ecteinascidin-743) in advanced pretreated myxoid liposarcomas: a retrospective study. Lancet Oncol. 2007;8(7):595–602.
27. Leu KM, Ostruszka LJ, Shewach D, Zalupski M, Sondak V, Biermann JS, Lee JS, Couwlier C, Palazzolo K, Baker LH. Laboratory and clinical evidence of synergistic cytotoxicity of sequential treatment with gemcitabine followed by docetaxel in the treatment of sarcoma. J Clin Oncol. 2004;22(9):1706–12.
28. Ohnstad HO, Bruland OS, Taksdal I, Bjerkehagen B, Nenadovic M, Saeter G, Jorgensen LH, Hall KS. Response to preoperative chemotherapy in patients undergoing resection of pulmonary metastasis from soft tissue sarcoma—a predictor of outcome? Acta Oncol. 2014;53(9):1180–7.
29. Temple LK, Brennan MF. The role of pulmonary metastasectomy in soft tissue sarcoma. Semin Thorac Cardiovasc Surg. 2002;14(1):35–44.
30. Stephens EH, Blackmon SH, Correa AM, Roth JA, Rice DC, Hofstetter W, Benjamin R, Mehran R, Swisher SG, Walsh GL, et al. Progression after chemotherapy is a novel predictor of poor outcomes after pulmonary metastasectomy in sarcoma patients. J Am Coll Surg. 2011;212(5):821–6.

4

Predictors of survival in patients with sarcoma admitted to the intensive care unit

Rohan Gupta[1], Neda Heshami[1], Chouhan Jay[1], Naveen Ramesh[2], Juhee Song[3], Xiudong Lei[3], Erfe Jean Rose[4], Kristen Carter[5], Dejka M. Araujo[5], Robert S. Benjamin[5], Shreyaskumar Patel[5], Joseph L. Nates[4] and Vinod Ravi[5*]

Abstract

Background: Advances in treatment of sarcoma patients has prolonged survival but has led to increased disease- or treatment-related complications resulting in greater number of admissions to the intensive care unit (ICU). Survival and long-term outcome information about such critically ill patients with sarcoma is unknown.

Methods: The primary objective of the study was to determine the ICU and post-ICU survival rates of critically ill sarcoma patients. Secondary objectives included determining the modifiable and non-modifiable predictors of poor survival. We performed a retrospective chart review of sarcoma patients admitted to the ICU at The University of Texas MD Anderson Cancer Center between January 1, 2005, and December 31, 2012. Main outcome measures were ICU mortality, in-hospital mortality and 1, 2, and 6-month survival rates. Covariates such as histological diagnosis, disease characteristics, chemotherapy use, Charlson comorbidity index, Sequential Organ Failure Assessment (SOFA) scores, and clinical findings leading to ICU admission were analyzed for their effects on survival.

Results: We identified 172 admissions over the 8-year study period hat met our inclusion criteria. The study population was 45.9 % males with a median age of 52 years. The most common sarcoma subgroups were high-grade unclassified sarcoma (25 %) and bone tumors (17.4 %). The ICU mortality rate was 23.3 % (95 % confidence interval [CI], 16.9–29.6 %), and an additional 6.4 % of patients died before hospital discharge (95 % CI, 22.9–37.1 %). 6-month OS rates were 41 %. The median SOFA scores on admission were 6 (inter quartile range (IQR), 3.5–9) in ICU survivors and 10 (IQR, 6.5–14) in ICU non-survivors. Increase in SOFA scores ≥6 led to poor outcomes (ICU survival 13.3 %, OS 6.7 %). Charlson comorbidity index (HR 1.139, 95 % CI 1.023–1.268, $p = 0.02$) and discharge SOFA scores (HR 1.210, 95 % CI 1.141–1.283, $p < 0.0001$) correlated with overall survival.

Conclusions: Our results suggest that patients that are admitted to the ICU for respiratory failure, cardiac arrest, septic shock, acute renal failure or acidosis and also have a high SOFA score with subsequent worsening in the ICU have poor prognosis. Based on the retrospective data which needs further validation we can recommend that judicious approach should be taken in patients with predictors of poor survival before subjecting them to aggressive treatment.

Keywords: Cancer, Sarcoma, ICU, Survival, SOFA

*Correspondence: vravi@mdanderson.org
[5] Department of Sarcoma Medical Oncology, The University of Texas MD Anderson Cancer Center, 1515 Holcombe Blvd # 450, Houston, TX 77030, USA

Background

Sarcomas are a rare, histologically and behaviorally diverse group of malignant connective tissue tumors that make up approximately 1 % of all adult malignancies and 12 % of pediatric cancers [1, 2]. As a result of the substantial progress made in the past 2 decades in understanding the behavior and molecular pathogenesis of sarcoma, new therapies have been developed. Advances in treatment may prolong survival but can lead to increased disease- or treatment-related complications requiring aggressive critical care. Due to the rarity of this class of tumors, the survival of critically ill sarcoma patients has not been well studied.

The treatment of such patients requires a multidisciplinary approach, with coordination among oncologists, critical care physicians, consulting services, ancillary staff, and patients' families. Despite the availability of advanced life support devices in intensive care centers in the United States, it is difficult for both patients and physicians to objectively determine the effect of such heroic measures on prognosis or quality of life. Studies up to the 1990s had shown that among all diseases, patients with cancer had the lowest intensive care unit (ICU) survival rates, and the majority of these patients died soon after their hospital discharge [3–5]. However, over the past two decades, the approach to treatment in such cases has been shifting. Some studies have shown that patients lacking predictors of poor survival outcomes are considered as good candidates for aggressive therapy [6–8].

The primary objective of our study was to determine the ICU and post-ICU survival rates of critically ill sarcoma patients. Secondary objectives included determining the modifiable and nonmodifiable predictors of poor survival.

Methods

Patient population

After obtaining institutional review board approval, we retrospectively reviewed the electronic medical records of 212 critically ill patients with sarcoma who had been admitted to the ICU at The University of Texas MD Anderson Cancer Center between January 1, 2006, and December 31, 2012. For the purpose of this analysis, we limited the study population to patient's first ICU admission only. We also excluded from the study population patients who had been admitted to the ICU for perioperative care.

Study design

This retrospective study was designed to identify predictors of poor survival that contribute to ICU mortality. ICU mortality was defined as the percentage of patients with sarcoma who died in the ICU among total number of patients admitted to the ICU with sarcoma during the study period. Secondary outcomes were in-hospital mortality and 1, 2, and 6-month survival rates, which were defined by similar means. Overall survival (OS) for each patient was measured from the time of initial ICU admission to the last date of contact or death. We defined *ICU survival* as short-term or acute survival and *6-month survival* as long-term survival. Median follow-up time was calculated from the date of ICU admission.

Patient's current and previous chemotherapy regimens were examined to evaluate the impact of various chemotherapy treatments on survival. Tumor burden was noted by recording the various sites of metastasis, such as head and neck, musculoskeletal, heart, lung, liver, gastrointestinal tract, and spleen. The Charlson comorbidities index (CCI) was used to assess the role of serious comorbid disease in the survival of patients in the study [9].

Clinical findings present at the time of ICU admission were recorded to assess acute illness (definitions in parentheses). Variables recorded included acute renal failure, anemia, thrombocytopenia, pancytopenia, hemorrhage (including bleeding from gastrointestinal tract), lactic acidosis, heart failure, pulmonary embolism, respiratory failure (use of noninvasive or invasive mechanical ventilation), cardiac arrest, atrial fibrillation, cardiac dysrhythmia, pneumonia, septic shock, hypotension (systolic blood pressure <100 or on vasopressors), hypertension, neutropenic fever (absolute neutrophil count <1500), altered mental status, and malnutrition (patient on feeding tube or total parental nutrition).

Severity of illness at the time of ICU admission was measured by Sequential Organ Failure Assessment (SOFA) scores. Maximum SOFA scores and discharge SOFA scores were also obtained to track the patients' progress while they were in the ICU. Change in SOFA scores were calculated by subtracting the admission SOFA scores from the maximum SOFA scores. Organ failure at the time of ICU admission was determined by an admission SOFA score ≥ 2 per organ system. The total number of organ failures was calculated for each patient.

Analysis

Patient characteristics were tabulated and compared between groups by using the Chi square test or Fisher exact test as appropriate for categorical variables and by the nonparametric Wilcoxon rank sum test for continuous variables. A multivariate logistic regression model was fitted to examine the relationship between death in the ICU and clinical characteristics. Patients who were lost to follow-up or alive were censored at their dates of last contact. The Kaplan–Meier product limit method was used to estimate the survival outcomes of all patients by groups; the log-rank statistic was used to compare groups.

Cox proportional hazards models were fitted to determine the association of patient and clinical characteristics with OS. Variables that had significant univariate log-rank p values were candidates for the multivariate model. Results were expressed in hazard ratios (HRs), odds ratios (ORs) and 95 % confidence intervals (CIs). p values of less than 0.05 were considered statistically significant; all tests were two-sided. Statistical analyses were carried out by using SAS 9.4 (SAS Institute Inc., Cary, NC) and S-Plus 8.2 (TIBCO Software Inc, Palo Alto, CA, USA).

Results

Patient characteristics

We identified a total of 212 sarcoma admissions to the ICU at MD Anderson between January 1, 2005, and December 31, 2012. We excluded 23 ICU admissions of patients who were admitted to the ICU multiple times during the study course. Of the remaining 189 admissions, 17 perioperative admissions were excluded, leaving a sample of 172 first-time ICU admissions. The study population was 45.9 % male with median age of 52 years (interquartile range [IQR] 38–62 years) (Supplemental Digital Content—Table 1). The most common sarcoma subgroups were unclassified high-grade sarcoma (25 %), bone sarcoma (Ewing sarcoma, osteosarcoma, and chondrosarcoma; 17.4 %), vascular sarcoma (angiosarcoma and epithelioid hemangioendothelioma; 9.9 %), and leiomyosarcoma (7.6 %). The ICU mortality rate was 23.3 % (95 % CI 16.9–29.6 %), and the hospital mortality rate was 29.7 % (95 % CI 22.9–37.1 %). The median Charlson comorbidity index was 6 (IQR 6–7) owing to presence of metastatic cancer in most of the patients at the time of admission.

Death in the ICU

There were 40 patient deaths (23.3 %) in the ICU. In the univariate logistic regression model for the death at the ICU, short-term mortality did not correlate with tumor site, histology, disease status, presence of metastatic disease, Charlson comorbidity index or neutropenia at the time of ICU admission. However, patients with clinical findings of acidosis, acute renal failure, cardiac arrest, hypotension (including septic shock), pneumonia, septic shock or respiratory failure at the time of ICU admission had worse outcomes than patients who lacked these findings on admission (Supplemental Digital Content—Tables 1, 2).

The median SOFA scores on admission were 6 (IQR 3.5–9) in ICU survivors and 10 (IQR 6.5–14) in non-survivors. In addition, the median maximum SOFA scores were 7 (IQR 4–9.5) in survivors and 14 (IQR 10–17) in non-survivors, and the median discharge SOFA scores were 4 (IQR 2–6) in survivors and 10 (IQR, 7.5–13.5) in non-survivors. Patients with admission SOFA scores of 11 or more had a lower ICU survival rate than did those with scores less than 11 (45.7 vs 80 % or more) (Table 2). An increase of 6 or more in the SOFA score from the time of admission significantly affected short- (ICU survival 13.3 %) and long-term outcomes (OS 6.7 %) (Table 3).

Multivariate logistic regression model for death in the ICU showed that SOFA admission score (OR 1.23, 95 % CI 1.12–1.35, $p < 0.0001$) was associated with death in the ICU. Variables that were initially included in the model and then reduced in a stepwise selection were SOFA admission score and number of metastatic sites.

OS from ICU admission

Median follow-up among all patients was 2.9 months (range 0.02–77.5 months). At the time of this analysis, 135 patients (78.5 %) had died. For the whole cohort, 1, 2, and 6-month OS rates were 64, 57, and 41 %, respectively (Table 4). The Kaplan–Meier curves for OS are shown in Fig. 1.

In multivariable Cox proportional hazards models (Table 5), patients with gastrointestinal stromal tumors (HR 0.281, 95 % CI 0.119–0.662, $p = 0.004$) and leiomyosarcoma (HR 0.375, 95 % CI 0.160–0.880, $p = 0.02$) had a lower risk of death than did patients with unclassified high-grade sarcoma. Patients with higher Charlson Comorbidity Index (HR 1.139, 95 % CI 1.023–1.268, $p = 0.02$) and those with higher SOFA scores at discharge (HR 1.210, 95 % CI 1.141–1.283, $p < 0.0001$) also had higher risk of death (Table 5). Median survival rates were lower in patients with acute renal failure, cardiac arrest, pneumonia, septic shock, and respiratory failure.

Discussion

Decisions about the intensive care treatment of critically ill cancer patients with poor prognoses are challenging and need to be evaluated on a patient-by-patient basis. Our study benefits both physicians and family members by providing objective data on ICU mortality, long-term survival, and objective predictors of survival. Our results showed that among sarcoma patients, the ICU mortality, in-hospital mortality, and long-term survival rates were 23.3, 29.7, and 41 %, respectively. Patients who were admitted due to acute renal failure, cardiac arrest, septic shock, or respiratory failure had poor ICU outcomes and median survival durations ranging from 1 to 21 days. The median SOFA scores at the times of admission and discharge were significantly lower in ICU survivors than in non-survivors. An increase in SOFA score during the ICU stay is an important predictor of poor survival outcomes. We also determined that a higher number of organ failures was associated with an increased risk of ICU mortality (Supplemental Digital Content—Table 1).

Table 1 Patient and clinical characteristics by Alive or Death at the Intensive Care Unit (ICU)

	All patients[a] (N = 172)	Alive at ICU discharge[b] (N = 132)	Death at ICU[b] (N = 40)	p*
Age (y)				
Median (IQR)	52 (38–62)	52 (38–62)	53.5(36–66)	0.65
Gender				
Female	93 (54.1 %)	71 (76.3 %)	22 (23.7 %)	
Male	79 (45.9 %)	61 (77.2 %)	18 (22.8 %)	0.89[†]
Histological diagnosis				
Unclassified high-grade sarcoma	43 (25.0 %)	36 (83.7 %)	7 (16.3 %)	
Bone sarcoma[c]	30 (17.4 %)	21 (70 %)	9 (30 %)	
Vascular[d]	17 (9.9 %)	16 (94.1 %)	1 (5.9 %)	
GIST[e]	11 (6.4 %)	10 (90.9 %)	1 (9.1 %)	
MFH[e]	11 (6.4 %)	6 (54.5 %)	5 (45.5 %)	
Muscle	10 (5.8 %)	7 (70 %)	3 (30 %)	
Leiomyosarcoma	13 (7.6 %)	12 (92.3 %)	1 (7.7 %)	
Liposarcoma	7 (4.1 %)	4 (57.1 %)	3 (42.9 %)	
Synovial sarcoma	9 (5.2 %)	5 (55.6 %)	4 (44.4 %)	
Others	21 (12.2 %)	15 (71.4 %)	6 (28.6 %)	0.09
Status of malignancy				
First course of chemotherapy	29 (16.9 %)	20 (69 %)	9 (31 %)	
Progression	59 (34.3 %)	45 (76.3 %)	14 (23.7 %)	
Stable disease or partial remission	61 (35.5 %)	50 (82 %)	11 (18 %)	
Complete remission	4 (2.3 %)	4 (100 %)	0 (0 %)	
Mixed response	6 (3.5 %)	4 (66.7 %)	2 (33.3 %)	
Unknown	13 (7.6 %)	9 (69.2 %)	4 (30.8 %)	0.57
Site of malignancy				
Head and neck	15 (8.7 %)	11 (73.3 %)	4 (26.7 %)	
Thoracic	43 (25 %)	34 (79.1 %)	9 (20.9 %)	
Abdomen	71 (41.3 %)	55 (77.5 %)	16 (22.5 %)	
Extremities	43 (25 %)	32 (74.4 %)	11 (25.6 %)	0.94
Organ metastasis				
Lung				
No	86 (50 %)	69 (80.2 %)	17 (19.8 %)	
Yes	86 (50 %)	63 (73.3 %)	23 (26.7 %)	0.28
Liver				
No	142 (82.6 %)	108 (76.1 %)	34 (23.9 %)	
Yes	30 (17.4 %)	24 (80 %)	6 (20 %)	0.64
Other				
No	79 (45.9 %)	57 (72.2 %)	22 (27.8 %)	
Yes	93 (54.1 %)	75 (80.6 %)	18 (19.4 %)	0.19
Number of organ metastasis				
0	42 (24.4 %)	32 (76.2 %)	10 (23.8 %)	
1	54 (31.4 %)	39 (72.2 %)	15 (27.8 %)	
≥2	76 (44.2 %)	61 (80.3 %)	15 (19.7 %)	0.56
Treatment				
Current chemotherapy regimen				
None	43 (25 %)	34 (79.1 %)	9 (20.9 %)	
Adriamycin-based	68 (39.5 %)	50 (73.5 %)	18 (26.5 %)	
Gemcitabine-based	20 (11.6 %)	13 (65 %)	7 (35 %)	
Targeted therapy	41 (23.8 %)	35 (85.4 %)	6 (14.6 %)	0.29

Table 1 continued

	All patients[a] (N = 172)	Alive at ICU discharge[b] (N = 132)	Death at ICU[b] (N = 40)	p*
No. cycles of current chemotherapy, median (IQR[e])	1 (0–3)	1 (0–3)	1 (1–2)	0.80†
No. cycles of prior chemotherapies, median (IQR)	1 (0–3)	1 (0–3)	0 (0–2)	0.037†
No. cycles of prior chemotherapies				
0–1	114 (66.3 %)	88 (77.2 %)	26 (22.8 %)	
≥2	58 (33.7 %)	44 (75.9 %)	14 (24.1 %)	0.85
Radiation				
No	109 (63.7 %)	80 (73.4 %)	29 (26.6 %)	
Yes	62 (36.3 %)	51 (82.3 %)	11 (17.7 %)	0.19
Clinical conditions present at ICU admission				
Anemia	144 (83.7 %)	110 (76.4 %)	34 (23.6 %)	0.80
Hypotension	92 (53.5 %)	63 (68.5 %)	29 (31.5 %)	0.006
Septic shock	53 (30.8 %)	33 (62.3 %)	20 (37.7 %)	0.003
Bacteremia	21 (12.2 %)	14 (66.7 %)	7 (33.3 %)	0.24
Thrombocytopenia	86 (5 %)	68 (79.1 %)	18 (20.9 %)	0.47
Respiratory failure	74 (43 %)	39 (52.7 %)	35 (47.3 %)	<0.0001
Acidosis	70 (40.7 %)	42 (60 %)	28 (40 %)	<0.0001
Altered mental status	65 (37 %)	42 (64.6 %)	23 (35.4 %)	0.003
Abnormal glucose	60 (34.9 %)	42 (70 %)	18 (30 %)	0.13
Acute renal failure	58 (33.7 %)	35 (60.3 %)	23 (39.7 %)	0.0003
Pancytopenia	58 (33.7 %)	47 (81 %)	11 (19 %)	0.34
Pneumonia	51 (29.7 %)	32 (62.7 %)	19 (37.3 %)	0.005
Neutropenia (ANC[e] <1500/mm^3)	51 (29.7 %)	40 (78.4 %)	11 (21.6 %)	0.73
Cardiac dysrhythmia	35 (20.3 %)	23 (65.7 %)	12 (34.3 %)	0.08
Heart failure	32 (18.6 %)	21 (65.6 %)	11 (34.4 %)	0.10
Hypertension	25 (14.5 %)	22 (88 %)	3 (12 %)	0.20*
Malnutrition (protein/calorie) NOS	23 (13.4 %)	15 (65.2 %)	8 (34.8 %)	0.16
Hemorrhage	15 (8.7 %)	12 (80 %)	3 (20 %)	1.0*
Gastrointestinal hemorrhage	13 (7.6 %)	12 (92.3 %)	1 (7.7 %)	0.30*
Cardiac arrest	11 (6.4 %)	3 (27.3 %)	8 (72.7 %)	0.0004*
Pulmonary embolism	11 (6.4 %)	8 (72.7 %)	3 (27.3 %)	0.72*
Atrial fibrillation	10 (5.8 %)	7 (70 %)	3 (30 %)	0.70*
Seizures/convulsions	9 (5.2 %)	8 (88.9 %)	1 (11.1 %)	0.69*
ICU admission data				
Mechanical v entilator	75 (43·6 %)	40 (30.3 %)	35 (87.5 %)	<0.0001
Charlson comorbidity index, median (IQR)	6 (6–7)	6 (6–7)	6 (4.5–7)	0.70†
≤2	26 (15.1 %)	19 (73.1 %)	7 (26.9 %)	
>2	146 (84.9 %)	113 (77.4 %)	33 (22.6 %)	0.63
SOFA admission score, median (IQR)	7 (4–10)	6 (3.5–9)	10 (6.5–14)	<0.0001†
Max SOFA admission score, median (IQR)	8 (5–12)	7 (4–9.5)	14 (10–17)	<0.0001†
SOFA discharge score, median (IQR)	5 (3–8)	4 (2–6)	10 (7.5–13.5)	<0.0001†
No. organ failures, median (IQR)	1 (0–2)	1 (0–2)	2 (1–3)	<0.0001

* Fisher exact p value

† Wilcoxon rank-sum test

[a] Count (column %—percent of admissions with that variable) are presented unless specified

[b] Count (row %—percent of N in column with All patients) are presented unless specified

[c] Ewing sarcoma, osteosarcoma, chondrosarcoma

[d] Angiosarcoma, epithelioid hemangioendothelioma

[e] Gastrointestinal stromal tumor, Malignant fibrous histiocytoma, Interquartile range, Sequential Organ Failure Assessment, Absolute Neutrophil Count

Table 2 Univariate logistic regression model for death at ICU

	Odds Ratio	95 % CI		p
Reason for ICU admission acidosis: yes v. no	5.000	2.317	10.788	<0.0001
Reason for ICU admission renal failure: yes v. no	3.750	1.795	7.831	0.0004
Reason for ICU admission cardiac arrest: yes v. no	10.750	2.699	42.824	0.0008
Reason for ICU admission cardiac dysrhythmia: yes v. no	2.031	0.902	4.575	0.0873
Reason for ICU admission hypotension: yes v. no	2.887	1.332	6.258	0.0072
Reason for ICU admission pneumonia: yes v. no	2.827	1.353	5.910	0.0057
Reason for ICU admission respiratory failure: yes v. no	16.691	6.086	45.775	<0.0001
Reason for ICU admission septic shock: yes v. no	3.000	1.439	6.253	0.0034
Number of organ failures	1.933	1.417	2.637	<0.0001
Number of mets	0.997	0.745	1.334	0.9835
Histology diagnosis				
Unclassified high grade sarcoma	1.000			
Bone (Ewing, Osteo, Chondrosarcoma)	2.204	0.716	6.788	0.1685
Vascular	0.321	0.036	2.833	0.3068
GIST	0.514	0.056	4.685	0.5552
MFH	4.286	1.019	18.029	0.0471
Muscle	2.204	0.456	10.661	0.3258
Leiomyosarcoma	0.429	0.048	3.848	0.4493
Liposarcoma	3.857	0.703	21.153	0.1200
Synovial sarcoma	4.114	0.878	19.270	0.0726
Others	2.057	0.592	7.149	0.2564

Table 3 Trends in Sequential Organ Failure Assessment (SOFA) scores and their impact on ICU and overall survival

Increase in SOFA score during ICU stay (Maximum SOFA- Admission SOFA)	No. patients in subgroup	Patients surviving ICU stay, %	Patients surviving till end of study, %	Median survival, d (range)
SOFA scores during ICU stay				
0 or less	103	86.4	22.3	187 (108–347)
1–3	43	81.4	27.9	96 (21–193)
4–5	10	60.0	10.0	12 (2–85)
≥6	15	13.3	6.7	17 (6–22)
Admission SOFA scores				
0–4	50	88.0	26.0	159 (49–289)
5–7	46	84.8	21.7	182 (38–347)
8–10	41	80.5	24.4	185 (58–494)
≥11	35	45.7	11.4	6 (2–19)
Change in SOFA scores of 35 patients with admission SOFA scores of 11 or more				
≤0	18	44.4	5.6	4.5 (0.5–9)
1	6	83.3	33.3	56 (4–NE)
2	3	66.7	33.3	13 (2–NE)
≥3	8	12.5	0.0	6 (1–46)

ADM SOFA SOFA score at the time of ICU admission, *MAXOFA* maximum SOFA score, *NE* not estimated

The ICU mortality rates observed in the study population were consistent with those in the existing medical literature and promote a case for a higher level of care with aggressive monitoring in patients who lack predictors of poor outcomes. Our data have shown that adequate cardiac, renal, and respiratory functions play a key role in acute survival. Serial SOFA scores may serve as an objective measure for short-term and long-term prognosis for

Table 4 Overall survival estimates by patients and clinical characteristics in percentages

	No of patients	No of deaths	1-month overall survival estimate (95 % CI)	2-month overall survival estimate (95 % CI)	6-month overall survival estimate (95 % CI)	p
All patients	172	135	64 (57–71)	57 (49–64)	41 (33–48)	
Age (years)						
<65	139	109	64 (56–72)	56 (47–64)	41 (33–50)	
≥65	33	26	64 (45–77)	61 (42–75)	37 (21–54)	0.91
Gender						
Female	93	72	66 (56–75)	60 (49–69)	45 (34–55)	
Male	79	63	62 (50–71)	48 (37–59)	36 (25–47)	0.33
Histological diagnosis						
Unclassified high-grade sarcoma	43	34	67 (51–79)	58 (42–71)	46 (30–60)	
Bones[a]	30	25	70 (50–83)	60 (40–75)	38 (21–55)	
Vascular[b]	17	16	64 (36–82)	51 (25–72)	32 (12–54)	
GIST	11	7	73 (37–90)	64 (30–85)	45 (17–71)	
MFH	11	8	55 (23–78)	55 (23–78)	36 (11–63)	
Muscle	10	9	60 (25–83)	60 (25–83)	20 (3–47)	
Leiomyosarcoma	13	7	84 (50–96)	84 (50–96)	75 (40–91)	
Liposarcoma	7	7	29 (4–61)	29 (4–61)	29 (4–61)	
Synovial sarcoma	9	6	56 (20–80)	56 (20–80)	56 (20–80)	
Others	21	16	56 (33–74)	45 (23–65)	28 (11–49)	0.07
Status of malignancy						
First course of chemotherapy	29	22	66 (45–8)	55 (35–71)	41 (22–59)	
Progression	59	56	49 (36–61)	37 (25–49)	17 (9–27)	
Stable disease or partial remission	61	41	75 (62–84)	72 (58–81)	61 (47–72)	
Complete remission	4	2	100	100	75 (13–96)	
Mixed response	6	5	67 (19–90)	67 (19–90)	67 (19–90)	
Unknown	13	9	68 (36–87)	68 (36–87)	29 (7–56)	<0.0001
Site of malignancy						
Head and neck	15	11	52 (25–73)	52 (25–73)	29 (9–53)	
Thoracic	43	33	67 (51–79)	60 (43–73)	46 (30–60)	
Abdomen	71	57	62 (49–72)	53 (41–64)	37 (26–48)	
Extremities	43	34	7 (54–81)	63 (47–75)	46 (31–60)	0.86
Organ metastasis						
Lung						
No	86	62	66 (55–75)	59 (48–69)	46 (35–56)	
Yes	86	73	62 (51–72)	55 (43–65)	36 (25–46)	0.02
Liver						
No	142	109	66 (58–73)	59 (51–67)	46 (37–54)	
Yes	30	26	56 (36–72)	45 (27–62)	17 (6–33)	0.0093
Other						
No	79	55	66 (54–75)	63 (51–73)	49 (38–60)	
Yes	93	80	63 (52–72)	52 (41–62)	33 (24–43)	0.0091
Number of organ metastases						
0	42	25	71 (55–83)	69 (53–81)	59 (43–72)	
1	54	43	59 (45–71)	53 (39–65)	40 (26–53)	
2+	76	67	64 (52–74)	53 (41–64)	31 (21–42)	0.001

Table 4 continued

	No of patients	No of deaths	1-month overall survival estimate (95 % CI)	2-month overall survival estimate (95 % CI)	6-month overall survival estimate (95 % CI)	p
Localized disease						
No	130	110	62 (53–7)	53 (44–61)	34 (26–43)	
Yes	42	25	71 (55–83)	69 (53–81)	59 (43–72)	<0.0001
Treatment						
Current chemotherapy regimen						
None	43	31	57 (41–7)	52 (36–66)	39 (24–53)	
Adriamycin-based chemotherapy	68	51	69 (56–78)	66 (53–76)	51 (38–63)	
Gemcitabine-based therapy	20	18	5 (27–69)	45 (23–65)	25 (9–45)	
Targeted therapy	41	35	71 (54–82)	54 (37–67)	34 (20–49)	0.31
Radiation						
No	109	85	63 (54–72)	59 (49–67)	39 (29–48)	
Yes	62	50	65 (52–76)	53 (40–65)	43 (30–55)	0.86
Clinical conditions present at ICU admission						
Anemia	144	113	66 (57–73)	59 (50–66)	43 (35–51)	0.60
Hypotension	92	73	57 (46–66)	51 (40–61)	42 (32–52)	0.96
Septic shock	53	44	49 (35–62)	45 (32–58)	33 (21–46)	0.10
Bacteremia	21	17	57 (34–75)	57 (34–75)	43 (22–62)	0.58
Thrombocytopenia	86	63	71 (60–79)	64 (52–73)	49 (37–59)	0.037
Respiratory failure	74	62	46 (34–56)	41 (30–52)	26 (16–37)	<0.0001
Acidosis	70	58	47 (35–58)	41 (30–53)	35 (24–46)	0.011
Altered mental status	65	57	52 (39–63)	42 (30–54)	25 (15–36)	0.001
Abnormal glucose	60	50	60 (46–71)	49 (36–61)	25 (14–37)	0.017
Acute renal failure	58	49	48 (35–60)	40 (27–52)	29 (18–41)	0.016
Pancytopenia	58	41	79 (66–88)	74 (61–83)	57 (43–69)	0.006
Respiratory abnormality	53	38	73 (59–83)	64 (49–75)	49 (35–62)	0.036
Pneumonia	51	42	53 (38–65)	49 (35–62)	35 (22–48)	0.41
Neutropenia (ANC <1500/mm^3)	51	36	78 (64–87)	70 (56–81)	58 (43–70)	0.013
Cardiac dysrhythmia	35	26	57 (39–72)	51 (34–66)	46 (29–61)	0.96
Heart failure	32	25	63 (44–77)	56 (37–71)	53 (34–68)	0.80
Hypertension	25	15	80 (58–91)	71 (48–85)	61 (39–78)	0.049
Malnutrition (protein/calorie) NOS	23	21	60 (37–77)	60 (37–77)	28 (11–47)	0.047
Hemorrhage (non–gastrointestinal)	15	9	64 (34–83)	64 (34–83)	47 (19–71)	0.44
Other pulmonary insufficiency	14	11	71 (41–88)	64 (34–83)	64 (34–83)	0.71
Gastrointestinal hemorrhage	13	9	62 (31–82)	54 (25–76)	38 (14–63)	0.51
Cardiac arrest	11	8	27 (7–54)	27 (7–54)	27 (7–54)	0.17
Pulmonary embolism	11	10	73 (37–90)	63 (29–84)	32 (8–59)	0.21
Atrial fibrillation	10	7	70 (33–89)	70 (33–89)	6 (25–83)	0.40
Seizures	9	8	67 (28–88)	44 (14–72)	30 (5–61)	0.54
ICU admission data						
Charlson comorbidity index						
≤2	26	15	69 (48–83)	69 (48–83)	54 (33–71)	
>2	146	120	63 (55–71)	55 (46–62)	38 (30–46)	0.0031

Table 4 continued

	No of patients	No of deaths	1-month overall survival estimate (95 % CI)	2-month overall survival estimate (95 % CI)	6-month overall survival estimate (95 % CI)	p
Charlson comorbidity index						
<6	42	25	71 (55–83)	69 (53–81)	59 (43–72)	
≥6	130	110	62 (53–70)	53 (44–61)	34 (26–43)	<0.0001
SOFA maximum score						
<8	79	60	82 (72–89)	71 (60–80)	49 (38–60)	
≥8	93	75	49 (39–59)	45 (34–55)	33 (24–43)	0.005
SOFA discharge score						
<5	77	59	80 (69–88)	71 (59–80)	47 (35–58)	
≥5	95	76	51 (41–61)	46 (36–56)	36 (26–45)	0.12
No. organ failures						
1	59	47	76 (63–85)	69 (56–79)	53 (40–65)	
≥2	113	88	58 (48–66)	50 (41–59)	34 (25–43)	0.12

ADM SOFA SOFA score at the time of ICU admission, *MAXOFA* maximum SOFA score, *NE* not estimated

[a] Ewing sarcoma, osteosarcoma, chondrosarcoma

[b] Angiosarcoma, epithelioid hemangioendothelioma

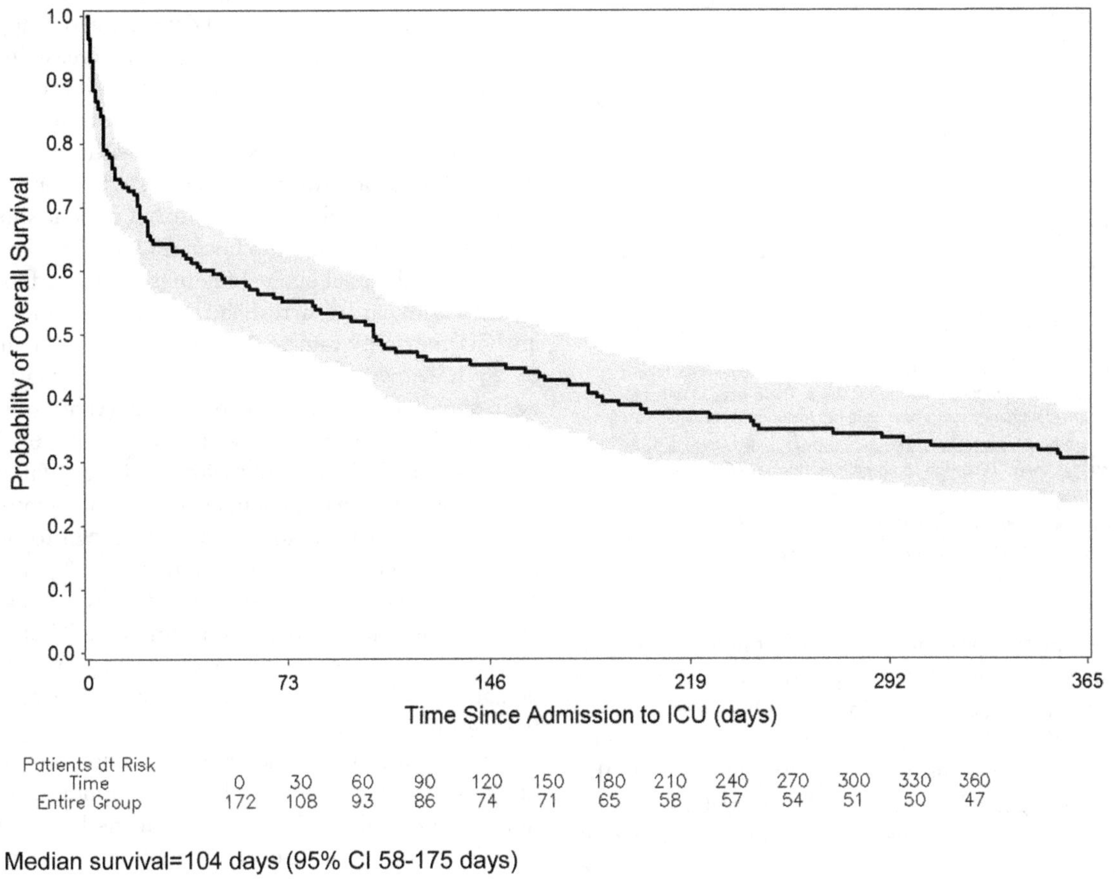

Fig. 1 Kaplan-Meier estimates of overall survival

Table 5 Multivariable cox proportional hazards model for overall survival

Variable	Hazard ratio	95 % CI P		p
Histological diagnosis				0.006
Unclassified high-grade sarcoma	1.000			
Bones[a]	0.881	0.516	1.506	0.64
Vascular[b]	1.657	0.862	3.185	0.13
GIST	0.281	0.119	0.662	0.004
MFH	0.674	0.236	1.929	0.46
Muscle	2.048	0.917	4.573	0.08
Leiomyosarcoma	0.375	0.160	0.880	0.02
Liposarcoma	1.412	0.575	3.468	0.45
Synovial sarcoma	0.793	0.293	2.143	0.65
Others	0.746	0.373	1.493	0.41
Status of malignancy				0.003
Complete remission	1.000			
First course of chemotherapy	2.323	0.473	11.425	0.30
Mixed response	2.720	0.444	16.677	0.28
Progression	5.172	1.075	24.874	0.04
Stable disease	2.262	0.501	10.218	0.29
Reason for ICU admission pancytopenia				
No				
Yes	0.351	0.226	0.546	<0.0001
Reason for ICU admission respiratory failure				
No				
Yes	1.703	1.125	2.579	01
CCI (continuous)	1.139	1.023	1.268	02
SOFA score at discharge (continuous)	1.210	1.141	1.283	<0.0001

Initially included in the model and then reduced by stepwise selection method: histology diagnosis, status of malignancy, number of organ metastasis, number of organ failures, and reason for ICU admission: acidosis, acute renal failure, pancytopenia, respiratory failure, and septic shock. There were 13 patients without known malignancy status who were not included in this analysis

CI confidence interval, *GIST* Gastrointestinal stromal tumor, *MFH* Malignant fibrous histiocytoma, *CCI* Charlson comorbidities index, *SOFA* Sequential Organ Failure Assessment

[a] Ewing sarcoma, osteosarcoma, chondrosarcoma

[b] Angiosarcoma, epithelioid hemangioendothelioma

sarcoma. There appears to be significant heterogeneity in ICU mortality among all cancer patients because of a lack of data comparing similar histologies. Our patient population had an ICU mortality rate of 23 %, which is comparable to the 20 % mortality in solid tumors [10]. The same study reported that ICU and in-hospital mortality rates for cancer patients were not significantly different from those of non-cancer patients [10]. However, among patients with multiple organ failures; mortality rates were higher in cancer patients than in non-cancer patients. This finding is consistent with our study, in which the number of organ failures was directly proportional to ICU mortality. Among mortality statistics reported for specific tumors, patients with head and neck cancer, lung cancer, and gynecological malignancies have been shown to have ICU mortality rates of 39, 36, and 17.3 %, respectively [11–13]. In contrast, patients with hematological cancers have been reported to have higher ICU mortality rates: 48.3 and 56 % in two separate studies [14, 15]. These higher rates may be attributed to increased severity of illness and higher incidence of sepsis due to associated leukopenia in these patients [10].

Several ICU scores; including MODS, APACHE II, SAPS II, and SOFA, have been used as objective ways to describe mild to severe organ dysfunction [16–19]. In our study, we used SOFA scores, which have been calibrated to predict ICU and in-hospital mortality rates in cancer patients by evaluating the combination of clinical conditions that lead to ICU admission [20–23].

We found out those patients who had high SOFA scores on admission did worse than patients with lower SOFA scores. Another important objective finding was that patients whose SOFA scores continued to rise following admission to the ICU had the worst outcomes, making these patients appropriate candidates for early supportive and palliative care. As a general guide, increase in scores of 6 or more since admission led to drastic changes in outcome and ICU survival decreased from 60 to 13.3 % (Table 3). A patient who is admitted with a SOFA score of 11 or higher and their score increases by 3 or more has dismal ICU survival of 12.5 %. Such a patient should be considered for transition to hospice (Table 3).

Among individual clinical findings on ICU admissions, patients with cardiac arrest had the worst prognosis, with an ICU mortality rate of 72 % (8/11) and a median OS of 24 h. However, cardiopulmonary resuscitation has been shown to be a non-beneficial intervention in more than 90 % of the patients with cancer [24–26]. In our univariate analysis, patients with respiratory failure had worse outcomes than patients with good respiratory status. Mechanical ventilation has been shown to be associated with increased mortality rates (73 %) in cancer patients, especially those with disseminated disease and poor performance status at the time of ICU admission [27]. Similar findings have been observed in patients with hematological, lung, and head and neck cancers in the ICU setting (64–74 %) [20, 28–30].

Hypotension and septic shock are additional clinical findings that correlated with higher ICU mortality in our multivariate analysis. Sepsis is one of the leading causes of ICU admission in cancer patients. However, patients with infections leading to shock and vasopressor use tend to do poorly and should be managed conservatively [10, 13, 15, 27]. Patients with acute kidney injury also have high acute mortality. This trend is more commonly seen in patients with hematological malignancies [31]. Furthermore, renal replacement therapy has been associated with high ICU mortality [24]. Given their bleak prognoses, patients with these individual or combinations of clinical findings should be triaged early so that inappropriate use of aggressive therapy can be avoided.

There are limited data evaluating long-term survival rates of critically ill cancer patients after their discharge from the ICU. Six-month OS in sarcoma patients was 41 % in our study, which is comparable to the 6-month mortality rates of 59.3 and 66 % reported in critically ill patients with hematological malignancies [28, 30]. However, long-term mortality rates of 63 to 98 % have been reported in patients with lung cancer. The major predictors of long-term prognosis in these patients were dependence on mechanical ventilation during the ICU stay and progression of cancer after discharge from the ICU [11]. In our study, we found that the status of malignancy, metastatic disease, Charlson comorbidity index and SOFA scores at discharge, and the presence of respiratory failure or cytopenia at the time of ICU admission were significant predictors of survival outcomes in both univariate and multivariate analyses (Table 4). Therefore, when looking at patterns of long-term survival after ICU stay, the above-mentioned clinical prognostic factors should be considered early in the clinical course.

There were a number of limitations to this study. First, this is a single-institution retrospective study covering a limited number of years. We are a tertiary care referral center for sarcomas, so the results of our study may not be applicable to smaller hospitals or low-volume centers. Each hospital has its own ICU admission and discharge policies which may bias the results of a single center study. Second, our study did not have a control group to compare the outcomes of critically ill sarcoma patients who were not admitted to the ICU and were managed conservatively. Even though it is a large collection of a rare tumor our study outcomes were limited to only 40 events in the ICU. Due to a small number of events and multiple risk factors, it is difficult to make a generalized presumption of which risk factor individually impacted the short term survival. In addition, quality-of-life measures and performance status scores could not be reliably collected in the retrospective setting.

In conclusion, our study is the largest study to date of OS in sarcoma patients admitted to the ICU. In our study span of 7 years, we have shown that OS in sarcoma is comparable with that of critically ill patients with other solid tumors. The admission SOFA scores and change in the SOFA scores during ICU stay are highly reliable indicators of probability of survival and should be used in decision making in critically ill patients. Our results suggest that patients with advanced malignancy that are admitted to the ICU for respiratory failure, cardiac arrest, septic shock, acute renal failure or acidosis and have high SOFA score with subsequent worsening in the ICU have very poor prognosis. Based on the retrospective data which needs further validation we can recommend that judicious approach should be taken in patients with predictors of poor survival before subjecting them to aggressive treatment.

Authors' contributions

RG, DA, RB, SP, JL, and VR were responsible for the study concept. All authors contributed to the study design. RG, NR, and EJR collected and assembled these data. NR, JS, and XL analyzed and interpreted these data. RG and NH wrote the initial draft, and all the authors approved the final draft of the report. All authors read and approved the final manuscript.

Author details

[1] The University of Texas at Houston Internal Medicine Residency Program, Houston, TX, USA. [2] The University of Texas Graduate School of Biomedical Sciences at Houston, Houston, TX, USA. [3] Division of Quantitative Sciences, The University of Texas MD Anderson Cancer Center, Houston, TX, USA. [4] Department of Critical Care, The University of Texas MD Anderson Cancer Center, Houston, TX, USA. [5] Department of Sarcoma Medical Oncology, The University of Texas MD Anderson Cancer Center, 1515 Holcombe Blvd # 450, Houston, TX 77030, USA.

Acknowledgements

We did not have any financial support. We thank critical care team for providing the initial data and SOFA scores. We thank statisticians Naveen Ramesh, Xiudong Lei and Juhee Song. The statistical analysis work was supported in part by the Cancer Center Support Grant (NCI Grant P30 CA016672). We thank scientific editors, Bryan Tutt and Tamara Locke, in Department of Scientific Publications at MD Anderson for manuscript editing.

Poster presented at 2014 American Society of Clinical Oncology National Meeting, Chicago, IL.

Competing interests

The authors declare that they have no competing interests.

References

1. Fletcher CDM, Bridge JA, Hogendoorn P, Mertens F. World Health Organization classification of tumors of soft tissue and bone. 4th ed. Lyon: IARC Press; 2013.
2. Mackall CL, Meltzer PS, Helman LJ. Focus on sarcomas. Cancer Cell. 2002;2:175–8.
3. Chassin MR. Costs and outcomes of medical intensive care. Med Care. 1982;20:165–79.
4. Turnbull A, Goldiner P, Silverman D, et al. The role of an intensive care unit in a cancer center. An analysis of 1035 critically ill patients treated for life-threatening complications editorial. Cancer. 1976;37:82–4.
5. Shapira DV, Studnicki J, Bradham DD. Intensive care, survival and expense of treating critically ill cancer patients. JAMA. 1993;269:783–6.
6. Azoulay E, Moreau D, Alberti C, et al. Predictors of short-term mortality in critically ill patients with solid malignancies. Intensive Care Med. 2000;26:1817–23.
7. Lecuyer L, Chevret S, Thiery G, et al. The ICU trial: a new admission policy for cancer patients requiring mechanical ventilation. Critical Care Med. 2007;35:808–14.
8. Azoulay E, Soares M, Darmon M, et al. Intensive care of the cancer patient: recent achievements and remaining challenges. Ann Intensive Care. 2011;1:5.

9. Charlson ME, Pompei P, Ales KL, et al. A new method of classifying prognostic comorbidity in longitudinal studies: development and validation. J Chronic Dis. 1987;40:373–83.
10. Taccone FS, Artigas AA, Sprung CL, et al. Caracteristics and outcomes of cancer patients in European ICUs. Crit Care. 2009;13:R15.
11. Soubani AO, Ruckdeschel JC. The outcome of medical intensive care for lung cancer patients: the case for optimism. J Thorac Oncol. 2011;6:633–8.
12. Namendys-Silva SA, González-Herrera MO, Texcocano-Becerra J, et al. Outcomes of critically ill gynecological cancer patients admitted to intensive care unit. Am J Hosp Palliat Care. 2013;30:7–11.
13. Soares M, Salluh JI, Ferreira CG, et al. Prognosis of lung cancer patients with life-threatening complications. Chest. 2007;131:840–6.
14. Pène F, Azoulay E, Blot F, et al. Outcome of critically ill allogeneic hematopoietic stem-cell transplantation recipients: a reappraisal of indications for organ failure supports. J Clin Oncol. 2006;24:643–9.
15. Geerse DA, Span LF, Pinto-Sietsma SJ, et al. Prognosis of patients with haematological malignancies admitted to the intensive care unit: sequential Organ Failure Assessment (SOFA) trend is a powerful predictor of mortality. Eur J Intern Med. 2011;22:57–61.
16. Marshall JC, Cook DJ, Christou NV, et al. Multiple organ dysfunction score: a reliable descriptor of a complex clinical outcome. Crit Care Med. 1995;23:1638–52.
17. Vincent JL, Moreno R, Takala J, et al. The SOFA (Sepsis-related Organ Failure Assessment) score to describe organ dysfunction/failure. On behalf of the Working Group on Sepsis-Related Problems of the European Society of Intensive Care Medicine. Intensive Care Med. 1996;22:707–10.
18. Knaus WA, Draper EA, Wagner DP, et al. APACHE II: a severity of disease classification system. Crit Care Med. 1985;13:818–29.
19. Le Gall JR, Lemeshow S, Saulnier F. A new simplified acute physiology score (SAPS II) based on a European/North American multicenter study. JAMA. 1993;270:2957–63.
20. Reichner CA, Thompson JA, O'Brien S, et al. Outcome and code status of lung cancer patients admitted to the medical ICU. Chest. 2006;130:719–23.
21. Soares M, Caruso P, Silva E, et al. Characteristics and outcomes of patients with cancer requiring admission to intensive care units: a prospective multicenter study. Crit Care Med. 2010;38:9–15.
22. Owczuk R, Wujtewicz MA, Sawicka W, et al. Patients with haematological malignancies requiring invasive mechanical ventilation differences between survivors and non-survivors in intensive care unit. Support Care Cancer. 2005;13:332–8.
23. Cárdenas-Turanzas M, Ensor J, Wakefield C, et al. Cross-validation of a sequential organ failure assessment score-based model to predict mortality in patients with cancer admitted to the intensive care unit. J Crit Care. 2012;27:673–80.
24. Heo SJ, Kim G, Lee CK, et al. Prediction of short- and long-term survival for advanced cancer patients after ICU admission. Support Care Cancer. 2014;1:1–9.
25. Wallace S, Ewer MS, Price KJ, et al. Outcome and cost implications of cardiopulmonary resuscitation in the medical intensive care unit of a comprehensive cancer center. Support Care Cancer. 2002;10:425–9.
26. Reisfield GM, Wallace SK, Munsell MF, et al. Survival in cancer patients undergoing in-hospital cardiopulmonary resuscitation: a meta-analysis. Resuscitation. 2006;71:152–60.
27. Azevedo LC, Caruso P, Silva UV, et al. Outcomes for patients with cancer admitted to the ICU requiring ventilatory support: results from a prospective multicenter study. Chest. 2014;146:257–66.
28. Bird GT, Farquhar-Smith P, Wigmore T, et al. Outcomes and prognostic factors in patients with hematological malignancy admitted to a specialist cancer intensive care unit: a 5 yr study. Br J Anesth. 2012;108:452–9.
29. Soares M, Salluh JI, Toscano L, et al. Outcomes and prognostic factors in patients with head and neck cancer and severe acute illnesses. Intensive Care Med. 2007;33:2009–13.
30. Benoit DD, Vandewoude KH, Decruyenaere JM, et al. Outcome and early prognostic indicators in patients with a hematologic malignancy admitted to the intensive care unit for a life-threatening complication. Crit Care Med. 2003;31:104–12.

5

Outcome and the effect of age and socioeconomic status in 1318 patients with synovial sarcoma in the English National Cancer Registry

Bernadette Brennan[1*], Charles Stiller[3], Robert Grimer[4], Nicola Dennis[2], John Broggio[3] and Matthew Francis[2]

Abstract

Background: The role of age as a prognostic factor has been examined in single institutional studies and in larger data sets from the SEER database, showing a survival advantage for younger versus adult patients with synovial sarcoma (SS). To further assess the role of age, socioeconomic status and other prognostic factors on outcome for SS, we analysed a contemporary all-age population-based cohort of patients with SS registered in England.

Methods: The data on 1318 synovial sarcomas diagnosed in England between 1985 and 2009 were retrospectively analysed for incidence, and the effect of age, patient characteristics and deprivation on outcome using both univariate and multivariate analysis.

Results: The incidence of SS increased to 1.4 per million over the time period, the numbers diagnosed in patients under 10 years of age were small. The site or incidence of metastases did not vary between age groups. There were, however, significant differences ($p < 0.05$) in the 5-year relative survival rates between patients aged 0–19 years and those ≥20 years of age, 76 % and 53 % respectively. Survival was better in localised tumours at an extremity site. In multivariate analysis higher mortality occurred in older patients, non-extremity site, presence of metastases, female adults and a higher deprivation score.

Conclusions: Synovial sarcoma in children/teenagers compared with adults, have a similar clinical presentation in this population-based series, but a superior outcome. The finding of socioeconomic deprivation affecting outcome in SS needs further exploration in a complete and contemporary dataset, where all prognostic variables are present.

Keywords: Synovial sarcoma, Age, Social deprivation

Background

In childhood and adolescence synovial sarcoma (SS) is rare with an annual incidence of 0.5 per million and only six new cases per year diagnosed in those less than 15 years of age in the UK [1]. The incidence, however, of SS differs across age groups. In the North American population-based surveillance epidemiology, and end results (SEER) cancer registry, the age-standardised incidence of SS was higher in adults at 1.42 per million [2] versus 0.81 per million in patients under 19 years of age [2]. Recorded incidence may have changed over time due to more accurate diagnosis, with the recognition of a characteristic translocation involving chromosome 18 and X, resulting in the detection of one of several types of fusion genes (SYT-SSX1, 2 and 4) in 90 % of cases [3, 4].

Surgery remains an important aspect of treatment for localised SS with radiation, which may facilitate surgical resection [5]. In paediatric practice, less radiotherapy is used in view of late effects [21]. The role of chemotherapy in SS is not completely defined, but is used more in paediatric patients [6, 7]. In adults, chemotherapy is not

*Correspondence: Bernadette.brennan@cmft.nhs.uk
[1] Department of Paediatric Oncology, Royal Manchester Children's Hospital, Oxford Road, Manchester M13 9WL, UK

standard of care, particularly in localised disease regardless of tumour size, but is used in high-risk patients and those with metastases [8] or as part of investigational trials [9].

The role of age as a prognostic factor has been examined in single-institutional studies and the SEER database; Ferrari et al. demonstrated that children had a better outcome than adults, asserting but not proving that this was due to the use of more chemotherapy [10]. Socioeconomic status has been shown to be a significant predictor of outcome in lung, colon and breast cancer, with those patients with lower socioeconomic status having a worse outcome [11–13]. The effect of socioeconomic status on the outcome of SS has not been studied. To further assess the role of age, socioeconomic status and other prognostic factors on outcome for SS, we analysed a contemporary all-age population-based cohort of patients with SS registered in England.

Methods

This study carried out a retrospective population-based analysis of the incidence, clinical characteristics, and survival of SS.

Source of data

The anonymised data were extracted from the National Cancer Data Repository (NCDR), a compilation of data collected by all regional cancer registry offices in England. The information includes age, sex, ethnicity, post code of residence, anatomical site of tumour, and some treatment data. Two different versions of the NCDR were utilised for the analyses. Incidence and survival data was utilised from the 1985–2009 version of the NCDR—containing 1318 SS. The 1990–2010 NCDR was utilised so that treatment data could be assessed as recently as possible, with 70 SS diagnosed in 2010.

All SS diagnosed in England between 1985 and 2009 classified by the 10th revision of the International Classification of Diseases (ICD-10 site code) and International Classification of Disease for Oncology, version 3 (ICD-0-3) morphology codes M9040-9043 were analysed [14, 15]. All incidence cases identified were included in the analysis except for four death certificate only (DCO) cases which were excluded for the purpose of survival analyses. This is in line with the recommended practice of data quality for conducting survival analyses [28] and none of the other quality controls were relevant to this cohort. Death certificates are provided by the Office of National Statistics (ONS).

Morphology subtype was not analysed since 1107 (84 %) of the 1318 patients were recorded as having SS not otherwise specified (NOS) [M9040].

Hospital Episode Statistics (HES) data is a record of all hospital admissions. HES data captures information on admission date, operations and procedures, and other co-morbidities. HES data was linked to the NCDR on the patient demographics—NHS number, date of birth and postcode.

Patient ethnicity is described in the analyses although not included in any statistics due to the incompleteness of this data item.

Metastatic status was derived from the HES data If a patient had a diagnosis of ICD-10 codes C77 (Secondary and unspecified malignant neoplasm of lymph nodes), C78 (Secondary malignant neoplasm of respiratory and digestive organs) or C79 (Secondary malignant neoplasm of other sites) recorded during an admission within 4 months following sarcoma diagnosis. OPCS Classification of Interventions and Procedures, version 4 (OPCS4) codes were extracted from the HES data for SS patients. Surgery was classified as the OPCS4 codes which relate to radical curative surgery, and occurred within 6 months of initial diagnosis. Patients for which no HES record could be identified were removed for this set of analyses. This resulted in 776 cases out of 819 diagnosed between 2000 and 2010 available for analysis.

Due to the low incidence of SS occurring outside of the extremities, cancer sites were classified as extremity or other for the purpose of statistical modelling.

Socioeconomic status

Socioeconomic status was assessed using the income domain (ID) of the index of multiple deprivation 2010 (IMD) [16]. The IMD uses information from the National Census to form a score from 7 measures of deprivation for a given area: income, employment, health, education, crime, access to services, and living environment. The scores are assigned to geographic areas within England, each with a local population of approximately 1500 so that each postal code can be allocated a score. The scores range from 1 (least deprived) to 5 (most deprived). For reasons of comparability with other parts of the United Kingdom, cancer data is analysed with respect to the income domain only.

Statistical methods and data analysis

Confidence intervals around incidence rates were calculated using the gamma method [17]. Significant differences for the incidence rates were inferred by comparing the confidence intervals (CI) for different rates. If the confidence intervals overlapped then the rates are not significantly different and if the confidence intervals did not overlap then the rates are significantly different. A p value of <0.05 was considered significant. All statistical tests were two-sided.

Relative survival was defined as the observed survival in the patient group divided by the expected survival of the general population, matched by age, sex and calendar year. Relative survival was estimated by the Ederer II method [18] using the STRS programme in STATA (version 13). National life tables were obtained from the Cancer Research UK Cancer Survival Group at the London School of Hygiene and Tropical Medicine. All patients were last followed up on 31 December 2013 and analysed in 2014. Therefore, patients diagnosed in 2009 were excluded from survival analyses because of lack of 5-year follow-up. Five-year relative survival was calculated using 5-year rolling averages. Cox proportional-hazard models were used to identify the prognostic factors most likely to result in death for people with SS and were calculated for patients diagnosed between 2000 and 2010. To assess the role of age as a prognostic factor a cut off of 19 years was chosen in view of the data from the SEER analysis (2).

Multivariable logistic regression models were used to assess the risk of metastases dependent on age at diagnosis, sex, site and ID score.

Results

Patient characteristics

Between 1985 and 2009, 1318 SS were registered. Age at diagnosis ranged from 8 months to 93 years, with only 25 cases reported under the age of 10 years. The largest numbers and highest age-specific rates occurred in males aged 30–34 years. (Fig. 1).

The age-standardised incidence rates (3-year rolling average) for all ages combined increased from 0.7 per million to 1.4 per million in males and from 0.5 per million to 1.4 per million in females between 1985 and 2009, with the steepest increase from 1997 onwards.

Among the population between 0 and 19 years the age-standardised incidence rates fluctuated between 0.08 per million and 1.1 per million. However, in the 20-years and over age group there was a statistically significant increase from 0.7 per million in 1985 to 1.4 per million in 2009 ($p < 0.05$).

Table 1 describes demographic and clinical characteristics for all ages combined and for the two age groups of 0–19 years and ≥20 years. Univariate analysis of the clinical characteristics in Table 1 showed there were no differences between children/adolescents and adults (all p values >0.07). The commonest site was extremity (65 %) followed by soft tissues of the trunk.

Among 776 of 819 patients diagnosed between 2000 and 2010 for which HES records were identified, whether distant metastases were found at diagnosis and whether the patient had any surgical intervention in the month preceding diagnosis or the 6 months following diagnosis were analysed, but there were no significant differences between the two age groups for either distant metastases or surgical intervention ($p > 0.1$) (Table 1).

The income domain of the IMD scores were equally distributed in the 5 groups, with a non-significant higher percentage in the most deprived group (score 5) for the 0–19 years cohort (all p values >0.06).

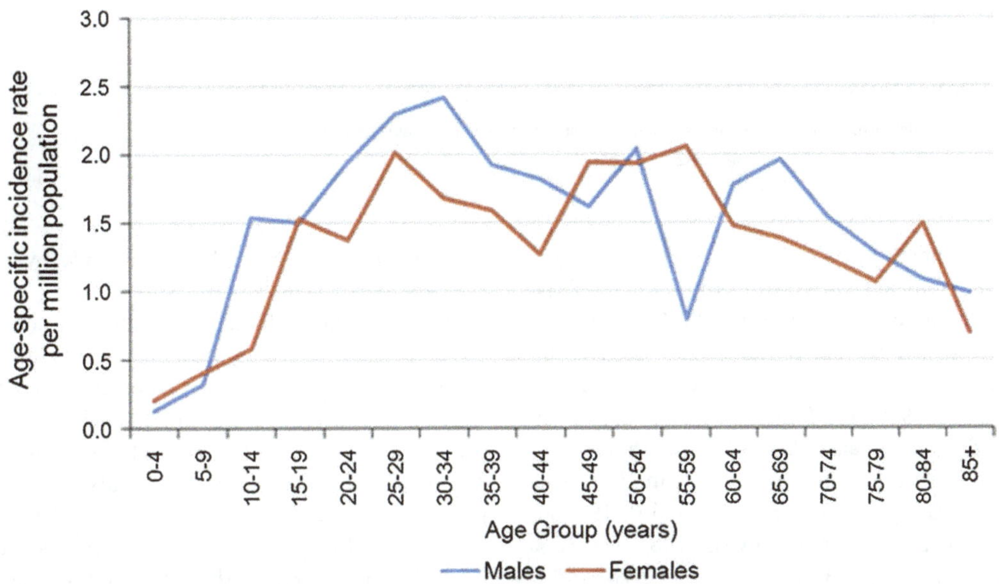

Fig. 1 Age specific incidence rates males and females, for the years 1985–2009 in England

Table 1 Patient characteristics in 1318 patients with synovial sarcoma

	All patients		Children and teenagers		Adults	
	No.	%	No	%	No.	%
Total	1318	–	182	–	1136	–
Age (years)						
0–9	25	2	25	14	0	0
10–19	157	12	157	86	0	0
20–29	237	18	0	0	237	21
30–39	239	18	0	0	239	21
40–49	207	16	0	0	207	18
50–59	189	14	0	0	189	17
60–69	130	10	0	0	130	11
≥ 70	134	10	0	0	134	12
Sex						
Female	628	48	79	43	549	48
Male	690	52	103	57	587	52
Location						
Head and neck	66	5	14	8	52	5
Extremity	861	65	114	63	747	66
Lungs and pleura	60	5	6	3	54	5
Trunk	190	14	27	15	163	14
Others	141	11	21	12	120	11
Quintile of the income domain of the index of multiple deprivation 2010						
Least deprived	257	19	36	20	221	19
2	256	19	30	16	226	20
3	261	20	29	16	232	20
4	278	21	41	23	237	21
Most deprived	266	20	46	25	220	19
Stage at diagnosis[a]						
Total known	776		109		667	
Localised	656	85	97	89	559	84
Metastatic	120	15	12	11	108	16
Did patients have surgery?						
Surgically treated	550	71	84	77	466	70
Not surgically treated	226	29	25	23	201	30

There were no significant differences in the proportions of children or adults having any of the tabulated characteristics

[a] Based on 2010 data to allow further inclusion of metastases

Survival and prognostic factors

There was no significant variation in the 5-year relative survival rates for SS over the period 1985–2008, regardless of age groups. (Figs. 2, 3). The 5-year relative survival rate was 56 % [CI: (47–64 %)] for patients diagnosed between 1985 and 1989, and 56 % [CI: (51–61 %)] in the most recent diagnosis years (2004–2008). There were, however, significant differences ($p < 0.05$) in the 5-year relative survival rates between patients aged 0–19 years and those ≥20 years of age, both in years 1985–89 [72 %, 95 % CI: (46–88 %)] vs. [53 %, 95 % CI: (44–62 %)] and in years 2004–08 [76 %, 95 % CI: (63–85 %)] vs. [53 %, 95 % CI: (47–58 %)]. (Fig. 3).

There was no difference in outcome among sex and ID of IMD. There was, however, a worse outcome for tumours at a non-extremity site compared to tumours of the extremity, 5-year relative survival 34 % [95 % CI: (27–42 %)] and 71 % [95 % CI: (64–76 %)] respectively, $p < 0.001$. Metastatic spread was also associated with a poorer outcome, 5-year relative survival was 7 % [95 % CI: (2, 15 %)] for those with distant metastases and 65 % [95 % CI: (59, 70 %)] for those without, $p < 0.001$.

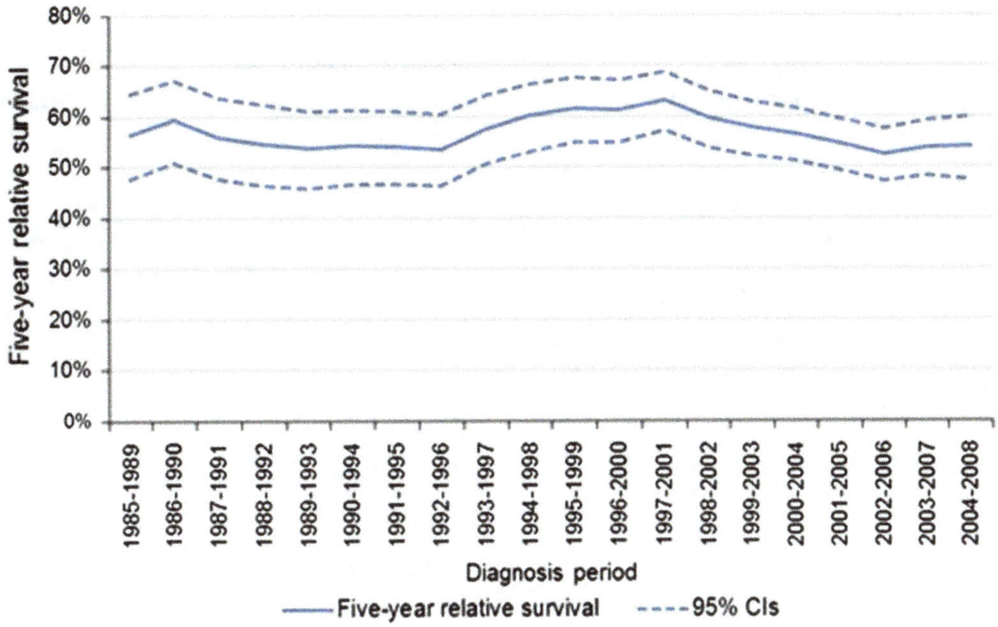

Fig. 2 Synovial sarcoma 5-year relative survival rates (5-year rolling average) (England: 1985–2008). *LCI* lower confidence interval, *UCI* upper confidence interval

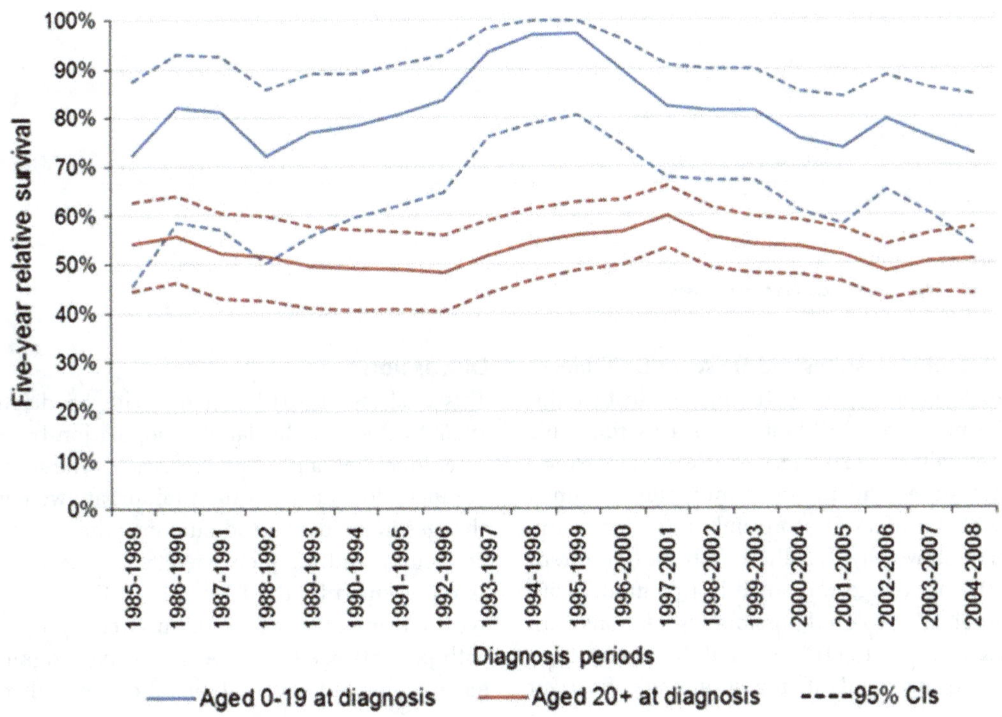

Fig. 3 5-year relative survival rates for synovial sarcoma (5-year rolling average) for the years 1985–2009 in England 0–19 years and 20+ years

For all patients in the multivariate analysis, age remained significant; the highest mortality was in those ≥70 years of age with a hazard ratio (HR) of 8.48 relative to those aged between 0–19 years (Table 2). For the whole population other factors associated with a higher mortality included non-extremity tumour site, female sex,

Table 2 Cox proportional hazards regression for mortality in 819 patients with synovial sarcoma diagnosed between 2000 and 2010

Variable	All patients Hazard ratio (95 % CI)	Children and adolescents Hazard ratio (95 % CI)	Adults Hazard ratio (95 % CI)
Age category, years			
0–19	1.00	–	–
20–29	1.39 (0.84–2.31)	–	–
30–39	1.92 (1.20–3.07)**	–	–
40–49	2.12 (1.32–3.43)**	–	–
50–59	2.73 (1.68–4.45)***	–	–
60–69	4.98 (3.08–8.05)***	–	–
≥ 70	8.48 (5.27–13.64)***	–	–
Sex			
Female	1.00	1.00	1.00
Male	0.67 (0.54–0.84)***	0.95 (0.40–2.23)	0.70 (0.56–0.88)**
Primary site			
Extremity	1.00	1.00	1.00
Other	2.25 (1.79–2.82)***	1.73 (0.68–4.36)	2.23 (1.76–2.82)***
Stage at diagnosis[a]			
Localised	1.00	1.00	1.00
Metastatic	6.15 (4.75–7.95)***	42.4 (12.53–143.70)***	4.86 (3.74–6.33)***
Quintile of the income domain of the index of multiple deprivation 2010			
Least deprived	1.11 (0.78–1.59)	2.39 (0.47–12.19)	1.17 (0.81–1.68)
2	1.34 (0.95–1.91)	1.68 (0.31–9.16)	1.33 (0.93–1.90)
3	1.00	1.00	1.00
4	1.18 (0.83–1.68)	0.61 (0.13–2.83)	1.22 (0.84–1.76)
Most deprived	1.48 (1.03–2.12)*	2.35 (0.54–10.16)	1.27 (0.88–1.84)
Time varying covariate			
Primary site	0.76 (0.64–0.91)**	–	0.73 (0.61–0.88)**

* Statistically significant at $p < 0.05$

** Statistically significant at $p < 0.01$

*** Statistically significant at $p < 0.001$

[a] Based on 2010 data to allow further inclusion of metastases

presence of distant metastases and ID score-5 (Table 2). For those <20 years of age non-extremity site lost significance but the presence of distant metastases remained significant. For adults (≥20 years), male sex, presence of distant metastases and non-extremity site remained significant, with ID of IMD score only just significant. (Table 2) It is noteworthy that the number of children/teenagers <20 years of age was small in this model with only 182 in total. We explored possible associations with the age at diagnosis and the ID score but did not find any significant results in several different groupings of patient age at diagnosis.

For patients with extremity SS, they were less likely to have distant metastases at diagnosis than those with SS at other sites with an odds ratio of 0.67 ($p < 0.05$). This was the only characteristic associated with a decreased risk of metastases (Table 3).

Discussion

This analysis of 1318 patients with SS diagnosed from 1985 to 2009 is the largest population-based study to date, including all stages of disease. The unusually large numbers for such a rare tumour allowed us to study changes in incidence and outcome, the effect of prognostic factors, and uniquely the effect of severe deprivation as represented by the ID of the IMD score on outcome. We confirmed that age is an important prognostic factor, with patients aged 0–19 years having a significantly better outcome but severe deprivation does affect outcome. As significant is the outcome for elderly patients the highest mortality was in those ≥70 years of age. Furthermore, the value of these findings is enhanced due to the quality of the national registrations and the high level of case ascertainment with minimal serious errors detected on regular completeness and validity checks [19].

Table 3 Multivariable logistic regression to assess the relative risk of being diagnosed with distant metastases dependent on age at diagnosis, sex, site and ID score in 819 patients with synovial sarcoma diagnosed between 2000 and 2010

Variable	Odds ratio (95 % CI)
Age 20–29	1.31 (0.60–2.83)
Age 30–39	2.14 (1.03–4.43)*
Age 40–49	1.20 (0.55–2.65)
Age 50–59	1.68 (0.76–3.71)
Age 60–69	1.57 (0.67–3.67)
Age 70+	1.52 (0.64–3.62)
Sex (male)	0.72 (0.49–1.08)
Primary site (extremity)	0.66 (0.49–0.98)*
Quintile of the income domain of the index of multiple deprivation 2010 (1)	0.76 (0.41–1.41)
(2)	0.71 (0.38–1.32)
(4)	0.93 (0.51–1.72)
(5)	0.87 (0.47–1.61)
Constant	0.20 (0.09–0.43)***

* Statistically significant at $p < 0.05$

*** Statistically significant at $p < 0.001$

There are, however, limitations to this study. Although data are available on the presence of metastases or not at diagnosis, which was similar in the two age groups, 0–19 years and ≥20 years, other factors explaining the better outcome in the younger age group, are missing. Data on tumour size, biology, chemotherapy and radiotherapy, were not routinely collected by the cancer registries in England until 2013. Therefore, the better outcome in children and adolescents maybe due to other factors unavailable in this series. Lastly, 77 % of children/adolescents and 70 % of adults were recorded as having surgery, compared with 98 and 88 % respectively in the SEER study [2], suggesting that surgery is incompletely recorded.

Two roughly contemporary Italian hospital-based series have contrasting results. At the Instituto Tumori, Milan, among the 255 patients with localised disease, more chemotherapy was given to younger patients suggesting that this accounted for their better outcome [10]. At Rizzoli, however, among patients with localised disease there was no difference in chemotherapy usage between age groups, but children had better survival than adults [22]. The lack of effect of treatment in particular chemotherapy has also been confirmed in a recent Netherlands cancer registry study in localised SS, furthermore they demonstrate that younger age is again important for outcome regardless of site or tumour size. [25].

The better outcome in children/adolescents compared to adults with SS was also found in the analysis of the SEER data [2]. Other similarities in our study included similar clinical presentation between adults and children/adolescents in terms of metastases and the site of the tumour. Our study also confirmed that those with limb primaries and no metastases had a superior outcome [2]. Poor outcome in SS arising in non-limb sites has also been demonstrated in a smaller Italian series and the SIOP MMT analysis [20, 21]. A possible explanation for the better outcome in younger patients with SS is biology, in particular the role of genomic index (GI) [26]. Increasing genomic instability as scored by GI is more frequent in adults compared to children with SS, and predicts for metastatic relapse and survival [26]. Furthermore GI is independent of response to neoadjuvant chemotherapy and remains an independent prognostic factor [27]. This factor could not be analysed in our series, and needs confirming in a prospective trial.

The overall 5-year relative survival at 57 % compared favourably with similar population-based series, in particular the SEER database [2]. Compared with series, which are institutionally based, our outcome seems superior, but it is likely that institutional series reflect a higher risk group, and contains patients from an earlier time period [10, 22]. It is disappointing that over time the survival in England has not improved. Recent paediatric series from the European Paediatric soft tissue group have a much better outcome, but they only included young patients with localised disease [24].

A novel feature of this study was the ability to assess the role of deprivation on outcome using the income domain of the Indices of Multiple Deprivation 2010. ID scores have been widely used to study the relationship between socioeconomic factors and outcome in cancer [11–13]. These studies demonstrated a worse outcome among patients with more deprivation and higher deprivation scores. For the whole cohort in our study, patients with the highest ID of IMD score 5 only, and hence the most deprived, had a worse outcome, this held in the adult cohort but was not significant in the younger age group, possible due the small numbers <19 years of age. This may be plausibly due to diagnostic delays (professional or patient), or to poor awareness of this tumour, but the lack of data on tumour size, treatment received and length of clinical pathway hampers any further interpretation. However, the ID score did not predict for increased metastases at diagnosis. The role of deprivation on survival from SS has not been studied previously, but in Ewing sarcoma survival was significantly lower in deprived groups [23].

Conclusion

Children/teenagers and adults with SS have a similar clinical presentation but children/teenagers have a superior outcome. The lack of complete data on treatment received makes it impossible to tell whether this or biological variables explain this difference, though the latter is more likely. The finding of severe socioeconomic deprivation as presented as the ID of IMD score affecting outcome in SS needs further exploration in a complete and contemporary dataset, where all prognostic variables are present. This may be possible in the current national cancer registry. The paucity of all-ages, large and international randomised studies in SS, with the testing of new targeted agents, may have contributed to the static outcome in this cohort over this time period.

Abbreviations

CI: confidence intervals; DCO: death certificate only; GI: genomic index; HES: hospital episode statistics; ID: income domain; IMD: index of multiple deprivation; NCDR: national cancer data repository; NOS: not otherwise specified; ONS: office of national statistics; SEER: surveillance epidemiology and end results; SS: synovial sarcoma; STS: soft tissue sarcoma.

Authors' contributions

BB and MF developed the concept and designed the study. BB, MF and JB performed the analysis and interpreted the results. BB, CS, RG, ND, JB and MF all contributed to the writing of the paper, corrections and final paper submitted.

Author details

[1] Department of Paediatric Oncology, Royal Manchester Children's Hospital, Oxford Road, Manchester M13 9WL, UK. [2] Knowledge and Intelligence Service West Midlands, Public Health England, Birmingham, UK. [3] National Cancer Registration and Analysis Service, Public Health England, Birmingham, UK. [4] Department of Orthopaedic Oncology, Royal Orthopaedic Hospital, Birmingham, UK.

Competing interests

The authors declare that they have no competing interests.

Acknowledgements

Not applicable.

Novelty and impact

This large population study's novelty is the completeness of registration of patients and the ability to look at the effect of deprivation and age on outcome in synovial sarcoma. This allows further stratification of synovial sarcoma for therapeutic intervention.

References

1. Stiller CA, Kroll ME, Eatock EM. Incidence of childhood cancer 1991–2000. In: Stiller C, editor. Childhood cancer in Britain: incidence, survival, mortality. Oxford: Oxford University Press; 2007. p. 23–105.
2. Sultan I, Rodriguez-Galindo C, Saab R, Yasir S, Casanova M, Ferrari A. Comparing children and adults with synovial sarcoma in the surveillance, epidemiology, and end results program, 1983 to 2005: an analysis of 1268 patients. Cancer. 2009;115:3537–47.
3. dos Santos NR, de Brujin DR, van Kessel AG. Molecular mechanisms underlying human synovial sarcoma development. Genes Chromosomes Cancer. 2001;30:1–14.
4. Ladanyi M. Fusion of the SYT and SSX genes in synovial sarcoma. Oncogene. 2001;20:5755–62.
5. Pollack A, Zagars GK, Goswitz MS, et al. Preoperative vs. postoperative radiotherapy in the treatment of soft tissue sarcomas: a matter of presentation. Int J Radiat Oncol Biol Phys. 1998;42:563–72.
6. Brecht IB, Ferrari A, Int-Veen C, et al. Grossly-resected synovial sarcoma treated by the german and italian pediatric soft tissue sarcoma cooperative groups: discussion on the role of adjuvant therapies. Pediatr Blood Cancer. 2006;46:11–7.
7. Okcu MF, Munsell M, Treuner J, et al. Synovial sarcoma of childhood and adolescence: a multicenter, multivariate analysis of outcome. J Clin Oncol. 2003;21:1602–11.
8. Eilber FC, Brennan MF, Eilber FR, et al. Chemotherapy is associated with improved survival in adult patients with primary extremity synovial sarcoma. Ann Surg. 2007;246:105–13.
9. Pervaiz N, Colterjohn N, Farrokhyar F, et al. A systematic meta-analysis of randomized controlled trials of adjuvant chemotherapy for localized resectable soft-tissue sarcoma. Cancer. 2008;3:573–81.
10. Ferrari A, Gronchi A, Casanova M, et al. Synovial sarcoma: a retrospective analysis of 271 patients of all ages treated at a single institution. Cancer. 2004;101:627–34.
11. Riaz SP, Horton M, Kang J, et al. Lung cancer incidence and survival in England: an analysis by socioeconomic deprivation and urbanization. J Thorac Oncol. 2011;6:2005–10.
12. Bharathan B, Welfare M, Borowski DW, et al. Impact of deprivation on short- and long-term outcomes after colorectal cancer surgery. Br J Surg. 2011;98:854–65.
13. Downing A, Prakash K, Gilthorpe MS, Mikeljevic JS, Forman D. Socioeconomic background in relation to stage at diagnosis, treatment and survival in women with breast cancer. Br J Cancer. 2007;96(5):836–40.
14. World Health Organisation, 2012. International Classification of Diseases (ICD). http://www.who.int/classifications/icd/en/ Accessed 24.07.2012.
15. World Health Organisation, 2012. International Classification of Diseases for Oncology, 3rd edition (ICD-O-3). http://www.who.int/classifications/icd/adaptations/oncology/en/ Accessed 24.07.2012.
16. Communities and local government: indices of deprivation. http://www.communities.gov.uk/corporate/researchandstatistics/statistics/subject/indicesdeprivation.
17. Fay MP, Feuer EJ. Confidence Intervals for directly standardised rates: a method based on the Gamma distribution. Stat Med. 1997;16(7):791–801.
18. Ederer F, Heise H. Instructions to Ibm 650 programmers in processing survival computations. Technical End Results Evaluation Section, National Cancer Institute: Bethesda; 1959.
19. Office for National Statistics. Cancer statistics registrations: registrations of cancer diagnosed in 2007, England. http://www.statistics.gov.uk/downloads/theme_health/MB1-38/MB1_No38_2007.pdf. Accessed Aug 30, 2010.
20. Ferrari A, Bisogno G, Alaggio G, et al. Synovial sarcoma of children and adolescents: the prognostic role of axial sites. Eur J Cancer. 2008;44:1202–9.

21. Orbach D, Mc Dowell H, Rey A, Bouvet N, et al. Sparing strategy does not compromise prognosis in pediatric localized synovial sarcoma: experience of the international society of pediatric oncology, malignant mesenchymal tumors (SIOP-MMT) working group. Pediatr Blood Cancer. 2011;57:1130–6.
22. Palmerini E, Staals EL, Alberghini M, et al. Synovial sarcoma: retrospective analysis of 250 patients treated at a single institution. Cancer. 2009;115:2988–98.
23. Lee J, Hoang BH, Ziogas A, et al. Analysis of prognostic factors in ewing sarcoma using a population-based cancer registry. Cancer. 2010;116:1964–73.
24. Ferrari A, De Salvo GL, Brennan B, et al. Synovial sarcoma in children and adolescents: the European pediatric soft tissue sarcoma study group prospective trial (EpSSG NRSTS 2005). Ann Oncol. 2014;26(3):567–72.
25. Vlenterie M, Ho VK, Kaal SE, et al. Age as an independent prognostic factor for survival of localised synovial sarcoma patients. Br J Cancer. 2015;113(11):1602–6.
26. Lagarde P, Przybyl J, Brulard C, et al. Chromosome instability accounts for reverse metastatic outcomes of pediatric and adult synovial sarcomas. J Clin Oncol. 2013;31:608–15.
27. Chakiba C, Lagarde P, Pissaloux D, et al. Response to chemotherapy is not related to chromosome instability in synovial sarcoma. Ann Oncol. 2014;25:2267–77.
28. Abdela L, Moore J, et al. Control of data quality for population-based cancer survival analysis. Cancer Epidemiology. 2014;38:314–20.

6

Retroperitoneal solitary fibrous tumor: surgery as first line therapy

Rahul Rajeev[1], Mohit Patel[1], Thejus T. Jayakrishnan[1], Fabian M. Johnston[1], Meena Bedi[2], John Charlson[3] and Kiran K. Turaga[1*]

Abstract

Background: Solitary fibrous tumors (SFT) of the retroperitoneum are rare spindle cell neoplasms, with a paucity of data on treatment outcomes. We hypothesized that surgical excision offered acceptable outcomes in SFTs.

Methods: The National Cancer Database (NCDB) was used to identify patients with SFT from 2004 to 2011. Primary outcome measures were 30 day mortality and overall survival. Descriptive analyses were performed. Furthermore, a systematic review of published literature was conducted after creating a pre-specified search strategy.

Results: Of 51 patients in the NCDB, 58.8 % (n = 30) were males, with a median age 60 years (IQR 49–72 years). Median tumor size was 16 cm (IQR 11–21 cm). Surgical resection was performed in 92.2 % (n = 47) with 63.8 % (n = 30) having a margin negative resection. Peri-operative mortality was 2.1 % (n = 1). Of survival outcomes available for 18 patients, the median OS was 51.1 months. From the systematic review, we identified 8 studies, with 24 patients. Median age and tumor size was similar to the NCDB [47.5 years (IQR 39–66.5 years), 12 cm (IQR 7–17 cm)]. Majority [91.7 % (n = 22)] underwent surgical excision alone while one received adjuvant chemotherapy and none received radiation. After median follow up of 54 months (IQR 28–144 months), 79.2 % (n = 19) were alive without disease. Three patients (12.5 %) died of disease, one was alive with disease and one was lost to follow up. Recurrence was reported in 16.7 % (n = 4) of patients.

Conclusion: Complete surgical excision is a viable treatment modality for retroperitoneal SFT leading to long term survival. Low recurrence rates would argue against the need for routine adjuvant radiation or chemotherapy.

Keywords: Solitary fibrous tumors, Retroperitoneal sarcoma, Adjuvant chemotherapy, Adjuvant radiotherapy, Surgical outcomes, Surgical Oncology

Background

Solitary fibrous tumors (SFT) are extremely rare spindle cell neoplasms with a varied presentation. First described as a pleural tumor by Klemperer et al. later they were identified in extra-thoracic sites, most commonly the adrenals, head and neck, retroperitoneum, kidneys, liver and skeletal muscle [1–3]. Existing literature on SFTs are limited to case reports that mostly describe pleural tumors [4, 5]. Owing to its rarity, extra-pleural SFTs have not been studied adequately.

Retroperitoneal SFTs are a distinct sub-group of extra-pleural SFTs, often incidentally discovered during imaging for an unrelated pathology and present with non-specific symptoms, mainly abdominal pain, hip pain and urinary symptoms [6]. Extra-thoracic SFTs have been classically described as benign tumors but recent studies with larger numbers of cases and longer follow up have demonstrated the existence of a subgroup of tumors that exhibit a malignant clinical course with local and distant recurrence even after surgical excision [4, 7, 8]. Adverse outcomes are usually associated with atypical histological features (nuclear pleomorphism, increased cellularity, necrosis or mitoses greater than 4/10 HPF) and size greater than 10 cm [9, 10]. Also, cases of extra-thoracic SFTs with benign features at initial presentation have

*Correspondence: kturaga@mcw.edu
[1] Division of Surgical Oncology, Department of Surgery, Medical College of Wisconsin, 9200 West Wisconsin Avenue, Milwaukee, WI 53226, USA

been reported to recur years after surgical excision with malignant features [9, 11, 12].

Surgical excision has been the standard treatment option for both benign and malignant SFTs but late recurrences have been observed [2, 13]. A multi-modality approach using adjunct radiotherapy and chemotherapy has been utilized in cases where complete excision is not achieved [14]. We hypothesized that surgical excision is an acceptable treatment modality with favorable outcomes for SFTs of retroperitoneal origin.

Methods

The National Cancer Database (NCDB) was surveyed for cases with a histological diagnosis of solitary fibrous tumors from 2004 to 2011. The NCDB was established in 1989 as a joint project of the American Cancer Society and the Commission on Cancer of the American College of Surgeons. It is a nationwide, facility-based, comprehensive clinical surveillance resource oncology data set that captures 70 % of all newly diagnosed malignancies in the US annually, covering more than 1500 commission-accredited cancer programs (http://www.ncdbpuf.facs.org). Cases diagnosed at autopsy were excluded. Demographic details, tumor characteristics, treatment and follow-up data were abstracted from the database. Primary outcome measures were 30-day mortality and overall survival. Descriptive statistical analysis was performed.

A systematic review of published literature on SFTs was conducted in the MEDLINE database using PubMed using a pre-specified search strategy (Fig. 1). Search terms used were "solitary fibrous tumor" and "retroperitoneum". Case reports and literature published in non-English languages were excluded from the study. The search strategy returned 55 articles and 8 studies satisfied the selection criteria. Bibliographies of the selected articles were further searched but no additional relevant articles were found. All the selected articles were retrospective cohort studies.

Statistical analysis was performed using Stata Software Version 12.1 (StataCorp, College Station, TX, USA).

Results

Patient characteristics

The NCDB database yielded 51 patients with 58.8 % (n = 30) males. Median age was 60 years (IQR 49–72 years). Clinical characteristics of the patients are shown in Table 1.

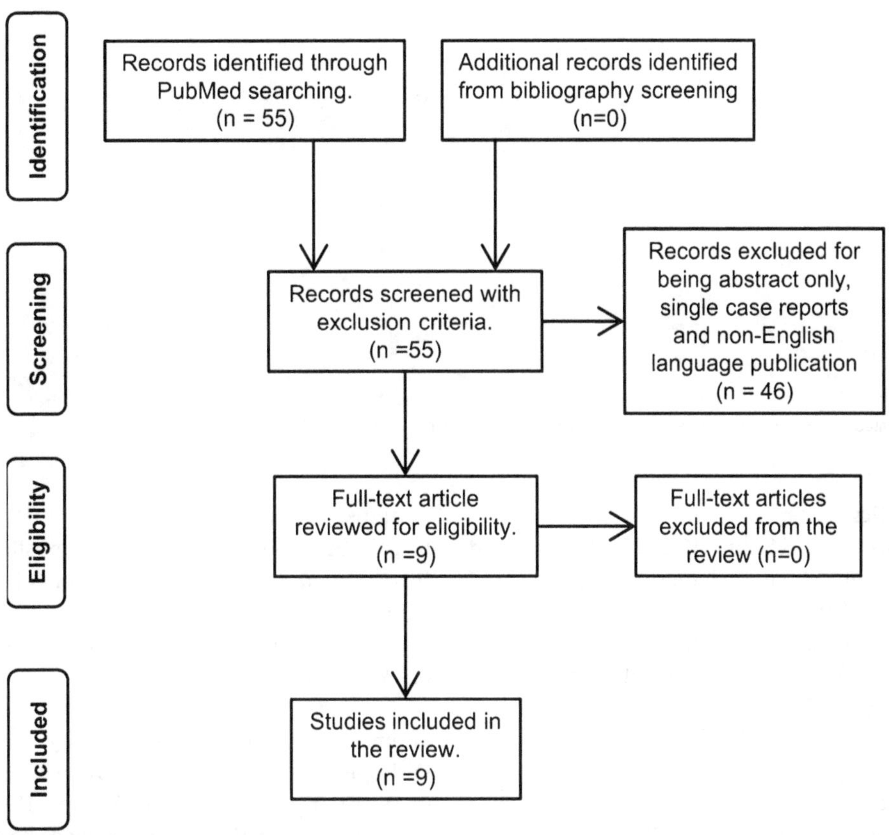

Fig. 1 Search strategy for selecting studies for the systematic review

Table 1 Baseline characteristics and therapies of solitary fibrous tumor (SFT) patients from National Cancer Database (NCDB) and systematic review

Characteristic	NCDB (51 pts)		Systematic review (24 pts)	
	Median (IQR)[a]	Frequency N (%)	Median (IQR)[a]	Frequency N (%)
(Age (years)	60 (49–72)		47.5 (39–66.5)	
Gender				
Male		30 (58.8)		14 (58.3)
Female		21 (41.2)		10 (41.7)
Tumor size (cm)	16 (11–21)		12 (7–17)	
<10 cm		12 (23.5)		7 (29.2)
≥10 cm		35 (68.6)		11 (45.8)
Tumor grade				
Well-differentiated		6 (11.76)		
Moderately differentiated		6 (11.76)		
Poorly differentiated		6 (11.76)		
Undifferentiated/anaplastic		5 (9.8)		
Distant metastasis at diagnosis		4 (9.09)		
Surgery		47 (92.2)		22 (91.7)
Surgical margins[b]				
Negative (R0)		30 (63.8)		
Microscopic positive (R1)		2 (4.3)		
Gross positive (R2)		3 (6.4)		
Unknown		12 (25.5)		
Unplanned 30-day readmission[b]		4 (8.5)		
30-day mortality[b]		1 (2.1)		
Radiation therapy		16 (31.4)		
Adjuvant		13 (25.5)		
Neo-adjuvant		3 (5.8)		
Chemotherapy		10 (19.6)		1 (4.2)
Adjuvant		5 (9.8)		
Neo-adjuvant		3 (5.8)		
Systemic		2 (3.9)		
Combination therapy		4 (7.8)		
Late recurrences				4 (16.7)
Follow-up (months)	45.2 (30.3–63.3)		54 (28–144)	
Mortality at last follow-up		10 (19.6)		3 (12.5)

[a] *IQR* inter-quartile range

[b] Percentages are calculated on the number of patients who had surgery for the tumor

Tumor characteristics

Median tumor size was 16 cm (IQR 11–21 cm) and 68.6 % of tumors were 10 cm or larger. When separated by tumor grade, 9.8 % (n = 5) were undifferentiated/anaplastic. Well-differentiated, moderately differentiated and poorly differentiated tumors were present in equal proportion of 11.8 % (n = 6). Distant metastases were present at diagnosis in 9.1 % (n = 4) of tumors.

Surgical treatment

Surgical excision was recorded in 92.2 % (n = 47) of patients. Among 35 patients with recorded surgical margins, microscopically negative (R0) accounted for 63.8 % (n = 30), microscopically positive (R1) in 4.3 % (n = 2) and gross positive (R2) in 6.4 % (n = 3). Peri-operative mortality was 2.1 % (n = 1). Unplanned readmissions within 30 days of surgery were observed in 8.5 % (n = 4) of patients.

Chemotherapy and radiation therapy

Peri-operative radiation therapy was given to 31.4 % (n = 16) of patients (3 neo-adjuvant, 13 adjuvant). Of the 19.6 % (n = 10) patients who received chemotherapy, 15.6 % (n = 8) were peri-operative (3 neo-adjuvant, 5 adjuvant) and

3.9 % (n = 2) did not undergo surgery. Both chemotherapy and radiation therapy were given to 7.8 % (n = 4) patients.

Survival analysis

Of the 18 patients with vital status recorded, median follow-up was 45.2 months (IQR 30.3–63.3 months) and overall median survival was 51.1 months (IQR 30.3–63.3 months). 10 patients died of disease with a median follow-up of 34.0 months, while 8 were alive with a median follow-up of 64.9 months. When stratified by therapy, median survival was not reached in patients undergoing surgery alone. Among patients with surgery and chemotherapy alone, only one patient had follow-up data.

Of the three patients who had both surgery and radiation and had follow-up data all three died with a median survival of 51.1 months (IQR 24.5–58.5 months). Median survival of patients undergoing surgery, chemotherapy and radiotherapy was 69.2 months (IQR 20.5–118 months) (Table 2). One patient who received surgery and chemotherapy alone died at 23 months.

Results of systematic review

The search strategy resulted in 55 articles of which 8 satisfied the inclusion criteria, with a total of 24 cases (Fig. 1; Table 3). 47 articles were excluded from the final analysis because these were published in non-English language, or were single patient case reports or were available as abstracts only. Median age was 47.5 years (IQR 39–66.5 years) and 58.3 % (n = 14) were male (Table 1). Mean tumor size was 12 cm (IQR 7–17 cm). Two of the identified cases were originally diagnosed as hemangiopericytomas while one was identified as deep fibrous histiocytoma. Of 21 cases with CD34 status available, 19 were positive. Similarly 12 cases were bcl-2 positive (of 12 avaialble reports) and 6 CD99 positive (of 7 available reports). 91.7 % (n = 22) patients underwent surgical excision (1 patient had positive surgical margins), while 1 patient also received adjuvant chemotherapy. Of the remaining two patients, only biopsies were performed for one case as multiple comorbidities precluded surgical excision and treatment information was not available in one patient. Median follow up was 54 months (IQR 28–144 months). Late recurrences were reported in 16.7 % (n = 4) cases (2 local and 2 distant recurrences). Recurrence free survival (RFS) ranged from 1 to 288 months. At last follow-up date, 79.2 % (n = 19) patients were alive without disease, 4.2 % (n = 1) alive with disease, 12.5 % (n = 3) died of the disease and one patient was lost to follow-up. Two of the deaths had late recurrences and one died within 30 days of surgery with a positive surgical margin.

Table 2 Survival outcomes of National Cancer Database patients stratified by therapy

	Median (IQR)
Median overall survival (months)	51.1 (30.3–63.3)
Median survival (months)	
Surgery alone (n = 10)	
Surgery + chemotherapy (n = 1)	
Surgery + radiotherapy (n = 3)	51.1 (24.5–58.5)
Surgery + chemotherapy + radiotherapy (n = 2)	69.2 (20.5–118)

IQR inter-quartile range

Discussion

In our study, we analyzed 51 cases of retroperitoneal SFTs from the National Cancer Database on their treatment modality and outcomes and compared it to published literature on retroperitoneal SFTs. To the authors' best knowledge, this is the largest and most comprehensive series on retroperitoneal SFTs till date and the first study to conduct a formal analysis of surgical outcomes.

Table 3 Summary of studies selected for literature review

Authors	Year	N	Average tumor size (cm)	Median follow-up (months)	Time to recurrence (months)
Decouvelaere et al. [9]	1998	3	10.5	120	12–168
Hasegawa et al. [3]	1999	8	10.25	57	
Morimitsu et al. [36]	2000	1	23	32	
Guillou et al. [37]	2000	3	18.17	39[b]	
Clayton et al. [35][a]	2001	2	10	36	
Takizawa et al. [6]	2007	4	15.9		
Mosquera et al. [17]	2009	1	20	1[c]	
Baldi et al. [2]	2013	2		228	156–276

[a] Adjuvant chemotherapy was given to one of the patients

[b] One patient was lost to follow-up

[c] Patient died within 30 days of surgery

Based on our study, surgery is a valid standard therapy for retroperitoneal SFTs.

Peri-operative morbidity and mortality rates were comparable with other retroperitoneal sarcomas [15, 16]. When stratified by therapy median survival of patients who underwent surgery and chemotherapy and radiation therapy was higher than patients with surgery and radiotherapy alone but it carries no statistical significance as the former group consisted of four patients of which follow-up information was available only for two. The efficacy of chemotherapy in retroperitoneal SFTs is questionable. When compared to patients who did not receive chemotherapy, chemotherapy group had a larger mean tumor size (18.2 cm vs. 15.8 cm), higher grade (40 % poorly differentiated/undifferentiated vs. 17 %) and more positive resection margins (20 vs. 17 %) and this might have confounded the results.

Retroperitoneal SFTs are different from other SFTs in their larger size at presentation. Retroperitoneal SFTs are mostly asymptomatic or present with vague non-specific symptoms of abdominal pain, increase in abdominal girth, weight loss and are often diagnosed incidentally when imaging for unrelated conditions, while SFTs of pleura, extremities and other sites present with signs and symptoms of mass lesion or are visible to the patient and is likely to be diagnosed early in their course [17]. Thus, the larger size at presentation could be explained by the delay in diagnosis due to lack of specific symptoms. Previous studies have reported a larger tumor size (>10–15 cm) as a predictor of worse outcome for metastasis [10, 18, 19]. Also, size greater than 10 cm is a component of England criteria for classifying SFTs into malignant and benign [5].

Management of retroperitoneal SFTs is not clearly defined. Data is lacking on treatment strategies owing to the orphan status of the tumor. Current therapy is drawn from data on therapy outcomes in similar tumors. Surgery is the standard treatment modality for retroperitoneal SFTs. A positive resection margin has been correlated with worse local recurrence free survival and metastasis free survival by Gold et al. and with local recurrence by van Houdt et al. [10, 19]. However, Wilky et al. has found no association of resection margins with recurrence and instead reported an association with malignant histology suggesting that histology may have confounded the association [20]. Regardless, the authors feel that it is safe to keep a high index of suspicion for recurrence in any tumor with positive resection margins as all the deaths due to disease in the systematic review had positive resection margins while all of the alive patients had negative margins. Recurrence rates in retroperitoneal SFTs are low compared to other retroperitoneal sarcomas (17 vs. 52–61 %) [15, 16]. This might argue against routine use of therapies to reduce recurrence rate unless validated by further evidence. However, the use of radiation therapy in the treatment of extra-abdominal SFT has been documented in case series with anecdotal effectiveness [2, 10].

The rates of peri-operative morbidity and mortality in NCDB data was minimal. Wignall et al. has reported technical complexity of the surgery due to the vascular nature of the tumor and the presence of collateral feeding vessels and recommends referral to a tertiary care center and use of techniques like embolization before surgery [21].

Solitary fibrous tumors may recur even after a prolonged latent period and retroperitoneal SFTs are no exception, as three of the recurrences in the review occurred after 10 years of surgery for primary tumor, as echoed by previous reports [9, 10, 18]. Furthermore, intra-abdominal and retroperitoneal SFTs have been reported to have a higher recurrence rate compared to extra-abdominal tumors [11]. These observations warrant a prolonged follow-up and surveillance for retroperitoneal SFTs. The authors recommend a minimum follow-up of 15 years with prolonged follow-up intervals after first 3 years.

The diagnosis of retroperitoneal SFTs requires histologic confirmation. The lack of a uniform nomenclature system in the past had led to SFTs being identified as localized fibrous tumor, localized fibrous mesothelioma, solitary fibrous mesothelioma, fibrous mesothelioma, subserosal fibroma and submesothelial fibroma [22]. Also, the absence of sensitive and specific markers and the nonspecific histologic pattern of the tumor prohibited an accurate diagnosis. However recent investigations into the genetics of the tumor has revealed the overexpression of STAT6 protein, a result of gene-fusion on chromosome 12q13 which leads to a NAB2-STAT6 fusion product. A highly sensitive and specific marker for SFTs has been developed based on a nuclear staining test for the STAT6 protein solving the diagnostic conundrum [23–26]. SFTs can be divided into benign and malignant categories based on its histological features, namely hyper cellularity, pleomorphism, necrosis/hemorrhage and mitoses (>4 mf/10 hpf). Different criteria have been developed to assign malignant or benign classification to SFTs based on histologic features, age, location, size, sessile/pedunculated nature [5, 18]. Nevertheless, SFTs classified as benign have been observed to undergo malignant transformation and recur at local and distant sites [8, 9, 12, 17, 27]. In view of this unpredictable behavior and the increased risk of retroperitoneal SFTs to recur than other SFTs, it is judicious to follow-up all cases of retroperitoneal SFTs irrespective of satisfying the criteria for benign tumors.

The treatment of recurrent SFTs is evolving. The uncommonness of the tumor prohibits a prospective trial. Anti-angiogenic drugs have been tried considering the vascular nature of the tumor. Interferon-alfa and bevacizumab–temozolomide combination has shown promise in disease stabilization in recurrent cases [28–30]. Tyrosine kinase inhibitors(TKI)s are another set of drugs being investigated for malignant and aggressive SFTs. Sunitinib, pazopanib and regorafenib has been shown to be efficacious in animal models and has been studied retrospectively [31–33]. Conventional chemotherapeutic agents like dacarbazine also has been shown to be effective against SFTs [28, 33]. Prospective studies on dacarbazine, TKIs and other investigational drugs are being conducted currently. Park et al. recommends targeted therapies/antiangiogenic drugs initially and stabilizing the disease later with conventional chemotherapy [34].

Given the rarity of solitary fibrous tumors of the retroperitoneum, studies that describe the management and outcomes of these tumors are limited in number. Available literature is focused on SFTs in the pleura due to its more common occurrence. Previous studies on retroperitoneal SFTs are mostly case reports and outcomes of surgery have not been studied.

Our study was limited by the number of cases, both in the NCDB registry and published literature. Number of patients was insufficient to perform a multi-variate subgroup analysis. Past studies on SFTs were heterogeneous in their reporting of surgeries. Treatment of recurrences was not recorded in some instances. The ambiguous pathologic terminology in practice for describing SFTs makes it possible that many tumors were misclassified and as a result not included in the literature review as our search strategy did not consider all available terms for SFTs. Three of the studies in the systematic review were from the United States and one of them is from a National Cancer Institute designated cancer center and this may lead to an overlap of two patients with the NCDB data [35].

Conclusions

Considering the orphan status of solitary fibrous tumors, it is impossible to conduct a study involving adequate number of cases. In this scenario, our analysis of NCDB and systematic review of published literature demonstrates that surgical excision is a feasible and reasonable first line of therapy for retroperitoneal solitary fibrous tumors with minimal perioperative morbidity and mortality and overall median survival above 4 years. The diagnosis may be confirmed by novel nuclear staining techniques if in doubt. For recurrent and aggressive tumors, a multimodality therapy incorporating surgery, chemotherapy and radiotherapy may be considered on a case to case basis. Anti–angiogenic drugs and TKIs are appropriate for initial therapy and conventional chemotherapy may be used later to stabilize the disease and the patient could be enrolled in ongoing clinical trials. Given the propensity for late recurrences even in clinically and histologically benign tumors, SFTs should be followed up for a prolonged period of 15 years, irrespective of nature of the tumor at initial presentation.

Authors' contributions

MP and RR carried out the literature search, analysis and drafted the manuscript. TTJ assisted with the literature search, data synthesis and manuscript preparation. FMJ, JC, MB and KKT supervised the study offering needful directions and expert opinion, and reviewed the manuscript at various stages of its preparation. All authors read and approved the final manuscript.

Author details

[1] Division of Surgical Oncology, Department of Surgery, Medical College of Wisconsin, 9200 West Wisconsin Avenue, Milwaukee, WI 53226, USA. [2] Department of Radiation Oncology, Medical College of Wisconsin, 8701 Watertown Plank Rd., Milwaukee, WI 53226, USA. [3] Section of Hematology and Oncology, Medical College of Wisconsin, 9200 West Wisconsin Avenue, Milwaukee, WI 53226, USA.

Acknowledgements

This study was funded by the Wadina Sarcoma Research Fund.

Competing interests

The authors have no financial or personal relationships with other people or organizations that could inappropriately influence this work. The authors report no proprietary or commercial interest in any product mentioned or concept discussed in this article. The authors declare that they have no competing interests.

Role of the funding source

The funding source had no role in study design, data collection and analysis, decision to publish, or preparation of the manuscript.

References

1. Klemperer PRC (1931) Primary neoplasms of the pleura. A report of five cases. Arch Pathol 11:385–412
2. Baldi GG, Stacchiotti S, Mauro V, Dei Tos AP, Gronchi A, Pastorino U et al (2013) Solitary fibrous tumor of all sites: outcome of late recurrences in 14 patients. Clin Sarcoma Res 3:4. doi:10.1186/2045-3329-3-4
3. Hasegawa T, Matsuno Y, Shimoda T, Hasegawa F, Sano T, Hirohashi S (1999) Extrathoracic solitary fibrous tumors: their histological variability and potentially aggressive behavior. Hum Pathol 30(12):1464–1473. doi:10.1016/S0046-8177(99)90169-7
4. Briselli M, Mark EJ, Dickersin GR (1981) Solitary fibrous tumors of the pleura: eight new cases and review of 360 cases in the literature. Cancer 47(11):2678–2689
5. England DM, Hochholzer L, McCarthy MJ (1989) Localized benign and malignant fibrous tumors of the pleura. A clinicopathologic review of 223 cases. Am J Surg Pathol 13(8):640–658
6. Takizawa I, Saito T, Kitamura Y, Arai K, Kawaguchi M, Takahashi K et al (2008) Primary solitary fibrous tumor (SFT) in the retroperitoneum. Urol Oncol Semin Ori 26(3):254–259. doi:10.1016/j.urolonc.2007.03.024
7. Kanthan R, Torkian B (2004) Recurrent solitary fibrous tumor of the pleura with malignant transformation. Arch Pathol Lab Med 128(4):460–462. doi:10.1043/1543-2165(2004)128<460:RSFTOT>2.0.CO;2

8. Tominaga N, Kawarasaki C, Kanemoto K, Yokochi A, Sugino K, Hatanaka K et al (2012) Recurrent solitary fibrous tumor of the pleura with malignant transformation and non-islet cell tumor-induced hypoglycemia due to paraneoplastic overexpression and secretion of high-molecular-weight insulin-like growth factor II. Intern Med 51(23):3267–3272
9. Vallat-Decouvelaere AV, Dry SM, Fletcher CD (1998) Atypical and malignant solitary fibrous tumors in extrathoracic locations: evidence of their comparability to intra-thoracic tumors. Am J Surg Pathol 22(12):1501–1511
10. Gold JS, Antonescu CR, Hajdu C, Ferrone CR, Hussain M, Lewis JJ et al (2002) Clinicopathologic correlates of solitary fibrous tumors. Cancer 94(4):1057–1068
11. Cranshaw IM, Gikas PD, Fisher C, Thway K, Thomas JM, Hayes AJ (2009) Clinical outcomes of extra-thoracic solitary fibrous tumours. Eur J Surg Oncol J Eur Soc Surg Oncol Br Assoc Surg Oncol 35(9):994–998. doi:10.1016/j.ejso.2009.02.015
12. Yokoi T, Tsuzuki T, Yatabe Y, Suzuki M, Kurumaya H, Koshikawa T et al (1998) Solitary fibrous tumour: significance of p53 and CD34 immunoreactivity in its malignant transformation. Histopathology 32(5):423–432
13. Robinson LA (2006) Solitary fibrous tumor of the pleura. Cancer Control J Moffitt Cancer Cent 13(4):264–269
14. de Perrot M, Kurt AM, Robert JH, Borisch B, Spiliopoulos A (1999) Clinical behavior of solitary fibrous tumors of the pleura. Ann Thorac Surg 67(5):1456–1459
15. Lee SY, Goh BK, Teo MC, Chew MH, Chow PK, Wong WK et al (2011) Retroperitoneal liposarcomas: the experience of a tertiary Asian center. World J Surg Oncol 9:12. doi:10.1186/1477-7819-9-12
16. Lochan R, French JJ, Manas DM (2011) Surgery for retroperitoneal soft tissue sarcomas: aggressive re-resection of recurrent disease is possible. Ann Roy Coll Surg 93(1):39–43. doi:10.1308/003588410x12771863936729
17. Mosquera JM, Fletcher CD (2009) Expanding the spectrum of malignant progression in solitary fibrous tumors: a study of 8 cases with a discrete anaplastic component—is this dedifferentiated SFT? Am J Surg Pathol 33(9):1314–1321
18. Demicco EG, Park MS, Araujo DM, Fox PS, Bassett RL, Pollock RE et al (2012) Solitary fibrous tumor: a clinicopathological study of 110 cases and proposed risk assessment model. Mod Pathol Off J US Can Acad Pathol Inc 25(9):1298–1306. doi:10.1038/modpathol.2012.83
19. van Houdt WJ, Westerveld CM, Vrijenhoek JE, van Gorp J, van Coevorden F, Verhoef C et al (2013) Prognosis of solitary fibrous tumors: a multicenter study. Ann Surg Oncol 20(13):4090–4095. doi:10.1245/s10434-013-3242-9
20. Wilky BA, Montgomery EA, Guzzetta AA, Ahuja N, Meyer CF (2013) Extrathoracic location and "borderline" histology are associated with recurrence of solitary fibrous tumors after surgical resection. Ann Surg Oncol 20(13):4080–4089. doi:10.1245/s10434-013-3241-x
21. Wignall OJ, Moskovic EC, Thway K, Thomas JM (2010) Solitary fibrous tumors of the soft tissues: review of the imaging and clinical features with histopathologic correlation. AJR Am J Roentgenol 195(1):W55–W62. doi:10.2214/AJR.09.3379
22. Langman G (2011) Solitary fibrous tumor: a pathological enigma and clinical dilemma. J Thorac Dis 3(2):86–87. doi:10.3978/j.issn.2072-1439.2011.03.04
23. Mohajeri A, Tayebwa J, Collin A, Nilsson J, Magnusson L, von Steyern FV et al (2013) Comprehensive genetic analysis identifies a pathognomonic NAB2/STAT6 fusion gene, nonrandom secondary genomic imbalances, and a characteristic gene expression profile in solitary fibrous tumor. Genes Chromosom Cancer 52(10):873–886. doi:10.1002/gcc.22083
24. Schweizer L, Koelsche C, Sahm F, Piro RM, Capper D, Reuss DE et al (2013) Meningeal hemangiopericytoma and solitary fibrous tumors carry the NAB2-STAT6 fusion and can be diagnosed by nuclear expression of STAT6 protein. Acta Neuropathol 125(5):651–658. doi:10.1007/s00401-013-1117-6
25. Robinson DR, Wu YM, Kalyana-Sundaram S, Cao X, Lonigro RJ, Sung YS et al (2013) Identification of recurrent NAB2-STAT6 gene fusions in solitary fibrous tumor by integrative sequencing. Nat Genet 45(2):180–185. doi:10.1038/ng.2509
26. Doyle LA, Vivero M, Fletcher CD, Mertens F, Hornick JL (2014) Nuclear expression of STAT6 distinguishes solitary fibrous tumor from histologic mimics. Mod Pathol Off J US Can Acad Pathol Inc 27(3):390–395. doi:10.1038/modpathol.2013.164
27. Law MK, Tung YW, Jinc JS (2014) Malignant transformation in solitary fibrous tumor of the pleura. Asian Cardiovasc Thorac Ann 22(8):981–983. doi:10.1177/0218492313498090
28. Park MS, Patel SR, Ludwig JA, Trent JC, Conrad CA, Lazar AJ et al (2011) Activity of temozolomide and bevacizumab in the treatment of locally advanced, recurrent, and metastatic hemangiopericytoma and malignant solitary fibrous tumor. Cancer 117(21):4939–4947. doi:10.1002/cncr.26098
29. Lackner H, Urban C, Dornbusch HJ, Schwinger W, Kerbl R, Sovinz P (2003) Interferon alfa-2a in recurrent metastatic hemangiopericytoma. Med Pediatr Oncol 40(3):192–194. doi:10.1002/mpo.10122
30. Kirn DH, Kramer A (1996) Long-term freedom from disease progression with interferon alfa therapy in two patients with malignant hemangiopericytoma. J Natl Cancer Inst 88(11):764–765
31. Stacchiotti S, Tortoreto M, Baldi GG, Grignani G, Toss A, Badalamenti G et al (2014) Preclinical and clinical evidence of activity of pazopanib in solitary fibrous tumour. Eur J Cancer 50(17):3021–3028. doi:10.1016/j.ejca.2014.09.004
32. Stacchiotti S, Negri T, Libertini M, Palassini E, Marrari A, De Troia B et al (2012) Sunitinib malate in solitary fibrous tumor (SFT). Ann Oncol Off J Eur Soc Med Oncol Esmo 23(12):3171–3179. doi:10.1093/annonc/mds143
33. Stacchiotti S, Tortoreto M, Bozzi F, Tamborini E, Morosi C, Messina A et al (2013) Dacarbazine in solitary fibrous tumor: a case series analysis and preclinical evidence vis-a-vis temozolomide and antiangiogenics. Clin Cancer Res Off J Am Assoc Cancer Res 19(18):5192–5201. doi:10.1158/1078-0432.CCR-13-0776
34. Park MS, Ravi V, Conley A, Patel SR, Trent JC, Lev DC et al (2013) The role of chemotherapy in advanced solitary fibrous tumors: a retrospective analysis. Clin Sarcoma Res 3(1):7. doi:10.1186/2045-3329-3-7
35. Clayton AC, Salomao DR, Keeney GL, Nascimento AG (2001) Solitary fibrous tumor: a study of cytologic features of six cases diagnosed by fine-needle aspiration. Diagn Cytopathol 25(3):172–176. doi:10.1002/Dc.2032
36. Morimitsu Y, Nakajima M, Hisaoka M, Hashimoto H (2000) Extrapleural solitary fibrous tumor: clinicopathologic study of 17 cases and molecular analysis of the p53 pathway. APMIS Acta Pathol Microbiol Immunol Scand 108(9):617–625
37. Guillou L, Gebhard S, Coindre JM (2000) Lipomatous hemangiopericytoma: a fat-containing variant of solitary fibrous tumor? Clinicopathologic, immunohistochemical, and ultrastructural analysis of a series in favor of a unifying concept. Hum Pathol 31(9):1108–1115. doi:10.1053/hupa.2000.9777

7

How a Clinical Trial Unit can improve independent clinical research in rare tumors: the Italian Sarcoma Group experience

Emanuela Marchesi[1*], Celeste Cagnazzo[2], Irene Quattrini[1], Martina Piccinni Leopardi[3], Chiara Villa[4], Giovanni Grignani[2], Lorenzo D'Ambrosio[2], Silvia Stacchiotti[4], Paolo Giovanni Casali[4] and Piero Picci[5]

Abstract

Background: The Italian Sarcoma Group (ISG) is a nonprofit group of professionals established in 1997 aimed to improve the quality of care and promote the independent research in sarcomas. The increased regulatory requirements, the chance to increase the number of trials with other cooperative groups and an interest from pharmaceutical companies in supporting independent research, generated the need of an internal service for research management.

Methods and results: In 2010, ISG implemented in its organization a Clinical Trial Unit (CTU). The CTU was appointed to fully manage Clinical Trial Operations, to guarantee regulation compliance and provide a central support to the investigators, fostering a collaboration both at national and international level. In 2016 ISG promoted 25 studies in about 120 centers, with a fivefold increase in the last 5 years: 68% were interventional and 32% observational. Nine of the 17 interventional studies (52%) were supported by pharmaceutical companies, while 4 (24%) were funded by European Commission within specific projects on sarcomas and 4 (24%) were supported by the ISG itself.

Conclusion: The contribution of ISG researchers to the international community was striking from the earliest years of the ISG creation. The challenges of the regulatory clinical research scenario, which imposes solid and hard-fast methodology with deep knowledge and expertise, highlighted the need to identify qualified and dedicated experts able to run and follow the multifaceted aspects of trials. Our analysis demonstrated how this model has led to a growth in competitiveness of the group. The collaboration between clinicians and CTU made possible to support the research with high scientific and ethical standards and to increase the number of trials, sites and overall enrolled patients. The reduced time for approvals, the continuous support to sites, the increased speed in data collection and analysis make the ISG research attractive for pharmaceutical industries, despite the problems that have characterized the independent research in the last years. The ability to fully manage and oversight Clinical Operations and the high quality of delivered services, have led the ISG to be recognized as a reliable partner and coordinator within the international sarcoma networks.

Background

Sarcomas are rare tumors of mesenchymal origin, accounting for nearly 21 and <1% of all pediatric and adult solid malignant tumors, respectively [1].

Clinical trial research in disease with a low incidence like sarcomas (<6 per 100,000 people per year) is crucial to guarantee to the affected population the opportunity to access new treatments and benefit from medical and scientific progresses [2, 3].

However, in rare diseases, clinical research is challenging: few clinical trials are available for these populations and patients encounter difficulties in accessing

*Correspondence: emanuela.marchesi@ior.it
[1] Italian Sarcoma Group, Istituto Ortopedico Rizzoli, Via Pupilli 1, 40136 Bologna, Italy

specialized centers where the most innovative clinical trials are run [4].

In addition, conventional clinical trial designs are not always applicable and the statistical design needs to be modulated in order to make the studies feasible also in small populations [5–9].

The management of sarcomas poses several problems and the need for reference centers to share their experiences let to the creation of networks and consortia of specialists [10, 11].

From the late eighties the Italian reference centers specialized in sarcoma treatment, began to collaborate within some national research programs and participated to the development of investigator-initiated clinical trials [12, 13].

From this experience, they felt the need to share their expertise and joint together in an Italian research network aimed to improve the academic research and committed to try to provide answers to unmet clinical questions, especially in the extremely rare sarcomas, or for peculiar sarcoma subtypes.

Thus in 1997, the Italian Sarcoma Group (ISG) was founded and, legally recognized as a scientific independent non-profit association in 2002, begun to promote independent clinical trials.

From the time the European Clinical Trials Directive 2001/20/CE [14] was fully adopted in Italy, at the end of 2007, its effects resulted in an increased in strictness and complexity of trial activities and trial oversight procedures.

This regulation, the chance to increase the number of trials conducted within international consortia [15, 16] and a greater interest of pharmaceutical companies in supporting independent research, imposed the need to introduce in the ISG organization, a Clinical Trial Unit (CTU) exclusively dedicated to Clinical Trial Operations to serve as an operative focal point for national and collaborative trials in sarcomas.

Methods

Development of the Clinical Trial Unit

The proposal to implement a CTU was presented to the ISG Directive Executive Board in 2009 that granted its approval for the initial financial support.

The source of funds was covered by the fundraising activities of the group and by the internal overheads derived from previous supported studies The main CTU office was established at central level and, under the central coordination, two satellites offices were introduced in other institutions.

The assigned mission to CTU was to promote high quality standard of the group promoted research, to guarantee the compliance with regulation, to provide central support to participating sites, to facilitate collaboration between them and to collaborate with the other European sarcoma cooperative groups, involved in common international studies.

Analysis

The impact of the CTU in ISG clinical research was assessed by comparing the number of clinical studies, the number of activated sites and of enrolled patients, the performance in data collection and the funds received to conduct the trials, in the time period from 2010 to the 3rd quarter of 2016.

The analysis included data of interventional, translational and observational studies as well as the educational activity promoted by the CTU.

Results

The first step toward the CTU creation was to implement the Clinical Operation (ClinOp) services, within the ISG secretariat by part-time personnel with a previous specific expertise in the management of clinical trials in sarcomas.

Among the first services offered were those related to study monitoring (site initiation, monitoring, and close-out visits) and to the development of specific Clinical Trial Monitoring Standard Operative Procedures, (CTM-SOPs) to be applied to all the ISG clinical trials, in full compliance with the regulatory requirements.

From 2010 to 2012 the number of interventional clinical trials and centers completely managed by ISG ClinOp, increased respectively of 75% (from 4 to 7 studies) and 158% (from 26 to 67 activated sites).

As consequence to these first positive results an internal budget analysis was performed.

The recorded increase of funds (+48%) allowed ISG to introduce a fully independent CTU, able to cover its own expenses with their services.

CTU was then formally recognized by ISG and, from mid-2013, the ISG ClinOp were no longer part of the secretariat services, but started to be delivered by the independent CTU.

Responsibility of the CTU is to oversight the trial management for interventional and observational multi-sites clinical studies where ISG is sponsor or national coordinator within international consortia networks programs.

As reporte d in Table 1, the services offered by CTU to the group are focused on 5 main domains: scientific support, project management, safety and regulatory management, educational and CTU administrative management.

From the beginning of 2014 the CTU also introduced an independent pharmacovigilance office and developed Standard Operative Procedures (SOP) to cover all the safety related activities.

Table 1 Clinical Operation Services offered by ISG CTU

Scientific support
Protocol development
Support to the coordinator physician within the study board, for the implementation of the ethical aspects and safety requirements of research
Study report, publication and result dissemination
Support to the final study report, publication submission and dissemination of the study results
Study project management
Study budget plan and budget negotiation
Evaluation of study costs, budget plan development and budget negotiation with pharma companies supporters of the independent research or with partners within consortium projects
Study feasibility
Support to sites selection through site feasibility development within the study board
Regulatory documentation
Preparation of the regulatory documents, preparation and maintenance of the study binders in accordance with Good Clinical Practices and ISG Clinical Trial Standard Operating Procedure (SOP)
Regulatory submission
Submission to the Competent Authorities and Independent Review Boards (IRB) of the regulatory (protocols, patient's information sheet and informed consents, Investigational Product information, safety information and all the others applicable documents)
Support activity in the preparation of the submission package for extra-Italian submission within international studies coordinated by ISG
Investigational Product (IP) activities
Management of the IP from labeling (if required) to supply and resupply activities
Database development
Support to the Case Report Form design
Investigators meetings
Support in the organization of the Investigators Meetings and logistics
Monitoring activities
Management and conduction, either remote and onsite, of the site activation, monitoring and close-out visits
Coordination of centralized activities
Development of procedures for centralized activities (samples management in case of centralized biological material analysis, centralized imaging review management)
Communication with the sites
Study state of art continuous monitoring
Regulatory and safety management
Safety regulatory activities conducted by the Pharmacovigilance Office
Communication of safety information (SUSAR, SAE line listing) to Competent Authorities and sites
Eudravigilance reporting activities
Educational
Protocol training activities
Training on GCP, regulatory and clinical operation
Administrative
Protocol budget plan
Site contract negotiation
External services contract negotiation

When the first ISG ClinOp services were implemented in 2010, 6 studies (4 interventional and 2 observational) were ongoing and were mainly managed by the coordinating investigators.

The trials promoted by ISG or in collaboration with other international sarcoma networks in mid-2016 were 25: 17 (68%) interventional and 8 (32%) observational (Table 2).

52% ($n = 9$) of the interventional have financial support from pharmaceutical companies, while 24% ($n = 4$) received funds within sarcoma European Commission projects and 24% ($n = 4$) are supported by ISG itself (Table 3). Taking into account only the interventional studies, whereof regulatory requirements impose stringent quality standards, a great improvement in the number of managed clinical sites and patients has been

Table 2 Number and type of studies managed by the CTU

Year	Interventional	Observational
2010	4 (71%)	2 (29%)
2011	7 (78%)	2 (22%)
2012	7 (78%)	2 (22%)
2013	7 (78%)	2 (22%)
2014	12 (66%)	6 (34%)
2015	13 (68%)	6 (32%)
2016	17 (68%)	8 (32%)

Table 3 Funding sources for interventional studies

Year	Supported by pharma companies	Supported within EC sarcomas' projects	Supported by ISG
2010	2/4 (50%)	0 (0%)	2 (50%)
2011	4/7 (57%)	1 (14%)	2 (29%)
2012	3/7 (43%)	1 (14%)	3 (43%)
2013	3/7 (43%)	1 (14%)	3 (43%)
2014	6/12 (50%)	3 (25%)	3 (25%)
2015	6/13 (46%)	4 (31%)	3 (23%)
2016	9/17 (52%)	4 (24%)	4 (24%)

recorded from 2010 to mid-2016, bringing the CTU to manage from 25 to 119 sites (+376%) and more than 800 active patients (+543%) with an mean increase, respectively, of 31 and 38% per year (Table 4).

Also a speed up in the time of ethical approval and in first patient enrollment have been recorded: a reduced mean time for approval of 4 months (and of 2 months for the First Patient First Visit).

During its 6 years of activity the high quality standard of clinical trial management, together with the capability of providing a comprehensive service for the ClinOp, brought the Italian Sarcoma Group to increase its collaborations within international cooperative groups (from 0 to 9 cooperative studies).

The services offered by the CTU had also impact on the supported research activity, with a more than sevenfold increase of funds from 2010 to 2016, and a mean number of new contracts for supported trials, in the last 3 years, of 3.3 (Table 5).

On the other hand, the increase of research management activities brought the need to potentiate the CTU personnel that, in mid-2016 account for 2 full time units and 5 partially dedicated units from satellites.

The key effort of the CTU in facilitating the collaboration within consortia trials led ISG to join as partner or leader in several European consortia studies.

This also permitted a direct collaborations with other European sarcoma CTU through the sharing of SOP and of the best ClinOp practices.

All the results of the ISG clinical studies, oversight by the CTU, are object of international meeting presentations and are published in the most important peer reviewed oncology journals.

The CTU is also committed in promoting educational and training activities, like periodic courses, addressed not only to Clinical Research Coordinators (CRC) and to the Investigators interested in clinical trial regulation and research methodology. As part of the educational mission of the CTU, from 2013 ISG introduced in its annual meeting, a parallel section dedicated to clinical trial coordination where regulatory and breaking news from trial regulation and methodology are presented.

The personnel of the CTU also collaborate with national groups in research methodology education and is involved in research in the field of clinical trial regulations [17, 18].

Discussion

In the last decade, ISG research network played a key role in the development of independent research in the sarcoma field, in Italy, promoting more than 30 clinical trials and managing over 100 sites with more than 800 patients. The number of clinical trials increased steadily from the

Table 4 Number of interventional CT studies, sites and patients managed by the CTU

Year	Nr of ongoing interventional trials	Nr. of sites	New sites/year	Nr. of active patients	New active patients/year
2010	4	26	NE	127	NE
2011	7	48	23	207	80
2012	7	67	18	323	116
2013	7	74	8	503	180
2014	12	91	17	601	98
2015	13	107	16	797	196
2016	17	119	12	816	19

NE not evaluated

Table 5 Number of new supported studies

Year	New supported studies
2010	0
2011	2
2012	1
2013	0
2014	5
2015	1
2016	4

CTU introduction, and the possibility to independently manage them, contributed to increase the number of consortia and pharmaceutical supported research.

This led to a significant annual income increase that resulted in a self-financing system where the CTU is able to provide to its own maintenance.

Reduced time for regulatory approvals, immediate and continuous support to sites, and speed up in data collection and analysis, are making the ISG clinical research attractive for pharmaceutical industries, despite the fact that independent research in this field has been extremely challenging in the last years.

Finally, the feedback received from the ISG investigators about the support provided by CTU is extremely positive and contributes to increase the network collaboration and involvement, not only in terms of recruitment and data quality, but also in terms of clinical trial coordination activities.

Conclusion

Contribution of ISG researchers to the international community was considered from the earliest years of ISG creation.

The regulatory trial scenario requires a more solid and hard-fast methodology with depth knowledge and expertise. These challenges highlighted the need to identify expert and dedica ted professionals able to run, manage and follow the multifaceted aspects of innovative clinical trials.

The proactive collaboration between clinicians and CTU professionals made possible to support the increasing research activity with high scientific and ethical standards.

The introduction of the CTU within the ISG organization represented an important a chievement in the group's research activity, by facilitating its conduction.

This allows the group to be competitive and be recognized as a reliable partner within the international sarcoma networks and to lead the conduction of consortia clinical trials.

Abbreviations

ISG: Italian Sarcoma Group; CTU: Clinical Trial Unit; SOP: Standard Operative Procedure; CTM-SOP: Clinical Trial Monitoring Standard Operative Procedure; ClinOp: Clinical Operation (ClinOp); FPFV: First Patient First Visit; FTE: full time equivalent; CRC: Clinical Research Coordinator.

Authors' contributions

EM collected, assembled and analyzed the data; review and drafted the manuscript. CC participated at the analysis and contributed to drafting of the manuscript. PP, GG, LDA, SS and CV offered conceptual advice. All reviewed and edited the manuscript. All the authors reviewed the final manuscript. All authors read and approved the final manuscript.

Author details

[1] Italian Sarcoma Group, Istituto Ortopedico Rizzoli, Via Pupilli 1, 40136 Bologna, Italy. [2] Division of Medical Oncology, Candiolo Cancer Institute-FPO, IRCCS, Candiolo, Italy. [3] Chemotherapy Unit, Orthopedic Rizzoli Institute, Bologna, Italy. [4] Adult Mesenchymal Tumour and Rare Cancer Medical Oncology Unit, Fondazione IRCCS Istituto Nazionale Tumori, Milan, Italy. [5] Laboratory of Experimental Oncology, Orthopedic Rizzoli Institute, Bologna, Italy.

Acknowledgements

All the authors would like thanks Alba Balladelli for the language revision of the final manuscript.

Competing interests

The authors declare that they have no competing interests.

References

1. Burningham Z, et al. The epidemiology of sarcoma. Clin Sarcoma Res. 2012;2:14.
2. Gatta G, van der Zwan JM, Casali PG, Siesling S, Dei Tos AP, Kunkler I, Otter R, Licitra L, Mallone S, Tavilla A, Trama A, Capocaccia R, RARECARE Working Group. Rare cancers are not so rare: the rare cancer burden in Europe. Eur J Cancer. 2011;47:2493–511.
3. Gatta G, Mallone S, van der Zwan JM, Trama A, Siesling S, Capocaccia R, EUROCARE Working Group. The burden of rare cancers in Europe. Adv Exp Med Biol. 2010;686:285–303.
4. Blay JY, Coindre JM, Ducimetiere F, Ray-Coquard I. The value of research collaboration and consortia in rare cancers. Lancet Oncol. 2016;17:e62–9.
5. Casali PG, Bruzzi P, Bogaerts J, Blay JY, on behalf of the Rare Cancers Europe (RCE) Consensus Panel. Rare Cancers Europe (RCE) methodological recommendations for clinical studies in rare cancers: a European consensus position paper. Ann Oncol. 2015;26(2):300–6.
6. Billingham L, Malottki K, Steven N. Research methods to change clinical practice for patients with rare cancers. Lancet Oncol. 2016;17:e70–80.
7. Tan SB, Dear KB, Bruzzi P, Machin D. Strategy for randomized clinical trials in rare cancers. BMJ. 2003;327:47–9.
8. Bogaerts J, Sydes MR, Keat N, et al. Clinical trial designs for rare diseases: studies developed and discussed by the International Rare Cancers Initiative. Eur J Cancer. 2015;51:271–81.
9. Gagne JJ, Thompson L, O'Keefe K, Kesselheim AS. Innovative research methods for studying treatments for rare diseases: methodological review. BMJ. 2014;349:g6802.
10. The ESMO/European Sarcoma Network Working Group. Soft tissue and visceral sarcomas: ESMO Clinical Practice Guidelines for diagnosis, treatment and follow-up. Ann Oncol. 2012;23(suppl_7):vii92–9.
11. The ESMO/European Sarcoma Network Working Group. Bone sarcomas: ESMO Clinical Practice Guidelines for diagnosis, treatment and follow-up. Ann Oncol. 2014;25(Suppl 3):iii113–23.

12. Bacci G, Avella M, Capanna R, Boriani R, Dallari S, Galletti S, Giunti A, Madon E, Mancini A, Mercuri M, Orlandi M, Padovani G, Picci P, Sudanese A, Campanacci M. Neoadjuvant chemotherapy in the treatment of osteosarcoma of the extremities: preliminary results in 131 cases treated preoperatively with methotrexate and cisdiamminoplatinum. Ital J Orthop Traumatol. 1988;14:23–39.
13. Picci P, Bacci G, Ruggieri P, Madon E, Paolucci G, Marangolo M, Mercuri M, Biagini R, Fabbri N, Casadei R, De Cristofaro R. The treatment of localized osteosarcoma of the extremities: the Italian experience (studies of the National Research Council). Ann Oncol. 1992;3(Suppl. 2):13–8.
14. European Commission. Directive 2001/20/EC of the European Parliament and of the Council of 4 April 2001 on the approximation of the laws, regulations and administrative provisions of the Member States relating to the implementation of good clinical practice in the conduct of clinical trials on medicinal products for human use. http://ec.europa.eu/health/files/eudralex/vol-1/dir_2001_20/dir_2001_20_en.pdf.
15. EuroSARC: European clinical trials in rare SARComas within an integrated translational trial network. Project funded by the European Commission through the Seventh Framework Programme under Grant Agreement. http://eurosarc.eu/.
16. Euro Ewing Consortium: International Clinical Trials to Improve Survival from Ewing Sarcoma. http://www.euroewing.eu/clinical-trials/reecur/index.
17. Cagnazzo C, Campora S, Arizio F, Marchesi E. The new European Clinical Trial Regulation: perception and expectations in Italy. Ann Oncol. 2016;27(suppl_16):321P.
18. Marchesi E, Monti M, Campora S, Gentili G, Frati P, Pirondi S, Taverniti C, Cagnazzo C. AIFA Determination 809/2015 on Phase I Clinical Trials: a new challenge for Italian Research. Ann Oncol. 2016;27(4):iv112.

8

Patterns of care for patients with advanced soft tissue sarcoma: experience from Australian sarcoma services

Susie Bae[1*], Philip Crowe[2], Raghu Gowda[3], Warren Joubert[4], Richard Carey-Smith[5], Paul Stalley[6] and Jayesh Desai[1]

Abstract

Background: There is a paucity of data on the current management of patients with advanced soft tissue sarcoma (STS) in the Australian health care setting. This study utilised the Australian sarcoma database to evaluate the patterns of care delivered to patients with advanced STS at Australian sarcoma services.

Methods: Prospectively collected data from six sarcoma centres in Australia were sourced to identify patients diagnosed with advanced STS between 1 January 2010 and 31 December 2012. Descriptive statistics were analysed for patient demographics, clinicopathological characteristics and treatment patterns. Overall survival was estimated using the Kaplan–Meier product limit method.

Results: Of 253 patients with advanced STS, four major STS subtypes were identified: undifferentiated pleomorphic sarcoma (23 %), leiomyosarcoma (17 %), liposarcoma (14 %), and synovial sarcoma (8 %); with the rest grouped as "other STS" (38 %). Approximately one-third of patients received palliative systemic therapy with the most common first-line therapy being doxorubicin alone (50 %). A small percentage of patients participated in clinical trials (20 %). Palliative radiotherapy was utilised mostly for treatment of symptomatic distant metastases and one-third of patients underwent metastasectomy, most commonly for pulmonary metastases. The median overall survival (OS) in this series was 18 months and no significant difference in OS was observed across different STS histological subtypes.

Conclusions: This is the first detailed study outlining patterns of care for Australian patients with advanced STS managed at sarcoma services. These data highlight a particular area of weakness in the lack of clinical trials for sarcoma patients and also serve as an important reference point for understanding how practice may change over time as treatment options evolve.

Keywords: Advanced soft tissue sarcoma, Metastatic sarcoma, Palliative-intent treatment, Patterns of care study, Chemotherapy, Radiotherapy, Metastasectomy

Background

Soft tissue sarcomas (STS) comprise a heterogeneous group of diseases, accounting for less than 1 % of adult malignancies [1]. Metastatic or locally advanced STS is generally considered incurable with the mainstay of treatment being systemic chemotherapy. For some patients with limited disease burden however, long-term remission can be achieved through a multimodality approach involving medical, surgical and radiation therapy. The goal of treatment here is to prolong survival whilst maintaining or improving quality of life and dealing with specific disease-related symptoms.

In clinical practice, the decision-making process regarding the choice of systemic therapy, the timing of treatment and the use of single versus combination therapy is highly complex. International guidelines such as the National Comprehensive

*Correspondence: Susie.Bae@petermac.org
[1] Department of Medical Oncology, Peter MacCallum Cancer Centre, St Andrews Place, East Melbourne, VIC 3002, Australia

Cancer Network and the European Society of Medical Oncology offer some consensus on the first-line treatment with anthracycline-based therapy [2, 3]. However, systemic therapy options remain limited beyond the first- and second-line therapy with a lack of evidence for improvement in overall survival with anthracycline-containing doublet chemotherapy [4–7]. Newer agents such as trabectedin and pazopanib with promising activity for certain histologic subtypes have been identified, but these remain a minority and access continues to be a challenge for the treating team and their patients. As novel agents are developed and approved by the regulatory authority, access is highly variable across geographical regions around the globe. Ostensibly these differences in access to effective drugs influence treatment choice but little is known about how treatment algorithms are modified accordingly in routine clinical practice.

A recent study by the North American and European colleagues described chemotherapy treatment patterns and clinical outcomes for patients with metastatic STS highlighting the poor overall survival for this group and the need for more therapeutic options [8]. There is a paucity of data on the current practice of managing patients with advanced STS in the Australian health care setting. The primary goal of this study was to utilise the Australian sarcoma database to evaluate the current patterns of care for patients with advanced STS, managed at sarcoma specialist centres.

Methods

A customised electronic database capturing clinical data considered most relevant to bone and soft tissue sarcomas were established at major sarcoma centres around Australia, with data collection commencing in 2009, approved by the governing ethics committee at each institution. Data from six sarcoma centres were sourced to identify patients diagnosed with advanced STS between 1st January 2010 and 31st December 2012, with a minimum follow up period of 12 months. Subjects aged 18 and above with locally advanced and/or metastatic STS were selected for inclusion into the study if they received care at sarcoma specialist centres with at least two visits during the study period. Data on all systemic therapies given with palliative-intent were collated. Information on palliative therapy other than systemic therapy, i.e. radiotherapy and/or surgery, was available in 89 % of the total study population (n = 225) for analysis. The BioGrid Australia platform was utilised to link the datasets for analysis. The study was approved by the Human Research Ethics Committee at Melbourne Health.

Definitions

- Advanced STS

We defined patients with advanced STS as patients with metastatic and/or locally advanced, unresectable histologically confirmed STS demonstrated by appropriate imaging and biopsy. For the purpose of this study, we excluded patients with gastrointestinal stromal tumour, bone sarcomas, dermatofibrosarcoma protuberans, or rhabdomyosarcomas. (Table 1)

- Palliative treatment modalities

We defined systemic chemotherapy, radiotherapy and surgery as palliative treatment modalities when they were used for the purpose of disease and symptom control in patients with advanced STS.

Statistical methods

Descriptive statistics were analysed for patients' demographics, clinicopathological characteristics and treatment patterns. Overall survival (OS) was estimated for the whole patient cohort using the Kaplan–Meier product limit method and separately for different STS subgroups. The prognostic impact of these variables was explored via the log-rank test. Statistical calculations were performed using SAS Enterprise Guide 6.1 (SAS institute Inc, Cary, NC, USA).

Results

A total of 942 individuals were identified as having histologically confirmed STS diagnosed between 1st January 2010 and 31st December 2012, of which 253 (27 %) were considered as having advanced STS. Of this group, 34 % (n = 86) had metastatic disease at diagnosis, with the remainder presenting with local recurrence that was unresectable and/or distant metastatic disease. The mean

Table 1 Soft tissue sarcoma WHO classification subtypes included and excluded in the study

Included histological subtypes	Excluded histological subtypes
Fibroblastic sarcoma	Rhabdomyosarcoma
Undifferentiated pleomorphic sarcoma	Chondrosarcoma
Leiomyosarcoma	Osteosarcoma
Adipocytic sarcoma	Ewing family tumour
Vascular sarcoma	Gastro-intestinal stromal tumour
Sarcomas of uncertain differentiation; including synovial sarcoma, malignant peripheral nerve sheath tumour, undifferentiated soft tissue sarcoma not otherwise specified	Dermatofibromatosis sarcoma protuberans
	Inflammatory myofibroblastic sarcoma
	Malignant mesothelioma
	Mixed mesodermal tumours of the uterus
	Kaposi's sarcoma
	Desmoid
	Giant cell tumour

age at diagnosis was 59 years (range; 18–95). There was a slight male preponderance with 149 males and 104 females represented in the cohort. The most frequent primary tumour sites were extremity (45 %), followed by retroperitoneum (15 %), intra-abdominal and intra-thoracic (11 % each). The lung was the most common site of distant metastasis (66 %), followed by intra-abdomen (28 %) and bone (19 %).

Based on tumour histology, the study cohort (n = 253) was classified into four major STS subtypes: undifferentiated pleomorphic sarcoma (n = 57; 23 %), leiomyosarcoma (n = 44; 17 %), liposarcoma (n = 34; 14 %), synovial sarcoma (n = 21; 8 %); with the rest grouped as "other STS" (n = 97; 38 %); consisting of 15 histologic subtypes, each with small sample sizes. The uptake of palliative-intent systemic therapy differed across the STS histological subtypes with patients with synovial sarcomas most likely to be treated with systemic therapy compared to other subtypes (Table 2).

Palliative treatment modalities

Palliative treatment other than conventional cytotoxic chemotherapy was reviewed in those with available data (n = 225). A total of 86 patients (34 %) were treated with systemic therapies for advanced STS. More than a third of patients underwent radiotherapy or metastasectomy for palliation (37 %; radiotherapy, 35 %; surgery).

Approximately 75 % of all patients diagnosed with advanced STS received at least one line of palliative-intent treatment modality. Fifty-five patients (22 %) underwent two or more lines of different modalities of treatment during their course of disease. There were 11 patients (4 %) who received all three treatment modalities. Those who were treated with systemic therapies tended to be younger (mean age 51 vs. 63 years) and were more likely to receive radiotherapy for palliation than those who were not treated with systemic therapies (49 vs. 33 % respectively). There was a similar male to female ratio in each group.

Table 2 Demographics and clinical characteristics of patients with advanced STS

Characteristic	Total (n = 253)	Treated group[a] (n = 86)	Not treated group[b] (n = 167)	*P*
Age at diagnosis				
Mean (range)	59 (18–91)	51 (18–85)	63 (22–95)	N/A
Number of patients				
<65 years, n (%)	147 (58)	68 (27)	79 (31)	0.0001
≥65 years, n (%)	106 (42)	18 (7)	88 (35)	
Gender, n (%)				
Female	104 (41)	37 (15)	67 (26)	0.687
Male	149 (59)	49 (19)	100 (40)	
Stage IV at diagnosis n (%)	86 (34)	32 (13)	51 (20)	0.323
Histological type, n (%)				
UPS[c]	57 (23)	21 (8)	36 (14)	N/A
Leiomyosarcoma	44 (17)	22 (9)	22 (9)	
Liposarcoma	34 (14)	9 (4)	25 (10)	
Synovial sarcoma	21 (8)	15 (6)	6 (2)	
Other	97 (38)	19 (7)	78 (31)	
Sites of metastases, n (%)[d]				
Lung	167 (66)	78 (31)	89 (35)	N/A
Intra-abdominal	70 (28)	32 (13)	38 (15)	
Bone	48 (19)	28 (11)	20 (8)	
Lymph node	44 (17)	16 (6)	18 (7)	
Head and neck	6 (2)	3 (1)	3 (1)	
Other	27 (11)	10 (4)	17 (7)	

[a] Group treated with palliative-intent systemic therapy

[b] Group not treated with palliative-intent systemic therapy

[c] UPS; undifferentiated pleomorphic sarcoma

[d] This value dose not add up to 100 % due to some having multiple sites of distant disease at different time points

Systemic treatment patterns

Of the 86 patients who received palliative-intent systemic therapy, 50 % (n = 43) received more than one line of systemic therapy (Table 3). In the first-line setting, the most common regimen used was doxorubicin alone (n = 43, 55 %) followed by combination therapy with doxorubicin (or epirubicin in one patient) and ifosfamide (n = 14, 16 %). The majority of patients (n = 62, 72 %) received single-agent chemotherapy as the first-line therapy. Patients receiving combination chemotherapy were younger than those receiving monotherapy (mean age, 46 vs. 53 years respectively); with synovial sarcoma the most common subtype to receive doublet chemotherapy with doxorubicin and ifosfamide (n = 5, 38 %). Other doublet regimens used as the first-line therapy included the combination of docetaxel and gemcitabine (n = 2), and that of gemcitabine and dacarbazine (n = 2). Fourteen patients (16 %) were enrolled in clinical trials for the first-line therapy. In the second-line setting, ifosfamide was the most frequently prescribed agent (n = 20, 53 %) with the majority of patients receiving it as monotherapy (n = 35, 92 %) and with three additional patients participating in clinical trials. In the third-line setting, various regimens of monotherapy and combination therapies were prescribed with dacarbazine, most commonly delivered as a single-agent (n = 7, 30 %). Newer systemic agents such as multi-targeted receptor tyrosine kinase inhibitor, pazopanib and marine alkaloid, trabectedin, were sporadically used as subsequent lines of therapy (pazopanib; n = 12, trabectedin; n = 3). Beyond the first-line treatment, the most commonly used combination regimen was gemcitabine and docetaxel. Eight patients were treated with oral cyclophosphamide at any given time period (first-line; n = 3, second-line; n = 1, third-line; n = 3, fourth-line; n = 1). No patients were enrolled in clinical trials beyond the second-line setting. Prior exposure to neoadjuvant or adjuvant chemotherapy (n = 41, 16 %) and STS histological subtype did not affect the subsequent use of systemic therapy for advanced disease.

Table 3 Summary of palliative systemic therapy in treated patients

Systemic therapy line, n (%[a])	Treatment details
First-line (n = 86, 100 %)	Single-agent chemtoherapy (n = 62, 72 %)
	Doxorubicin (n = 43)
	Clinical trial (n = 7)
	Ifosfamide (n = 4)
	Paclitaxel (n = 3)
	Other (n = 5)
	Combination therapy (n = 24, 28 %)
	Doxorubicin[b] and ifosfamide (n = 13)
	Clinical trial (n = 7)
	Other combination (n = 4)
Second-line (n = 38, 44 %)	Single-agent chemtoherapy (n = 35, 92 %)
	Ifosfamide (n = 20)
	Dacarbazine (n = 5)
	Pazopanib (n = 3)
	Clinical trial (n = 3)
	Other (n = 4)
	Combination therapy (n = 3, 8 %)
Third-line (n = 20, 23 %)	Single-agent chemtoherapy (n = 18, 90 %)
	Pazopanib (n = 6)
	Dacarbazine (n = 6)
	Cyclophophamide (n = 3)
	Other (n = 3)
	Combination therapy (n = 2, 10 %)
Fourth-line (n = 6, 7 %)	Single-agent chemtoherapy (n = 6, 100 %)
	Pazopanib (n = 2)
	Doxorubicin (n = 1)
	Ifosfamide (n = 1)
	Cyclophophamide (n = 1)
	Trabectedin (n = 1)
Fifth-line (n = 1, 1 %)	Pazopanib (n = 1)

[a] The percentage refers to the proportion of patients who received the corresponding line treatment out of the total number treated with systemic therapy (n = 86)

[b] One patient had epirubicin and ifosfamide

Other treatment patterns

Details of palliative-intent radiotherapy delivery and metastasectomy were available in 89 % of patients in this study (n = 225). The majority of patients received palliative-intent radiotherapy for symptoms arising from distant metastases (n = 81, 36 %), of which the most common sites included bone, followed by lung/mediastinum and intra-abdominal metastases. A further 34 % of patients with advanced STS underwent resection of metastases, of which pulmonary metastasectomy was the most common procedure performed. Approximately 10 % of patients underwent more than one metastasectomies.

Survival analysis

There were 110 deaths captured in this series, accounting for 43 % of the patients with advanced STS in this study cohort. The median overall survival in this series was 18 months (Fig. 1). Younger age at diagnosis of advanced STS (<65 years) conferred a statistically significant higher probability of survival than older age (≥65 years; log rank test p value 0.032). There was no statistically significant difference in overall survival stratified by STS histological

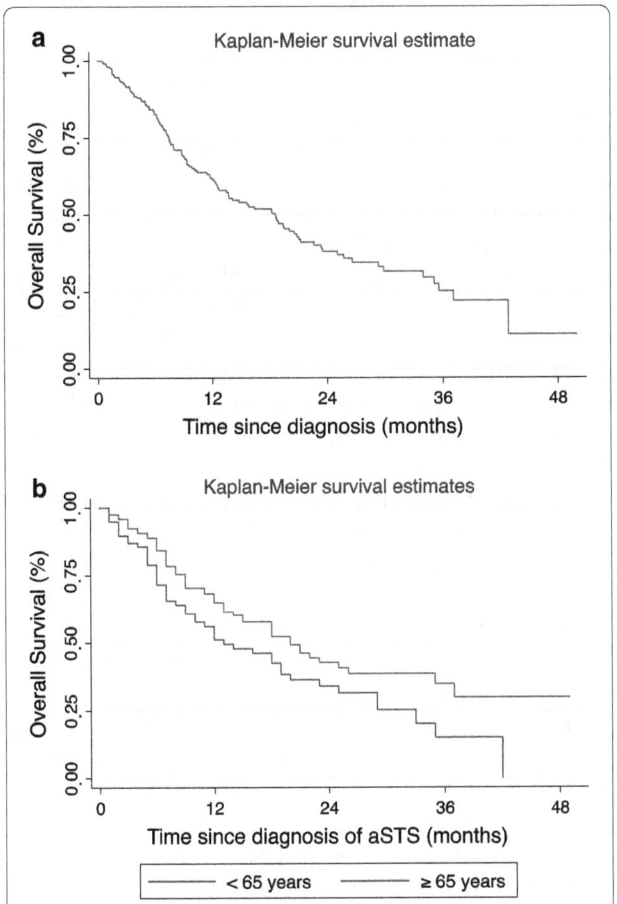

Fig. 1 **a** Kaplan–Meier curves for overall survival. Overall survival for the whole patient cohort. **b** Kaplan–Meier curves for overall survivsl. Overall survival stratified by age group, <65 years versus ≥65 years

subtypes. In the subgroup of patients who had one or more lines of systemic therapy, the median overall survival was 11 months from the time of diagnosis with advanced STS.

Discussion

To our knowledge, this is the first detailed study outlining patterns of care for patients with advanced STS in Australian sarcoma centres using a prospectively maintained sarcoma-specific database. The STS histological subtypes represented in this series were comparable to other studies on patients with STS [8, 9]. Although each subtype was small in number, the study findings provide valuable insights into how patients with advanced STS are routinely managed in real-world clinical practice. Consistent with the literature, the most common site of distant metastasis was lung, and this was also reflected by a high uptake of pulmonary metastasectomy.

Over three quarters of all patients diagnosed with advanced STS received at least one modality of palliative-intent treatment. Systemic treatment, surgery and radiotherapy were used with almost equal distribution during the course of disease. A higher proportion of patients treated with systemic therapy also received palliative-intent radiotherapy than those who did not receive systemic therapy (49 vs. 33 %). The process involved in treatment decision-making is often complex and there may be several reasons for not recommending treatment for some patients with advanced STS. This may reflect the natural history of STS, which may exhibit more indolent course of disease with a lack of or minimal symptoms requiring intervention. Soft tissue sarcomas are generally considered less responsive to systemic chemotherapy than bone sarcomas such as osteosarcoma or Ewing's sarcoma. As a result, depending on the overall disease burden, it may be appropriate to delay starting chemotherapy until it is required. Patients' performance status and comorbidities should also be weighed against potential treatment toxicities. Little is known about how these variables influence the treatment decision and the patients' overall outcome. It would be valuable to explore these further in subsequent studies.

Therapeutic options for many solid tumours have rapidly expanded and evolved over the last decades, however, patients with STS continue to experience difficulties with limited therapeutic options. Traditionally, doxorubicin-based regimens have been the standard of care [4–7, 10] and this was similarly observed in our practice with doxorubicin monotherapy or doxorubicin-containing combination chemotherapy as the most frequently prescribed first-line systemic therapy (n = 56, 65 %). In cases where other agents were administered, this was largely due to enrolment in clinical trials or the use of subtype-specific agents such as paclitaxel in angiosarcomas or gemcitabine and docetaxel in uterine leiomyosarcomas [11–13]. Interestingly, the uptake of doublet chemotherapy with gemcitabine and docetaxel was low at 7 % in Australia. This compares to approximately 30 % reported from the SABINE study and another single-institution North American study [8, 9]. This discrepancy may be related to differences in drug reimbursement available at the time of the study and a subsequent follow-up study will be of value to further characterise chemotherapy prescribing patterns impacted by changes in reimbursement over time. The uptake of doublet chemotherapy was also commonly seen, mostly in the younger patient groups with locally advanced STS. Given the evidence supporting the use of doxorubicin-based combination chemotherapy in improving the response rate at the expense of increased toxicities, this seems appropriate [2, 4–7].

It is well recognised that certain histological subtypes may have higher rates of chemo-sensitivity which may factor into the decision-making process for timing and type of treatment. Examples include ifosfamide with synovial sarcoma, taxanes with angiosarcoma and trabectedin with myxoid/round cell liposarcomas [11, 12, 14–16]. A closer review of treatment according to STS histological subtypes revealed a trend for an increased use of systemic therapy in patients with leiomyosarcoma and synovial sarcoma compared to the rest of histological subtypes including those with liposarcoma and undifferentiated pleomorphic sarcoma (Table 2). However, the small sample size of each histological subtype was insufficient to allow conclusive results.

Another salient finding from this study was the poor participation rate of patients with advanced STS in clinical trials. Approximately 20 % of patients treated with chemotherapy were enrolled in clinical trials during their course of disease with the majority participating in Phase III studies as the first-line therapy. This represents a strikingly small number of participants in contrast to 56–67 % of patients accessing clinical trials in European and North American settings [8, 9]. Australian medical oncologists are actively engaged in local and international cancer clinical trials. However, the heterogeneity and the rarity of soft tissue sarcoma, combined with the relative geographical isolation of Australia pose significant challenges in developing and opening clinical trials. Enhancing clinical trial access is critical, not only to improve cancer outcomes, but also to empower patients to play an active role in their management and to gain access to new treatments before they become widely available. Recent efforts by the Australian Sarcoma Study Group have facilitated multiple Australian and New Zealand sites to participate in investigator-initiated research as well as internationally-led cooperative group trials [17]. This is an important step forward in fostering relationship with future partners for sarcoma initiatives and research projects.

Access to new emerging agents continues to be a barrier to Australian patients. A total of 15 patients accessed novel agents, pazopanib (n = 12) and trabectedin (n = 3), for various STS subtypes, via compassionate access schemes. Although benefit in progression-free survival was not assessed in this series, these agents serve as additional active agents, which are important for patients with advanced STS. In general, timelines for access to new agents in Australia is lagging behind that of Europe and the United States. It is worth noting that it took seven more years for trabectedin to obtain a seal of approval by the Food and Drug Administration of the United States since its first approval in Europe in 2007. Trabectedin is yet to be approved by the Australian regulatory authority. On the other hand, pazopanib, has been added to the Pharmaceutical Benefits Scheme listing in March 2014 in Australia for the indication of non-adipocytic STS and will assist patients' access to this targeted option at a Government-subsidised price [18].

The median overall survival of patients in our cohort was 18 months, which is longer than previous studies reporting approximately 12 months in this setting [19, 20]. However, long-term survival has been described in a subset of patients with limited disease burden and certain STS histologic subtypes are well recognised for their slow and indolent natural history. It is worth noting that the SABINE study evaluating a highly selected group of patients with a favourable response to chemotherapy reported the median overall survival as 23 months [8]. Interestingly, the group of patients who received palliative-intent systemic therapy in our study had the overall survival of only 11 months, which is more consistent with the historical control [19, 20]. This may represent the clinician's decision in selecting patients with symptomatic and larger disease burden to receive systemic therapy. Not surprisingly in the setting of advanced or metastatic disease, the cause of death in most patients was disease-related.

There are several strengths to our data including the prospective nature of comprehensive data collection from the time of diagnosis through to recurrence and death. Details on clinic-pathological data as well as treatments were complete for analysis in most patients. Given the intrinsic heterogeneity of STS and its rarity, a considerable level of complexity exists in capturing an accurate dataset. However, a high quality, well-maintained database can be utilised as an important resource for research, including many questions not adequately addressed by clinical trials. Some limitations are worth noting. Data on multiple STS histological subtypes were combined together for this analysis, as they are commonly done in other studies. This renders interpretation of results difficult in treatment uptake and survival, as certain histological subtypes are inherently different from one another.

Conclusions

In this retrospective study, we reviewed the patterns of care in managing patients with locally advanced and/or metastatic STS at sarcoma specialist services, providing a valuable insight into the current practice in the Australian health care setting. The presented data highlight varying practice in delivering palliative-intent treatment modalities at different time points and the ongoing need for addressing lack of clinical trials for sarcoma patients in Australia. The study will serve as an important reference point for understanding how practice may change over time as treatment options continue to evolve.

Abbreviations

PFS: progression-free survival; OS: overall survival; STS: soft tissue sarcoma.

Authors' contributions

SB and JD designed the study and performed data analysis. All authors participated in manuscript writing and editing. All authors read and approved the final manuscript.

Author details

[1] Department of Medical Oncology, Peter MacCallum Cancer Centre, St Andrews Place, East Melbourne, VIC 3002, Australia. [2] Department of Surgery, Prince of Wales Hospital, Barker St, Randwick, NSW 2031, Australia. [3] Department of Radiation Oncology, Royal Adelaide Hospital, North Terrace, Adelaide, SA 5000, Australia. [4] Department of Medical Oncology, Princess Alexandra Hospital, 199 Ipswich Rd, Woolloongabba, QLD 4102, Australia. [5] Department of Orthopaedic Surgery, Sir Charles Gardner Hospital, Hospital Ave, Nedlands, WA 6009, Australia. [6] Department of Orthopaedic Surgery, Royal Prince Alfred Hospital, Missenden Rd, Camperdown, NSW 2050, Australia.

Acknowledgements

The authors wish to acknowledge the Australian Sarcoma Study Group for supporting database collection at sarcoma services in Australia and BioGrid Australia for providing data linkage platform. The following data managers are acknowledged for their work in data retrieval; Jasmine Mar, Diane Schipp, Sonya Stephens, Kim Matten, Jenny Woodhouse and Rebecca Da Silva.

Competing interests

The authors declare that they have no other competing interests.

Ethics approval and consent to participate

This study utilised de-identified data of patients in the sarcoma databases at Peter MacCallum Cancer Centre, Prince of Wales Hospital, Royal Adelaide Hospital, Princess Alexandra Hospital, Sir Charles Gardiner Hospital, and Royal Prince Alfred Hospital. Sarcoma data collection is approved by ethics committee at each institution with a waiver of consent on the basis of low risk and negligible risk research purpose for ethically approved studies. This research activity is supported by the Australian Sarcoma Study Group and is reviewed regularly by each governing state for renewal of ethics approval. The present study was approved on 14 February 2014 by the Melbourne Health Human Research Ethics Committee (Project Number: 201301/5).

Funding

This work was supported through an unrestricted research grant from GlaxoSmithKline, who participated from the concept of the study through final approval for submission

References

1. Jemal A, Siegel R, Xu J, Ward E. Cancer statistics, 2010. CA Cancer J Clin. 2010;60(5):277–300.
2. National Comprehensive Cancer Network. Soft Tissue Sarcoma. NCCN Clinical Practice Guidelines in Oncology. 2015, https://www.nccn.org/professionals.physician-gls/pdf/sarcoma.pdf.
3. Group EE. Soft tissue and visceral sarcomas: ESMO clinical practice guidelines for diagnosis, treatment and follow-up. Ann Oncol ESMO. 2012;23(Suppl 7):vii92–9.
4. Borden EC, Amato DA, Rosenbaum C, Enterline HT, Shiraki MJ, Creech RH, et al. Randomized comparison of three adriamycin regimens for metastatic soft tissue sarcomas. J Clin Oncol. 1987;5(6):840–50.
5. Edmonson JH, Ryan LM, Blum RH, Brooks JS, Shiraki M, Frytak S, et al. Randomized comparison of doxorubicin alone versus ifosfamide plus doxorubicin or mitomycin, doxorubicin, and cisplatin against advanced soft tissue sarcomas. J Clin Oncol. 1993;11(7):1269–75.
6. Antman K, Crowley J, Balcerzak SP, Rivkin SE, Weiss GR, Elias A, et al. An intergroup phase III randomized study of doxorubicin and dacarbazine with or without ifosfamide and mesna in advanced soft tissue and bone sarcomas. J Clin Oncol. 1993;11(7):1276–85.
7. Judson I, Verweij J, Gelderblom H, Hartmann JT, Schoffski P, Blay JY, et al. Doxorubicin alone versus intensified doxorubicin plus ifosfamide for first-line treatment of advanced or metastatic soft-tissue sarcoma: a randomised controlled phase 3 trial. Lancet Oncol. 2014;15(4):415–23.
8. Leahy M, Garcia Del Muro X, Reichardt P, Judson I, Staddon A, Verweij J, et al. Chemotherapy treatment patterns and clinical outcomes in patients with metastatic soft tissue sarcoma. The SArcoma treatment and Burden of Illness in North America and Europe (SABINE) study. Annal Oncol. 2012;23(10):2763–70.
9. Wagner MJ, Amodu LI, Duh MS, Korves C, Solleza F, Manson SC, et al. A retrospective chart review of drug treatment patterns and clinical outcomes among patients with metastatic or recurrent soft tissue sarcoma refractory to one or more prior chemotherapy treatments. BMC Cancer. 2015;15:175.
10. Patel SR, Vadhan-Raj S, Burgess MA, Plager C, Papadopolous N, Jenkins J, et al. Results of two consecutive trials of dose-intensive chemotherapy with doxorubicin and ifosfamide in patients with sarcomas. Am J Clin Oncol. 1998;21(3):317–21.
11. Fata F, O'Reilly E, Ilson D, Pfister D, Leffel D, Kelsen DP, et al. Paclitaxel in the treatment of patients with angiosarcoma of the scalp or face. Cancer. 1999;86(10):2034–7.
12. Penel N, Bui BN, Bay JO, Cupissol D, Ray-Coquard I, Piperno-Neumann S, et al. Phase II trial of weekly paclitaxel for unresectable angiosarcoma: the ANGIOTAX Study. J Clin Oncol. 2008;26(32):5269–74.
13. Hensley ML, Maki R, Venkatraman E, Geller G, Lovegren M, Aghajanian C, et al. Gemcitabine and docetaxel in patients with unresectable leiomyosarcoma: results of a phase II trial. J Clin Oncol. 2002;20(12):2824–31.
14. Grosso F, Jones RL, Demetri GD, Judson IR, Blay JY, Le Cesne A, et al. Efficacy of trabectedin (ecteinascidin-743) in advanced pretreated myxoid liposarcomas: a retrospective study. Lancet Oncol. 2007;8(7):595–602.
15. Rosen G, Forscher C, Lowenbraun S, Eilber F, Eckardt J, Holmes C, et al. Synovial sarcoma. Uniform response of metastases to high dose ifosfamide. Cancer. 1994;73(10):2506–11.
16. Spurrell EL, Fisher C, Thomas JM, Judson IR. Prognostic factors in advanced synovial sarcoma: an analysis of 104 patients treated at the Royal Marsden Hospital. Annal Oncol. 2005;16(3):437–44.
17. Bae S, Caruso D, Desai J. An Australasian perspective on sarcoma research, translational biology and clinical trials: the Australasian Sarcoma Study Group (ASSG). Pathology. 2014;46(2):160–3.
18. Australian Government Department of Health. Pharmaceutical Benefits Scheme. Pazopanib, accessed September 2015, [http://www.pbs.gov.au/medicine/item/10052C-2201W].
19. Karavasilis V, Seddon BM, Ashley S, Al-Muderis O, Fisher C, Judson I. Significant clinical benefit of first-line palliative chemotherapy in advanced soft-tissue sarcoma: retrospective analysis and identification of prognostic factors in 488 patients. Cancer. 2008;112(7):1585–91.
20. Van Glabbeke M, van Oosterom AT, Oosterhuis JW, Mouridsen H, Crowther D, Somers R, et al. Prognostic factors for the outcome of chemotherapy in advanced soft tissue sarcoma: an analysis of 2,185 patients treated with anthracycline-containing first-line regimens–a European Organization for Research and Treatment of Cancer Soft Tissue and Bone Sarcoma Group Study. J Clin Oncol. 1999;17(1):150–7.

9

UK clinical practice guidelines for the management of gastrointestinal stromal tumours (GIST)

Ian Judson[1*], Ramesh Bulusu[2], Beatrice Seddon[3], Adam Dangoor[4], Newton Wong[5] and Satvinder Mudan[6]

Abstract

Background: Soft tissue sarcomas (STS) are rare tumours arising in mesenchymal tissues. Gastrointestinal stromal tumour (GIST) is the commonest STS and arises within the wall of the gastrointestinal (GI) tract. While most GISTs occur in the stomach they do occur in all parts of the GI tract. As with other STS, it is important that GISTs are managed by expert teams, to ensure consistent and optimal treatment, as well as recruitment to clinical trials, and the ongoing accumulation of further knowledge of the disease. The development of appropriate guidance, by an experienced panel referring to the evidence available, is therefore a useful foundation on which to build progress in the field.

Methodology: British Sarcoma Group guidelines for the management of GIST were initially developed by a panel of physicians experienced in the management of GIST. This current version has been updated and amended with reference to other European and US guidance. We have received input from representatives of all diagnostic and treatment disciplines as well as patient representatives. Levels of evidence and strength of recommendation gradings are those used by ESMO adapted from those published by the Infectious Disease Society of America.

Conclusions: The guidelines cover aetiology, genetics and underlying molecular mechanisms, diagnosis and initial investigations, staging and risk stratification, surgery, neoadjuvant and adjuvant therapy, the management of advanced disease and follow-up. The importance of mutational analysis in guiding treatment is highlighted, since this can indicate the most effective treatment and avoid administration of ineffective drugs, emphasising the need for management in specialist centres.

Background

British Sarcoma Group guidelines for the management of GIST were initially developed in 2004 by a panel of physicians experienced in the management of GIST representing all diagnostic and treatment disciplines. These Clinical Practice Guidelines update reflect the improvements in our knowledge of the disease and developments that have taken place since then [1]. Levels of evidence and strength of recommendation gradings are those used by ESMO adapted from those published by the Infectious Disease Society of America (Table 1) [2].

*Correspondence: Ian.Judson@icr.ac.uk
[1] The Institute of Cancer Research, Royal Marsden NHS Foundation Trust, Fulham Road, London SW3 6JJ, UK
Full list of author information is available at the end of the article

Incidence

Gastrointestinal stromal tumours (GISTs) are rare cancers, with an estimated unadjusted incidence of 1.5/100,000/year [3]. Data from the Rhône-Alpes region of France [4] and "NHS England Cancer Registry" (personal communication) suggest an incidence of just under 11 per million per annum, equating to 650 clinically meaningful new cases a year in the UK, approximately 900 in total. Accurate data on prevalence in the UK are not yet available.

The median age at diagnosis is around 60–65 years, with a wide range. Occurrence in children, adolescents and younger patients is very rare, although paediatric GISTs represent a distinct subset, marked by female predominance, absence of *KIT*/platelet-derived growth factor alpha (*PDGFRA*) mutations, usually gastric origin,

Table 1 Levels of evidence and Grades of recommendation

Levels of evidence
I Evidence from at least one large randomised, controlled trial of good methodological quality (low potential for a bias) or meta-analyses of well-conducted randomised trials without heterogeneity
II Small randomised trials or large randomised trials with a suspicion of bias (lower methodological quality) or meta-analyses of such trials or of trials with demonstrated heterogeneity
III Prospective cohort studies
IV Retrospective cohort studies or case–control studies
V Studies without control group, case reports, and experts' opinions
Grades of recommendation
A Strong evidence for efficacy with a substantial clinical benefit, strongly recommended
B Strong or moderate evidence for efficacy but with a limited clinical benefit, generally recommended
C Insufficient evidence for efficacy or benefit does not outweigh the risk or the disadvantages (adverse events, costs,...), optional
D Moderate evidence against efficacy or for adverse outcome, generally not recommended
E Strong evidence against efficacy or for adverse outcome, never recommended

often multifocal, and with possible lymph node metastases [5].

Aetiology

In most cases the aetiology is unknown, although it is reported that patients with GIST are more likely to be diagnosed with another cancer than the general population [6, 7], suggesting a likely link with inherited increased susceptibility to cancer in some patients. In the majority of cases GIST is associated with an activating mutation in either the *KIT* or *PDGFRA* (platelet derived growth factor receptor alpha) gene. However, other rare drivers may include mutations in *NF1* (neurofibromatosis type 1, loss of function) or *BRAF* (gain of function). Tumours lacking mutations in *KIT* or *PDGFRA* are often called "wild-type", and those lacking mutations in not only these genes but also *BRAF* and *NF1* have been dubbed "quadruple wild-type" [8]. Specific advice concerning the management of patients with paediatric, "wild-type" and syndromic GIST can be obtained from a UK based alliance of medical specialists via the web site http://www.pawsgistclinic.org.uk.

A number of genetic syndromes are linked to GIST:

- The Carney triad syndrome, comprising gastric GIST, paraganglioma and pulmonary chondroma (these may occur at different ages) [9].
- Carney–Stratakis syndrome, marked by germ-line mutations of one of the SDH subunits A, B, C or D, leading to a dyad of GIST and paraganglioma [10, 11].
- Type-1 neurofibromatosis, i.e. associated with loss of function of *NF1*, whether sporadic or inherited, and absence of mutations in *KIT or PDGFRA*, the GISTs are often multifocal, predominantly located in the small bowel [12].
- Familial GIST, i.e. families with a germ-line autosomal dominant mutation of *KIT*, are extremely rare, presenting with multiple GISTs at an early age.

Diagnosis

Clinical presentation and investigation

The most common symptoms of GIST include upper gastrointestinal bleeding and anaemia, whilst larger tumours may present with abdominal pain/discomfort and a palpable mass. Small bowel GISTs may remain silent for a long period before presenting with an acute event such as haemorrhage or rupture. Symptomatic colorectal GISTs may present with abdominal pain, obstruction and lower gastrointestinal bleeding; oesophageal and gastro-oesophageal junction GISTs with dysphagia. Some patients may have non-specific systemic symptoms such as weight loss, night sweats and fever. Lack of awareness of the presenting features may lead to delayed diagnosis of GIST in some patients. Small GISTs may be asymptomatic and are often diagnosed incidentally during investigation for other conditions.

Small lesions below 2 cm in diameter may safely be followed by endoscopic ultrasound on an annual basis and biopsied or excised if they continue to grow. For larger lesions it is necessary to make a histological diagnosis. The standard approach for small nodules of 2 cm or above is excisional biopsy, as GISTs of this size carry a higher risk. For gastric lesions it is preferable to perform a fine needle aspirate or core needle biopsy under endoscopic ultrasound (EUS) guidance. If this is not feasible, and limited surgery is possible, primary resection may be appropriate. However, the differential diagnosis of intra-abdominal tumours may include leiomyosarcoma, germ cell tumour, lymphoma, benign and malignant neurogenic tumours, and fibromatosis. Given that the management of these conditions differs substantially, and primary excision is not always appropriate, it is sometimes necessary to do a percutaneous core needle biopsy to confirm the diagnosis. This however carries a very small risk of contaminating the peritoneal cavity, especially if bleeding were to occur. If surgery would require multi visceral resection, or is likely to be morbid, e.g. total gastrectomy, then multiple core needle biopsies are definitely required, again ideally under EUS guidance, or alternatively using an ultrasound/computed tomography (CT)-guided percutaneous approach. Depending on the histological diagnosis initial treatment may be with systemic therapy, e.g., lymphomas, mesenteric fibromatosis, germ cell tumours and GIST, or alternatively surveillance for benign entities such as non-malignant neurogenic tumours. Lesions at risk of rupture, such as cystic masses, should only be biopsied in specialised centres. If a patient presents with obvious metastatic disease, then a biopsy of an easily accessible metastatic focus should be performed and a laparotomy for diagnostic purposes is usually unnecessary.

Pathologically, the diagnosis of GIST relies on morphological assessment and immunohistochemistry, the diagnosis being supported by CD117 immunopositivity [13, 14]. More recently DOG1 has been added to the diagnostic armamentarium [15, 16]. About 5% of GISTs are CD117 immunonegative, about 5% of GISTs are DOG1 immunonegative and about 1% of GISTs are immunonegative for both. The mitotic count has prognostic value and although several risk assessment tools use an index of mitoses per 50 high-power fields, it would be more accurate and reproducible to express this as the number of mitoses in a total area of 5 mm^2, which is therefore recommended. If there is some diagnostic doubt, particularly in CD117 and/or DOG1 immunonegative suspected GIST, molecular analysis for activating mutations in *KIT* or *PDGFRA* may help confirm the diagnosis. Mutational analysis has predictive value for sensitivity to molecular-targeted therapy, and also prognostic value. If initial treatment is with imatinib, mutational analysis is particularly critical, since some GISTs are insensitive to the drug (e.g. *PDGFRA* exon 18 mutation D842V). The inclusion of mutational analysis in the diagnostic work-up of all GISTs should be considered standard practice, with the possible exclusion of sub 2 cm non-rectal GISTs, which are very unlikely ever to need medical treatment. It is strongly recommended that mutational analysis is performed in centralised laboratories which are enrolled in an external quality assurance program, and which have expertise in GIST analysis. In *KIT/PDGFRA* mutation negative, or "Wild-Type" GIST, immunohistochemistry for succinate dehydrogenase B (SDHB), and, if negative, SDHA, should be performed if available, since loss of expression may assist the diagnosis and may help to guide therapy. In the absence of mutations in *KIT* or *PDGFRA* it is also important to look for mutations in *BRAF*, a rare, but important finding from a treatment perspective, since BRAF inhibitors are available, and also in *NF1*. Patients with neurofibromatosis, who have a germline mutation in *NF1*, are at increased risk of GIST and this finding may indicate occult neurofibromatosis. The optimal treatment for advanced GIST with *NF1* mutation has yet to be determined. Collection of fresh/frozen tissue is encouraged, because new molecular pathology assessments can then be made at a later stage in the patient's interest. Informed consent for tumour banking should be sought, so that the tissue is available for later analyses and research, provided that local ethical approval is in place. Consent forms for the National GIST Tissue Bank based at the Royal Marsden Hospital can be found at http://www.givemysample.org/gist.

Key recommendations:

1. Lesions larger than 2 cm in diameter need to be investigated and a diagnosis made. Often this can be done by endoscopic ultrasound and needle biopsy, particularly if the lesion is in the stomach.
2. The diagnosis should be made by a pathologist experienced in the disease and include the use of immunohistochemistry and mutational analysis, which should be performed by an accredited laboratory.
3. If neoadjuvant treatment with imatinib is planned, it is vital to confirm the diagnosis, since there is a wide differential. It may be necessary to perform a percutaneous core needle biopsy if the tumour is inaccessible to endoscopic ultrasound-guided biopsy. Mutational analysis is obligatory, since some GISTs are insensitive to imatinib (e.g. those with D842V mutation in exon 18 of *PDGFRA*).

Risk assessment for primary tumours with no evidence of metastatic disease

The TNM classification for staging has several limitations and its use is not recommended in this disease. Prognostic factors of proven value are the mitotic rate, tumour size, tumour site, and presence or absence of tumour rupture. Gastric GISTs have a better prognosis than small bowel or rectal GISTs. Tumour rupture through a serosal surface is an adverse prognostic factor and should be recorded, whether it took place before or during surgery. Mutational status has not been incorporated in any risk classification so far, although some genotypes have a distinct natural history, for example *KIT/PDGFRA* wild type GISTs tend to exhibit more indolent behaviour than *KIT* exon 11 mutant disease.

It is possible to assess risk of recurrence after resection of a localised GIST. This can be especially useful in deciding the role of adjuvant therapy in individual patients. Several risk classifications have been proposed. An initial risk classification developed at a consensus meeting convened by the National Institute of Health (NIH) [13] was useful but only considered size and mitotic index. Although the 'high-risk' category based on the NIH criteria has a much worse prognosis than the others, with both 'very low-risk' and 'low-risk' categories having a very favourable prognosis, the 'intermediate-risk' category did not reliably identify patients with an unfavourable prognosis. A risk classification was proposed by the Armed Forces Institute of Pathology, which incorporates

Table 2 Modified NIH risk classification for primary GIST

Risk category	Tumour size (cm)	Mitotic index (per 50 HPFs)	Primary tumour site
Very low risk	<2.0	≤5	Any
Low risk	2.1–5.0	≤5	Any
Intermediate risk	2.1–5.0	>5	Gastric
	<5.0	6–10	Any
	5.1–10.0	≤5	Gastric
High risk	Any	Any	Tumour rupture
	>10	Any	Any
	>5.0	>5	Any
	2.1-5.0	>5	Non gastric
	5.1–10.0	≤5	Non gastric

After Joensuu [18]

the primary tumour site, in addition to mitotic count and tumour size, i.e. three of the main prognostic factors in localized GISTs [17]. There are also problems with the application of this risk classification tool since mitotic index and tumour size are non-linear continuous variables, so that the risk thresholds, especially based on number of mitoses, need to be interpreted with care. A modification to the NIH criteria has been proposed that incorporates tumour site and additionally tumour rupture, an important risk factor, [18] see Table 2. Prognostic contour maps have been generated through a number of series of GIST patients not treated with adjuvant therapy. These maps incorporate the mitotic index and tumour size as continuous non-linear variables, while tumour rupture is considered in addition to tumour site. They have been validated against pooled data from 10 series and 2560 patients from the literature [19]. Several nomograms and web or mobile phone applications are available to enable rapid risk category calculations to be made, which may assist multidisciplinary planning of patient management.

Staging procedures

Staging procedures take into account the fact that most relapses affect the peritoneum and the liver. Contrast-enhanced abdominal and pelvic CT scan is the investigation of choice for staging and follow-up. Magnetic resonance imaging (MRI) or contrast-enhanced ultrasound may be alternatives, especially in younger patients where exposure to radiation should be limited. MRI provides better preoperative staging information for rectal GISTs. Chest CT scan or X-ray and routine laboratory testing complement the staging work-up of the asymptomatic patient, but are not routinely required during follow-up. Evaluation of ^{18}F-fluorodeoxyglucose (FDG) uptake using an FDG-positron emission tomography (PET) scan, or FDG-PET–CT/MRI, can sometimes be useful, mainly when early assessment of response to tyrosine kinase inhibitor therapy is of special interest, for example after initiation of neo-adjuvant imatinib therapy.

Treatment

When small oesophago-gastric or duodenal nodules less than 2 cm in size are detected, endoscopic biopsy may be difficult and laparoscopic/laparotomic excision may be the only way to make a histological diagnosis. Many of these small nodules, if diagnosed as GIST, will be low risk, or entities whose clinical significance remains unclear. Therefore, the standard approach to these patients is endoscopic ultrasound assessment, usually with fine needle aspiration or core needle biopsy, then annual follow-up, reserving excision for patients whose tumour increases in size or becomes symptomatic. Alternatively, the decision about a treatment plan can be discussed with the patient. This may depend on age, life expectancy and comorbidities. If follow-up is the choice, definitive evidence regarding an optimal surveillance policy is lacking, but annual follow-up is reasonable. For a small histologically proven GIST of 2 cm or greater, the standard treatment is excision, unless major morbidity is expected. Alternatively, in the case of a low-risk GIST, the possibility of surveillance could be discussed with the patient. Rectal (or recto-vaginal space) nodules should be biopsied and preferably excised after ultrasound assessment, regardless of tumour size. This is because GISTs at these sites have a higher risk of local recurrence after surgery, and the local implications for surgery in relation to morbidity are more critical. In specific clinical contexts, if the tumour is small, a follow-up policy without surgery could be adopted, but such an approach should be discussed in detail with the patient.

Multidisciplinary treatment planning is needed. This should involve histopathologists, radiologists, surgeons, and oncologists, as well as gastroenterologists, nuclear medicine specialists and others, as applicable. Such teams are available in reference centres for sarcomas and GISTs, which treat a large number of GIST patients annually. Support staff, such as clinical nurse specialists, play a vital role and are not likely to be available, or have the appropriate expertise, outside specialist centres.

Localised disease—surgery

Standard treatment of localized GISTs is complete surgical excision of the lesion, with no dissection of clinically negative lymph nodes [III, A]. Surgery should be performed by a sub speciality surgeon who is fully trained and experienced in radical anatomic site specific cancer surgery. When adjacent organs are involved, *en bloc* resection is recommended wherever possible. If laparoscopic excision is planned, the technique needs to follow the principles of oncological surgery [20] [III, A]. A laparoscopic approach is clearly discouraged in patients with large tumours, because of the risk of tumour rupture, which is associated with a very high risk of relapse. R0 excision is the goal (i.e., an excision whose margins are clear of tumour cells). When R0 surgery is likely to result in major functional sequelae, e.g. total gastrectomy or abdomino-perineal resection of rectum, neoadjuvant imatinib should be regarded as standard therapy [21–24] [IV, A]. Treatment is given to reduce the size of the tumour and to limit subsequent surgical morbidity. This may also be the case if surgery will be safer following cyto-reduction (e.g. the risk of bleeding and tumour rupture is likely to be decreased). After maximal tumour response, generally after 6–12 months, surgery is performed. Prior mutational analysis is crucial to prevent patients with less sensitive or resistant tumours (e.g. *PDGFRA* D842 V mutations) from receiving therapy with imatinib, and to allow appropriate dosing for patients with *KIT* exon 9 mutated tumours. Early tumour response assessment is mandatory, so that surgery is not delayed in the case of non-responding disease. Functional imaging, such as PET-CT, makes it possible to assess the tumour response very rapidly, within a few weeks. There are limited data to guide the physician on when to stop imatinib before surgery, but it can safely be stopped a few days, or even 1 day, before surgery and it can be resumed promptly when the patient has recovered from the acute effects of surgery.

If preoperative medical treatment has not helped or cannot be used, there should be a discussion with the patient about accepting a possible R1 resection with microscopically positive margins (i.e. excision margins containing tumour cells) [IV, B]. This may be more acceptable for low-risk lesions, with the lack of any formal demonstration that R1 surgery is associated with worse overall survival [25]. If an unplanned R1 excision has already been carried out, re-excision may be an option, provided the original site of lesion can be found, and major functional sequelae are not foreseen.

Localised disease—adjuvant therapy

The risk of relapse following surgery can be substantial, as defined by available risk classifications. Adjuvant treatment with imatinib for 3 years was associated with improved relapse-free and overall survival compared with 1 year of therapy in a randomized trial in high-risk patients [26]. Previously, a placebo-controlled trial demonstrated that imatinib given for 1 year prolongs relapse-free survival in localized GISTs larger than 3 cm with a macroscopically complete resection [27]. Therefore, adjuvant therapy with imatinib for 3 years is standard treatment for patients with a significant risk of relapse [I, A] and was approved by the National Institute for Care and Health Excellence (NICE) in their recent re-appraisal (https://www.nice.org.uk/guidance/ta326). Mutational analysis is critical to making a clinical decision regarding adjuvant therapy. In fact, there is a consensus that *PDGFRA* D842 V-mutated GISTs should not be treated with any adjuvant therapy, given the lack of sensitivity of this genotype to imatinib both in vitro and in vivo [IV, A]. Given the data supporting the use of a higher dose of imatinib (800 mg daily) in the presence of an exon 9 *KIT* mutation in advanced GIST, clinicians might consider using this dose in the adjuvant setting for this genotype [28–31]. However, this is not supported by any controlled trial data in the adjuvant setting and use of the higher dose is not approved by NICE in the UK. There is consensus on avoiding adjuvant treatment in NF-1 related GISTs, which are insensitive to imatinib in the advanced setting. On the other hand, a consensus is lacking among experts about whether *KIT/PDGFRA* wild-type SDH-negative GIST should be treated with adjuvant therapy. This reflects their lower sensitivity to imatinib, as well as their peculiar natural history, which is often more indolent; subgroup analyses of available randomized trials are too limited to provide sufficient evidence.

If there has been tumour rupture before or during surgery, there will have been spillage of tumour cells into the peritoneal cavity, and therefore occult peritoneal disease can be assumed to exist. This puts the patient at a very high risk of peritoneal relapse. Therefore, these patients should be considered for adjuvant imatinib therapy. The optimal duration of treatment in these cases is unknown, given the uncertainty as to whether they should be viewed as essentially having metastatic disease, but should be at least 3 years, as for high risk resected GIST.

Key recommendations

1. GIST should be managed by an experienced multidisciplinary team.
2. Pre-operative imatinib should be considered for those large gastric or rectal primaries where immediate resection is likely to be morbid, e.g. total gastrectomy or abdomino-perineal resection. In this situation mutational analysis is mandatory prior to the initiation of imatinib therapy.
3. Patients at high risk of recurrence or distant relapse should receive 3 years of adjuvant imatinib, provided their tumour is not likely to be resistant to therapy (*PDGFRA* exon 18 mutation D842V).

Metastatic disease—systemic treatment

In patients with inoperable and metastatic disease, imatinib is the standard treatment [32, 33] [III, A], including patients who had previously received the drug as adjuvant therapy without relapse during this treatment. This also applies to metastatic patients whose disease has been completely removed surgically, although surgery as a primary approach to metastatic GIST is not recommended. The standard dose of imatinib is 400 mg daily [I, A]. However, data have shown that patients with *KIT* exon 9 mutations fare better in terms of progression-free survival (PFS) on a higher dose of 800 mg daily, which is therefore the standard treatment in this subgroup [31] [III, A], albeit not recommended by a NICE appraisal which only assessed dose escalation in the context of disease progression. A report on the long term follow-up of the European/Australasian clinical trial which compared 400 mg with 800 mg imatinib in patients with advanced GIST has shown a survival advantage for the initial use of the 800 mg dose in those with exon 9 mutations in *KIT* (Casali P et al., in press) indicating a need to review this issue in the UK. Treatment should be continued indefinitely, since treatment interruption is generally followed by relatively rapid tumour progression, even when lesions have previously been surgically excised [34] [II, B]. At the start of treatment the patient should be alerted to the importance of adherence to therapy, and of possible interactions with concomitant medications and foods. They should also be given guidance about the best ways to handle any possible side effects. Dose intensity should be maintained by effective management of side effects, and a rational policy of dose reductions and interruptions should be applied if there is excessive, persistent toxicity. Retrospective data suggest that suboptimal plasma levels of imatinib are associated with a worse outcome, though a correlation with outcome has not been established prospectively [35]. A recent report confirmed that patients with imatinib trough levels of less than 760 ng/ml, taken after a minimum of 3 months' treatment, which equates to steady state [36], had a worse outlook in terms of progression-free survival, which applied in the case of both gastric and small bowel GIST [37]. Aside from its potential use to tailor the imatinib dose, plasma level assessment may be useful in the case of: (i) patients receiving concomitant medications that put them at a risk of major interactions; (ii) unexpected observed toxicities; (iii) progression on 400 mg. Dose adaptation according to inadequate imatinib trough level is being studied in the Netherlands, and is a standard approach in a number of institutions. However, the use of a higher dose of imatinib in patients with progressive disease is not approved by NICE.

Close monitoring of the tumour response should be carried out in the early phases of treatment. Follow-up should be continued throughout the treatment, since the risk of secondary progression persists over time. Complete excision of residual metastatic disease has been shown to be related to a good prognosis, provided the patient is responding to imatinib, but whether this is due to surgery or to patient selection [38–40] has never been demonstrated prospectively. Conducting a randomised trial did not prove feasible; thus, at the present time surgery can be discussed with the patient but not recommended on the basis of a definitive proof of benefit [III, C]. Surgical excision of progressive disease is not recommended, given the poor results in published series, but surgery of limited progression, such as the 'nodule within a mass', has been associated with a progression-free interval in the same range as for second-line treatment with sunitinib. So, this may be a palliative option in the individual patient with limited progression, while continuing imatinib [V, C]. Non-surgical procedures, such as radiofrequency ablation of liver metastases may also be used. Prior to performing such interventions PET-CT can be useful to confirm the location of imatinib-resistant disease.

Dose escalation of imatinib to 800 mg in the case of a GIST with a *KIT* exon 9 mutation showing disease progression could be considered if the higher dose was not used initially, since the higher dose is significantly more effective in this setting [31]. Higher doses, though not necessarily 800 mg, could be useful if satisfactory plasma levels of imatinib are not being achieved, but the use of higher doses is not approved by NICE. The potential misinterpretation of the images produced by the complex tumour response patterns to TKIs can lead to a false diagnosis of progression, which must be considered. Patient non-compliance and drug interactions with concomitant medications must also be ruled out as the possible cause of progression.

If there is confirmed progression, or rare intolerance to imatinib after all attempts to manage side effects have failed, the standard second-line treatment is the tyrosine kinase inhibitor (TKI) sunitinib [41] [I, B]. This drug was proven to be effective in terms of PFS using a regimen of 50 mg daily 4 weeks on/2 weeks off. Data have been published showing that continuous treatment with a lower daily dose of 37.5 mg is also effective and well tolerated, although no formal comparison has been performed within a randomized clinical trial. This schedule can therefore be considered an alternative on an individualized basis [42] [III, B]. However, not all patients resistant to imatinib respond to sunitinib particularly those with secondary mutations affecting the activation loop domain of KIT and the *PDGFRA* exon 18 D842V mutation, which is always resistant.

A prospective placebo-controlled randomized trial demonstrated that regorafenib, at a dose of 160 mg daily on a 3 weeks on/1 week off schedule, significantly prolonged PFS in patients progressing after both imatinib and sunitinib [43]. Regorafenib is regarded as standard therapy for the third-line treatment of patients progressing on or failing to respond to imatinib and sunitinib [I, B]. It is currently available in England via the National Cancer Drugs Fund and is also available in Scotland, Wales and Northern Ireland as standard 3rd line therapy. The key distinction between sunitinib and regorafenib, as also previously shown with the analogue sorafenib, is its ability to inhibit tumours with secondary mutations in the activation loop of KIT, especially in exon 17 [44, 45]. These mutations are known to confer resistance both to imatinib and sunitinib, hence the value of regorafenib in this setting.

Patients with metastatic GIST failing all three standard agents should be considered for participation in clinical trials of new agents. These studies are only likely to be available in major centres treating GIST. There is limited evidence that patients who have already progressed on imatinib may benefit for a limited period when re-challenged with the drug [46]. Likewise, there is anecdotal evidence that maintaining treatment with a TKI even in the case of progressive disease, as opposed to stopping it, may slow down progression if no other option is available at the time. Therefore, re-challenging or continuing treatment with a TKI, to which the patient has already been exposed, is an option which may be considered for symptom control in patients with progression [V, B].

Metastatic disease—local therapy

Selected patients with limited liver metastatic disease may be amenable to surgery or radiofrequency ablation (RFA) after maximum response to imatinib, or if there is evidence of localised disease progression. The use of RFA is restricted to tumours in the region of 3 cm in maximum diameter and is less likely to be a suitable approach for lesions adjacent to large vessels or superficial lesions, especially if displacing the liver capsule. However, larger isolated lesions and superficial lesions may still be suitable for surgical resection, either by partial hepatectomy or wedge resection. Dedicated liver MRI scans and when appropriate PET-CT scans may be required to determine whether this is a legitimate approach by excluding other occult active disease.

Radiotherapy can be a useful local therapy in GIST under certain circumstances in the advanced disease setting. If there is a single site of disease that is progressing on a TKI and can be encompassed within a radiotherapy treatment field, then radiotherapy delivered to a moderate or high dose can offer local tumour control, and possibly prolong the use of the TKI [47]. Radiotherapy can also be used at lower doses to palliate symptomatic disease, for example to relieve pain or bleeding.

Response assessment

Response assessment is complex and early progression in particular should be confirmed by a team experienced in treating GIST. Anti-tumour activity translates into tumour shrinkage in most patients, but some patients may show only changes in tumour "density" on imaging, these changes sometimes precede a reduction in tumour volume. Such changes in tumour radiological appearance should be considered as indicative of tumour response. Tumour size may even increase in the short term but if tumour density on CT scan is decreased this may still indicate tumour response [48, 49]. Even the apparent 'appearance' of new lesions may be due to them becoming less dense, or cystic, especially in the liver. Therefore, both tumour size and tumour density on CT scan, or consistent changes on MRI or contrast-enhanced ultrasound, should be considered when determining tumour response. ^{18}F-FDG-PET has proved useful in the early assessment of tumour response, for example when prediction of the response is valuable, for example in the case of preoperative therapy, or when response is in doubt. However, a small proportion of GISTs have no FDG uptake. The absence of tumour progression at 6 months [50] is also equivalent to a tumour response. Conversely, tumour progression may not always be accompanied by changes in tumour size. For example, an increase in the tumour density shown by contrast enhancement within a previously responding low density tumour lesion, may be indicative of tumour progression. A typical progression pattern is the 'nodule within the mass', in which a portion of a responding lesion becomes hyper-dense [51].

Key recommendations

1. Imatinib is the treatment of choice for patients with unresectable or metastatic disease and is given until progression at the standard dose of 400 mg daily. Data suggest that patients whose tumours have an exon 9 mutation in *KIT* benefit from a larger dose, though this is not currently recommended by NICE.
2. Isolated progression may be amenable to surgery or other local measures, such as radiofrequency ablation.
3. Standard second line treatment is sunitinib, which may be given at the recommended dose of 50 mg daily for 4 weeks every 6 weeks, or 37.5 mg daily continuously.
4. Standard 3rd line treatment is regorafenib.

Follow-up

The optimal follow-up policy for surgically treated patients with localized disease is unclear. Relapses occur most often in the liver and/or the peritoneal cavity. Other sites of metastases, including bone and brain are uncommon, but may be less unusual following prolonged treatment with several lines of therapy. The mitotic rate most likely affects the frequency with which relapses occur. Risk assessment based on the mitotic count, tumour size and tumour site may be useful in choosing the routine follow-up policy. High-risk patients generally relapse within 1–3 years from the end of adjuvant therapy. Low-risk patients may relapse later, given that the disease is likely to be slower growing.

The issue of follow-up has been addressed by Joensuu and colleagues based on the currently available evidence [52]. High-risk patients who have undergone resection of their primary generally undergo a routine follow-up with abdominal CT or MRI scan every 3–6 months during adjuvant therapy, for 3 years. This frequency of follow up is because of the need to manage the side effects of the therapy. On cessation of adjuvant therapy follow up is every 3 months for 2 years, then every 6 months for another 3 years, after which follow up is annually for another 5 years. Patients with high-risk tumours not given adjuvant therapy, for whatever reason, should be followed up 3 monthly for 2 years, 6 monthly for 3 years and then annually for a further 5 years.

For low to intermediate risk tumours, the optimal frequency of follow-up is less clear. If follow-up is performed, it will usually be an abdominal CT or MRI scan, or ultrasound, every 6–12 months for 5 years.

Very low-risk GISTs do not require routine follow-up, provided excision was complete, although one must be aware that the risk of progression is not zero.

Radiation exposure is a factor to consider when selecting the imaging modality for long term follow-up. Abdominal MRI is an acceptable alternative to CT which could be used at selected intervals.

Key recommendations

1. Patients with high risk disease on adjuvant therapy should be followed up by cross-sectional imaging every 3–6 months during their 3 years of treatment, 3 monthly for 2 years following cessation of treatment and thereafter every 6 months for 3 years and annually for 5 years.
2. Patients with high risk disease not receiving adjuvant treatment should follow the post-adjuvant treatment scheme.
3. For patients with lesser levels of risk less frequent follow-up is generally recommended, although the clinical benefits are unclear. For intermediate risk patients 6 monthly scans for 5 years followed by annual scans and for low risk patients shorter duration follow-up would be considered reasonable.

Authors' contributions

All authors contributed to the content of the manuscript and consent to its publication. IJ adapted the guideline from the previous version published in 2010, with reference to the ESMO Guidelines from 2014 of which he was a co-author. Amendments and suggestions from the co-authors were incorporated. All authors read and approved the final manuscript.

Author details

[1] The Institute of Cancer Research, Royal Marsden NHS Foundation Trust, Fulham Road, London SW3 6JJ, UK. [2] Addenbrooke's Hospital, Cambridge University Hospitals, Cambridge, UK. [3] University College Hospital, University College London Hospitals NHS Foundation Trust, London, UK. [4] Bristol Cancer Institute, University Hospitals, Bristol NHS Trust, Bristol, UK. [5] Southmead Hospital, North Bristol NHS Trust, Bristol, UK. [6] Royal Marsden NHS Foundation Trust London, London, UK.

Acknowledgements

The authors would also like to thank the following on behalf of the British Sarcoma Group for valuable review, suggestions and amendments: Dr. Robin Jones (Consultant Medical Oncologist, Royal Marsden Hospital, London), Dr. Palma Dileo (Consultant Medical Oncologist, University College Hospital, London), Mrs. Judith Robinson (GIST Support UK), Jayne Bressington (GIST Support UK), Dr. Nicholas Carroll (Consultant Radiologist, Addenbrooke's Hospital, Cambridge).

Competing interests

IJ has received honoraria for attending advisory boards and speaking engagements from GSK, Ariad, Amgen, Clinigen, Lilly and Bayer; BS has received honoraria for attending advisory boards from Ariad, Novartis, Clinigen, Lilly and Daichi. NW has received honoraria from Novartis for speaking engagements; RB has received honoraria for attending advisory boards and speaking engagements from Novartis, Pfizer, Ariad, Pierre Fabre, Bristol Myers Squibb, Astra Zeneca, and Bayer Pharmaceuticals. AD & SM have no competing interests to report.

References

1. Group ESESNW. Gastrointestinal stromal tumours: ESMO clinical practice guidelines for diagnosis, treatment and follow-up. Ann Oncol. 2014;25 Suppl 3:iii21–6.
2. Dykewicz CA, Centers for Disease C, Prevention, Infectious Diseases Society of A, American Society of B, Marrow T. Summary of the guidelines for preventing opportunistic infections among hematopoietic stem cell transplant recipients. Clin Infect Dis. 2001;33(2):139–44.
3. Gatta G, van der Zwan JM, Casali PG, Siesling S, Dei Tos AP, Kunkler I, et al. Rare cancers are not so rare: the rare cancer burden in Europe. Eur J Cancer. 2011;47(17):2493–511.
4. Cassier PA, Ducimetiere F, Lurkin A, Ranchere-Vince D, Scoazec JY, Bringuier PP, et al. A prospective epidemiological study of new incident GISTs during two consecutive years in Rhone Alpes region: incidence and molecular distribution of GIST in a European region. Br J Cancer. 2010;103(2):165–70.
5. Pappo AS, Janeway KA. Pediatric gastrointestinal stromal tumors. Hematol Oncol Clin N Am. 2009;23(1):15–34.

6. Agaimy A, Wunsch PH, Sobin LH, Lasota J, Miettinen M. Occurrence of other malignancies in patients with gastrointestinal stromal tumors. Semin Diagn Pathol. 2006;23(2):120–9.
7. Ballinger ML, Goode DL, Ray-Coquard I, James PA, Mitchell G, Niedermayr E, et al. Monogenic and polygenic determinants of sarcoma risk: an international genetic study. Lancet Oncol. 2016;17:1261–71.
8. Pantaleo MA, Nannini M, Corless CL, Heinrich MC. Quadruple wild-type (WT) GIST: defining the subset of GIST that lacks abnormalities of KIT, PDGFRA, SDH, or RAS signaling pathways. Cancer Med. 2015;4(1):101–3.
9. Zhang L, Smyrk TC, Young WF Jr, Stratakis CA, Carney JA. Gastric stromal tumors in Carney triad are different clinically, pathologically, and behaviorally from sporadic gastric gastrointestinal stromal tumors: findings in 104 cases. Am J Surg Pathol. 2010;34(1):53–64.
10. Pasini B, McWhinney SR, Bei T, Matyakhina L, Stergiopoulos S, Muchow M, et al. Clinical and molecular genetics of patients with the Carney–Stratakis syndrome and germline mutations of the genes coding for the succinate dehydrogenase subunits SDHB, SDHC, and SDHD. Eur J Hum Genet. 2008;16(1):79–88.
11. Gaal J, Stratakis CA, Carney JA, Ball ER, Korpershoek E, Lodish MB, et al. SDHB immunohistochemistry: a useful tool in the diagnosis of Carney–Stratakis and Carney triad gastrointestinal stromal tumors. Mod Pathol. 2011;24(1):147–51.
12. Miettinen M, Fetsch JF, Sobin LH, Lasota J. Gastrointestinal stromal tumors in patients with neurofibromatosis 1: a clinicopathologic and molecular genetic study of 45 cases. Am J Surg Pathol. 2006;30(1):90–6.
13. Fletcher CD, Berman JJ, Corless C, Gorstein F, Lasota J, Longley BJ, et al. Diagnosis of gastrointestinal stromal tumors: a consensus approach. Hum Pathol. 2002;33(5):459–65.
14. Rubin BP, Cooper K, Fletcher CD, Folpe AL, Gannon FH, Hunt JL, et al. Protocol for the examination of specimens from patients with tumors of soft tissue. Arch Pathol Lab Med. 2010;134(4):e31–9.
15. Miettinen M, Wang ZF, Lasota J. DOG1 antibody in the differential diagnosis of gastrointestinal stromal tumors: a study of 1840 cases. Am J Surg Pathol. 2009;33(9):1401–8.
16. Lopes LF, West RB, Bacchi LM, van de Rijn M, Bacchi CE. DOG1 for the diagnosis of gastrointestinal stromal tumor (GIST): comparison between 2 different antibodies. Appl Immunohistochem Mol Morphol. 2010;18(4):333–7.
17. Miettinen M, Lasota J. Gastrointestinal stromal tumors: pathology and prognosis at different sites. Semin Diagn Pathol. 2006;23(2):70–83.
18. Joensuu H. Risk stratification of patients diagnosed with gastrointestinal stromal tumor. Hum Pathol. 2008;39(10):1411–9.
19. Joensuu H, Vehtari A, Riihimaki J, Nishida T, Steigen SE, Brabec P, et al. Risk of recurrence of gastrointestinal stromal tumour after surgery: an analysis of pooled population-based cohorts. Lancet Oncol. 2012;13(3):265–74.
20. Novitsky YW, Kercher KW, Sing RF, Heniford BT. Long-term outcomes of laparoscopic resection of gastric gastrointestinal stromal tumors. Ann Surg. 2006;243(6):738–45 **(discussion 45–7)**.
21. Eisenberg BL, Harris J, Blanke CD, Demetri GD, Heinrich MC, Watson JC, et al. Phase II trial of neoadjuvant/adjuvant imatinib mesylate (IM) for advanced primary and metastatic/recurrent operable gastrointestinal stromal tumor (GIST): early results of RTOG 0132/ACRIN 6665. J Surg Oncol. 2009;99(1):42–7.
22. Cananzi FC, Judson I, Lorenzi B, Benson C, Mudan S. Multidisciplinary care of gastrointestinal stromal tumour: a review and a proposal for a pre-treatment classification. Eur J Surg Oncol. 2013;39(11):1171–8.
23. Wilkinson MJ, Fitzgerald JE, Strauss DC, Hayes AJ, Thomas JM, Messiou C, et al. Surgical treatment of gastrointestinal stromal tumour of the rectum in the era of imatinib. Br J Surg. 2015;102(8):965–71.
24. Rutkowski P, Gronchi A, Hohenberger P, Bonvalot S, Schoffski P, Bauer S, et al. Neoadjuvant imatinib in locally advanced gastrointestinal stromal tumors (GIST): the EORTC STBSG experience. Ann Surg Oncol. 2013;20(9):2937–43.
25. McCarter MD, Antonescu CR, Ballman KV, Maki RG, Pisters PW, Demetri GD, et al. Microscopically positive margins for primary gastrointestinal stromal tumors: analysis of risk factors and tumor recurrence. J Am Coll Surg. 2012;215(1):53–9 **(discussion 9–60)**.
26. Joensuu H, Eriksson M, Sundby Hall K, Hartmann JT, Pink D, Schutte J, et al. One vs three years of adjuvant imatinib for operable gastrointestinal stromal tumor: a randomized trial. JAMA. 2012;307(12):1265–72.
27. Dematteo RP, Ballman KV, Antonescu CR, Maki RG, Pisters PW, Demetri GD, et al. Adjuvant imatinib mesylate after resection of localised, primary gastrointestinal stromal tumour: a randomised, double-blind, placebo-controlled trial. Lancet. 2009;373(9669):1097–104.
28. Debiec-Rychter M, Sciot R, Le Cesne A, Schlemmer M, Hohenberger P, van Oosterom AT, et al. KIT mutations and dose selection for imatinib in patients with advanced gastrointestinal stromal tumours. Eur J Cancer. 2006;42(8):1093–103.
29. Heinrich MC, Owzar K, Corless CL, Hollis D, Borden EC, Fletcher CD, et al. Correlation of kinase genotype and clinical outcome in the North American Intergroup Phase III Trial of imatinib mesylate for treatment of advanced gastrointestinal stromal tumor: CALGB 150105 Study by Cancer and Leukemia Group B and Southwest Oncology Group. J Clin Oncol. 2008;26(33):5360–7.
30. Heinrich MC, Corless CL, Demetri GD, Blanke CD, von Mehren M, Joensuu H, et al. Kinase mutations and imatinib response in patients with metastatic gastrointestinal stromal tumor. J Clin Oncol. 2003;21(23):4342–9.
31. Gastrointestinal Stromal Tumor Meta-Analysis G. Comparison of two doses of imatinib for the treatment of unresectable or metastatic gastrointestinal stromal tumors: a meta-analysis of 1640 patients. J Clin Oncol. 2010;28(7):1247–53.
32. Verweij J, Casali PG, Zalcberg J, LeCesne A, Reichardt P, Blay JY, et al. Progression-free survival in gastrointestinal stromal tumours with high-dose imatinib: randomised trial. Lancet. 2004;364(9440):1127–34.
33. Blanke CD, Rankin C, Demetri GD, Ryan CW, von Mehren M, Benjamin RS, et al. Phase III randomized, intergroup trial assessing imatinib mesylate at two dose levels in patients with unresectable or metastatic gastrointestinal stromal tumors expressing the kit receptor tyrosine kinase: S0033. J Clin Oncol. 2008;26(4):626–32.
34. Le Cesne A, Ray-Coquard I, Bui BN, Adenis A, Rios M, Bertucci F, et al. Discontinuation of imatinib in patients with advanced gastrointestinal stromal tumours after 3 years of treatment: an open-label multicentre randomised phase 3 trial. Lancet Oncol. 2010;11(10):942–9.
35. Demetri GD, Wang Y, Wehrle E, Racine A, Nikolova Z, Blanke CD, et al. Imatinib plasma levels are correlated with clinical benefit in patients with unresectable/metastatic gastrointestinal stromal tumors. J Clin Oncol. 2009;27(19):3141–7.
36. Eechoute KFM, Reyners AK, de Jong FA, Sparreboom A, van der Graaf WTA, et al. A long-term prospective population pharmacokinetic study on imatinib plasma concentrations in GIST patients. Clin Cancer Res. 2012;18:5780–7.
37. Bouchet S, Poulette S, Titier K, Moore N, Lassalle R, Abouelfath A, et al. Relationship between imatinib trough concentration and outcomes in the treatment of advanced gastrointestinal stromal tumours in a real-life setting. Eur J Cancer. 2016;57:31–8.
38. Raut CP, Posner M, Desai J, Morgan JA, George S, Zahrieh D, et al. Surgical management of advanced gastrointestinal stromal tumors after treatment with targeted systemic therapy using kinase inhibitors. J Clin Oncol. 2006;24(15):2325–31.
39. Gronchi A, Fiore M, Miselli F, Lagonigro MS, Coco P, Messina A, et al. Surgery of residual disease following molecular-targeted therapy with imatinib mesylate in advanced/metastatic GIST. Ann Surg. 2007;245(3):341–6.
40. Mussi C, Ronellenfitsch U, Jakob J, Tamborini E, Reichardt P, Casali PG, et al. Post-imatinib surgery in advanced/metastatic GIST: is it worthwhile in all patients? Ann Oncol. 2010;21(2):403–8.
41. Demetri GD, van Oosterom AT, Garrett CR, Blackstein ME, Shah MH, Verweij J, et al. Efficacy and safety of sunitinib in patients with advanced gastrointestinal stromal tumour after failure of imatinib: a randomised controlled trial. Lancet. 2006;368(9544):1329–38.
42. George S, Blay JY, Casali PG, Le Cesne A, Stephenson P, Deprimo SE, et al. Clinical evaluation of continuous daily dosing of sunitinib malate in patients with advanced gastrointestinal stromal tumour after imatinib failure. Eur J Cancer. 2009;45(11):1959–68.
43. Demetri GD, Reichardt P, Kang YK, Blay JY, Rutkowski P, Gelderblom H, et al. Efficacy and safety of regorafenib for advanced gastrointestinal stromal tumours after failure of imatinib and sunitinib (GRID): an international, multicentre, randomised, placebo-controlled, phase 3 trial. Lancet. 2013;381(9863):295–302.
44. Heinrich MC, Marino-Enriquez A, Presnell A, Donsky RS, Griffith DJ, McKinley A, et al. Sorafenib inhibits many kinase mutations associated

with drug-resistant gastrointestinal stromal tumors. Mol Cancer Ther. 2012;11(8):1770–80.

45. Hsueh YS, Lin CL, Chiang NJ, Yen CC, Li CF, Shan YS, et al. Selecting tyrosine kinase inhibitors for gastrointestinal stromal tumor with secondary KIT activation-loop domain mutations. PLoS ONE. 2013;8(6):e65762.
46. Kang YK, Ryu MH, Yoo C, Ryoo BY, Kim HJ, Lee JJ, et al. Resumption of imatinib to control metastatic or unresectable gastrointestinal stromal tumours after failure of imatinib and sunitinib (RIGHT): a randomised, placebo-controlled, phase 3 trial. Lancet Oncol. 2013;14(12):1175–82.
47. Joensuu H, Eriksson M, Collan J, Balk MH, Leyvraz S, Montemurro M. Radiotherapy for GIST progressing during or after tyrosine kinase inhibitor therapy: a prospective study. Radiother Oncol. 2015;116(2):233–8.
48. Benjamin RS, Choi H, Macapinlac HA, Burgess MA, Patel SR, Chen LL, et al. We should desist using RECIST, at least in GIST. J Clin Oncol. 2007;25(13):1760–4.
49. Choi H, Charnsangavej C, Faria SC, Macapinlac HA, Burgess MA, Patel SR, et al. Correlation of computed tomography and positron emission tomography in patients with metastatic gastrointestinal stromal tumor treated at a single institution with imatinib mesylate: proposal of new computed tomography response criteria. J Clin Oncol. 2007;25(13):1753–9.
50. Le Cesne A, Van Glabbeke M, Verweij J, Casali PG, Findlay M, Reichardt P, et al. Absence of progression as assessed by response evaluation criteria in solid tumors predicts survival in advanced GI stromal tumors treated with imatinib mesylate: the intergroup EORTC-ISG-AGITG phase III trial. J Clin Oncol. 2009;27(24):3969–74.
51. Shankar S, vanSonnenberg E, Desai J, Dipiro PJ, Van Den Abbeele A, Demetri GD. Gastrointestinal stromal tumor: new nodule-within-a-mass pattern of recurrence after partial response to imatinib mesylate. Radiology. 2005;235(3):892–8.
52. Joensuu H, Martin-Broto J, Nishida T, Reichardt P, Schoffski P, Maki RG. Follow-up strategies for patients with gastrointestinal stromal tumour treated with or without adjuvant imatinib after surgery. Eur J Cancer. 2015;51(12):1611–7.

10

Zoledronic acid in metastatic osteosarcoma: encouraging progression free survival in four consecutive patients

Robert M. Conry[1*], Michael G. Rodriguez[2] and Joseph G. Pressey[3,4]

Abstract

Background: Zoledronic acid (ZA) is a third-generation bisphosphonate in widespread clinical use to reduce pain and skeletal events in patients from a variety of malignancies with bone metastases. Pre-clinical studies indicate that ZA inhibits osteosarcoma through direct anti-proliferative effects, immune activation and anti-angiogenic activity.

Methods: The purpose of this study was to evaluate the antitumor efficacy of ZA at standard dose until progression in patients with stage IV osteosarcoma lacking a standard of care treatment option proven to influence survival. Researchers retrospectively reviewed medical records of all patients at our institution with high-grade osteosarcoma presumed to be incurable due to metastases progressive after primary combination chemotherapy who received single agent ZA in an effort to delay progression.

Results: In our four-patient cohort following initiation of ZA, the median progression-free survival was 19 months, and median overall survival was 56+ months. Two of four patients have remained progression-free since starting ZA. The other two initially progressed after 18–20 months on ZA followed by metastasectomy of lung or dural metastases and further stability for over a year following resumption of ZA. After a 20-month progression-free interval on ZA alone, one patient had partial response following addition of pazopanib to ZA that likely contributed to long term disease control. The four patients experienced no significant toxicities despite protracted dosing of ZA for up to 5 years, and none have required chemotherapy since beginning ZA.

Conclusions: Single agent ZA was associated with encouraging progression-free survival in four consecutive patients with metastatic osteosarcoma. Prospective trials of single agent ZA are warranted as protracted maintenance therapy in surgically incurable osteosarcoma relapsed or refractory to first line combination chemotherapy with radiographically measurable metastases.

Keywords: Zoledronic acid, Bisphosphonates, Osteosarcoma, Metastatic, Survival, Human

Background

Osteosarcoma is the most common malignant bone tumor in children and young adults. Despite aggressive surgical and medical therapy, the estimated 5-year event-free survivals of patients presenting with localized or metastatic disease are 50–70 % and less than 20 %, respectively [1]. Patients with either unresectable primary tumors or distant metastases progressing after conventional primary chemotherapy have dismal outcomes, little changed over the past 30 years [2]. There is no "standard" second-line systemic therapy for inoperable osteosarcoma progressing after conventional chemotherapy. Results of three cooperative group experiences in this population reveal median survival of 6 months [3], median time to progression of 2 months with only 6 % event-free survival at 6 months [4], and a 2-year post-relapse survival <2 % [5]. Thus, novel systemic treatment approaches are urgently needed.

Zoledronic acid (ZA) is a third-generation, nitrogen-containing bisphosphonate analog of endogenous

*Correspondence: rconry@uabmc.edu
[1] Division of Hematology Oncology, University of Alabama at Birmingham, 2145 Bonner Way, Birmingham, AL 35243, USA

pyrophosphate that strongly binds to calcium-containing hydroxyapatite bone mineral. Although the plasma half-life of ZA is less than 24 h, bisphosphonates are stable in bone with a skeletal half-life of more than 300 days [6]. Osteosarcoma is characterized by the production of osteoid or immature bone containing focal calcium deposits of hydroxyapatite crystals [7]. Thus, ZA may preferentially concentrate in primary osteosarcomas as well as their lung and bone metastases and persist for years. ZA inhibits farnesyl diphosphate synthase, a key enzyme in the mevalonate pathway, and thus reduces protein prenylation essential for normal cell function and survival [8, 9]. Bone-resorbing osteoclasts internalize relatively large quantities of ZA and are thus particularly vulnerable to functional inhibition, underlying the widespread use of this drug to reduce pain and skeletal-related events in adults with bone metastases [10]. However, nitrogen-containing bisphosphonates appear to have direct anti-proliferative and pro-apoptotic effects against normal osteoblasts and a variety of tumor cells, including breast, myeloma, pancreatic and prostate cancers [11–15]. ZA has been shown to reduce primary tumor growth, decrease lung metastases and prolong survival in animal models of osteosarcoma [16–18]. ZA also acts synergistically with mTOR inhibition to decrease proliferation of murine and human osteosarcoma cell lines in vitro and to reduce osteosarcoma tumor growth in two distinct syngeneic murine modals [19]. Ewing's sarcoma is the second most frequent malignant bone tumor in adolescents and young adults. ZA inhibits Ewing's sarcoma cell invasion through down regulation of matrix metalloproteinase and significantly reduces development of spontaneous lung metastases in a nude mouse model of human Ewing's sarcoma cells injected into the tibia [20].

The Children's Oncology Group (COG) performed a phase I feasibility trial of monthly ZA for eight cycles with concurrent conventional multi-agent chemotherapy in 24 children with previously untreated, high-grade metastatic osteosarcoma [21]. The maximum tolerated dose (MTD) was equivalent to the standard adult dose for bone metastases, and there was a trend toward improved event-free survival at 2 years compared to historical data from intergroup study INT 0133 ($p = 0.079$). This manuscript is the first reported clinical experience with ZA as single agent therapy for osteosarcoma.

Methods

With approval from The University of Alabama at Birmingham institutional review board, the researchers retrospectively reviewed medical records of all patients at our institution with high-grade osteosarcoma treated from December 2010 to January 2015. This timeframe was selected for analysis to allow a minimum of 8 months of follow-up for progression-free survival prior to this report. Twenty-seven such patients were identified; four of whom were presumed to be incurable due to metastatic osteosarcoma progressive after primary combination chemotherapy and received off-label ZA in an effort to delay progression. Those four consecutive patients so treated are the basis of this report. To provide details of each clinical situation and response to ZA, individual patient histories are briefly described in case report format. Treatment outcomes for the four patient cohort are summarized in Table 1.

Results

All four patients presented with high-grade osteosarcoma without detectable metastases. All received neoadjuvant and/or adjuvant chemotherapy with conventional doses of doxorubicin and cisplatin with or without high-dose methotrexate and ifosfamide. All underwent definitive surgical resection of the primary tumor using a limb-sparing approach in the three extremity cases. Patients 2 and 4 had microscopically positive soft tissue margins treated with post-operative external beam radiotherapy. All patients subsequently developed stage IV osteosarcoma involving the lungs that was treated with ZA. Patients 1 and 2 received ZA as consolidative treatment following metastasectomies and a likely transient

Table 1 Treatment outcomes with zoledronic acid

Patient	Sites of disease[a]	PFS[b] (months)	Additional therapy	Status at last visit	OS[b] (months)
1	Lung	20	Pazopanib/surgery	NED	63+
2	Lung	54+	None	NED	54+
3	Lung and hilum	18	Radiation to hilum/neurosurgery	SD	59+
4	Lung	14+	None	SD	14+
		Median 19			Median 56+

PFS progression-free survival; *OS* overall survival; *NED* no evidence of disease; *SD* stable disease

[a] sites of osteosarcoma active during or immediately preceding ZA

[b] calculated from start of ZA

response to salvage chemotherapy in the case of patient 2. Patients 3 and 4 received ZA for treatment of persistently measurable metastases to the lung and other sites. The University of Alabama at Birmingham Department of Anatomical Pathology histologically confirmed the diagnosis of high-grade osteosarcoma from the primary site of all four patients as well as from resection specimens from lung metastases in patient 1 before and after ZA and patient 2 before ZA. Histological confirmation of metastatic high-grade osteosarcoma was also obtained at our academic center from bronchoscopic biopsy of a hilar lymph node and subsequent resection of a brain metastasis in patient 3.

Case #1

A 20-year-old male presented with osteosarcoma of the left tibia, and 16 months after completion of primary therapy a solitary metastasis of high-grade osteosarcoma was wedge resected from the right upper lobe. Over the subsequent 5 years prior to treatment with ZA, he required bilateral pulmonary metastasectomies on four occasions with no objective response to multiple intervening combination chemotherapy regimens including cyclophosphamide with topotecan, ifosfamide with etoposide, gemcitabine with docetaxel and cisplatin with vinorelbine. During that 5-year period, the longest progression-free interval was 6 months and the interval between metastasectomies progressively shortened from 20 months to 17 to 11 and ultimately to 9 months. A new subpleural 6 mm left upper lobe metastasis was seen on chest CT performed in June 2010 (Fig. 1a) and markedly enlarged on chest CT in December 2010 (Fig. 1b) prior to his fifth metastasectomy. In an attempt to delay further recurrence, ZA was initiated at 4 mg every 6 weeks rather than a 4-week interval indicated for bone metastases due to lengthy travel to clinic. Chest computed tomographies (CTs) were performed at 3-month intervals. After a 20-month progression-free interval, a solitary 8 mm metastasis to the left lung was detected (Fig. 1c). The patient continued ZA with the addition of oral pazopanib at 600 mg daily. The solitary metastasis responded to the combination of pazopanib and ZA, decreasing to 3 mm following 2 months of therapy. After 7 months, pazopanib was reduced to 400 mg daily due to plateaued response (Fig. 1d) as well as mild to moderate anorexia, insomnia and hypertension. After 14 months of combined pazopanib and ZA, chest computed tomography (CT) showed a stable 3 mm solitary left lung nodule, and ZA was discontinued to facilitate dental procedures related to advanced caries predating ZA use with no evidence of osteonecrosis. Pazopanib was also discontinued 4 months later to facilitate dental work with the lung nodule remaining stable after 18 months of pazopanib

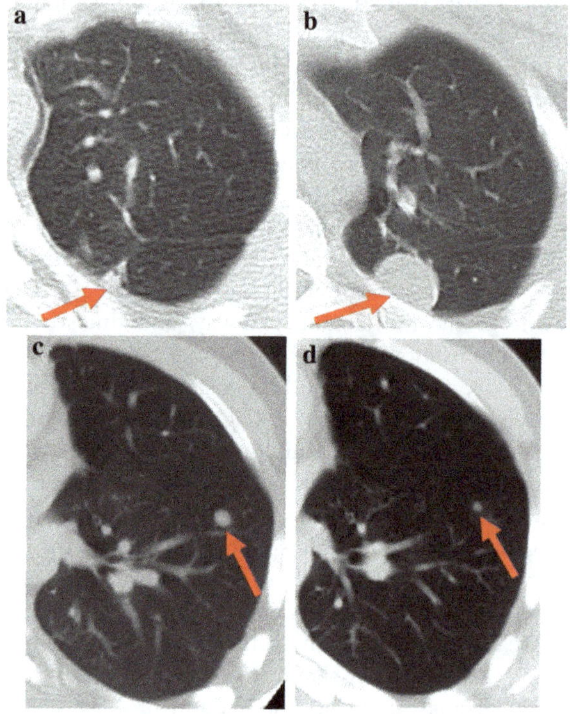

Fig. 1 **a** Axial CT scan performed on 6/10/10 shows a new subpleural 6 mm *left upper lobe* nodule. **b** Follow-up CT performed on 12/10/10 shows interval increase in size of the pleural based *left upper lobe* nodule representing metastatic osteosarcoma at resection. **c** Axial CT performed on 3/28/11 shows a new 8 mm nodule in the *left lower lobe*. **d** Follow-up axial CT performed on 11/7/12 showed interval decrease in size of the *left lower lobe* nodule to 3 mm, confirmed to be osteosarcoma at subsequent resection

therapy. Chest CT after 3 months off therapy revealed enlargement of the left lung nodule from 3 to 17 mm, and positron emission tomography (PET) showed no disease elsewhere. The solitary left lung metastasis was wedge resected, and single agent ZA was resumed at the prior dose. The patient remains progression-free 20 months after surgery with overall survival 63+ months from the start of ZA.

Case #2

A 63-year-old male underwent left radical parotidectomy and neck dissection to resect an extraosseous osteosarcoma with no lymph node involvement. Two years after completion of primary therapy a CT scan of the chest revealed a new right lung metastasis which was wedge resected. Repeat chest CT scan 3 months later demonstrated five new pulmonary metastases. He was considered incurable due to rapid progression of multiple, bilateral pulmonary metastases 2 years after completion of optimal adjuvant chemotherapy for a man of his age. He received salvage chemotherapy with four cycles of doxorubicin and dacarbazine since he was unable to tolerate additional cisplatin due to peripheral neuropathy. Chest CT scan showed a complete radiographic response which was followed by three cycles of vinorelbine with oral cyclophosphamide. Since the prognosis was dismal, the patient began ZA at 4 mg every 6 weeks due to lengthy travel to clinic as consolidative therapy. He continued this schedule for 18 months followed by dosing every 3 months for 36 additional months without apparent toxicity or relapse of osteosarcoma as determined by chest CT scans at 3-month intervals. He has been on ZA for 54+ months.

Case #3

A 48-year-old female presented with osteosarcoma of the right femur, and 38 months after completion of primary therapy a chest CT scan revealed an enlarging 11 mm right lung nodule, new calcified left hilar adenopathy and narrowing of the lingular bronchus. Bronchoscopic biopsy confirmed metastatic osteosarcoma. Over the subsequent 19 months, she had no objective response to multiple chemotherapy regimens including ifosfamide with etoposide, cyclophosphamide with vinorelbine, gemcitabine, cisplatin and ridaforolimus. Bilateral pulmonary metastases increased in size and number, and left hilar adenopathy increased from 1.9 to 4.1 cm with distal atelectasis, cough and dyspnea on exertion (Fig. 2a, b). Since standard treatment options had been exhausted, ZA was initiated at 3.5 mg every 4 weeks due to an abnormal glomerular filtration rate at baseline. After 18 months of ZA, bilateral lung metastases remained stable, and the left hilar adenopathy increased modestly to 5 cm with progressive atelectasis. Although she was stable by RECIST 1.1 criteria, palliative radiation to 40 Gy in 8 fractions was delivered to the hilar mass to reduce dyspnea, and ZA was continued. After 26 additional months of ZA, the hilar adenopathy and multiple, bilateral pulmonary metastases remained stable by RECIST 1.1 criteria. A 5 cm intracranial dural-based calcified falcine mass was incidentally detected on sinus films, and neurosurgical resection revealed metastatic osteosarcoma. She has remained on monthly ZA for 59+ months and is stable 16 months after resection of the intracranial metastasis (Fig. 2c, d).

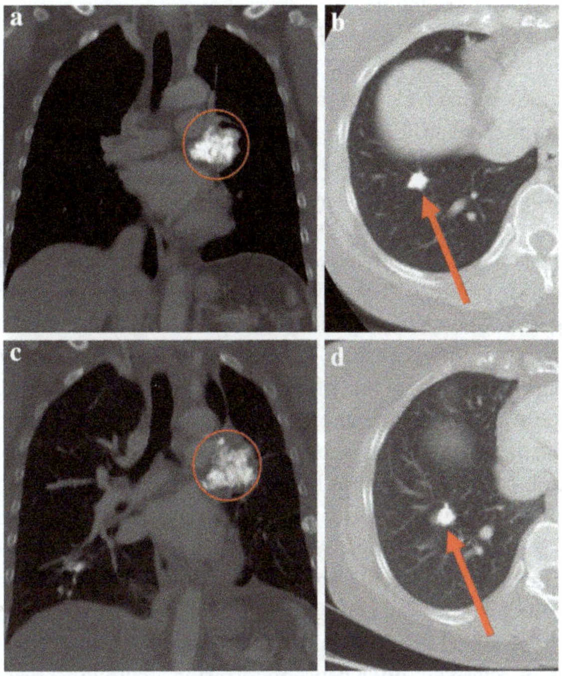

Fig. 2 **a** Coronal CT image on 3/31/11 showing a calcified *left hilar mass* with metastatic osteosarcoma biopsy confirmed. **b** Axial CT image performed on 3/31/11 showing a calcified nodule in the *right lower lobe* consistent with metastatic disease. **c** Coronal CT image performed on 12/11/15 shows grossly stable appearance of the calcified *left hilar mass*. **d** Axial CT image performed on 12/11/15 shows a grossly stable appearance of the *right lower lobe* nodule

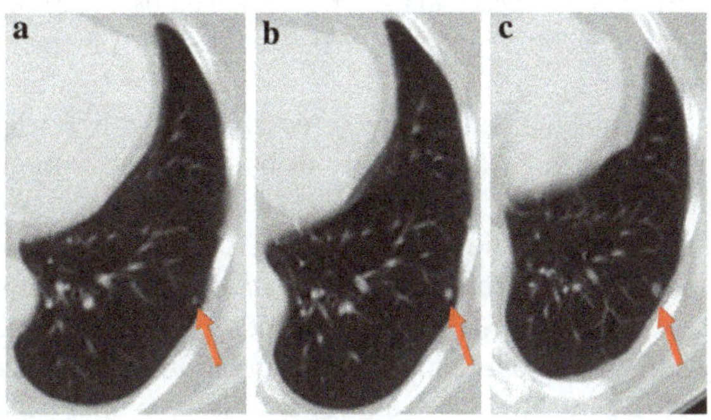

Fig. 3 Axial CT images performed on 12/11/14 (**a**) and 1/23/15 (**b**) show interval growth of a *left lower lobe* nodule from 3 to 6 mm. Follow-up axial CT image performed on 2/1/16 (**c**) shows a grossly stable 6 mm *left lower lobe* nodule

Case #4

A 65-year-old male presented with chondroblastic osteosarcoma of the left femur and multiple new bilateral lung metastases measuring up to 1 cm diameter developed during the fourth cycle of adjuvant chemotherapy. These were confirmed to be progressive by two CT scans of the chest performed 6 weeks apart (Fig. 3a, b). Chemotherapy was discontinued, and ZA was initiated at 4 mg every 4 weeks. After 14 months of follow-up, the patient remains stable with no local recurrence, pulmonary metastases stable by RECIST 1.1 criteria (Fig. 3c) and no new lesions as determined by MRI and chest CT, respectively at 3 month intervals.

Summary of outcomes

All patients had stage IV osteosarcoma and lacked a standard of care treatment option proven to significantly influence survival. The treatment outcomes with ZA are summarized in Table 1. Following initiation of ZA, the median progression free survival was 19 months, and median overall survival was 56+ months. At the time of this report, two of the four patients have no evidence of disease, and the other two have stable disease. None of the four patients have required chemotherapy since starting ZA. The case of patient 1 is particularly compelling since ZA dramatically extended the progression-free interval following his fifth pulmonary metastasectomy to 20 months. Once another metastasis became detectable, it objectively responded to the addition of pazopanib to ZA for 14 months followed by resection, and he remains progression-free 20 months later on single agent ZA. Patient 3 demonstrated stable hilar and pulmonary metastases for a remarkable 44 months on ZA allowing her to survive long enough to develop a very uncommon metastasis to the dura possibly representing a sanctuary site of relatively poor drug penetration. Following resection of the intracranial metastasis, she has remained stable for an additional 16 months on ZA.

Discussion

Bisphosphonates are relatively well tolerated with side effects including electrolyte disturbances, flu-like symptoms, nausea and less commonly osteonecrosis of the jaw and renal dysfunction [22, 23]. The four patients reported herein receiving ZA for advanced osteosarcoma experienced no significant toxicities despite protracted dosing for up to 5 years. ZA is a convenient treatment for patients with incurable osteosarcoma with far less detrimental impact on quality of life than conventional chemotherapy.

Pre-clinical studies indicate that ZA inhibits osteosarcoma through direct anti-proliferative effects, immune activation and anti-angiogenic activity. ZA directly inhibits human osteosarcoma cell proliferation and induces apoptosis in vitro [24–26]. γδ T cells recognize small phosphoantigens associated with metabolites of bacterial isoprenoid biosynthesis or the mevalonate pathway in eukaryotes [27]. ZA sensitizes tumor cells to γδ T cell cytotoxicity through accumulation of mevalonate pathway intermediates within bisphosphonate-treated cells [28]. ZA promotes γδ T cell proliferation from peripheral blood mononuclear cells of osteosarcoma patients and enhances γδ T cell cytotoxicity against human osteosarcoma cells [29, 30]. Vascular endothelial growth factor-A (VEGF-A) and vascular endothelial growth factor receptor-1 (VEGFR-1) are highly expressed by aggressive osteosarcoma cells, but not in clonally-related less aggressive cell lines [31]. Plasma levels of VEGF-A are elevated in osteosarcoma patients, and ZA decreases circulating levels of VEGF-A in these patients [32, 33]. ZA inhibits tumor-associated angiogenesis not only via direct inhibition of endothelial cells, but also by decreasing VEGF-A expression in osteosarcoma. Furthermore, evidence indicates that ZA induces apoptosis in aggressive osteosarcoma cells at least partly by inhibiting autocrine stimulation via VEGF-A and VEGFR signaling [31]. Thus, nitrogen-containing bisphosphonates have pleiotropic inhibitory effects on osteosarcoma and tumor-associated endothelial cells.

Inherent limitations in this study include the retrospective nature of the review and the small cohort of patients analyzed. However, this report does include all patients receiving single agent ZA to delay osteosarcoma progression at our institution during the specified timeframe.

COG has demonstrated the feasibility of co-administering ZA with conventional chemotherapy for first line treatment of metastatic osteosarcoma, but the small trial was underpowered to detect efficacy of ZA, particularly in the presence of highly active chemotherapy. A large, randomized French trial of conventional adjuvant chemotherapy with or without ZA for resectable primary osteosarcoma was stopped early due to futility with hazard ratios for event-free survival and death exceeding unity in the ZA cohort. Although not statistically significant, these data suggests that ZA in this context may increase mortality [34]. However, this trial may likewise have been suboptimally designed to evaluate efficacy of ZA in this disease. Direct antiproliferative effects of ZA could actually protect osteosarcoma cells from tumoricidal effects of chemotherapy. Enhancement of antitumor immune responses by ZA could be undermined by concurrent cytotoxic chemotherapy, and antiangiogenic actions of ZA may have little relevance in treating micrometastases in the adjuvant setting. ZA may actually have greater efficacy against surgically incurable macroscopic osteosarcoma used as a single agent or in combination with the mTOR inhibitor everolimus or the VEGFR tyrosine kinase inhibitor pazopanib, targeting tumor cell proliferation and angiogenesis, respectively [19, 35]. The combination of ZA and sirolimus has recently been demonstrated to be effective and tolerable therapy for a young adult with aggressive lymphatic malformations associated with Gorham-Stout disease [36]. Intriguing results from a recent study of the multi-tyrosine kinase inhibitor sorafenib with activity against VEGFR in combination with everolimus further support the use of such agents in recurrent or refractory osteosarcoma [37]. In fact, this trial represents the first positive study in at least 25 years in patients with relapsed osteosarcoma [38]. Interestingly, patient 1 in this report experienced disease control for 20 months on single agent ZA followed by emergence of another lung metastasis that objectively responded for over 14 months to the addition of pazopanib to ZA. We have also observed objective response of multiple pulmonary metastases to combined ZA and pazopanib for over 9 months in a patient with relapsed osteosarcoma not included here due to lack of single agent ZA use.

Conclusions

Zoledronic acid represents a convenient, well tolerated therapy which may provide durable control of incurable osteosarcoma. Therefore, prospective trials of single agent ZA are warranted in surgically incurable osteosarcoma relapsed or refractory to first line conventional combination chemotherapy with radiographically measurable metastases.

Abbreviations

ZA: zoledronic acid; mTOR: mammalian target of rapamycin; CT: computed tomography; PET: positron emission tomography; RECIST: response evaluation criteria in solid tumors; MRI: magnetic resonance imaging; VEGF: vascular endothelial growth factor; VEGFR: vascular endothelial growth factor receptor; COG: Children's Oncology Group.

Authors' contributions

Dr. RMC was involved in conception of the study, treating patients and monitoring their antitumor response and toxicities. He was actively involved in writing the manuscript. Dr. MGR comprehensively reviewed patient imaging and provided Figs. 1, 2, and 3. Dr. JGP assisted with study conception, data interpretation and manuscript writing. All authors read and approved the final manuscript.

Author details

[1] Division of Hematology Oncology, University of Alabama at Birmingham, 2145 Bonner Way, Birmingham, AL 35243, USA. [2] Department of Radiology, University of Alabama at Birmingham, 619 19th St South, Birmingham, AL 35249, USA. [3] Department of Pediatrics, University of Alabama at Birmingham, 1600 7th Avenue South, Birmingham, AL 35233, USA. [4] Present Address: Cancer & Blood Disorders Institute, Cincinnati Children's Hospital Medical Center, Cincinnati, OH, USA.

Acknowledgements

The authors thank Kendra Gilpin for expert preparation of the manuscript.

Competing interests

The authors declare that they have no competing interests.

References

1. Bacci G, Ferrari S, Bertoni F, Ruggieri P, Picci P, Longhi A, et al. Long-term outcome for patients with nonmetastatic osteosarcoma of the extremity treated at the istituto ortopedico rizzoli according to the istituto ortopedico rizzoli/osteosarcoma-2 protocol: an updated report. J Clin Oncol Off J Am Soc Clin Oncol. 2000;18:4016–27.
2. Grignani G, Palmerini E, Dileo P, Asaftei SD, D'Ambrosio L, Pignochino Y, et al. A phase II trial of sorafenib in relapsed and unresectable high-grade osteosarcoma after failure of standard multimodal therapy: an Italian Sarcoma Group study. Ann Oncol Off J Eur Soc Med Oncol ESMO. 2012;23:508–16.
3. Kempf-Bielack B, Bielack SS, Jurgens H, Branscheid D, Berdel WE, Exner GU, et al. Osteosarcoma relapse after combined modality therapy: an analysis of unselected patients in the Cooperative Osteosarcoma Study Group (COSS). J Clin Oncol Off J Am Soc Clin Oncol. 2005;23:559–68.
4. Leary SE, Wozniak AW, Billups CA, Wu J, McPherson V, Neel MD, et al. Survival of pediatric patients after relapsed osteosarcoma: the St. Jude Children's Research Hospital experience. Cancer. 2013;119:2645–53.
5. Ferrari S, Briccoli A, Mercuri M, Bertoni F, Picci P, Tienghi A, et al. Postrelapse survival in osteosarcoma of the extremities: prognostic factors for long-term survival. J Clin Oncol Off J Am Soc Clin Oncol. 2003;21:710–5.
6. Fleisch H. Bisphosphonates. Pharmacology and use in the treatment of tumour-induced hypercalcaemic and metastatic bone disease. Drugs. 1991;42:919–44.
7. Mierau GW, Weeks DA, Hicks MJ. Role of electron microscopy and other special techniques in the diagnosis of childhood round cell tumors. Hum Pathol. 1998;29:1347–55.
8. Perry CM, Figgitt DP. Zoledronic acid: a review of its use in patients with advanced cancer. Drugs. 2004;64:1197–211.
9. Green JR. Skeletal complications of prostate cancer: pathophysiology and therapeutic potential of bisphosphonates. Acta Oncol. 2005;44:282–92.
10. Rodan GA, Fleisch HA. Bisphosphonates: mechanisms of action. J Clin Invest. 1996;97:2692–6.
11. Wittrant Y, Theoleyre S, Chipoy C, Padrines M, Blanchard F, Heymann D, et al. RANKL/RANK/OPG: new therapeutic targets in bone tumours and associated osteolysis. Biochim Biophys Acta. 2004;1704:49–57.
12. Nakajima H, Magae J, Tsuruga M, Sakaguchi K, Fujiwara I, Mizuta M, et al. Induction of mitochondria-dependent apoptosis through the inhibition of mevalonate pathway in human breast cancer cells by YM529, a new third generation bisphosphonate. Cancer Lett. 2007;253:89–96.
13. Baulch-Brown C, Molloy TJ, Yeh SL, Ma D, Spencer A. Inhibitors of the mevalonate pathway as potential therapeutic agents in multiple myeloma. Leuk Res. 2007;31:341–52.
14. Tassone P, Tagliaferri P, Viscomi C, Palmieri C, Caraglia M, D'Alessandro A, et al. Zoledronic acid induces antiproliferative and apoptotic effects in human pancreatic cancer cells in vitro. Br J Cancer. 2003;88:1971–8.
15. Iguchi K, Nakano T, Usui S, Hirano K. Incadronate inhibits aminopeptidase N expression in prostatic PC-3 cells. Cancer Lett. 2006;237:223–33.
16. Dass CR, Choong PF. Zoledronic acid inhibits osteosarcoma growth in an orthotopic model. Mol Cancer Ther. 2007;6:3263–70.
17. Labrinidis A, Hay S, Liapis V, Ponomarev V, Findlay DM, Evdokiou A. Zoledronic acid inhibits both the osteolytic and osteoblastic components of osteosarcoma lesions in a mouse model. Clin Cancer Res Off J Am Assoc Cancer Res. 2009;15:3451–61.
18. Ory B, Heymann MF, Kamijo A, Gouin F, Heymann D, Redini F. Zoledronic acid suppresses lung metastases and prolongs overall survival of osteosarcoma-bearing mice. Cancer. 2005;104:2522–9.
19. Moriceau G, Ory B, Mitrofan L, Riganti C, Blanchard F, Brion R, et al. Zoledronic acid potentiates mTOR inhibition and abolishes the resistance of osteosarcoma cells to RAD001 (Everolimus): pivotal role of the prenylation process. Cancer Res. 2010;70:10329–39.
20. Odri G, Kim PP, Lamoureux F, Charrier C, Battaglia S, Amiaud J, et al. Zoledronic acid inhibits pulmonary metastasis dissemination in a preclinical model of Ewing's sarcoma via inhibition of cell migration. BMC Cancer. 2014;14:169.
21. Goldsby RE, Fan TM, Villaluna D, Wagner LM, Isakoff MS, Meyer J, et al. Feasibility and dose discovery analysis of zoledronic acid with concurrent chemotherapy in the treatment of newly diagnosed metastatic osteosarcoma: a report from the Children's Oncology Group. Eur J Cancer. 2013;49:2384–91.
22. Bamias A, Kastritis E, Bamia C, Moulopoulos LA, Melakopoulos I, Bozas G, et al. Osteonecrosis of the jaw in cancer after treatment with bisphosphonates: incidence and risk factors. J Clin Oncol Off J Am Soc Clin Oncol. 2005;23:8580–7.
23. Perazella MA, Markowitz GS. Bisphosphonate nephrotoxicity. Kidney Int. 2008;74:1385–93.

24. Chang J, Wang W, Zhang H, Hu Y, Yin Z. Bisphosphonates regulate cell proliferation, apoptosis and pro-osteoclastic expression in MG-63 human osteosarcoma cells. Oncol Lett. 2012;4:299–304.
25. Ory B, Blanchard F, Battaglia S, Gouin F, Redini F, Heymann D. Zoledronic acid activates the DNA S-phase checkpoint and induces osteosarcoma cell death characterized by apoptosis-inducing factor and endonuclease-G translocation independently of p53 and retinoblastoma status. Mol Pharmacol. 2007;71:333–43.
26. Hirbe AC, Roelofs AJ, Floyd DH, Deng H, Becker SN, Lanigan LG, et al. The bisphosphonate zoledronic acid decreases tumor growth in bone in mice with defective osteoclasts. Bone. 2009;44:908–16.
27. Todaro M, D'Asaro M, Caccamo N, Iovino F, Francipane MG, Meraviglia S, et al. Efficient killing of human colon cancer stem cells by gammadelta T lymphocytes. J Immunol. 2009;182:7287–96.
28. D'Asaro M, La Mendola C, Di Liberto D, Orlando V, Todaro M, Spina M, et al. V gamma 9 V delta 2 T lymphocytes efficiently recognize and kill zoledronate-sensitized, imatinib-sensitive, and imatinib-resistant chronic myelogenous leukemia cells. J Immunol. 2010;184:3260–8.
29. Li Z, Tang J, Sun L, Ye Z. Effect of zoledronate on the cytotoxicity of gammadelta T cells from PBMCs of osteosarcoma patients against osteosarcoma. Chin J Cell Mol Immunol. 2013;29:6–9.
30. Li Z. Potential of human gammadelta T cells for immunotherapy of osteosarcoma. Mol Biol Rep. 2013;40:427–37.
31. Ohba T, Cates JM, Cole HA, Slosky DA, Haro H, Ichikawa J, et al. Pleiotropic effects of bisphosphonates on osteosarcoma. Bone. 2014;63:110–20.
32. Santini D, Vincenzi B, Galluzzo S, Battistoni F, Rocci L, Venditti O, et al. Repeated intermittent low-dose therapy with zoledronic acid induces an early, sustained, and long-lasting decrease of peripheral vascular endothelial growth factor levels in cancer patients. Clin Cancer Res Off J Am Assoc Cancer Res. 2007;13:4482–6.
33. Savitskaya YA, Rico-Martinez G, Linares-Gonzalez LM, Delgado-Cedillo EA, Tellez-Gastelum R, Alfaro-Rodriguez AB, et al. Serum tumor markers in pediatric osteosarcoma: a summary review. Clin Sarcoma Res. 2012;2:9.
34. Battaglia S, Dumoucel S, Chesneau J, Heymann MF, Picarda G, Gouin F, et al. Impact of oncopediatric dosing regimen of zoledronic acid on bone growth: preclinical studies and case report of an osteosarcoma pediatric patient. J Bone Miner Res Off J Am Soc Bone Miner Res. 2011;26:2439–51.
35. Safwat A, Boysen A, Lucke A, Rossen P. Pazopanib in metastatic osteosarcoma: significant clinical response in three consecutive patients. Acta Oncol. 2014;53:1451–4.
36. Cramer SL, Wei S, Merrow AC, Pressey JG. Gorham-Stout disease successfully treated with sirolimus and zoledronic acid therapy. J Pediatr Hematol Oncol. 2016;38:e129–32.
37. Grignani G, Palmerini E, Ferraresi V, D'Ambrosio L, Bertulli R, Asaftei SD, et al. Sorafenib and everolimus for patients with unresectable high-grade osteosarcoma progressing after standard treatment: a non-randomised phase 2 clinical trial. Lancet Oncol. 2015;16:98–107.
38. Wagner MJ, Livingston JA, Patel SR, Benjamin RS. Chemotherapy for bone sarcoma in adults. J Oncol Pract Am Soc Clin Oncol. 2016;12:208–16.

11

Perioperative chemotherapy in the treatment of osteosarcoma

G M O'Kane[1*], K A Cadoo[2], E M Walsh[1], R Emerson[1], P Dervan[3], C O'Keane[3], B Hurson[4], G O'Toole[4], S Dudeney[4], E Kavanagh[5], S Eustace[5] and D N Carney[1]

Abstract

Background: Chemotherapy in the multimodality treatment of osteosarcoma has improved survival. Reported outcomes on adult patients are limited. Poor necrosis rates post neoadjuvant chemotherapy (NAC) is considered an adverse prognostic factor and attempts have been made to improve survival in this group.

Patients and methods: Adult and young adult patients diagnosed with osteosarcoma between January 1986 and August 2012 were retrospectively reviewed. Patients identified were stratified according to stage (localised or metastatic) and age (≤40 and >40 years). Event free survival (EFS) and overall survival (OS) outcomes were determined. In patients with localised disease ≤40 years, survival was assessed according to necrosis rates post NAC (<90 and ≥90%). NAC consisted of two cycles of methotrexate alternating with doxorubicin/cisplatin (MAP) followed by definitive surgery. Those with ≥90% tumour necrosis continued on MAP. Patients with <90% necrosis received ifosfamide and etoposide (IE) post operatively.

Results: A total of 108 patients were reviewed and 97 were included. Median age was 23 years (range 16–75) and 70% of patients were male. Five year EFS and OS across all groups was 57% and 63% respectively. Of the patients with localised disease ($N = 81$), 5-year overall survival (OS), with a median follow up of 7 years (2–26) was 70% ($p < 0.0001$). Patients aged 16–40 ($N = 68$) with localised osteosarcoma had a significantly improved 5-year OS (74%) compared to those >40 years ($N = 13$) (42%) ($p = 0.004$). Of the 68 patients with localised osteosarcoma ≤40 years, 62 were evaluated according to necrosis rates post MAP. In 33 patients who achieved ≥90% necrosis and continued MAP, 5-year OS was 82%. In 29 patients who had <90% tumour necrosis and received adjuvant IE, 5-year OS was 68% ($p = 0.15$). Multivariate analysis confirmed age and stage as prognostic factors but not poor necrosis rates in our treated population.

Conclusions: Long-term survival outcomes in a predominantly adult Irish population are similar to large reported trials. Age and stage at diagnosis are prognostic. Postoperative ifosfamide/etoposide alone in patients with poor necrosis rates is a feasible regimen, but its role in the adjuvant setting remains uncertain.

Keywords: Adult osteosarcoma, Neoadjuvant chemotherapy, Poor necrosis rates, MAP, Ifosfamide/etoposide

Background

Osteosarcoma is a rare tumour type occurring with an incidence of 0.2–3/1,00,000 per year in Europe [1]. Despite this, it is the most common primary tumour of bone (excluding multiple myeloma), which occurs with a bimodal age distribution. The first peak, in adolescents and young adults, possibly coincides with the pubertal growth spurt. The second peak in patients over 65 years may result from the development of osteosarcoma as a secondary malignancy [2, 3]. The metaphyses of long bones are the most commonly affected site [3] with more than 50% of occurrences adjacent to the knee joint [4].

*Correspondence: okaneg@tcd.ie
[1] Department of Medical Oncology, Mater Misericordiae University Hospital, Eccles Street, Dublin 7, Ireland

Prior to the 1970s surgery alone cured <20% of patients; the majority of deaths resulted from the rapid development of lung metastases [5]. Since the incorporation of chemotherapy, multimodality treatment has improved survival to approximately 70% at 5 years with little improvement in the last two decades [4, 6, 7]. Trials demonstrating this survival have largely included paediatric patients and outcomes in adult patients alone are limited.

Where feasible, the standard of care for patients with localised extremity osteosarcoma involves NAC followed by definitive surgical resection and adjuvant chemotherapy [8]. Although NAC versus immediate surgery and adjuvant chemotherapy has not been shown to improve OS [6], it does allow for optimal surgical planning [9] and avoids the need for amputation in most patients. Chemotherapy protocols have generally incorporated four active agents: Methotrexate with leucovorin rescue, doxorubicin, cisplatin and ifosfamide [10]. The most appropriate combination of these drugs however, continues to be debated [8].

NAC also provides prognostic information on tumour necrosis rates, which has been used to tailor postoperative treatment. Based on the Huvos grading system, patients with ≥90% necrosis are considered good responders and those with <90% necrosis as poor responders [11]. Large trials have demonstrated inferior 5-year survival rates in patients with a poor response versus those with a good response (45–56% versus 71–80% respectively) [4, 12–14]. Attempts in the past have failed to improve survival by modifying adjuvant treatment in poor responders and a recent meta-analysis found no benefit in switching or intensifying drugs [7, 15, 16]. Ifosfamide/etoposide (IE) has been shown to have efficacy in the metastatic setting [17] and is considered safe when added to MAP [18]. MAPIE formed the adjuvant arm of poor responders in the EURAMOS-1 trial and provisional results reveal no improvement in survival [19]. At our institution patients with poor necrosis rates have been receiving postoperative IE alone since 1986.

In this article we review the outcomes of a predominantly adult population over a 26-year period and assess the impact of switching chemotherapy to IE in patients with <90% necrosis rates post neoadjuvant MAP.

Patients and methods

Patient population

A retrospective review was undertaken of patients with a diagnosis of osteosarcoma seen by the oncology department at the Mater Misericordiae University Hospital from January 1986 to August 2012. This hospital has been a tertiary referral centre for the systemic treatment of adult osteosarcoma, collaborating with Cappagh Hospital, the national orthopaedic hospital, where the majority of bone tumour surgeries are performed. All pathology was reviewed at our institution. During the period analysed, three orthopaedic surgeons performed 98% of the surgeries and the same oncologist delivered systemic treatment in all patients.

Patient details were obtained from the pathology department database and corroborated with the hospital information system search for patients with a diagnosis of osteosarcoma. Medical records of the patients collected were then appraised. Data was obtained on all patients with a histological diagnosis of high-grade osteosarcoma. We included patients with extremity or truncal high-grade osteosarcoma who received systemic treatment. Patients with craniofacial osteosarcoma, which is considered less aggressive, and those who did not receive chemotherapy were excluded. Patients were stratified according to stage: localised and metastatic disease at presentation and then further classified by age: ≤40 and >40 years. Those patients with localised disease ≤40 years, who received NAC were subsequently assessed according to necrosis rates based on the Huvos grading system [11]: poor responders(<90% necrosis, grade I–II) and good responders (≥90% necrosis, grade III–IV).

Staging and treatment details

Staging was performed using a plain film, radionuclide bone scan and/or magnetic resonance imaging (MRI) of the affected limb. Computed tomography (CT) thorax, abdomen and pelvis (TAP) and Chest X-Ray (CXR) completed radiological staging. More recently FDG PET/CT has been incorporated into routine work up. Full blood count and biochemical analyses were also measured at diagnosis and throughout treatment. The intended operating surgeon performed diagnostic biopsies where possible. All patients were discussed at our institutional multidisciplinary team meeting (MDT) at diagnosis, post NAC and post resection.

The systemic treatment of resectable osteosarcoma at our institution consists of two cycles of high dose methotrexate 8 g/m^2 alternating with doxorubicin 25 mg/m^2 days 1–3 and cisplatin 100 mg/m^2 on day 1 (MAP), followed by definitive surgery and adjuvant chemotherapy (Additional file 1: Table S1). Patients with tumours which upon histological review demonstrate ≥90% necrosis continue MAP for a further two alternating cycles while those who have <90% necrosis rates switch to ifosfamide 1,800 mg/m^2 with mesna 1,800 mg/m^2 days 1–5 and etoposide 100 mg/m^2 days 1–5 for a total of four cycles (Additional file 1: Table S1). Dosing and scheduling of chemotherapy administered was confirmed with the pharmacy department.

Patients with metastases at diagnosis who were considered resectable were treated with the same protocol and at surgery had resection of the primary lesion and metastases where applicable.

Close surveillance was initiated upon completion of adjuvant treatment. Patients were seen 3 monthly for the first 2 years with a CXR; a CT Thorax was performed every 6 months. Thereafter patients were reviewed 4–6 monthly with a CXR until year 5 at which point annual follow-up was commenced.

Data collection

Demographic and clinical details were extracted from the patient's medical records. Information on histology was obtained from the laboratory report system. Data collected included age, sex, stage at diagnosis, tumour site, type of operation, percentage necrosis, chemotherapy regimen used and number of cycles administered. Relapse date and site, together with survival and follow up information was also recorded.

Statistical analysis

Demographic details and treatment variables are reported by descriptive statistics. EFS and OS were computed from time of tissue biopsy until first recurrence or death respectively. Time of cut off for analyses was July 31st 2014. The Kaplan–Meier survival analysis method and the log rank test were used to estimate survival probability and compare survival within stratified groups. The Cox Regression model was used to assess the prognostic impact of age, stage and necrosis rates on survival. Analyses were conducted using SPSS 20.0

Results

Patient characteristics

Between January 1st 1986 and July 31st 2012 108 adult patients with a diagnosis of osteosarcoma were reviewed by medical oncology. Eight patients who did not receive chemotherapy due to poor performance status (median age 73 years, range 46–81) and three patients with craniofacial disease were excluded. A total of 97 patients were included. Detailed baseline patient demographics and tumour characteristics are available in Additional file 2: Table S2. Specific high-grade subtypes were incompletely reported during the time period and not available for analysis. Five patients were under 18 years (16–17 years) with the majority (95%) ≥18 years. Median age overall was 23 years (16–73). Seventy percent of patients were male. The most common site of tumour was the femur (54%) followed by the tibia (20%). Of the total patients included ($N = 97$) 81 (84%) had localised disease and 16 (16%) had metastatic osteosarcoma at diagnosis. In patients with localised disease, 68/81 (84%) were ≤40 years (16–40) and in patients with metastatic disease at diagnosis, 11/16 (68%) were ≤40 years (17–40). Follow-up for all patients ranged from 2 to 28.6 years with a median of 7 years.

Surgical treatment

Limb-salvage surgery was performed in 70% of patients with disease of the extremities ($N = 90$). Of these 90 patients 77 had localised disease and 13 metastatic disease. Limb-salvage was possible in 77% of patients with localised disease and was performed in only 31% of patients with metastatic disease (4/13) (Additional file 2: Table S2). Notably the period of this review from 1986 to 2012 has seen changes in approaches to the surgical management of extremity osteosarcoma with the increasing use of limb-salvage techniques in recent years [20, 21].

Chemotherapy

In patients with localised disease ($N = 81$), 618 of planned 648 chemotherapy cycles were completed (95%). Eight patients (10%) did not complete the intended cycles of treatment. Four patients ≥40 years with localised disease, developed grade 3–4 toxicities, as did three patients ≤40 years. One further patient ≤40 years refused two final cycles of adjuvant treatment. Of the 16 patients with metastatic disease 11 (70%) completed intended first line treatment.

Survival outcomes

The 5-year EFS and OS across all groups was 57 and 63% respectively. Stage at diagnosis was prognostic. Patients with localised disease ($N = 81$) had a significantly improved 5-year OS compared to those with metastatic disease at diagnosis ($N = 16$), 70 versus 25% $p < 0.0001$ (all age groups) (Figure 1a). EFS was 65 versus 13% $p < 0.0001$ (Figure 1b). Despite unbalanced numbers in each group age was also prognostic. EFS in localised disease ≤40 years ($N = 68$) was 70% compared to 30% in those >40 years ($N = 13$) ($p = 0.009$). Corresponding 5-year OS was 74% compared to 42%. ($p = 0.004$) (Figure 2a, b). Seven of the 13 patients >40 years (median age 54 years, range 44–74) with localised disease have died. Of these four were unable to complete chemotherapy due to toxicity. Multivariate analysis using the Cox Regression model confirmed the prognostic impact of age and stage for EFS ($p = 0.001$ and $p = 0.001$ respectively) and for OS ($p = 0.002$ and $p = 0.001$ respectively).

Relapsed disease in patients with localised osteosarcoma at diagnosis

Of the 81 patients with localised disease, 32 (40%) experienced recurrences. This included seven patients >40 years (54% of all patients >40 years). The lung was site

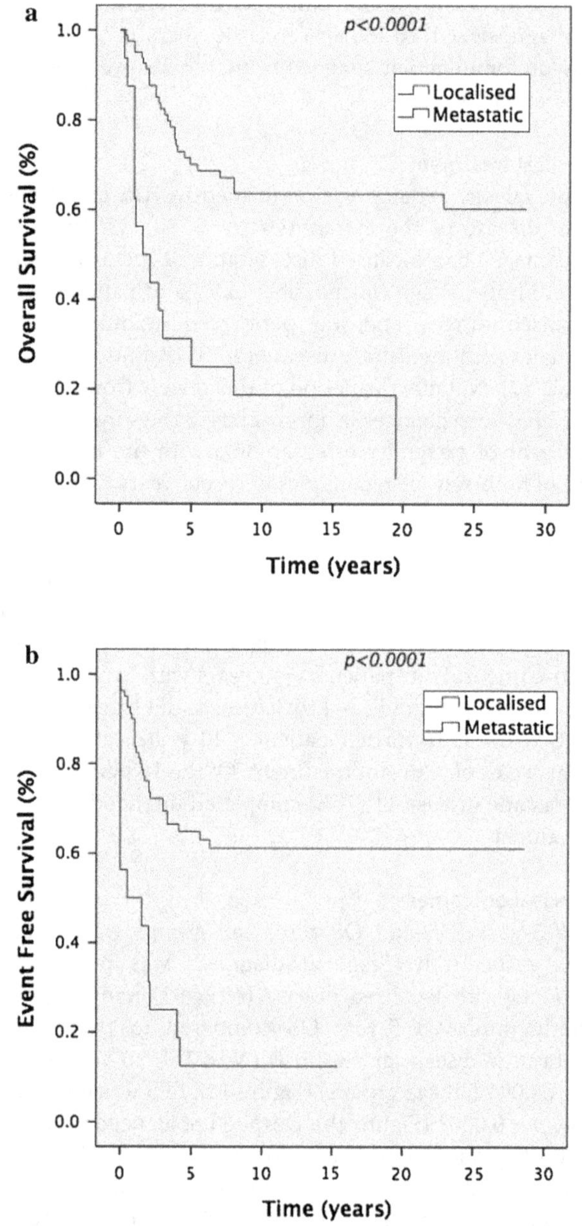

Figure 1 **a** Overall survival in patients with localised disease versus metastatic disease. **b** Event free survival in patients with localised disease versus metastatic disease.

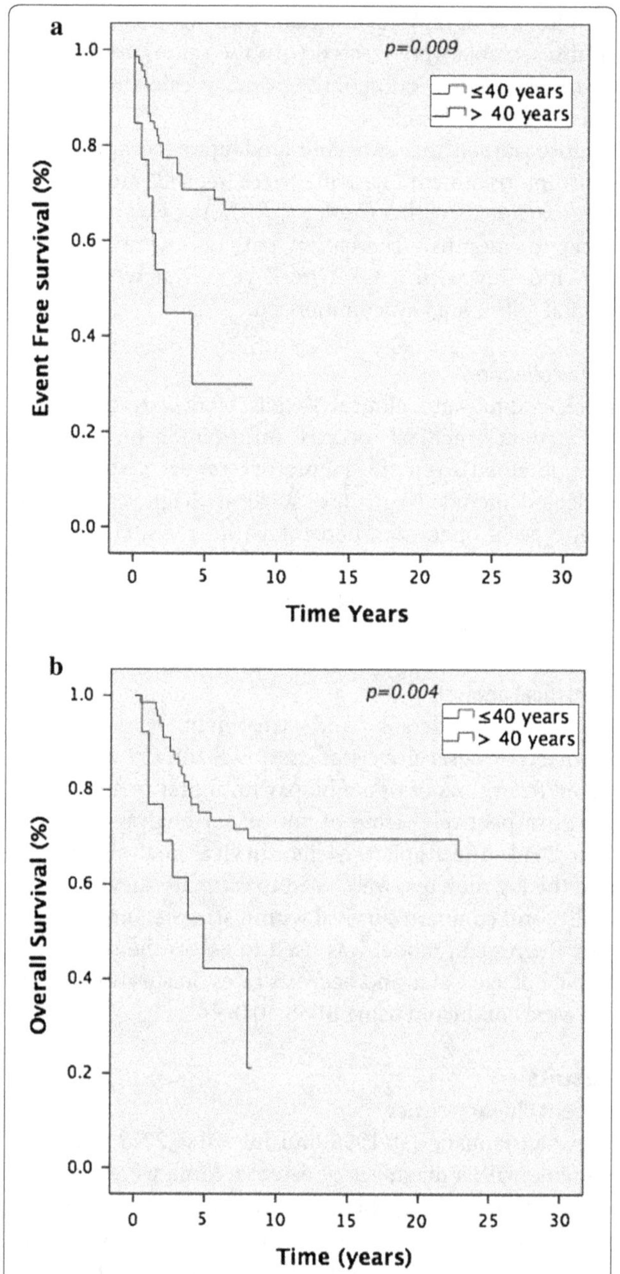

Figure 2 **a** EFS and **b** OS in localised disease according to age.

of first recurrence in 22/32 (69%) patients, with locally recurrent disease in nine patients. Three of these nine patients developed lung metastases within 1 year and one patient developed lung metastases 4 years later. One patient developed brain metastases as first documented recurrence but was also found to have lung metastases post complete imaging. Of the 32 patients who recurred, 11 patients (9 ≤ 40 years and 2 > 40 years) are alive and disease free with a median follow-up of 10.3 years (range 4.8–27.1). Four of these 11 patients developed local recurrences and were treated with surgery including one amputation; the remaining seven patients had thoracotomies for lung metastases (median number of thoracotomies 1; range 1–3).

Impact of switching chemotherapy in patients with poor necrosis (localised ≤40 years)

Of the 68 patients with localised disease ≤40 years, 62 were eligible for assessment of survival according to necrosis rates. The remaining six patients had upfront surgery without NAC and were thus excluded. Five of these six patients were initially thought to have parosteal osteosarcoma and one patient a chondrosarcoma. Pathological review of tumour specimens post resection revealed high-grade osteosarcoma. These six patients all received eight cycles of chemotherapy in the adjuvant setting and five are still alive with a median follow up of 3.8 years (2.2–14.4).

The 62 patients included all had initial biopsies and post NAC histology reviewed at our institution. Median follow-up time in this group was 9.4 years (range 2–28.6). 33 patients demonstrated ≥90% necrosis post MAP and 29 patients <90% necrosis. There was no significant difference in 5 year-EFS in good responders (81%) and in poor responders (64%) ($p = 0.18$) (Figure 3a). Five year OS was 82% in those with ≥90% necrosis versus 68% in those with <90% necrosis; this result was again not statistically significant $p = 0.15$ (Figure 3b). When included in multivariate analysis, necrosis rates post NAC was not prognostic for EFS ($p = 0.9$) or OS ($p = 0.62$) in our cohort (Additional file 3: Table S3).

Outcomes in patients with metastatic disease at diagnosis

Sixteen patients (16%) had evidence of metastases at diagnosis and 5-year OS was 25%. Lung metastases were present in 13 patients and 3 patients had multifocal disease. Of the 13 patients with lung metastases 7 had thoracotomies, 2 at primary resection and 5 at recurrence. The median number of thoracotomies was 1 (range 1–4). Two patients with metastases at presentation, 1 with multifocal disease and 1 with lung metastases are still alive 8.3 and 15.4 years later.

Discussion

This is a retrospective study of predominantly adult osteosarcoma patients treated systemically at a single institution over 26 years. We have established that long term overall survival outcomes in this Irish population are comparable to previously reported large clinical trials. This study has also demonstrated the feasibility of IE postoperatively in patients with a poor response to neoadjuvant MAP.

Adult patients are generally underrepresented in osteosarcoma trials despite approximately half of patient diagnoses occurring in those over 20 years. [22] The median age in our study was 23 years with 95% of patients ≥18 years and 70% of patients included were male. The male preponderance in osteosarcoma is well documented and although the proportion is slightly higher than reported ratios [3, 23] this may be explained by the older age of the patients included, as peak incidence in the female population occurs earlier [23].

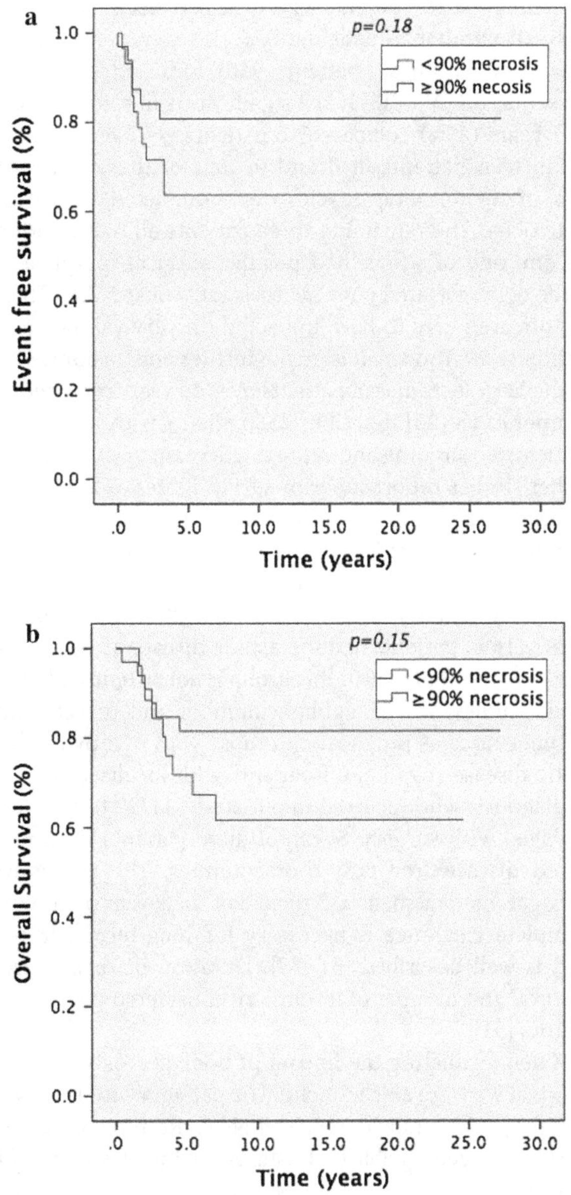

Figure 3 **a** EFS and **b** OS in patients with localised disease <40 years according to necrosis rates.

Inferior outcomes have been reported in patients over 40 [24, 25] and over 65 years [26]. A meta-analysis reported by Harting et al. investigating age as a prognostic factor in osteosarcoma, revealed that patients aged 21–40 ($N = 110$) had the same outcomes as that of the paediatric population with inferior survival in those >40 years ($N = 56$) [27]. This study acknowledges however that age alone is unlikely to contribute to inferior outcomes, but rather site, size and tumour necrosis rates in this group. In our study 5-year OS for all 97 patients included was 64%, improving to 74% when selecting patients aged 16–40 years with localised disease ($N = 68$). A small number of patients ($N = 18$) were >40 years at diagnosis. Of these, patients with localised disease at presentation ($N = 13$) had a significantly inferior survival at 5 years (45%) compared to patients ≤40 years. Seven of thirteen patients died and in four of these less than 50% of chemotherapy cycles were completed as a result of toxicity. The remaining three patients all had tumours >8 cm, one of whom had positive surgical margins; all three demonstrated poor necrosis rates post NAC. These factors are likely to have impacted on survival, however numbers are too small to make further conclusions. One of the largest studies in patients over 40 years reported by Grimer et al. [25] describes 238 patients with non metastatic osteosarcoma and reports a 5-year survival of 46%. Other studies report superior survival rates of 55–62% at 5 years [4, 28]. It is therefore likely that other patient and tumour characteristics contribute to outcomes.

Less than 20% of patients with osteosarcoma will present with de novo metastatic disease [29]. In our cohort 16/97 (16%) patients had metastatic disease at diagnosis. The 5-year OS of 25% in this group is consistent with previous studies, which highlight number and resectability of metastases as prognostic in those with de novo metastatic disease [29, 30]. Of patients with localised disease at diagnosis who recurred in our study, 11/32 (34%) were salvaged with surgery. Seven of these patients were rendered disease free post thoracotomies. The aggressive surgical management of recurrent osteosarcoma with complete clearance is necessary for long-term survival and is well described [31–33]. Duration of relapse free interval and number of lesions are considered prognostic factors [31].

When evaluating the impact of poor necrosis rates on survival we were able to include 62 patients with localised disease ≤40 years who received NAC. Responsiveness to NAC has been established as a predictor of survival [4, 12–14, 34].

The COSS, EOI and IOR groups have reported 5-year survival rates of 55.5, 45 and 56% respectively for poor responders with localised osteosarcoma [4, 12, 35]. Multiple studies have attempted to improve outcomes in this poor prognostic group by switching drugs or intensifying treatment, however a meta-analysis published by Anninga et al. [16] showed no benefit to either method.

MAP as a neoadjuvant regimen has been used since the 1980s and is considered standard of care in the United States [36]. This combination formed the backbone of the international multi-group EURAMOS-1 trial [37], the largest trial conducted in osteosarcoma. Survival outcomes in osteosarcoma have plateaued in recent decades and this group attempted to improve outcomes in both good and poor responders. The addition of IFN alpha-2b to MAP in good responders has recently been reported and failed to enhance survival [38]. Patients with poor necrosis rates were randomized to remain on MAP post-operatively or switch to MAP and IE.

The role of ifosfamide in osteosarcoma has been controversial. It has been shown to be active in the metastatic setting [17, 39] and has shown improvements in recurrence free survival and overall survival in patients at first recurrence [32]. The use of ifosfamide as a fourth drug in the neoadjuvant setting however does not improve histologic response and increases hematological toxicity [40]. When IE is added to MAP in poor responders post operatively results have differed. The IOR group have found favorable outcomes with use of ifosfamide [41] however the Scandinavian Sarcoma Group (SSG) failed to show a benefit of the addition of IE to MAP adjuvantly in poor responders [42]. Early results from EURAMOS-1 have also failed to show a benefit of additional IE to MAP in poor necrosis patients. It should be noted that fewer patients in this group received the intended doses and more toxicities were experienced [19]. In our patients survival at 5 years was 82% in good responders versus 68% in those treated with IE alone postoperatively. This difference was not statistically significant but suggests that IE is an acceptable adjuvant regimen in patients with poor necrosis rates.

Conclusions

Adult and young adult osteosarcoma patients under 40 years with localised osteosarcoma treated at our institution have equivalent outcomes compared to paediatric patients. Patients over 40 years are more challenging and are more likely to experience toxicity. Switching chemotherapy to ifosfamide/etoposide alone in patients with poor necrosis rates post neoadjuvant methotrexate, doxorubicin, cisplatin is a feasible regimen, but where these drugs fit in the treatment paradigm remains to be established.

Additional files

Additional file 1: Table S1. Chemotherapy protocol for resectable disease.

Additional file 2: Table S2. Patient characteristics.

Additional file 3: Table S3. Multivariate Cox-regression analysis of prognostic factors for event free survival and overall survival.

Authors' contributions

KC participated in data collection, study design and data interpretation. EW participated in data collection, study design and data interpretation. RE participated in data collection and analysis. PD participated in study design. COK participated in study design and manuscript revision. BH participated in study design. GOT participated in study design and manuscript revision. SD participated in study design. EK participated in study design and data interpretation. SE participated in study design and data interpretation. DC participated in study design, data collection and interpretation and manuscript revision. All authors read and approved the final manuscript.

Author details

[1] Department of Medical Oncology, Mater Misericordiae University Hospital, Eccles Street, Dublin 7, Ireland. [2] Gynaecologic Medical Oncology Service, Memorial Sloan-Kettering Cancer Centre, 300 East 66th Street, New York, NY 10065, USA. [3] Department of Histopathology, Mater Misericordiae University Hospital, Eccles Street, Dublin 7, Ireland. [4] Department of Orthopaedic Surgery, Cappagh National Orthopaedic Hospital, Finglas, Dublin 11, Ireland. [5] Department of Radiology, Mater Misericordiae University Hospital, Eccles Street, Dublin 7, Ireland.

Competing interests

The authors declare that they have no competing interests.

References

1. Bielack S, Carrle D, Casali PG, Group EGW (2009) Osteosarcoma: ESMO clinical recommendations for diagnosis, treatment and follow-up. Ann Oncol 20(Suppl 4):137–139
2. Huvos AG (1986) Osteogenic sarcoma of bones and soft tissues in older persons. A clinicopathologic analysis of 117 patients older than 60 years. Cancer 57(7):1442–1449
3. Ottaviani G, Jaffe N (2009) The epidemiology of osteosarcoma. Cancer Treat Res 152:3–13
4. Bielack SS, Kempf-Bielack B, Delling G, Exner GU, Flege S, Helmke K et al (2002) Prognostic factors in high-grade osteosarcoma of the extremities or trunk: an analysis of 1,702 patients treated on neoadjuvant cooperative osteosarcoma study group protocols. J Clin Oncol Off J Am Soc Clin Oncol 20(3):776–790
5. Marcove RC, Miké V, Hajek JV, Levin AG, Hutter RV (1970) Osteogenic sarcoma under the age of twenty-one. A review of one hundred and forty-five operative cases. J Bone Joint Surg Am 52(3):411–423
6. Goorin AM, Schwartzentruber DJ, Devidas M, Gebhardt MC, Ayala AG, Harris MB et al (2003) Presurgical chemotherapy compared with immediate surgery and adjuvant chemotherapy for nonmetastatic osteosarcoma: Pediatric Oncology Group Study POG-8651. J Clin Oncol 21(8):1574–1580
7. Provisor AJ, Ettinger LJ, Nachman JB, Krailo MD, Makley JT, Yunis EJ et al (1997) Treatment of nonmetastatic osteosarcoma of the extremity with preoperative and postoperative chemotherapy: a report from the Children's Cancer Group. J Clin Oncol Off J Am Soc Clin Oncol 15(1):76–84
8. Hogendoorn PC, Athanasou N, Bielack S, De Alava E, Dei Tos AP, Ferrari S et al (2010) Bone sarcomas: ESMO clinical practice guidelines for diagnosis, treatment and follow-up. Ann Oncol 21(Suppl 5):v204–v213
9. Rosen G (1985) Preoperative (neoadjuvant) chemotherapy for osteogenic sarcoma: a 10 year experience. Orthopedics 8(5):659–664
10. Ta HT, Dass CR, Choong PF, Dunstan DE (2009) Osteosarcoma treatment: state of the art. Cancer Metastasis Rev 28(1–2):247–263
11. Rosen G, Marcove RC, Huvos AG, Caparros BI, Lane JM, Nirenberg A et al (1983) Primary osteogenic sarcoma: eight-year experience with adjuvant chemotherapy. J Cancer Res Clin Oncol 106(Suppl):55–67
12. Bacci G, Bertoni F, Longhi A, Ferrari S, Forni C, Biagini R et al (2003) Neoadjuvant chemotherapy for high-grade central osteosarcoma of the extremity. Histologic response to preoperative chemotherapy correlates with histologic subtype of the tumor. Cancer 97(12):3068–3075
13. Hauben EI, Weeden S, Pringle J, Van Marck EA, Hogendoorn PC (2002) Does the histological subtype of high-grade central osteosarcoma influence the response to treatment with chemotherapy and does it affect overall survival? A study on 570 patients of two consecutive trials of the European Osteosarcoma Intergroup. Eur J Cancer 38(9):1218–1225
14. Bacci G, Longhi A, Versari M, Mercuri M, Briccoli A, Picci P (2006) Prognostic factors for osteosarcoma of the extremity treated with neoadjuvant chemotherapy: 15-year experience in 789 patients treated at a single institution. Cancer 106(5):1154–1161
15. Smeland S, Müller C, Alvegard TA, Wiklund T, Wiebe T, Björk O et al (2003) Scandinavian Sarcoma Group Osteosarcoma Study SSG VIII: prognostic factors for outcome and the role of replacement salvage chemotherapy for poor histological responders. Eur J Cancer 39(4):488–494
16. Anninga JK, Gelderblom H, Fiocco M, Kroep JR, Taminiau AH, Hogendoorn PC et al (2011) Chemotherapeutic adjuvant treatment for osteosarcoma: where do we stand? Eur J Cancer 47(16):2431–2445
17. Goorin AM, Harris MB, Bernstein M, Ferguson W, Devidas M, Siegal GP et al (2002) Phase II/III trial of etoposide and high-dose ifosfamide in newly diagnosed metastatic osteosarcoma: a pediatric oncology group trial. J Clin Oncol Off J Am Soc Clin Oncol 20(2):426–433
18. Schwartz CL, Wexler LH, Devidas M, Goorin A, Grier H, Meyers P et al (2004) P9754 therapeutic intensification in non-metastatic osteosarcoma: a COG trial. In J Clin Oncol (meeting abstracts) July 2004, vol. 22, no. 14_suppl8514
19. Marina N, Smeland S, Bielack SS, Bernstein M, Jovic G, Hook JM et al (2014) MAPIE vs MAP as postoperative chemotherapy in patients with a poor response to preoperative chemotherapy for newly-diagnosed osteosarcoma: results from EURAMOS-1 (Paper 032). Presented at Connective Tissue Oncology Society (CTOS) 2014.
20. Simon MA, Aschliman MA, Thomas N, Mankin HJ (1986) Limb-salvage treatment versus amputation for osteosarcoma of the distal end of the femur. J Bone Joint Surg Am 68(9):1331–1337
21. Rougraff BT, Simon MA, Kneisl JS, Greenberg DB, Mankin HJ (1994) Limb salvage compared with amputation for osteosarcoma of the distal end of the femur. A long-term oncological, functional, and quality-of-life study. J Bone Joint Surg Am 76(5):649–656
22. Ries LA, Smith M, Gurney JG et al (eds) (1999) Cancer incidence and survival among children and adolescents: United States SEER Program 1975–1995
23. Mirabello L, Troisi RJ, Savage SA (2009) International osteosarcoma incidence patterns in children and adolescents, middle ages and elderly persons. Int J Cancer 125(1):229–234
24. Carsi B, Rock MG (2002) Primary osteosarcoma in adults older than 40 years. Clin Orthop Relat Res 397:53–61
25. Grimer RJ, Cannon SR, Taminiau AM, Bielack S, Kempf-Bielack B, Windhager R et al (2003) Osteosarcoma over the age of forty. Eur J Cancer 39(2):157–163
26. Longhi A, Errani C, Gonzales-Arabio D, Ferrari C, Mercuri M (2008) Osteosarcoma in patients older than 65 years. J Clin Oncol Off J Am Soc Clin Oncol 26(33):5368–5373
27. Harting MT, Lally KP, Andrassy RJ, Vaporciyan AA, Cox CS, Hayes-Jordan A et al (2010) Age as a prognostic factor for patients with osteosarcoma: an analysis of 438 patients. J Cancer Res Clin Oncol 136(4):561–570
28. Bacci G, Ferrari S, Donati D, Longhi A, Bertoni F, Di Fiore M et al (1998) Neoadjuvant chemotherapy for osteosarcoma of the extremity in patients in the fourth and fifth decade of life. Oncol Rep 5(5):1259–1263
29. Kager L, Zoubek A, Pötschger U, Kastner U, Flege S, Kempf-Bielack B et al (2003) Primary metastatic osteosarcoma: presentation and outcome of patients treated on neoadjuvant Cooperative Osteosarcoma Study Group protocols. J Clin Oncol Off J Am Soc Clin Oncol 21(10):2011–2018
30. Aljubran AH, Griffin A, Pintilie M, Blackstein M (2009) Osteosarcoma in adolescents and adults: survival analysis with and without lung metastases. Ann Oncol 20(6):1136–1141
31. Bielack SS, Kempf-Bielack B, Branscheid D, Carrle D, Friedel G, Helmke K et al (2009) Second and subsequent recurrences of osteosarcoma: presentation, treatment, and outcomes of 249 consecutive cooperative osteosarcoma study group patients. J Clin Oncol Off J Am Soc Clin Oncol 27(4):557–565
32. Chou AJ, Merola PR, Wexler LH, Gorlick RG, Vyas YM, Healey JH et al (2005) Treatment of osteosarcoma at first recurrence after contemporary therapy: the Memorial Sloan-Kettering Cancer Center experience. Cancer 104(10):2214–2221
33. Bacci G, Briccoli A, Longhi A, Ferrari S, Mercuri M, Faggioli F et al (2005) Treatment and outcome of recurrent osteosarcoma: experience at Rizzoli in 235 patients initially treated with neoadjuvant chemotherapy. Acta Oncol 44(7):748–755
34. Bielack SS, Kempf-Bielack B, Winkler K (1996) Osteosarcoma: relationship of response to preoperative chemotherapy and type of surgery to local recurrence. J Clin Oncol Off J Am Soc Clin Oncol 14(2):683–684

35. Lewis IJ, Nooij MA, Whelan J, Sydes MR, Grimer R, Hogendoorn PC et al (2007) Improvement in histologic response but not survival in osteosarcoma patients treated with intensified chemotherapy: a randomized phase III trial of the European Osteosarcoma Intergroup. J Natl Cancer Inst 99(2):112–128
36. Jaffe N, Gorlick R (2008) High-dose methotrexate in osteosarcoma: let the questions surcease—time for final acceptance. J Clin Oncol Off J Am Soc Clin Oncol 26(27):4365–4366
37. Marina N, Bielack S, Whelan J, Smeland S, Krailo M, Sydes MR et al (2009) International collaboration is feasible in trials for rare conditions: the EURAMOS experience. Cancer Treat Res 152:339–353
38. Bielack SS, Smeland S, Whelan JS, Marina N, Jovic G, Hook JM et al (2015) Methotrexate, doxorubicin, and cisplatin (map) plus maintenance pegylated interferon Alfa-2b versus MAP alone in patients with resectable high-grade osteosarcoma and good histologic response to preoperative MAP: first results of the EURAMOS-1 good response randomized controlled trial. J Clin Oncol. doi:10.1200/JCO.2014.60.0734
39. Carli M, Passone E, Perilongo G, Bisogno G (2003) Ifosfamide in pediatric solid tumors. Oncology 65(Suppl 2):99–104
40. Ferrari S, Ruggieri P, Cefalo G, Tamburini A, Capanna R, Fagioli F et al (2012) Neoadjuvant chemotherapy with methotrexate, cisplatin, and doxorubicin with or without ifosfamide in nonmetastatic osteosarcoma of the extremity: an Italian sarcoma group trial ISG/OS-1. J Clin Oncol Off J Am Soc Clin Oncol 30(17):2112–2118
41. Bacci G, Briccoli A, Ferrari S, Longhi A, Mercuri M, Capanna R et al (2001) Neoadjuvant chemotherapy for osteosarcoma of the extremity: long-term results of the Rizzoli's 4th protocol. Eur J Cancer 37(16):2030–2039
42. Bruland Ø, Bauer H, Alvegaard T, Smeland S (2009) Treatment of osteosarcoma. The Scandinavian Sarcoma Group experience. Cancer Treat Res 152:309–318

12

Histone 3.3 hotspot mutations in conventional osteosarcomas: a comprehensive clinical and molecular characterization of six H3F3A mutated cases

Christian Koelsche[1,2*†], Daniel Schrimpf[1,2†], Lars Tharun[3], Eva Roth[4], Dominik Sturm[4,5], David T. W. Jones[4,5], Eva-Kristin Renker[6], Martin Sill[7], Annika Baude[8], Felix Sahm[1,2], David Capper[1,2], Melanie Bewerunge-Hudler[9], Wolfgang Hartmann[10], Andreas E. Kulozik[4], Iver Petersen[11], Uta Flucke[12], Hendrik W. B. Schreuder[13], Reinhard Büttner[3], Marc-André Weber[14], Peter Schirmacher[15], Christoph Plass[8], Stefan M. Pfister[4,5], Andreas von Deimling[1,2*‡] and Gunhild Mechtersheimer[15*‡]

Abstract

Background: Histone 3.3 (H3.3) hotspot mutations in bone tumors occur in the vast majority of giant cell tumors of bone (GCTBs; 96%), chondroblastomas (95%) and in a few cases of osteosarcomas. However, clinical presentation, histopathological features, and additional molecular characteristics of H3.3 mutant osteosarcomas are largely unknown.

Methods: In this multicentre, retrospective study, a total of 106 conventional high-grade osteosarcomas, across all age groups were re-examined for hotspot mutations in the H3.3 coding genes *H3F3A* and *H3F3B*. H3.3 mutant osteosarcomas were re-evaluated in a multidisciplinary manner and analyzed for genome-wide DNA-methylation patterns and DNA copy number aberrations alongside H3.3 wild-type osteosarcomas and *H3F3A* G34W/L mutant GCTBs.

Results: Six osteosarcomas (6/106) carried *H3F3A* hotspot mutations. No mutations were found in *H3F3B*. All patients with *H3F3A* mutant osteosarcoma were older than 30 years with a median age of 65 years. Copy number aberrations that are commonly encountered in high-grade osteosarcomas also occurred in *H3F3A* mutant osteosarcomas. Unlike a single osteosarcoma with a *H3F3A* K27M mutation, the DNA methylation profiles of *H3F3A* G34W/R mutant osteosarcomas were clearly different from H3.3 wild-type osteosarcomas, but more closely related to GCTBs. The most differentially methylated promoters between *H3F3A* G34W/R mutant and H3.3 wild-type osteosarcomas were in *KLLN/PTEN* ($p < 0.00005$) and *HIST1H2BB* ($p < 0.0005$).

*Correspondence: christian.koelsche@med.uni-heidelberg.de; Andreas.vonDeimling@med.uni-heidelberg.de; Gunhild.Mechtersheimer@med.uni-heidelberg.de
†Christian Koelsche and Daniel Schrimpf shared first authorship
‡Andreas von Deimling and Gunhild Mechtersheimer shared last authorship
[1] Department of Neuropathology, Institute of Pathology, University Hospital Heidelberg, Im Neuenheimer Feld 224, 69120 Heidelberg, Germany
[15] Department of General Pathology, Institute of Pathology, University Hospital Heidelberg, Im Neuenheimer Feld 224, 69120 Heidelberg, Germany

Conclusions: H3.3 mutations in osteosarcomas may occur in *H3F3A* at mutational hotspots. They are overall rare, but become more frequent in osteosarcoma patients older than 30 years. Osteosarcomas carrying *H3F3A* G34W/R mutations are associated with epigenetic dysregulation of *KLLN/PTEN* and *HIST1H2BB*.

Keywords: Mutation, H3.3, H3F3A, HIST1H2BB, KLLN, PTEN, Osteosarcoma, Giant cell tumor of bone, DNA methylation, Copy number alteration

Background

Osteosarcoma is a malignant bone forming neoplasm with a broad spectrum of morphologies [1]. Conventional high-grade osteosarcoma is the most common subtype and typically arises in the long bones of the extremities with a predilection to the metaphysis, although any bone of the skeleton may be affected. The incidence of osteosarcomas has a bimodal age distribution with a first peak in the second decade of life and a second smaller peak in older adults [1, 2].

The etiology of osteosarcomas is still largely unknown. However, several genetic syndromes (e.g. Li-Fraumeni and hereditary retinoblastoma) greatly increase the risk of developing osteosarcomas, especially in younger patients [3, 4]. Osteosarcomas in older patients often develop from a precursor bone lesion that is prone for malignant transformation (i.e. Paget disease) or may occur after radiation treatment for other diseases, typically after a latency period of several years [1, 5, 6].

The genomic landscape of osteosarcomas is complex [7]. A remarkable attribute of primary and secondary conventional osteosarcomas is their chromosomal instability leading to high aneuploidy [8]. Chromosomal regions frequently affected by somatic structural variations and copy number alterations often contain cell-cycle regulating genes such as *TP53*, *RB1*, or c-*MYC* [9, 10]. Sequencing studies revealed recurrent mutations affecting these genes, supporting their major role in osteosarcoma development [8]. However, the mutational make-up of osteosarcomas is versatile, as some osteosarcomas also present with molecular signatures reminiscent of BRCA1/2 deficient tumors [10]. *Chromothripsis*, a single cellular catastrophic event resulting in extensive DNA rearrangements and DNA copy number changes, has been observed in roughly one-third of osteosarcomas [11].

Alternative lengthening of telomeres (ALT), a telomere maintaining mechanism compensating progressive telomere attrition by homologous recombination of telomere sequences, is associated with chromosomal instability in osteosarcomas [12]. Almost all osteosarcomas utilize ALT, highlighting its particular importance in these tumors [8, 13]. Somatic mutations in the H3.3-ATRX-DAXX chromatin-remodeling pathway have been linked to ALT in different tumor entities [14, 15]. *ATRX* (α-thalassaemia/mental retardation syndrome X-linked) mutations, which result in a loss of its nuclear expression, were found in osteosarcomas at a frequency of 20–30% [8, 16]. Loss of DAXX (death-domain associated protein) expression has not yet been observed in any sarcoma [17]. However, a high frequency of mutations in the two genes encoding histone 3 variant 3 (H3.3) was revealed in certain bone tumors. Giant cell tumors of bone (GCTBs) almost always carry mutations in *H3F3A* at codon 34, whereas chondroblastomas are characterized by a high frequency of *H3F3B* mutations at codon 36 [18–20]. Little is known about H3.3 mutations in osteosarcomas. Previous studies described single high-grade osteosarcomas carrying H3.3 mutations, whereas other series did not. So the question arises whether osteosarcomas carrying H3.3 mutations really exist or might rather be malignant variants of GCTBs [8, 18–21].

The present study addresses these issues by determining the frequency of H3.3 mutations across the entire age spectrum in de novo high-grade osteosarcomas of the conventional type. Genome-wide DNA methylation and DNA copy number profiling was applied to gain further molecular insight into osteosarcomas carrying H3.3 mutations.

Methods

Tissues specimens

Tissue samples of 106 de novo high-grade osteosarcomas of the conventional type (86 primary tumors, 3 recurrences, 17 metastases) and 14 GCTBs, one of them with signs of malignancy in the local relapse two years after surgical treatment, serving as H3.3 G34 mutant bone tumor control group were collected from the Institutes of Pathology of the University Hospital Heidelberg, Cologne, Jena (Germany), and Nijemegen (the Netherlands). Patients' characteristics are outlined in Additional file 1: Table S1. Tissue samples were banked in the archives of the Department of Pathology and administered by the tissue bank of the National Center for Tumor Diseases (NCT), Heidelberg. Initial diagnoses were established by interdisciplinary oncology boards and were based on radiological findings, standard histopathological criteria in conjunction with immunohistochemical and molecular analyses according to the current WHO classification [1]. H3.3 mutant osteosarcomas were correlated with clinical information and were histologically and radiologically re-evaluated where available. The local ethics committee approved these analyses.

DNA extraction and Sanger sequencing of *H3F3A/B* mutational hotspots

Source material for DNA extraction was formalin-fixed and paraffin-embedded (FFPE) tumor tissue. Representative tumor tissue with highest available tumor content was chosen for genomic DNA isolation, as microscopically documented on H&E stained paraffin sections. In GCTBs, which are known for their prominent non-tumoral giant cell component, areas with predominant tumor cells (at least 70%) were selected for DNA extraction. The Maxwell® 16FFPE Plus LEV DNA Kit was applied on the automated Maxwell device (Promega, Madison, WI, USA) according to the manufacturer's instructions. Polymerase chain reaction was performed with 20 ng of DNA under conditions as previously described [19]. Two microliters of the amplification product were submitted to bidirectional sequencing using the BigDye Terminator v3.1 Sequencing Kit (Applied Biosystems, Foster City, CA, USA). Sequences were determined using an ABI 3500 Genetic Analyzer (Applied Biosystems) and the Sequence Pilot version 3.1 (JSI-Medisys, Kippenheim, Germany) software.

Genome-wide DNA methylation data generation and pre-processing

The Illumina Infinium HumanMethylation450 (450 k) array was used to assess the DNA methylation status of 482,421 CpG sites (Illumina, San Diego, USA), according to the manufacturer's instructions at the Genomics and Proteomics Core Facility of the German Cancer Research Center (DKFZ) Heidelberg. DNA methylation data were normalized by performing background correction and dye bias correction (shifting of negative control probe mean intensity to zero and scaling of normalization control probe mean intensity to 10,000, respectively). Probes targeting sex chromosomes, probes containing multiple single nucleotide polymorphism and those that could not be uniquely mapped were removed. In total, 438,370 probes were kept for analysis.

Unsupervised clustering, copy number profiling and identification of differentially methylated regions

For unsupervised hierarchical clustering, we selected 20,000 probes that showed the highest standard deviation (SD) of beta values across the entire dataset. Samples were hierarchically clustered using the 1-Pearson correlation coefficient as distance measure and average linkage. DNA methylation probes were reordered using Euclidian distance and complete linkage.

Copy number profiles were generated from the 450 k raw data using the 'conumee' R package and assessed manually. The dmpFinder method of the R package minfi was used for the identification of differentially methylated regions [22]. Both packages are available from the Bioconductor repository (http://www.bioconductor.org).

Statistical analysis

A two-sided t test was used to test for differences between the mean values for continuous variables. P values of less than 0.05 were considered significant.

Results

H3F3A mutations occur in high-grade osteosarcomas of elderly patients

Targeted sequencing of the two genes encoding histone 3 variant 3 (*H3F3A* and *H3F3B*) in 106 de novo high-grade osteosarcomas revealed six *H3F3A* mutant cases (Fig. 1a). One case carried a c.80A>T heterozygous mutation leading to an amino acid exchange of lysine by methionine at codon 27 (K27M). Another osteosarcoma presented with a c.100G>C heterozygous mutation leading to an exchange of glycin (G) by arginine (R) at codon 34. Four cases carried a c.100G>T mutation, one hemizygous and three heterozygous, leading to an exchange of glycin (G) by tryptophan (W). No mutation was detected in *H3F3B*. Patients with *H3F3A* mutant osteosarcomas were diagnosed at higher age (median age 65 years; range 34–75 years vs median age 18 years; range 2–86 years) and were significantly older ($p < 0.05$) compared to the control group of *H3F3A* mutant GCTBs (median age 29 years, range 18–75 years). Hence, the incidence increased from overall 5% (6/106) to 15% (6/40) in osteosarcoma patients over 30 years of age (Fig. 1b, c). The six *H3F3A* mutant osteosarcomas affected the long bones and were distributed similar to H3.3 wild-type osteosarcomas and GCTBs. They occurred in the proximal and distal femur, proximal tibia, proximal fibula, or the distal radius (Fig. 1c; Table 1).

Radiological features and histological patterns are indistinguishable between *H3F3A* mutant and H3.3 wild-type osteosarcomas

Radiological data was available for re-evaluation in five of six *H3F3A* mutant osteosarcomas (Fig. 2; Additional file 2: Figure S1). At radiographic examination, the tumors to a variable extent demonstrated a mixed pattern of sclerotic opacities with mineralization and lytic areas violating the cortex. The infiltrative growth pattern was associated with expansive growth into the surrounding soft tissue. Some cases presented with prominent soft-tissue masses (e.g. Fig. 2b). On MR imaging, where available, these masses partly wrapped around the circumference of the affected bone (Additional file 2: Figure S1).

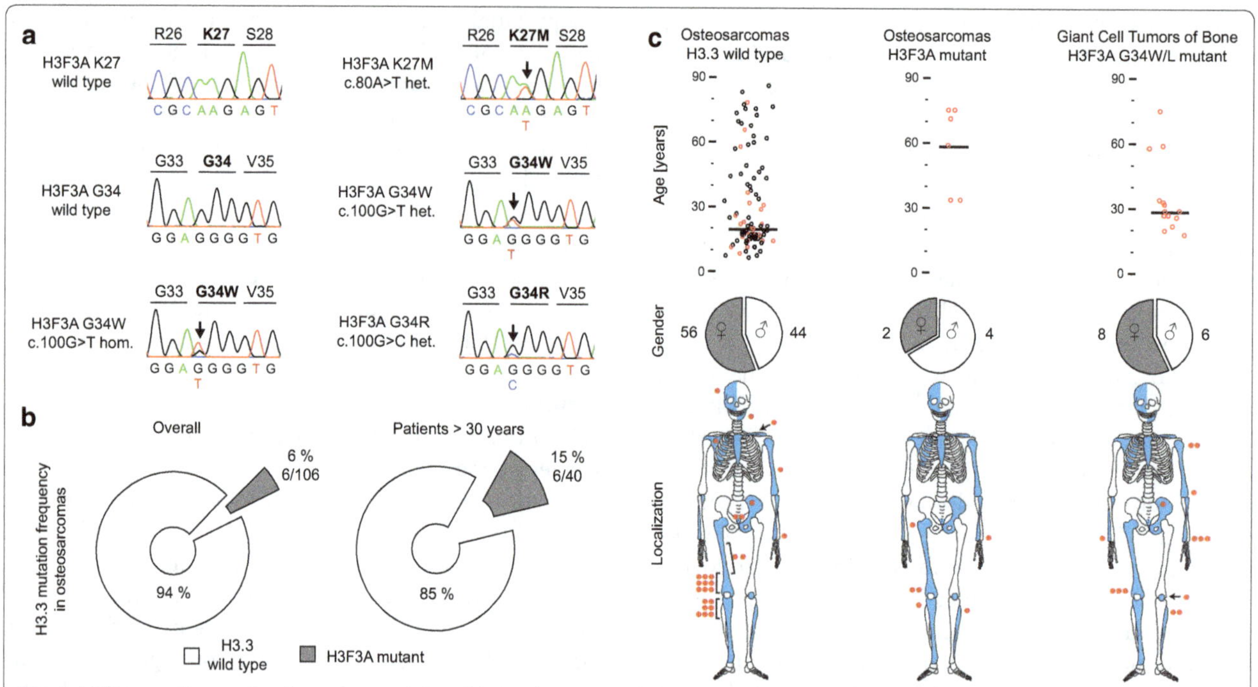

Fig. 1 *H3F3A* mutations and patients characteristics of the study group. **a** Chromatograms showing the *H3F3A* sequence spanning codon 27 and 34 illustrate the wild-type status and mutations that exchange either the amino acid lysine with methionine (K27M), glycin (G34) with tryptophan (G34W) or with arginine (G34R) **b** *Charts* show the overall incidence of *H3G3A* G34W mutations in our series of osteosarcomas over all age groups and in the group of patients older than 30 years. **c** Osteosarcomas are separated in wild-type and mutant regarding their *H3F3A* status. Giant cell tumors of bone act as control. The age distribution is demonstrated for each case. The *black bar* indicates the median age. Gender distribution is illustrated in the form of a diagram. The site of occurrence is only shown for cases that were further analysed for methylome and copy number profiling. Each *ring/dot* represents a case. *Red color codes* for cases that were further analyzed for methylome and copy number profiling

All six *H3F3A* mutant cases showed histological features indistinguishable from other conventional high-grade osteosarcomas (Fig. 2; Additional file 3: Figure S2). Mitotic activity was variable with presence of atypical mitotic figures. Neoplastic bone formation was observed in all *H3F3A* mutant osteosarcoma, although to a variable extent. Of note, giant cells were sparse to absent in all six *H3F3A* mutant osteosarcomas.

DNA methylation profiling separates *H3F3A* G34 mutant osteosarcomas from H3.3 wild-type counterparts

We next investigated the six *H3F3A* mutant and 28 H3.3 wild-type osteosarcomas and 14 *H3F3A* G34W/L mutant GCTBs for genome-wide DNA methylation patterns applying the 450 k DNA methylation array (Fig. 3). Unsupervised hierarchical clustering identified two distinct DNA methylation clusters (Fig. 3, upper panel). The first cluster was composed of H3.3 wild-type osteosarcomas and the single osteosarcoma carrying a *H3F3A* K27M mutation. This particular case was indistinguishable from that of H3.3 wild-type osteosarcomas. The second methylation cluster was composed of the five *H3F3A* G34 mutant osteosarcomas and the *H3F3A* G34 mutant GCTB control cases. Within this cluster, the 14 GCTBs showed the most homogeneous DNA methylation patterns and accordingly grouped together (Fig. 3, heatmap with dendrogram).

We next analyzed copy number data derived from the DNA methylation arrays (Fig. 3, lower panel). *H3F3A* mutant osteosarcomas frequently showed a gain of chromosome arm 8q involving the c-*MYC* locus (3/6) and a distinct deletion of 3q13.31 involving *LSAMP* (2/6). However, c-*MYC* amplification, 6p12–21 amplification or *chromothripsis*, both hallmark copy number alterations in osteosarcomas, were absent in all six *H3F3A* mutant osteosarcomas. GCTBs lacked any copy number alterations except for the single GCTB with a secondary malignant transformation (Additional file 4: Figure S3).

H3F3A G34 mutant osteosarcomas present with a promoter methylation phenotype

Given the distinct DNA methylation patterns of *H3F3A* G34 mutated osteosarcomas we next examined differences in DNA methylation in specific genomic regions (Fig. 4). *H3F3A* G34 mutant and H3.3 wild-type osteosarcomas showed widespread hypomethylation across the whole genome, especially in non-promoter regions, which was particularly prominent at centromeres and

Table 1 Clinical characteristics of the six H3.3 mutant osteosarcomas

#	H3.3 status	Age at Dx (years)	Gender	Tumor location	Histology	Therapy protocol	Follow-up (months)	Status	Comments
77896	H3F3A G34W	59	Male	Distal radius	Osteoblastic	According to EUROBOSS	52	Progressive disease	Local recurrence, lung, pleura and liver metastases 49 months after Dx
79428	H3F3A G34W	75	Male	Proximal tibia	Osteoblastic/fibroblastic	Unknown	–	Unknown	No further clinical documentation available
84676	H3F3A G34W	71	Male	Distal femur	Osteoblastic/fibroblastic	According to EUROBOSS	–	Unknown	No further clinical documentation available
84712	H3F3A G34W	34	Female	Proximal fibula	Osteoblastic	According to euramos	17	Complete remission	Initially dx of an aneurysmal bone cyst treated by excochleation with bone grafting, continuous progress, re-biopsy 1 year later with dx osteosarcoma
94316	H3F3A G34R	75	Male	Distal femur	Osteoblastic/fibroblastic	No further treatment	28	Death of disease	Local recurrence and lung metastases 19 months after Dx
94314	H3F3A K27M	34	Female	Proximal femur	Osteoblastic/fibroblastic	According to EURAMOS	27	Death of disease	Traumatic fracture of the proximal femur treated with nail osteosynthesis 7 years before Dx, bone and lung metastases, bone infection

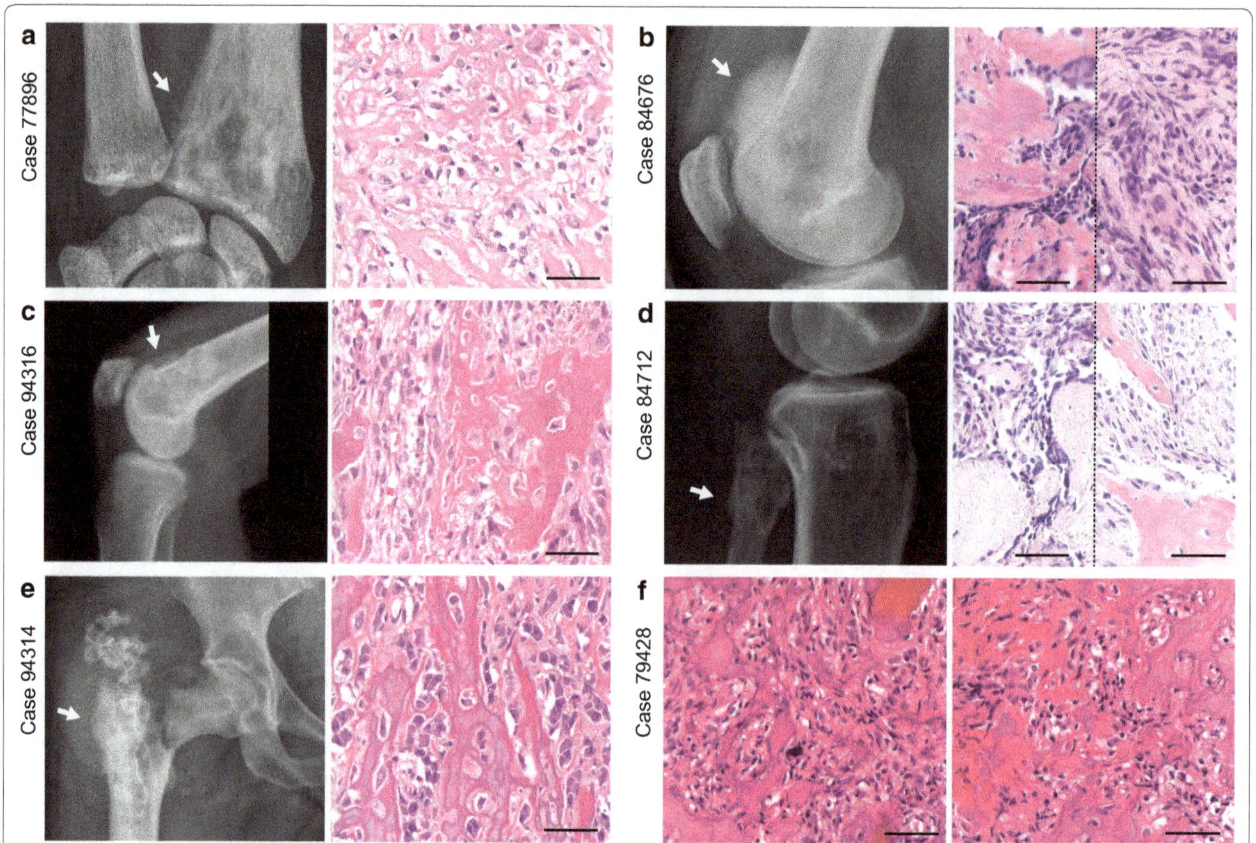

Fig. 2 Radiologic appearance and morphological phenotypes of *H3F3A* mutant osteosarcomas. **a** Anteroposterior radiograph of the left wrist shows a lesion in the epi- and metaphysis of the distal radius (*left*). Histology revealed an osteoblastic osteosarcoma with pronounced nuclear atypia, brisk mitotic activity and a compact, extensive sclerosing osteoid matrix. **b** Lateral radiograph of the right knee shows a lesion in the distal femoral metaphysis with infiltration of the epiphysis and prominent extension into the soft tissue. The tumor was composed of pleomorphic, relatively plump and focally spindle-shaped tumor cells depositing osteoid in plaques (mixed osteoblastic/fibroblastic osteosarcoma). **c** Lateral radiograph of the right knee shows a lesion in the distal femoral meta- and epiphysis with subchondral extension and infiltration of the joint. The tumor (mixed osteoblastic/fibroblastic osteosarcoma) was predominantly composed of plump tumor cells producing coarse plaque-like osteoid. **d** Lateral radiograph of the right knee shows a lesion in the proximal fibula (caput fibulae). Histology revealed an osteoblastic osteosarcoma with highly pleomorphic tumor cells focally producing coarse and lace-like osteoid deposits. **e** Anteroposterior radiograph of the hip joint shows a lesion in the intertrochanter and subtrochanter region of the proximal femur. Histology revealed a mixed osteoblastic/fibroblastic osteosarcoma with coarse osteoid production. **f** X-ray imaging of the proximal tibia was not available in case 79,428. Histologically this bone lesion presented as osteosarcoma (mixed osteoblastic/fibroblastic subtype) with neoplastic bone production that was focally arranged in a coarse lace-like pattern. Foci with necrosis and dystrophic calcification were noted. *White arrows* indicate the corresponding lesion (**a**–**e**). *Scale bars* equal 50 μm (**a**–**f**)

telomeres (Fig. 4a). However, *H3F3A* G34 mutant osteosarcomas had higher methylation levels in promoter regions compared with their H3.3 wild-type counterparts. Specifically, we found that the promoter region of the genes *HIST1H2BB* ($p < 0.00005$) and *KLLN/PTEN* ($p < 0.0005$) showed significantly higher methylation levels in *H3F3A* G34 mutant osteosarcomas (Fig. 4b).

Discussion

H3.3 mutations in bone tumors occur with an exceedingly high frequency in GCTBs and chondroblastomas [18, 19]. We herein present for the first time a clinical and molecular characterization of six *H3F3A* mutant de novo osteosarcomas and suggest that H3.3 mutations might define a distinct molecular subtype in the heterogeneous group of osteosarcomas.

Looking at the *H3F3A* G34 mutational status and the age distribution alone raises the possibility that the group of H3.3 mutant osteosarcomas may be composed of GCTBs presenting with Denosumab-therapy induced changes mimicking an osteosarcoma-like histology, may have undergone malignant progression or may represent the very rare de novo malignant variant of GCTBs, the latter two of which are known for their occurrence in elderly [23–25]. It is also evident that osteosarcomas in elderly are often of secondary origin, which would further argue in this direction [1].

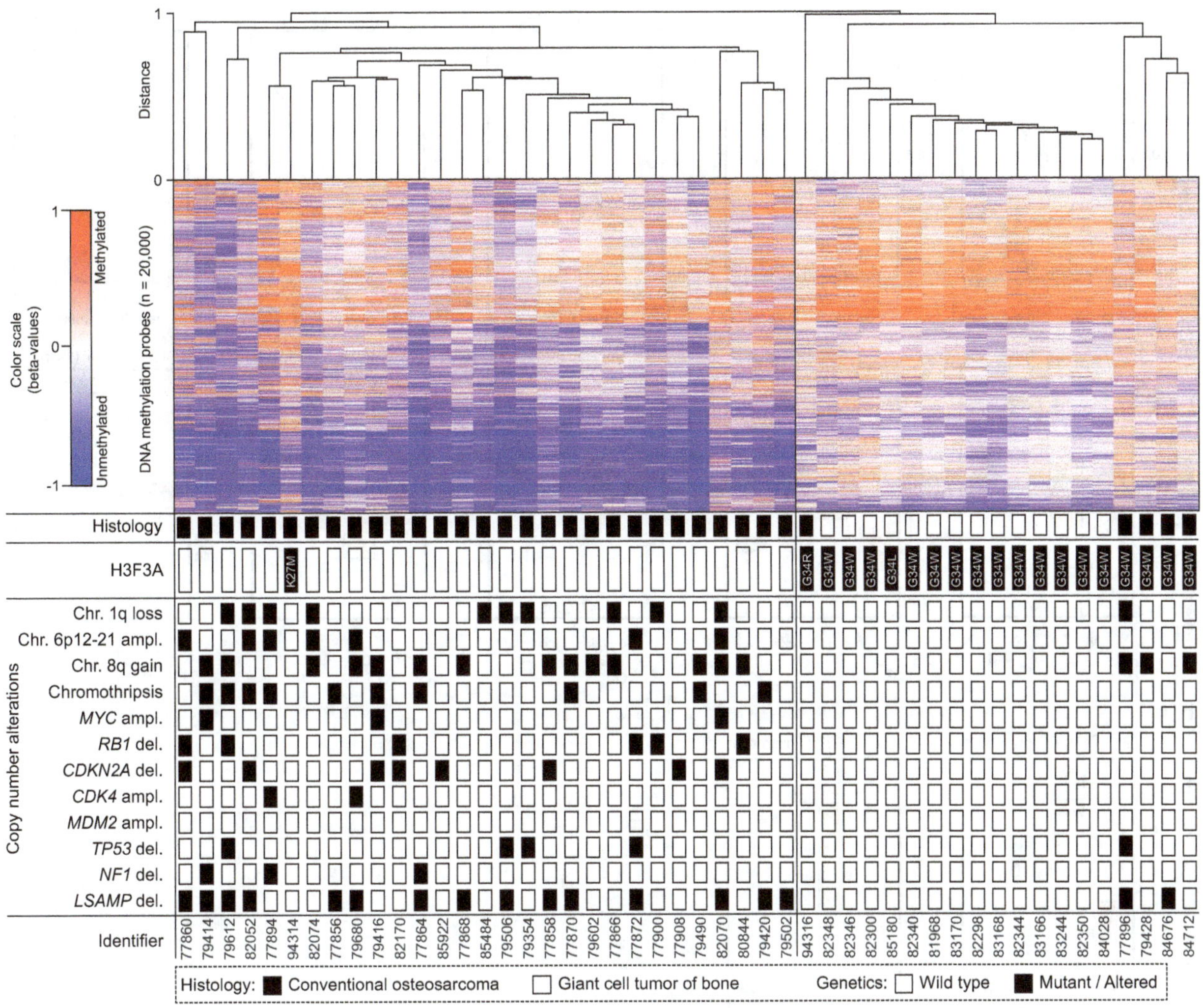

Fig. 3 Methylome and copy number profiling. The heatmap depicts unsupervised hierarchical clustering of methylation levels of the top 20,000 most variant probes (highest standard deviation). Each *row* represents a probe and each *column* a sample. The level of DNA methylation (beta value) is represented with a *colour scale* as depicted. Fourteen giant cell tumors of bone carrying H3F3A G34 mutations served as control group. For each sample ($n = 48$), histological diagnosis, mutational status of H3F3A and selected chromosomal copy number alterations are indicated

Indeed, at least for the *H3F3A* G34 mutant osteosarcoma cases presented here, there is no absolute certainty that they might not represent the most undifferentiated end in a spectrum of GCTB differentiation. However, none of the *H3F3A* mutant osteosarcomas presented with distinct radiological and histological features resembling GCTBs or its malignant variant, even though the radiologic appearance of malignant GCTBs may be challenging to distinguish from osteosarcomas [26]. We also cannot preclude with absolute certainty that areas reminiscent for a GCTB were missed due to a sampling bias in the *H3F3A* mutant osteosarcomas, which would argue for the extremely rare de novo malignant variant of GCTBs. However, this can be considered very unlikely. Furthermore, the patients were treated according to standard treatment protocols for osteosarcoma, thereby excluding Denosumab-induced changes. It is also unlikely that a precursor lesion underwent malignant transformation, since medical records were empty in this regard (Table 1). Therefore, taking all information into account, the diagnosis conventional osteosarcoma has been retained in all six H3.3 mutant cases. The *H3F3A* mutant osteosarcoma cases of this study predominantly occurred at higher patient age. This finding might explain why other osteosarcoma studies focusing on pediatric patients alone did not find H3.3 mutations at all [8]. However, larger future studies will be required to confirm that *H3F3A* mutant osteosarcomas are rare or even

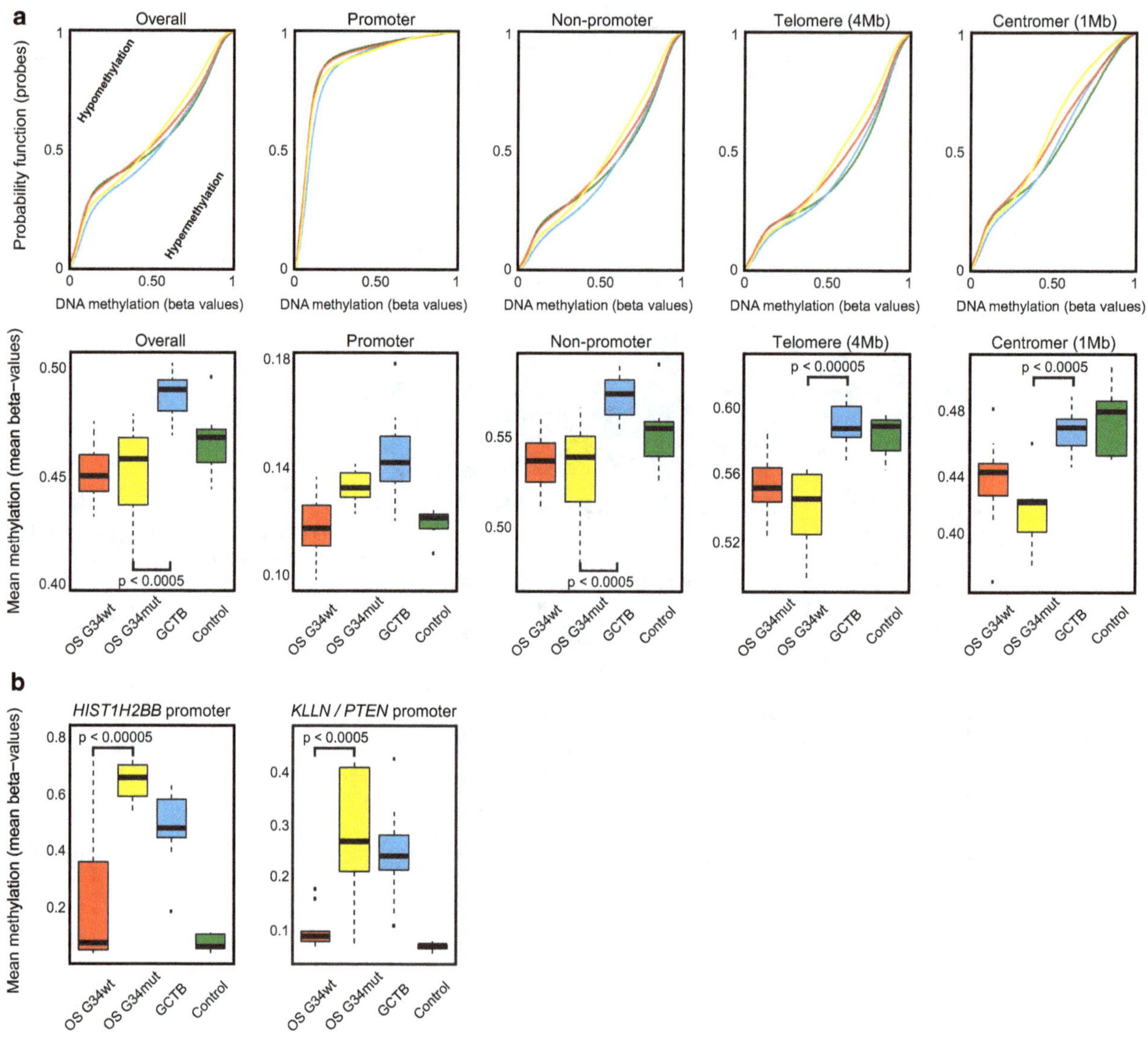

Fig. 4 Distinct DNA methylation patterns in osteosarcoma subgroups and giant cell tumors of bone. **a** *Upper part* the empirical cumulative distribution function for DNA methylation levels (beta-values) is plotted individually for each subgroup. *Lower part* DNA methylation levels (mean beta values) regarding different genomic regions of individual osteosarcoma methylation subgroups. **b** Further DNA methylation analyses identified the *HIST1H2BB* and *KLNN*/PTEN promoter as the most differentially methylated region when comparing the *H3F3A* G34 mutant osteosarcoma subgroup (OS G34) with the H3.3 wild-type osteosarcoma group (OS H3.3 wt). Significant difference to the *H3F3A* G34 mutant osteosarcoma subgroup (OS G34) is indicated

absent in children and adolescent patients. Interestingly, the age distribution of the H3.3 mutant osteosarcomas is in contrast to H3.3 mutant brain tumors, which typically present at younger age than their wild-type adult counterparts [15, 27]. This observation coupled with evidence from studies about *H3F3A* G34 mutant GCTBs might suggest an entity dependent age distribution of H3.3 mutant tumors [18, 19].

Our integrated approach revealed several molecular alterations in *H3F3A* mutant osteosarcomas that are typical for high-grade osteosarcomas. A homozygous deletion of 3q13.31 carrying the *LSAMP* gene was seen in two of the six *H3F3A* mutant osteosarcomas. One of them additionally carried a *TP53* deletion, a prominent tumor suppressor gene known to be involved in the development of osteosarcomas [8]. *LSAMP* is a tumor suppressor that is frequently inactivated in conventional osteosarcomas and linked to increased proliferation. It is also a predictor for an unfavorable biological behavior [28]. Thus, an aggressive biological behavior typically seen in conventional osteosarcomas might also be assumed for osteosarcomas with *H3F3A* mutations. Accordingly, three of four *H3F3A* mutant osteosarcoma patients with follow-up data available showed an unfavorable clinical course. Two patients died of the disease shortly after diagnosis. One patient presented with widespread metastases and progressive disease (Table 1).

A gain of chromosome 8q bearing the c-*MYC* locus was detected in three of six *H3F3A* mutant osteosarcomas. Amplification of c-*MYC*, a member of the *MYC* transcription factor family tightly involved in the modulation of gene expression and a strong oncogene, has been frequently observed in osteosarcomas [7, 8, 10]. It has also been shown in mice that c-*MYC* overexpression in mesenchymal bone stem cells may induce osteosarcomas [29]. The gain of 8q might confer a tumor propagating gene dosage effect, although c-*MYC* is not amplified in the six *H3F3A* mutant osteosarcomas presented here. In this context, other *MYC* gene family members may also be pivotal in the development of *H3F3A* mutant osteosarcomas. Brain tumors with *H3F3A* G34 mutations have been associated with an increased expression of *MYCN*, another transcription factor well known for its oncogenic capacity [30]. Expression analysis might give further insights whether c-*MYC*, *MYCN*, and/or other oncogenes orchestrate together in *H3F3A* G34 mutant osteosarcomas. The *H3F3A* G34 mutation alone will probably not be sufficient to induce osteosarcomas, since GCTBs carrying such mutations usually do not undergo malignant transformation [1].

We also detected one osteosarcoma with a *H3F3A* K27M mutation. This mutation was initially found in diffuse pontine midline gliomas and has recently been described also in other brain tumor entities [27, 31]. The *H3F3A* K27M mutation has been demonstrated leading to an enzymatic inhibition of EZH2 in brain tumors, a catalytic subunit of Polycomb Repressor Complex 2 [32]. EZH2 catalyzes methylation of histone H3 at lysine 27 and mediates gene silencing of target genes via local chromatin reorganization. Dysregulated EZH2 activity is seen in many cancer types [33]. We here report the first H3 K27M mutant tumor outside the nervous system. It therefore remains to be determined whether the underlying molecular mechanisms of H3.3 K27M mutation described in brain tumors may be adapted to other cancer types.

Interestingly, the DNA methylation analysis revealed several differing aspects in *H3F3A* mutant osteosarcomas compared to their H3.3 wild-type counterparts. Our data indicate that the DNA methylation signature of G34 mutant osteosarcomas is different to their conventional wild-type counterparts, but more closely related to GCTBs. However, this difference was only seen for G34 mutant cases, since the single K27M mutant osteosarcoma of this series was indistinguishable from H3.3 wild-type cases. On the one hand, the close relation between *H3F3A* G34 mutant osteosarcomas and *H3F3A* G34W/L mutant GCTBs might suggest a similar cell of origin. On the other hand, their close relation at the methylation level might reflect similar changes in the epigenetic landscape caused by the *H3F3A* G34 mutation or a responsible higher order mechanism. However, the DNA methylation profile of a dedifferentiated chondrosarcoma, in which we detected a *H3F3A* G34L mutation, was neither related to GCTBs, nor related to *H3F3A* G34W/R mutant osteosarcomas (data not shown).

In-depth analysis of the methylome data revealed widespread DNA hypomethylation in both, *H3F3A* G34 mutant and wild-type osteosarcomas. DNA hypomethylation is generally more pronounced with increased aggressiveness, which might explain this pattern [34]. However, the hypomethylation phenotype was less pronounced within the promoter regions in *H3F3A* G34 mutant osteosarcomas compared to their wild-type counterparts. The most differentially methylated promoter regions involved the *HIST1H2BB* and *KLNN/PTEN* genes. Both showed significantly higher methylation in *H3F3A* G34 mutant osteosarcomas. The role of *HIST1H2BB* in cancer is largely unknown. *HIST1H2BB* is an integral element of the nucleosome complex and hence, impaired expression could disrupt the physiological status and affect nucleosome remodelling [35]. *KLNN* is located juxtaposed to *PTEN* on chromosome 10q23 and both genes share the same promoter site [36]. Accordingly, both genes probably might be affected in *H3F3A* G34 mutant osteosarcomas. An important role of *PTEN* in the development of osteosarcomas has not been described yet, although *PTEN* alteration has been observed [8, 10, 37]. The neighboring gene *KLLN* functions at the pericentric region of chromosomes. *KLLN* organizes the heterochromatin by maintaining the H3K9 trimethylation and thereby contributes to chromosomal stability. Loss of *KLLN* resulted in the dysregulation of pericentric heterochromatin with consequent chromosomal instability and numerical chromosomal aberrations in vitro [38]. Interestingly, hypomethylation was significantly pronounced around the pericentric region in *H3F3A* G34 mutant osteosarcomas compared with GCTBs. Whether the hypomethylation phenotype may be a surrogate for pericentric instability and the role of *KLLN* in context of H3.3 mutations will be subject of future projects.

Conclusions

Taken together, our data confirm that detection of *H3F3A* mutations in bone tumors does not exclude malignancy in individual cases, especially in older patients. *H3F3A* mutant conventional high-grade osteosarcomas may radiologically, histologically and karyotypically be indistinguishable from conventional high-grade osteosarcomas, but present with distinct epigenetic features.

Additional files

Additional file 1: Table S1. Clinical information of the entire study cohort.

Additional file 2: Figure S1. Radiological data of *H3F3A* mutant osteosarcomas. (A) Case 77896: anteroposterior and lateral radiograph of the left wrist. Arrows indicate toward the lesion with permeated growth pattern (moth-eaten) and periosteal reaction. (B) Case 84676: anteroposterior and lateral radiograph (upper panel) with arrows indicating a large soft tissue mass with prominent mineralization and corresponding sagittal T1- and fat-saturated proton-weighted MR image (lower panel) of the right knee. The tumor involves the adjacent epiphyses through the epiphyseal growth plate (arrow). (C) Case 94316: anteroposterior and lateral radiograph (upper panel) and corresponding sagittal T1-weighted MR image (lower panel left) of the right knee. The MR image shows the intact bone cortex in the cranial part of the lesion (white arrows), but cortical disruption with "wrap-around" sign in the caudal part of the lesion. Anteroposterior radiograph (lower panel right) shows the local recurrence in the soft tissue adjacent to the knee joint prosthesis. (D) Case 84712: anteroposterior and lateral radiograph (upper panel) and corresponding axial T1-weighted and sagittal fat-saturated proton-weighted MR image (lower panel) of the right knee. Arrows indicate periosteal reaction and cortical disruption. (E) Case 94314: anteroposterior radiograph (upper panel, left), coronal fat-saturated T1-weighted MR image after administration of gadolinium contrast agent (upper panel, right) and coronal T1-weighted MR image (lower panel, left) of the right hip. Thickened bone cortex (arrow-heads, hypointense fibrous structure) is wrapped by the lesion. Anteroposterior radiograph (lower panel, right) after hip joint replacement.

Additional file 3: Figure S2. Histological data of the six *H3F3A* mutant osteosarcomas (A–F) and the single giant cell tumor of bone with malignant transformation (G).

Additional file 4: Figure S3. Copy number plots of the six *H3F3A* mutant osteosarcomas (A–F), one prototypic H3.3 wild-type osteosarcoma with an scattered chromosome arm 2q and the entire chromosome 3 indicating chromothripsis (G), one prototypical giant cell tumor of bone with a flat profile, (H) and one malignant giant cell tumor of bone with hints for a segmental loss of chromosome arm 2q and segmental gain of 7q (I). Abbreviations: OS = osteosarcoma; GCTB = giant cell tumor of bone.

Abbreviations

OS: osteosarcoma; GCTB: giant cell tumor of bone; H3.3: histone 3.3; ALT: alternative lengthening of telomeres; ATRX: α-thalassaemia/mental retardation syndrome X-linked; DAXX: death-domain associated protein; H3F3A/B: histone 3 family 3 A/B; DKFZ: german cancer research center; SD: standard deviation; MR: magnetic resonance.

Authors' contributions

CK conceived the project. DaS performed the bioinformatic. CK, LT, EKR, IP, UF, HWBS, RB, PS, SMP, AVD and GM collected the cases. CK, ER, AK and HWBS collected clinical data. CK, LT, WH, IP, UF, RB, PS, AVD and GM classified the cases. MAW re-evaluated the radiological data. CK, FS, AB, DC, MBH and CP performed the molecular analyses. CK, DoS, DTJ, MS, AVD and GM analysed the generated data. The manuscript was prepared by CK, AVD and GM. All authors read and approved the final manuscript.

Author details

[1] Department of Neuropathology, Institute of Pathology, University Hospital Heidelberg, Im Neuenheimer Feld 224, 69120 Heidelberg, Germany. [2] German Cancer Consortium (DKTK), CCU Neuropathology, German Cancer Research Center (DKFZ), Heidelberg, Germany. [3] Institute of Pathology, University Hospital Cologne, Cologne, Germany. [4] Department of Pediatric Oncology, Hematology and Immunology, University Hospital Heidelberg, Heidelberg, Germany. [5] Division of Pediatric Neurooncology, German Cancer Consortium (DKTK), German Cancer Research Center (DKFZ), Heidelberg, Germany. [6] Department of Orthopedics and Traumatology, University Hospital Heidelberg, Heidelberg, Germany. [7] Division of Biostatistics, German Cancer Research Center (DKFZ), Heidelberg, Germany. [8] Division of Epigenomics and Cancer Risk Factors, German Cancer Research Center (DKFZ), Heidelberg, Germany. [9] Genomics and Proteomics Core Facility, Microarray Unit, German Cancer Research Center (DKFZ), Heidelberg, Germany. [10] Gerhard Domagk Institute of Pathology, University Hospital, Muenster, Germany. [11] Institute of Pathology, University Hospital, Jena, Germany. [12] Department of Pathology, Radboud University Hospital, Nijmegen, The Netherlands. [13] Department of Orthopedics, Radboud University Hospital, Nijmegen, The Netherlands. [14] Clinic of Diagnostic and Interventional Radiology, University Hospital Heidelberg, Heidelberg, Germany. [15] Department of General Pathology, Institute of Pathology, University Hospital Heidelberg, Im Neuenheimer Feld 224, 69120 Heidelberg, Germany.

Acknowledgements

We thank the Tissue Bank of the National Center for Tumor Diseases Heidelberg for providing samples, and the Microarray unit of the Genomics and Proteomics Core Facility, German Cancer Research Center (DKFZ), for providing excellent methylation services. We also acknowledge financial support by Deutsche Forschungsgemeinschaft and Ruprecht-Karls-Universität Heidelberg within the funding program. The work was supported by the German Cancer Aid (70112499).

Competing interests

The authors declare that they have no competing interests.

References

1. Fletcher CDM, Bridge JA, Hogendoorn PCW, Mertens F. WHO classification of tumours of soft tissue and bone. Lyon: IARC Press; 2013.
2. Ducimetiere F, Lurkin A, Ranchere-Vince D, Decouvelaere AV, Peoc'h M, Istier L, Chalabreysse P, Muller C, Alberti L, Bringuier PP, Scoazec JY, Schott AM, Bergeron C, Cellier D, Blay JY, Ray-Coquard I. Incidence of sarcoma histotypes and molecular subtypes in a prospective epidemiological study with central pathology review and molecular testing. PLoS ONE. 2011;6:e20294.
3. Ognjanovic S, Olivier M, Bergemann TL, Hainaut P. Sarcomas in TP53 germline mutation carriers: a review of the IARC TP53 database. Cancer. 2012;118:1387–96.
4. MacCarthy A, Bayne AM, Brownbill PA, Bunch KJ, Diggens NL, Draper GJ, Hawkins MM, Jenkinson HC, Kingston JE, Stiller CA, Vincent TJ, Murphy MF. Second and subsequent tumours among 1927 retinoblastoma patients diagnosed in Britain 1951-2004. Br J Cancer. 2013;108:2455–63.
5. Hansen MF, Nellissery MJ, Bhatia P. Common mechanisms of osteosarcoma and Paget's disease. J Bone Miner Res. 1999;14(Suppl 2):39–44.
6. Huvos AG, Woodard HQ, Cahan WG, Higinbotham NL, Stewart FW, Butler A, Bretsky SS. Postradiation osteogenic sarcoma of bone and soft tissues. A clinicopathologic study of 66 patients. Cancer. 1985;55:1244–55.
7. Kansara M, Teng MW, Smyth MJ, Thomas DM. Translational biology of osteosarcoma. Nat Rev Cancer. 2014;14:722–35.
8. Chen X, Bahrami A, Pappo A, Easton J, Dalton J, Hedlund E, Ellison D, Shurtleff S, Wu G, Wei L, Parker M, Rusch M, Nagahawatte P, Wu J, Mao S, Boggs K, Mulder H, Yergeau D, Lu C, Ding L, Edmonson M, Qu C, Wang J, Li Y, Navid F, Daw NC, Mardis ER, Wilson RK, Downing JR, Zhang J, et al. Recurrent somatic structural variations contribute to tumorigenesis in pediatric osteosarcoma. Cell Rep. 2014;7:104–12.

9. Atiye J, Wolf M, Kaur S, Monni O, Bohling T, Kivioja A, Tas E, Serra M, Tarkkanen M, Knuutila S. Gene amplifications in osteosarcoma-CGH microarray analysis. Genes Chromosomes Cancer. 2005;42:158–63.
10. Kovac M, Blattmann C, Ribi S, Smida J, Mueller NS, Engert F, Castro-Giner F, Weischenfeldt J, Kovacova M, Krieg A, Andreou D, Tunn PU, Durr HR, Rechl H, Schaser KD, Melcher I, Burdach S, Kulozik A, Specht K, Heinimann K, Fulda S, Bielack S, Jundt G, Tomlinson I, Korbel JO, Nathrath M, Baumhoer D. Exome sequencing of osteosarcoma reveals mutation signatures reminiscent of BRCA deficiency. Nat Commun. 2015;6:8940.
11. Stephens PJ, Greenman CD, Fu B, Yang F, Bignell GR, Mudie LJ, Pleasance ED, Lau KW, Beare D, Stebbings LA, McLaren S, Lin ML, McBride DJ, Varela I, Nik-Zainal S, Leroy C, Jia M, Menzies A, Butler AP, Teague JW, Quail MA, Burton J, Swerdlow H, Carter NP, Morsberger LA, Iacobuzio-Donahue C, Follows GA, Green AR, Flanagan AM, Stratton MR, et al. Massive genomic rearrangement acquired in a single catastrophic event during cancer development. Cell. 2011;144:27–40.
12. Scheel C, Schaefer KL, Jauch A, Keller M, Wai D, Brinkschmidt C, van Valen F, Boecker W, Dockhorn-Dworniczak B, Poremba C. Alternative lengthening of telomeres is associated with chromosomal instability in osteosarcomas. Oncogene. 2001;20:3835–44.
13. Heaphy CM, Subhawong AP, Hong SM, Goggins MG, Montgomery EA, Gabrielson E, Netto GJ, Epstein JI, Lotan TL, Westra WH, Shih Ie M, Iacobuzio-Donahue CA, Maitra A, Li QK, Eberhart CG, Taube JM, Rakheja D, Kurman RJ, Wu TC, Roden RB, Argani P, De Marzo AM, Terracciano L, Torbenson M, Meeker AK. Prevalence of the alternative lengthening of telomeres telomere maintenance mechanism in human cancer subtypes. Am J Pathol. 2011;179:1608–15.
14. Heaphy CM, de Wilde RF, Jiao Y, Klein AP, Edil BH, Shi C, Bettegowda C, Rodriguez FJ, Eberhart CG, Hebbar S, Offerhaus GJ, McLendon R, Rasheed BA, He Y, Yan H, Bigner DD, Oba-Shinjo SM, Marie SK, Riggins GJ, Kinzler KW, Vogelstein B, Hruban RH, Maitra A, Papadopoulos N, Meeker AK. Altered telomeres in tumors with ATRX and DAXX mutations. Science. 2011;333:425.
15. Schwartzentruber J, Korshunov A, Liu XY, Jones DT, Pfaff E, Jacob K, Sturm D, Fontebasso AM, Quang DA, Tonjes M, Hovestadt V, Albrecht S, Kool M, Nantel A, Konermann C, Lindroth A, Jager N, Rausch T, Ryzhova M, Korbel JO, Hielscher T, Hauser P, Garami M, Klekner A, Bognar L, Ebinger M, Schuhmann MU, Scheurlen W, Pekrun A, Fruhwald MC, et al. Driver mutations in histone H3.3 and chromatin remodelling genes in paediatric glioblastoma. Nature. 2012;482:226–31.
16. Koelsche C, Renner M, Johann P, Leiss I, Sahm F, Schimmack S, Wardelmann E, Renker EK, Schirmacher P, Korshunov A, von Deimling A, Mechtersheimer G. Differential nuclear ATRX expression in sarcomas. Histopathology. 2016;68:738–45.
17. Liau JY, Lee JC, Tsai JH, Yang CY, Liu TL, Ke ZL, Hsu HH, Jeng YM. Comprehensive screening of alternative lengthening of telomeres phenotype and loss of ATRX expression in sarcomas. Mod Pathol. 2015;28:1545–54.
18. Behjati S, Tarpey PS, Presneau N, Scheipl S, Pillay N, Van Loo P, Wedge DC, Cooke SL, Gundem G, Davies H, Nik-Zainal S, Martin S, McLaren S, Goody V, Robinson B, Butler A, Teague JW, Halai D, Khatri B, Myklebost O, Baumhoer D, Jundt G, Hamoudi R, Tirabosco R, Amary MF, Futreal PA, Stratton MR, Campbell PJ, Flanagan AM. Distinct H3F3A and H3F3B driver mutations define chondroblastoma and giant cell tumor of bone. Nat Genet. 2013;45:1479–82.
19. Presneau N, Baumhoer D, Behjati S, Pillay N, Tarpey PS, Campbell PJ, Jundt G, Hamoudi R, Wedge DC, Van Loo P, Hassan AB, Khatri B, Ye H, Tirabosco R, Amary MF, Flanagan A. Diagnostic value of H3F3A mutations in giant cell tumour of bone compared to osteoclast-rich mimics. J Pathol. 2015;1:113–23.
20. Amary MF, Berisha F, Mozela R, Gibbons R, Guttridge A, O'Donnell P, Baumhoer D, Tirabosco R, Flanagan AM. The H3F3 K36M mutant antibody is a sensitive and specific marker for the diagnosis of chondroblastoma. Histopathology. 2016;69:121–7.
21. Joseph CG, Hwang H, Jiao Y, Wood LD, Kinde I, Wu J, Mandahl N, Luo J, Hruban RH, Diaz LA Jr, He TC, Vogelstein B, Kinzler KW, Mertens F, Papadopoulos N. Exomic analysis of myxoid liposarcomas, synovial sarcomas, and osteosarcomas. Genes Chromosomes Cancer. 2014;53:15–24.
22. Aryee MJ, Jaffe AE, Corrada-Bravo H, Ladd-Acosta C, Feinberg AP, Hansen KD, Irizarry RA. Minfi: a flexible and comprehensive bioconductor package for the analysis of Infinium DNA methylation microarrays. Bioinformatics. 2014;30:1363–9.
23. Nascimento AG, Huvos AG, Marcove RC. Primary malignant giant cell tumor of bone: a study of eight cases and review of the literature. Cancer. 1979;44:1393–402.
24. Gong L, Liu W, Sun X, Sajdik C, Tian X, Niu X, Huang X. Histological and clinical characteristics of malignant giant cell tumor of bone. Virchows Arch. 2012;460:327–34.
25. Wojcik J, Rosenberg AE, Bredella MA, Choy E, Hornicek FJ, Nielsen GP, Deshpande V. Denosumab-treated giant cell tumor of bone exhibits morphologic overlap with malignant giant cell tumor of bone. Am J Surg Pathol. 2016;40:72–80.
26. Chakarun CJ, Forrester DM, Gottsegen CJ, Patel DB, White EA, Matcuk GR Jr. Giant cell tumor of bone: review, mimics, and new developments in treatment. Radiographics. 2013;33:197–211.
27. Sturm D, Witt H, Hovestadt V, Khuong-Quang DA, Jones DT, Konermann C, Pfaff E, Tonjes M, Sill M, Bender S, Kool M, Zapatka M, Becker N, Zucknick M, Hielscher T, Liu XY, Fontebasso AM, Ryzhova M, Albrecht S, Jacob K, Wolter M, Ebinger M, Schuhmann MU, van Meter T, Fruhwald MC, Hauch H, Pekrun A, Radlwimmer B, Niehues T, von Komorowski G, et al. Hotspot mutations in H3F3A and IDH1 define distinct epigenetic and biological subgroups of glioblastoma. Cancer Cell. 2012;22:425–37.
28. Pasic I, Shlien A, Durbin AD, Stavropoulos DJ, Baskin B, Ray PN, Novokmet A, Malkin D. Recurrent focal copy-number changes and loss of heterozygosity implicate two noncoding RNAs and one tumor suppressor gene at chromosome 3q13.31 in osteosarcoma. Cancer Res. 2010;70:160–71.
29. Shimizu T, Ishikawa T, Sugihara E, Kuninaka S, Miyamoto T, Mabuchi Y, Matsuzaki Y, Tsunoda T, Miya F, Morioka H, Nakayama R, Kobayashi E, Toyama Y, Kawai A, Ichikawa H, Hasegawa T, Okada S, Ito T, Ikeda Y, Suda T, Saya H. c-MYC overexpression with loss of Ink4a/Arf transforms bone marrow stromal cells into osteosarcoma accompanied by loss of adipogenesis. Oncogene. 2010;29:5687–99.
30. Bjerke L, Mackay A, Nandhabalan M, Burford A, Jury A, Popov S, Bax DA, Carvalho D, Taylor KR, Vinci M, Bajrami I, McGonnell IM, Lord CJ, Reis RM, Hargrave D, Ashworth A, Workman P, Jones C. Histone H3.3. mutations drive pediatric glioblastoma through upregulation of MYCN. Cancer Discov. 2013;3:512–9.
31. Gessi M, Capper D, Sahm F, Huang K, von Deimling A, Tippelt S, Fleischhack G, Scherbaum D, Alfer J, Juhnke BO, von Hoff K, Rutkowski S, Warmuth-Metz M, Chavez L, Pfister SM, Pietsch T, Jones DT, Sturm D. Evidence of H3 K27 M mutations in posterior fossa ependymomas. Acta Neuropathol. 2016;132:635–7.
32. Bender S, Tang Y, Lindroth AM, Hovestadt V, Jones DT, Kool M, Zapatka M, Northcott PA, Sturm D, Wang W, Radlwimmer B, Hojfeldt JW, Truffaux N, Castel D, Schubert S, Ryzhova M, Seker-Cin H, Gronych J, Johann PD, Stark S, Meyer J, Milde T, Schuhmann M, Ebinger M, Monoranu CM, Ponnuswami A, Chen S, Jones C, Witt O, Collins VP, et al. Reduced H3K27me3 and DNA hypomethylation are major drivers of gene expression in K27M mutant pediatric high-grade gliomas. Cancer Cell. 2013;24:660–72.
33. Volkel P, Dupret B, Le Bourhis X, Angrand PO. Diverse involvement of EZH2 in cancer epigenetics. Am J Transl Res. 2015;7:175–93.
34. Ehrlich M. DNA hypomethylation in cancer cells. Epigenomics. 2009;1:239–59.
35. Zink LM, Hake SB. Histone variants: nuclear function and disease. Curr Opin Genet Dev. 2016;37:82–9.
36. Bennett KL, Mester J, Eng C. Germline epigenetic regulation of KILLIN in Cowden and Cowden-like syndrome. JAMA. 2010;304:2724–31.
37. Freeman SS, Allen SW, Ganti R, Wu J, Ma J, Su X, Neale G, Dome JS, Daw NC, Khoury JD. Copy number gains in EGFR and copy number losses in PTEN are common events in osteosarcoma tumors. Cancer. 2008;113:1453–61.
38. Nizialek EA, Sankunny M, Niazi F, Eng C. Cancer-predisposition gene KLLN maintains pericentric H3K9 trimethylation protecting genomic stability. Nucleic Acids Res. 2016;44:3586–94.

13

UK guidelines for the management of bone sarcomas

Craig Gerrand[1*], Nick Athanasou[2], Bernadette Brennan[3], Robert Grimer[4], Ian Judson[5], Bruce Morland[6], David Peake[7], Beatrice Seddon[8], Jeremy Whelan[8] and On behalf of the British Sarcoma Group

Abstract

This document is an update of the British Sarcoma Group guidelines published in 2010. The aim is to provide a reference standard for the clinical care of patients in the UK with bone sarcomas. Recent recommendations by the European Society of Medical Oncology, The National Comprehensive Cancer Network and The National Institute for Health and Care Excellence have been incorporated, and the literature since 2010 reviewed. The standards represent a consensus amongst British Sarcoma Group members in 2015. It is acknowledged that these guidelines will need further updates as care evolves. The key recommendations are that bone pain or a palpable mass should always lead to further investigation and that patients with clinico-radiological findings suggestive of a primary bone tumour at any site in the skeleton should be referred to a specialist centre and managed by a fully accredited bone sarcoma multidisciplinary team. Treatment recommendations are provided for the major tumour types and for localised, metastatic and recurrent disease. Follow up schedules are suggested.

Background

Rationale and objective of guidelines

Bone sarcomas are uncommon malignancies and it was recognised more than 30 years ago that their management should be centralized. Following various NHS reforms, the diagnosis and surgical treatment of primary bone sarcomas is now commissioned by the NHS England Highly Specialized Commissioning Group [1] in five centres in England. However, other treatments such as chemotherapy and radiotherapy may be delegated to other centres. Arrangements in Scotland and Northern Ireland differ. The surgical treatment of patients in Wales takes place in specialist centres in England, with other modalities of treatment delivered within Wales.

This reference document aims to improve the quality of care for patients with bone tumours by identifying and informing key management decisions and is an update of the 2010 British Sarcoma Group (BSG) guidelines [2].

*Correspondence: Craig.Gerrand@nuth.nhs.uk

[1] Newcastle upon Tyne Hospitals NHS Foundation Trust, Freeman Hospital, Newcastle upon Tyne NE7 7DN, UK

Methods

In developing these guidelines, the following were consulted: The National Comprehensive Cancer Network (NCCN) Clinical Practice Guidelines [3]; ESMO/European Network Working Group, Clinical Practice Guidelines for Bone Sarcomas [4]; National Institute for Health and Care Excellence (NICE) Quality Standard [QS78] Sarcoma [5] and Suspected cancer: recognition and referral guideline [NG12] [6] and the published literature from 2010 to 2015. The authors considered the applicability to UK practice and reached consensus on the content. The document was then circulated widely within the British Sarcoma Group for comment and approval.

Scope of guidelines

The guidelines apply to all primary bone sarcomas (and giant cell tumours of bone) arising in any skeletal location. These guidelines consider clinical effectiveness, and include treatments to which a specialist bone sarcoma multidisciplinary team (MDT) in the UK should have access. While representing a broad consensus in 2015, these guidelines will require updating as treatment evolves. Haemopoietic tumours of bone, rehabilitation, prosthetic services and palliative care are not included.

Classification of bone sarcomas

Primary malignant bone tumours comprise 0.2 % of all cancers diagnosed in England and have an annual incidence of around 7.9 per million [7]. On average, 380 people were diagnosed with primary bone sarcomas each year in England between 1985 and 2009. Therefore, a General Practitioner (GP) is unlikely to see a patient with a bone sarcoma in a working lifetime. Delays in diagnosis are common. Reducing delays would almost certainly lead to improved survival outcomes and less extensive surgery [8].

Despite their rarity, primary malignant bone tumours comprise approximately 5 % of all childhood cancers in European Countries [7, 9] and include two major cancers of children and young adults: osteosarcoma and Ewing sarcoma [7]. In children under 5 years of age, a destructive bone lesion is more likely to be metastatic neuroblastoma or eosinophilic granuloma [4, 10]. Chondrosarcoma is more common in middle aged and elderly people [7].

In adults, especially those over 40 years of age, metastatic carcinomas (usually from lung, breast, thyroid, kidney or prostate) and haemopoietic malignancies (e.g. plasma cell tumour or lymphoma) in bone considerably outnumber primary bone tumours. At any age the possibility of a benign lesion or infection must be considered [11]. If there is diagnostic uncertainty, it should be assumed the patient has a primary bone sarcoma until proven otherwise [12].

There has been no significant improvement in 5-year overall survival rates for patients with bone sarcomas over the past 25–30 years, with rates static at between 53 and 55 % [7, 13].

A classification of bone sarcomas adapted from the World Health Organization (WHO) classification of primary bone tumours is shown in Table 1 [14].

Table 1 Classification of malignant primary bone tumours (adapted from WHO classification [14])

Chondrogenic tumours	(1) Atypical cartilaginous tumour/ chondrosarcoma (grade I) (2) Chondrosarcoma (grades II/III) (3) Dedifferentiated chondrosarcoma (4) Mesenchymal chondrosarcoma (5) Clear cell chondrosarcoma
Osteogenic tumours	(1) Low-grade central osteosarcoma (2) Conventional (high-grade) osteosarcoma (chondroblastic fibroblastic osteoblastic) (3) Telangiectatic osteosarcoma (4) Small cell osteosarcoma (5) Secondary osteosarcoma (6) Parosteal osteosarcoma (7) Periosteal osteosarcoma (8) High-grade surface osteosarcoma
Notochordal tumours	Chordoma
Vascular tumours	(1) Epithelioid haemangioendothelioma (2) Angiosarcoma
Other malignant mesenchymal tumours	Fibrosarcoma, Leiomyosarcoma, Liposarcoma etc.
Miscellaneous tumours	(1) Ewing sarcoma (2) Adamantinoma (3) Undifferentiated high-grade pleomorphic sarcoma of bone

Although some inherited and acquired factors are associated with the development of primary bone tumours, a cause cannot be identified in the majority of patients [15, 16].

The 5-year relative survival for patients diagnosed in England in 1985–2004 is considerably lower than that reported within the US Surveillance, Epidemiology and End Results (SEER) programme (66 %) [17]. This may reflect the fact that patients in the SEER programme are younger (30 % of NCIN patients were >65 years, compared with 21 % of SEER patients: 22 % of NCIN patients were <19 years, compared with 29 % of SEER patients). Furthermore, the SEER programme does not specify which morphological sub-types are included. Further investigation is required [7].

Osteosarcoma

Osteosarcoma is the second most frequent primary cancer of bone and accounts for over 10 % of all solid cancers in adolescents (age 15–19). Another peak in incidence occurs in the seventh and eighth decades of life [7, 13]. It is slightly more common in males (male to female ratio 1.4:1.0) [7]. Survival rates are significantly higher in younger patients (5-year survival, <40 years 53 % vs. >40 years 22 %; $p < 0.0001$) [7, 13].

Osteosarcoma usually arises in the metaphysis of an extremity long bone, most commonly around the knee [18, 19]. Some tumours (predominantly in adults) arise in the axial skeleton, pelvis or craniofacial bones. Risk factors for osteosarcoma include previous radiation therapy, Paget's disease of bone and germline abnormalities such as Li-Fraumeni syndrome, Werner syndrome, Rothmund -Thomson syndrome and familial retinoblastoma [20, 21]. The temporal association of osteosarcoma with the pubertal growth spurt and the location in the metaphysis of long bones suggest an association with rapid bone growth.

Ewing sarcoma

Ewing sarcoma is the second most common primary malignant bone tumour in children and adolescents, but is also seen in adults. The median age at diagnosis is around 15 years and in the UK there is a male preponderance of 1.5:1 [7]. It is less common in people of Chinese or Black African origin. Identification of chromosomal translocations specific to Ewing sarcoma e.g. (t11;22) have provided a useful diagnostic criterion. In recent years undifferentiated bone sarcomas with morphological features of Ewing sarcoma but with uncharacteristic translocations e.g. CIC-DUX have been described. Although clinical information is limited these appear to respond less well than Ewing sarcoma to chemotherapy and may have an unfavourable prognosis [22].

The most frequent anatomical sites of involvement of Ewing sarcoma are the long bones, pelvis, ribs and vertebral column. All forms of Ewing Sarcoma are high grade [23, 24].

Chondrosarcoma

Chondrosarcoma most commonly presents between 30 and 60 years of age [7]. The ageing UK population means that chondrosarcoma has become the most common bone sarcoma, ahead of osteosarcoma [25]. Differentiating between an atypical enchondroma and a low grade chondrosarcoma can be extremely difficult and has led to these tumours being categorised together in the WHO classification as atypical cartilaginous tumour/chondrosarcoma grade I. It is considered to be a tumour of intermediate malignancy, most often behaving in a locally aggressive fashion and rarely metastasising. Care must be taken not to overtreat benign tumours or undertreat malignant ones [26].

Most chondrosarcomas are located in long bones but they also arise in flat bones (e.g. pelvis, rib and scapula). Chondrosarcomas arising in pre-existing benign lesions such as osteochondromas and enchondromas are known as secondary peripheral chondrosarcomas and secondary central chondrosarcomas respectively. The risk of developing chondosarcoma in solitary osteochondromas and enchondromas is uncertain, but is increased when there are multiple lesions or when lesions are located in the axial skeleton, particularly the pelvis [27].

The majority of primary chondrosarcomas are low- rather than high-grade [28] and are of the conventional subtype. Rare subtypes include mesenchymal chondrosarcoma and clear cell chondrosarcoma. In rare circumstances, conventional chondrosarcomas "dedifferentiate" into very high-grade tumours (so-called de-differentiated chondrosarcoma) [29–31] with a poor prognosis.

Undifferentiated pleomorphic sarcoma of bone

Undifferentiated pleomorphic sarcoma (UPS) of bone is a relatively recent term for sarcomas that do not exhibit a specific line or pattern of differentiation (previously termed malignant fibrous histiocytoma of bone) [32, 33]. UPS of bone is typically high-grade with metastatic rates of at least 50 % [33]. Treatment usually involves neoadjuvant therapy followed by wide excision. Its chemosensitivity and survival rate are similar to osteosarcoma [34]. Occasionally, an undifferentiated pleomorphic sarcoma is found to be a dedifferentiated chondrosarcoma or osteosarcoma after resection.

Chordoma

Chordomas develop from persistent notochordal elements, and originate from the sacrum (50 %), skull base (30 %), and mobile spine (20 %). Extraskeletal tumours are very rare. Chordoma is a locally invasive, typically low-grade tumour but infrequently (around 5 %) highly malignant dedifferentiated cases occur [35]. Metastases develop in 30–40 % of patients, typically late in the disease trajectory and usually after local recurrence. Metastases can occur in lung, liver, bone, subcutis, lymph nodes and other sites.

Adamantinoma

Adamantinoma is a rare, low-grade malignant neoplasm that arises in the tibia, fibula or both bones, although it has rarely been reported in other bones [36]. Adamantinoma accounts for 0.3–1 % of all malignant bone tumours and occurs mostly in young to middle-aged adults (20–40 years of age), with a male-to female ratio of 1.3:1. The tibial shaft (medial or distal) is most commonly affected. The tumour has lytic and sometimes destructive areas which can lead to fracture [37]. Recurrence is late (can be >20 years) but frequent (about 30 %) after incomplete excision. The rate of metastasis is 10 % to 20 %, usually to lung [36].

Giant cell tumour of bone

Giant cell tumours of bone are generally considered benign but locally aggressive tumours; there is a low risk of metastasis, particularly after local recurrence [38]. Giant cell tumours rarely appear before skeletal maturity and most often affect patients between 20 and 30 years of age [39]. Tumours characteristically occur at the end of a long bone in a juxtaarticular location. Histologically tumours contain a proliferation of mononuclear stromal cells amongst which are scattered numerous multinucleated giant cells that have been identified as osteoclasts recruited by the RANK-ligand expressing stromal cells. Tumours cause local destruction of bone and may be associated with a soft tissue mass or pathological fracture [40].

Other malignant mesenchymal tumours

Very rarely malignant mesenchymal tumours that more commonly arise in soft tissues can present as a primary (often spindle cell) sarcoma of bone. These include spindle cell malignancies such as leiomyosarcoma and fibrosarcoma. In general, spindle cell sarcomas are thought to represent between 2 and 5 % of primary bone malignancies. Spindle cell sarcomas arise in a similar age group to chondrosarcoma but the skeletal distribution is similar to osteosarcoma. There is a high incidence of fracture at presentation. Associations with pre-existing conditions (e.g. Paget's disease or bone infarct) or previous irradiation have been reported [41].

Presentation and referral

The most common symptom of a primary malignant bone tumour is pain, which may gradually increase in intensity [42]. Bone pain at night should always be considered a 'red flag' symptom requiring further investigation. Pain levels may vary and a bone swelling or soft tissue mass may develop later. Even high-grade tumours do not usually cause systemic symptoms; when present these may indicate metastatic disease [42]. The average duration of symptoms is 3 months, although 6 months or longer is not uncommon [8, 43, 44].

A plain x-ray is the first investigation of choice. The presence of any of the following X-ray features is suggestive, but not diagnostic, of a primary bone tumour and should be investigated further, usually following urgent referral to a bone sarcoma MDT:

- Bone destruction
- New bone formation
- Periosteal swelling
- Soft tissue swelling

Additionally, it must be remembered that a 'normal' x-ray does not rule out bone sarcoma; persistent bone pain/night pain should still require urgent MRI scan/referral to a sarcoma centre. Hip and knee pain in children is often attributed to sporting injury with early 'normal' looking x-rays.

In all patients a full clinical history should be taken (including duration, intensity and diurnal variation of pain, prior benign or malignant tumours, family history and previous radiotherapy) and examination performed (with specific attention to the size, consistency, mobility, and location in relation to bone of any mass and palpation of regional and local lymph nodes), considering the most likely diagnosis for a patient of a given age. Recent injury does not rule out a primary bone tumour and should not prevent further examination.

In patients under 40 years of age, investigations prior to referral should include X-ray of the affected bone (in two planes) and simple blood tests [full blood count (FBC), erythrocyte sedimentation rate (ESR), biochemical profile including alkaline phosphatase (ALP)]. Further urgent imaging of the local site with magnetic resonance imaging (MRI) or computed tomography (CT) is usually required, prior to or after referral [8].

In patients over 40 years of age more extensive investigation before referral is appropriate (if it can be done quickly) as the most likely diagnosis is of metastatic carcinoma in bone. Appropriate investigations include CT of chest, abdomen and pelvis, isotope bone scan, and myeloma screen. If the bone lesion is solitary the patient should be referred to a reference centre to exclude a primary malignant bone tumour.

All patients with a possible diagnosis of a primary bone tumour should be referred urgently under the 2 week wait pathway to a fully accredited bone sarcoma MDT [4, 45, 46]. This core principle is embedded in the NICE 'Improving Outcomes for People with Sarcomas' guidance [47], 'Children and Young People with Cancer' guidance [48] and the NICE Quality Standard QS78 Sarcoma [5].

Referral before biopsy is essential to ensure optimal diagnosis and management [49, 50] since poorly planned or executed biopsies can compromise future treatment [42].

Networks should ensure GPs are aware of and comply with the urgent referral criteria in the NICE Suspected cancer: recognition and referral guideline NG12 [6] and that GPs and hospital doctors are aware of the local diagnostic pathways for patients with suspected primary bone tumours. There are also referral guidelines specific to Scotland which can be found at healthcare improvements Scotland [51].

UK reference centres

Royal National Orthopaedic Hospital Stanmore, London

rno-tr.LondonSarcomaService@nhs.net

Royal Orthopaedic Hospital Northfield, Birmingham

Nuffield Orthopaedic Centre Oxford

North of England Bone and Soft Tissue Tumour Service,
Freeman Hospital
Newcastle upon Tyne

Greater Manchester and Oswestry Sarcoma Service,
Robert Jones and Agnes Hunt Hospital
Oswestry

Scotland: The Scottish Sarcoma Network,
Glasgow Royal Infirmary
Glasgow G4 0SF

In Scotland sarcomas are managed under the umbrella of the Scottish Sarcoma Network, which includes centres in Edinburgh, Glasgow and Aberdeen with a shared MDT. Links to the three national networks can be found at the West of Scotland Cancer Network (WoSCAN) [52].

Northern Ireland Sarcoma Network
Musgrave Park Hospital
Stockmans Lane
Belfast
BT9 7JB

Key recommendations

- The most common symptom of a primary bone tumour is pain which may gradually increase or vary in intensity. Bone pain at night should always be considered a 'red flag' symptom requiring further investigation.
- The presence of pain or a palpable mass arising from any bone requires further investigation. A plain X-ray is the first investigation of choice.
- The presence of radiological features including bone destruction, new bone formation, periosteal swelling and/or soft tissue swelling are suggestive, but not diagnostic, of a bone tumour and require further investigation.
- Networks should ensure that GPs are aware of and comply with the urgent referral criteria in the NICE 'Suspected cancer: recognition and referral guidlines' and 'Cancer referral guidelines for Scotland' and that GPs and hospital doctors are aware of the diagnostic pathways for patients with suspected primary bone tumours.
- All patients with a provisional histological and/or radiological diagnosis of bone sarcoma should have their diagnosis reviewed by a specialist sarcoma pathologist and/or radiologist, both of whom should be part of a bone sarcoma MDT.

Investigation

Imaging

All patients should have X-rays in two planes at presentation.

Further local site imaging should be with MRI [42], including the whole anatomical compartment, the involved bone and adjacent joints [53]. CT is helpful if there is diagnostic uncertainty or MRI is contraindicated, and may better visualise areas of microcalcification, periosteal bone formation and cortical destruction. CT is routinely used in addition to MRI for pelvic tumours. Dynamic contrast enhanced MRI may identify high-grade areas within a chondrosarcoma, and therefore guide biopsy.

Staging investigations for patients with confirmed primary malignant bone tumours should include chest radiography and/or CT. CT is the technique of choice for imaging the chest, pelvis and mandible [53–55]. If indeterminate nodules are detected in the lungs, an interval scan may be indicated. All suspicious chest CTs should be reported by a radiologist experienced in bone sarcoma or sent to an MDT for review.

Whole body bone scintigraphy will detect lesions elsewhere in the skeleton [24]. Whole body MRI and positron emission tomography (PET) may be considered for staging and treatment response evaluation [54, 56–58]. A recent retrospective study of 91 patients with Ewing sarcoma [57], concluded that F-18-deoxy-D-glucose positron emission tomography (^{18}FDG-PET) may be sufficient for initial screening of osseous metastases and also identified all patients with bone marrow metastases.

During chemotherapy clinical assessment (pain and clinical measurement) and imaging of the local site and lungs by MRI, chest X-ray and CT may be helpful to evaluate response to chemotherapy [53, 59].

Staging systems

Two staging systems are in widespread use, the Enneking [60] and the TNM system (American Joint Committee on Cancer–AJCC/International Union against cancer–UICC) [61].

The Enneking system is based on histological grade (I = low and II = high grade) and extent in relation to the anatomical compartments of the limb (a = intracompartmental, b = extracompartmental). If the bone cortex is intact and there is no soft tissue mass, the tumour is considered intracompartmental. Stage III tumours have metastases, but can be high or low grade. The TNM (AJCC/UICC) system is based on tumour grade, size and the presence of metastases (Table 2).

Laboratory tests

There are no specific laboratory tests for the diagnosis of bone sarcoma. However, the following are of prognostic value: erythrocyte sedimentation rate (ESR), alkaline phosphatase (ALP) and lactate dehydrogenase (LDH) [62, 63].

Table 2 AJCC/UICC Staging [61]

Stage	Grade	Size (cm)	Metastases
1°	Low grade	≤8	None
1b	Low grade	>8	None
2°	High grade	≤8	None
2b	High grade	>8	None
3	Any grade	Any	Skip metastases
4	Any grade	Any	Distant metastases at diagnosis

Other baseline assessments

Around 10 % of Ewing sarcomas metastasise to bone marrow, and therefore bone marrow biopsy should be routinely performed as a staging investigation [42].

Chemotherapy treatment can result in renal, cardiac and auditory dysfunction [64]. Pretreatment evaluation should therefore include baseline renal function testing (e.g. urea, creatinine, glomerular filtration rate) and assessment of cardiac function (e.g. echocardiogram, MUGA [multi-gated acquisition scan]). An audiogram is recommended for patients due to receive cisplatin.

Sperm storage is recommended for male patients of reproductive age. For female patients, a fertility physician may be consulted to discuss options for fertility preservation.

Biopsy

Biopsy is the definitive diagnostic test. Biopsy of a suspected primary malignant bone tumour should be carried out at a specialist sarcoma reference centre by, or in consultation with, the surgical team who will perform definitive tumour resection [47]. This improves access to modern molecular diagnostic techniques and ensures the biopsy track can be excised at the time of definitive surgery. Inappropriate biopsy can compromise limb salvage or even cure. The principles of biopsy [49] are:

- Biopsy should only be done after local imaging of the affected bone to allow planning of the approach and most representative area to biopsy.
- There should be minimal contamination of normal tissues.
- In many situations, core needle biopsy will be adequate, often guided by ultrasound, X-ray or CT.
- Samples should always be taken for microbiological assessment as well as histology and cytogenetic/molecular genetic studies.
- Where possible, samples should be snap frozen for storage in a tumour bank for future research studies with patient consent.
- Samples must be interpreted by an experienced bone tumour pathologist.
- The pathology request form should ensure sufficient detail to make a diagnosis, including anatomical site, patient age and the radiological differential diagnosis.

CT-guided biopsies [65, 66] are most appropriate for deeper locations (e.g. pelvis) or to target a particular area of concern within the tumour (e.g. a possibly dedifferentiated area in a chondrosarcoma). Frozen sections can help to confirm that lesional tissue has been obtained, but they should not be relied upon for a definitive diagnosis and may use up a significant volume of potentially diagnostic material. Biopsy tracks should be clearly marked with a small incision or tattoo to ensure they are excised at the definitive procedure.

Biopsy of other indeterminate lesions should always be considered if management might change as a result (e.g. entry into a trial or a decision to amputate).

Laminectomy or decompression for spinal tumours should be avoided at diagnosis unless necessary to relieve spinal cord compression, and after consultation with a member of the bone sarcoma MDT.

Pathology

Pathologists reporting biopsies and/or resections of bone sarcomas should be accredited bone tumour pathologists and members of a bone sarcoma MDT.

Reports should comply with Royal College of Pathologists guidance [67].

The biopsy report should include a description of the specimen, the microscopic findings and the histological diagnosis.

The pathology report relating to the definitive resection specimen should include a gross description recording the location and size (measured in three dimensions in mm) of the tumour. It should note the extent of local tumour spread and involvement of specific anatomical compartments. Resection margins should be reported as clear or involved by tumour. The distance (in mm) of infiltrating tumour from the nearest resection margin and the nature of tissue at this margin should be specified. The histological features of the tumour and results of relevant further investigations (e.g. immunohistochemistry or molecular genetics) should be recorded. The tumour type (and subtype) should be recorded in keeping with the latest WHO criteria [14]. The tumour type should be coded using the systematized nomenclature of medicine—clinical terms (SNOMED-CT) codes [68].

Molecular genetics and pathology

Tissue banks are essential for diagnostic and translational research in cancer; therefore, informed consent for tumour banking, analysis and research should be sought according to local practice wherever possible. In specialist centres, storage of fresh frozen tissue should be undertaken in every case where consent has been given.

Although most Ewing sarcomas can be recognised morphologically and by immunohistochemical identification of the surface glycoprotein CD99, molecular genetic confirmation of a Ewing sarcoma translocation is recommended, particularly if the clinicopathological presentation is unusual or the histological diagnosis is doubtful. A reference laboratory for Ewing sarcoma diagnosis should have both interphase fluorescence in situ hybridisation (FISH) and reverse transcription—polymerase chain reaction (RT-PCR) technology available [69] and should participate in an external quality assurance programme.

Confirmation of diagnosis

To confirm the diagnosis and minimise the risk of diagnostic and management errors, all patients with suspected bone tumours should be discussed by a bone sarcoma MDT with a surgeon, radiologist, pathologist and oncologist who have access to the relevant information and biopsy material [47].

Key recommendations

- Patients with suspected primary bone tumours should have access to timely and appropriate imaging.
- The definitive diagnostic test is a biopsy, which should be carried out at or in consultation with the team in a reference centre.
- All patients should have tissue stored for subsequent investigation with appropriate consent, including frozen tissue, when possible.
- Both the diagnostic and resection specimens should be examined by an accredited bone tumour pathologist who is part of a bone sarcoma MDT. The pathology report should comply with the Royal College of Pathologists guidance.
- In every case the diagnosis must be confirmed by reference to clinical findings, laboratory investigation and radiological imaging at a bone sarcoma MDT.
- Patients with a confirmed diagnosis should be staged according to AJCC criteria.
- Where treatment may have an impact on fertility, patients should be referred to the appropriate reproductive medicine service before commencing treatment.

Overview of management

As well as having care delivered or supervised by a specialist bone sarcoma MDT, patients should be allocated a key worker. Children, teenagers and young adults should also be discussed at the relevant children's or TYA (young adult) MDT. This requires sufficient specialist staff to ensure age-appropriate care. A bone sarcoma MDT should be properly constituted, adhering to the requirements for core membership of the relevant specialties, and meeting minimum criteria for the number of patients treated each year; they should collect data on patients, tumours, treatment and outcomes as agreed nationally and participate in national audit.

Where possible and where trials are available, patients should be supported to participate in clinical trials. Lists of clinical trials in the National Institute for Health Research portfolio can be found on the UK Clinical Research Network Study Portfolio website [70] and the National Cancer Research Institute Clinical Trials website [71].

Chemotherapy

Chemotherapy is part of standard treatment for osteosarcoma, Ewing sarcoma, undifferentiated pleomorphic sarcoma and spindle cell sarcoma. Treatment of chondrosarcoma remains predominantly surgical, although chemotherapy may have a role in dedifferentiated and mesenchymal subtypes.

Management usually comprises preoperative neoadjuvant systemic combination chemotherapy, local surgery and post-operative adjuvant chemotherapy [64]. While the main aim of neoadjuvant chemotherapy is to decrease the incidence of a subsequent distant relapse [72, 73], it may also help control the primary tumour.

Surgery

Decisions about the optimal surgical procedure for the primary tumour (i.e. limb salvage or amputation) require MDT discussion, considering tumour size and involvement of anatomical structures, response to neoadjuvant therapies and patient preference. Surgical reconstruction may be influenced by patient and surgeon choice and should follow open discussion of the risks and benefits of available options and expected functional outcomes.

The aim of curative surgery is to resect the whole tumour with adequate margins. Where possible, wide *en-bloc* resection of the affected part of the bone and involved soft tissue should be performed. Close surgical margins may be marked with (MRI-inert) haemo-clips placed in the surgical field. In Ewing sarcoma, surgery should involve removal of all anatomical structures involved in the original prechemotherapy tumour volume where feasible. The specimen should be orientated to allow the pathologist to describe the anatomical location and thickness of surgical margins.

Surgical excision of local recurrence or metastatic disease requires discussion in a bone sarcoma MDT.

Requirements for the surgical report

The surgeon should describe the procedure performed and the tissues resected. The planned surgical margin should be identified, along with areas of concern where the resection was close to tumour or gross tumour was encountered. The type of reconstruction should be described as well as postoperative care, including expected rehabilitation. The use of prophylactic antibiotics and thromboprophylaxis (e.g. mechanical and/or chemical agents) should be clearly stated.

Radiotherapy

Radiotherapy is frequently used in the definitive management of the primary tumour for Ewing sarcoma, but the relative radio-resistance of osteosarcoma and chondrosarcoma means it is only used as definitive treatment if there is no surgical option. Radiotherapy is not given routinely post-operatively, although it may be used in selected high-risk cases. However, radiotherapy has a palliative role in all tumour types.

Although considered exploratory, heavy particle therapy with protons or carbon ions, often in combination with photons, is increasingly used to treat unresectable primary bone sarcomas [74–76]. Excellent outcomes are reported for skull base chondrosarcomas or chordomas in which proton beam radiotherapy combined with surgery can achieve local control rates of approximately 70–90 % [77–79]. In unresectable or incompletely resectable osteosarcoma the five-year disease free survival (DFS) was 65 %, and the 5-year overall survival (OS) was 67 % [80]. High local control rates have also been achieved in sacral chordomas [81, 82].

At present there is no proton facility in the United Kingdom, but cases can be submitted to the UK Proton Panel to consider funding for treatment overseas. Referral guidelines can be found at the UK NHS England Commissioning website [83].

Prevention and management of pathological fracture

Patients with an existing or impending pathological fracture associated with a suspected primary bone tumour should be managed with external splintage or immobilisation and appropriate pain control until a diagnosis is established by local imaging (MRI and/or CT) and biopsy. Internal fixation is contraindicated.

Although pathological fracture is an adverse prognostic factor for survival in osteosarcoma, and is likely to be associated with an increased risk of local recurrence [84], it does not preclude limb sparing surgery [85].

Fractures often heal during neoadjuvant chemotherapy and allow subsequent resection of the tumour and involved soft tissues. Amputation may still be indicated if tumours fail to show a radiological response and/or resection of the tumour and the contaminated area cannot safely leave a useful limb [86]. Adjuvant radiotherapy may decrease the risk of local recurrence in osteosarcoma and may have a role in other tumour types after pathological fracture [87].

Thoracotomy

Pulmonary metastatectomy may be indicated in the presence of oligometastatic disease where the patient can be rendered disease free. Thoracotomy with manual exploration of both lungs is strongly recommended, even when imaging studies suggest unilateral disease. Thoracoscopic techniques are strongly discouraged, as they lack sensitivity and may be associated with an increased risk of intraoperative tumour dissemination [88].

Key recommendations

- All patients with a confirmed diagnosis of bone sarcoma should have their care supervised by a bone sarcoma MDT and be allocated a key worker. Children, teenagers and young adults should also be discussed at the relevant children's or TYA (young adult) MDT.
- Networks should ensure that they meet the needs of children and young people with cancer with sufficient specialist staff and care and facilities appropriate to the child or young person's age.
- A bone sarcoma MDT should meet minimum criteria for the number of patients treated in each year and adhere to the requirements for core membership of the relevant specialties.
- All bone sarcoma MDTs should collect data on patients, tumours, treatment and outcomes as agreed nationally.
- Patients should undergo definitive resection of their sarcoma by a surgeon who is a core or extended member of a bone sarcoma MDT or by a surgeon with tumour site specific or age appropriate skills in consultation with the bone sarcoma MDT.
- When considering the local treatment of bone tumours, options for amputation or limb sparing surgery should be tailored to the needs of the patient.
- Chemotherapy and radiotherapy are important components of the treatment of some patients and should be carried out at designated centres by appropriate specialists as recommended by a bone sarcoma MDT.
- For pulmonary metastatectomy, open thoracotomy is recommended over endoscopic techniques.

Specific treatment

Osteosarcoma

Adverse prognostic factors for osteosarcoma include detectable metastases at presentation, axial or proximal extremity tumour site, large tumour volume, elevated ALP or LDH, older age, high body mass index (BMI) at diagnosis, poor histological response to preoperative chemotherapy or pathological fracture [62, 89–91]. There is some evidence that females may have better outcomes than males [91] and patients >18 years may have poorer outcomes than younger patients [92].

Localised disease

Curative treatment for high-grade osteosarcoma consists of surgery and chemotherapy [88, 93]. Compared with surgery alone, multimodal treatment of high-grade osteosarcoma increases survival from only 10–20 % to around 60 % [94, 95]. Whenever possible, patients with osteosarcoma should receive chemotherapy within a prospective trial. Chemotherapy is also recommended for older patients with osteosarcoma using adapted protocols [96].

Treatment commonly takes 6–9 months, comprising 10 weeks of neoadjuvant therapy, surgical resection and adjuvant chemotherapy.

Although neoadjuvant treatment is not proven to add survival benefit over postoperative chemotherapy alone, advantages include: rapid improvement in symptoms; early treatment of micrometastatic disease; facilitation of resection in responsive tumours; it allows time to manufacture customised endoprosthesis and provides prognostic information about histological response [42, 45, 97].

The most accepted regimen is induction therapy with MAP (high-dose methotrexate (HDMTX), doxorubicin and cisplatin). This is recommended in the UK for patients with potentially resectable tumours [98] and was chosen for the EURAMOS study[1] (Table 3).

If not tolerated, the regimen may be modified to AP alone for patients >40 years old. Impaired renal function can cause delayed clearance of methotrexate resulting in mucositis and nephrotoxicity and therefore close monitoring is required. Combination regimens without methotrexate can be effective in patients intolerant of HDMTX or where pharmacokinetic monitoring is not available [99].

The goal of surgery is to safely remove the whole tumour whilst preserving as much function as possible. Most patients with extremity tumours are candidates for limb salvage if adequate surgical margins can be achieved. Where possible, wide surgical margins should be achieved to reduce the risk of recurrence [100]. It is accepted that a good (>90 %) histological necrosis rate after chemotherapy may allow a closer margin of excision to be considered safe. In patients with a poor response to chemotherapy and 'close' margins there is insufficient evidence to advise as to whether amputation offers a better outcome even accepting the increased rate of local recurrence with limb salvage [86].

The benefit of adjuvant therapy compared with surgery alone was demonstrated many years ago [104] and long-term (>25 years) follow-up has shown that a statistically significant survival benefit is maintained [105]. Adjuvant therapy may involve the same regimen as the induction phase or may be modified, but the ideal combination regimen and the optimal treatment duration for certain clinical situations are yet to be defined [93, 106].

Immune modulation has been proposed as a possible treatment in bone sarcomas. The immune modulator liposomal muramyl tripeptide (mifamurtide) added to postoperative chemotherapy demonstrated a statistically significant advantage in overall survival and a trend in event-free survival in a large randomised trial [101] and has been approved in Europe for patients under 30 with completely resected localised osteosarcoma.

Interferon has also been investigated in in vitro and xenograft models [107] but its evaluation in the EURAMOS-1 trial showed no apparent advantage [108, 109].

Histological response to induction therapy has been accepted as a robust prognostic indicator [62, 91, 100, 110]. Imaging techniques to identify response preoperatively, such as FDG-PET [111] and dynamic (diffusion weighted) MRI [112] are under investigation.

Changing postoperative chemotherapy on the basis of response has not been shown to improve outcome, and is not recommended at present [42].

The use of haematopoietic growth factors to increase dose intensity has not consistently resulted in improved survival of osteosarcoma patients [95] but may limit morbidity associated with myelosuppression. Prophylactic antibiotics are now recommended for cancer patients at risk of neutropenic sepsis [113].

Central, parosteal and craniofacial osteosarcomas

Low-grade central and parosteal osteosarcoma are variants with lower malignant potential, for which treatment is surgical. Histological examination of the resected tumour may show high grade areas in which case treatment should be with chemotherapy as for conventional osteosarcoma.

The exact role of chemotherapy has not been defined for periosteal and jaw osteosarcoma but experience shows that standard chemotherapy can be given and should be considered for all patients at presentation as part of evaluation by an experienced MDT. Jaw and other

[1] EURAMOS is a collaboration of the Children's Oncology Group (US) the Co-operative Osteosarcoma Study Group (European) the European Osteosarcoma Intergroup and the Scandinavian Sarcoma Group. Collectively these groups represent the largest ever clinical experience in osteosarcoma.

Table 3 Sarcoma advisory group guidelines for osteosarcoma

Category	1st line	2nd line	3rd line and other
Resectable <30 years	Doxorubicin, cisplatin methotrexate ± mifamurtide [101]	Ifosfamide and etoposide [102]	Gemcitabine and docetaxel [103] or oral etoposide
Other	Doxorubicin, cisplatin ± methotrexate [101]	Ifosfamide, etoposide ± methotrexate	Gemcitabine and docetaxel [103] or oral etoposide

Taken from: London and South East Sarcoma Network (LSESN) Guidelines [98]

craniofacial osteosarcomas present specific problems for management, especially to achieve local control, and must always be referred to a bone sarcoma MDT before surgery. ^{18}FDG PET is more reliable than standard imaging in evaluating response to neoadjuvant chemotherapy in craniofacial bone sarcomas and may correlate better with outcome than histological response [114].

Metastatic disease

Patients presenting with metastatic osteosarcoma are a heterogeneous group and may be treated using the same regimens as for non-metastatic osteosarcomas, provided that surgical resection of all disease sites is deemed feasible [115]. Approximately 30 % of patients with primary metastatic osteosarcoma and over 40 % of those who achieve complete surgical remission become long-term survivors [93].

Recurrent disease

The prognosis for recurrent disease is poor, with long-term post-relapse survival of less than a third [93]. Early relapse and distant non-lung metastases are associated with a poorer prognosis [116].

Treatment for locally recurrent or metastatic osteosarcoma is primarily surgical, if possible. Pulmonary metastatectomy can lead to long term survival if all metastases can be completely removed [117]. More than a third of patients with a second surgical remission survive for over 5 years, and patients with multiple recurrences may be cured as long as recurrences are resectable: repeated thoracotomies are often warranted [118]. However, if pulmonary metastases are inoperable the disease is almost universally fatal.

The role of second-line chemotherapy for recurrent osteosarcoma is less well defined than that of surgery and there is no accepted standard regimen [93, 115]. The choice of agents may take into account the prior disease-free interval; suggested regimens are shown in Table 3 [98].

Second-line chemotherapy is associated with limited prolongation of survival in patients with inoperable metastases, but a positive benefit in operable disease was observed in one series [119–121]. Radiotherapy, including samarium, may palliate inoperable sites [4, 122].

Agents targeting the epidermal growth factor receptor are investigational in patients with unresectable disease failing first-line therapy [123].

Treatment evaluation

Assessment of response is usually only possible after several cycles of chemotherapy. Changes in the size and ossification of the tumour do not reliably reflect response to neoadjuvant chemotherapy. However, reduction in peritumoural oedema seen on MRI indicates a good treatment response [124]. A small study showed PET/CT is more accurate than MRI for following bone lesions [58, 125] but confirmation in larger prospective studies is needed.

Key recommendations

- Treatment for osteosarcoma involves chemotherapy and surgery under the care of a specialist bone sarcoma MDT.
- Patients should be informed about relevant clinical trials and supported to enter them.
- First line standard treatment is MAP chemotherapy for patients under 40 years.
- Mifamurtide may be offered to patients without metastases after surgery.
- Treatment of the primary tumour should be surgical removal of the tumour with negative surgical margins where feasible.
- The adequacy of local clearance should be assessed by considering the response to chemotherapy and the surgical margin.
- Radiotherapy can be offered for local control where surgical removal is not possible.
- Where pulmonary metastases are present successful excision may prolong survival.
- The primary treatment of recurrent disease is surgical although there is a role for chemotherapy.

Ewing sarcoma

Prognostic factors for Ewing sarcoma include axial location, tumour volume, raised serum LDH, and older age (>15 years). A poor histological response to preoperative chemotherapy and incomplete or no surgery for local therapy are further adverse prognostic factors [89, 126–128].

Ewing Sarcoma is a radiosensitive tumour. Radiotherapy may be used in combination with surgery, where there is a poor response to chemotherapy (radiological or histological), if there are concerns about surgical resection margins [129, 130] or if the anatomical site makes complete resection impossible. Radiotherapy may be given to the primary tumour site preoperatively, postoperatively or as definitive local therapy where surgery is not possible.

With surgery or radiotherapy alone, 5-year survival for Ewing sarcoma is <10 %. With treatment in current multimodality trials including chemotherapy, 5-year survival is between 60 and 70 % in localized and 20 to 40 % in metastatic disease [4].

Localised disease

All current trials employ 10 to 12 months of treatment comprising three to six cycles of neoadjuvant chemotherapy, followed by local therapy and a further six to ten cycles of chemotherapy usually given at 2 or 3 week intervals and based on current agreed national or international protocols. Agents considered most active include doxorubicin, cyclophosphamide, ifosfamide, vincristine, dactinomycin and etoposide [23, 89, 127, 130–139]. The LSEN guidelines [98] are summarized in Table 4. Virtually all active protocols are based on four to six drug combinations of these agents. Chemotherapy intensity is positively associated with outcome: superior outcome has been demonstrated with compressed 2 weekly chemotherapy [140]. High dose chemotherapy with blood stem cell transplantation is still investigational [141].

Local treatment may comprise surgery or radiotherapy or both. Individual decisions about local therapy are frequently complex and should only be made by a bone sarcoma MDT in conjunction with the patient and their family if appropriate. It is also recommended that the MDT's treatment plan is then discussed at the UK National Ewings MDT (ROH-tr.ewingsMDT@nhs.net) and entry into a clinical trial considered. At the time of writing (2015), the EE2012 trial is still open [151].

Complete surgery is regarded as the best treatment for local control but may not always be feasible. There is increasing recognition of the importance of treating all tissue initially involved by tumour, even if there has been a good response to chemotherapy. If this volume cannot confidently be removed surgically then radiotherapy should be used.

Indications for planned preoperative radiotherapy include poor response to induction chemotherapy, expected marginal resection, or if radiotherapy is anticipated to be required and the bone sarcoma MDT judges there is a technical advantage to preoperative radiotherapy.

Preoperative radiotherapy may also be useful in particular anatomical locations (e.g. pelvis, rib) when preoperative treatment allows the tumour volume to be defined more easily, or when treatment volumes will be smaller than in the post-operative setting. Radiotherapy alone should be considered if complete surgery is impossible or would be very disabling, (e.g. for sacral tumours crossing the midline) [152, 153]. If standard conformal radiotherapy will not achieve an adequate dose to the tumour, techniques such as IMRT (intensity modulated radiotherapy) may deliver a higher dose [154–156]. Insertion of pelvic spacers can displace bowel away from pelvic tumours, facilitating delivery of a higher dose and preventing long term bowel toxicity [157]. Proton beam radiotherapy may be considered when there is a dosimetric advantage over photon radiotherapy in achieving the optimal radiotherapy dose due to proximity to critical structures such as spinal cord, and for younger patients having curative treatment in order to reduce the risk of radiation-induced second malignancy. Applications for treatment are made via the UK Proton Panel [83]).

Toxicities leading to death have been observed in some patients who received high dose large volume radiotherapy following busulpan-melphalan high dose chemotherapy (BuMel HDT). BuMel HDT may therefore compromise the delivery of effective radiation doses to central axial sites. In patients with an indication for radiotherapy, the patient should not be offered BuMel HDT if there are critical organs such as gut, spinal cord, brain or significant volumes of lung in the fields, unless the technique used can limit the dose to critical organs.

Specific indications for post-operative radiotherapy include (Taken from: Euro-Ewing-2012 radiotherapy guidelines [158]):

- positive surgical margins with microscopic residual disease (R1 excision; <1 mm or tumour up to edge of resection specimen) if further surgery to achieve negative margins is not possible.
- positive surgical margins with macroscopic residual disease (R2 excision), if further surgery to achieve negative margins is not possible (this should be an unusual situation).
- if all tissues involved by the original pre-chemotherapy tumour volume have not been excised, even if the surgical margins are negative.
- if there is a poor histological response (≤90 % necrosis) to pre-operative chemotherapy, even if the surgical margins are negative.
- a displaced pathological fracture of bone at primary site (unless it is possible to excise all contaminated tissue).

Table 4 Sarcoma advisory group guidelines—ewing sarcomas

Category	1st line	2nd line	3rd line and other
Localised or metastatic disease with lung or pleural metastases only	VIDE 6 cycles VAC or VAI × 8 cycles [142]	High dose ifosfamide [144] or Ifosfamide and etoposide or cyclophosphamide and topotecan [145] or irinotecan and temozolamide [146] ± High dose chemotherapy (busulphan/lmelphalan or treosulphan/melphalan) with peripheral blood stem cell rescue [147] N.B. Choice of 2nd line therapy will depend on patient/disease specific factors (e.g. if chemo being given with curative intent) and/or patient choice	Cyclophosphamide and topotecan [145] or Irinotecan and temozolamide [146] or gemcitabine and docetaxel [148, 149] or oral etoposide [150] or cisplatin and etoposide
Metastatic disease with bone or bone marrow involvement	VIDE × 6 cycles → VAC or VAI × 8 cycles [142, 143] or VDC/IE interval compressed regimen × 14 cycles [140]		

Taken from: London and South East Sarcoma Network (LSESN) Guidelines [98]

V vincristine; *I* ifosfamide; *D* doxorubicin; *E* etoposide; *A* actinomycin *D* (dactinomycin); *C* cyclophosphamide

- certain tumour sites where local control is judged to be more difficult to achieve e.g.:
  - Spine and paraspinal sites—in these sites excision is rarely complete, and is often intra-lesional.
  - Pelvis and sacrum—in these sites it is frequently difficult or impossible to be sure that the entire pre-chemotherapy tumour volume has been excised.
  - Rib tumours when presenting with a pleural effusion.

Reasons for deciding *against* radiotherapy may include:

- Concerns about impaired healing of the wound or biological reconstruction following surgery and radiotherapy.
- Concerns about morbidity of radiotherapy in young patients.
- Concerns about the increased risk of infection of a metallic prosthesis following radiotherapy.
- Concerns about the risk of a radiation-induced malignancy.

Definitive radiotherapy is advised only for inoperable lesions. Inoperability is determined during bone sarcoma MDT discussion. Inoperable tumours are those which cannot be resected completely, or are in anatomical sites where complete surgery would result in unacceptable morbidity or have a high risk of significant complications. Suggested radiotherapy doses are given in Table 5.

Metastatic and recurrent disease

Around 26 % of patients with Ewing sarcoma have metastatic disease at presentation (10 % lung, 10 % bones/bone marrow, 6 % combinations or others) [159]. Bone metastases confer a poorer outcome than lung/pleural metastases (<21 % compared with 55 % 5-year relapse free survival) [143].

Patients with metastases at diagnosis are treated similarly to those with localised disease but have a poorer prognosis. Several non-randomised trials have evaluated more intensive, time compressed or high-dose chemotherapy approaches, followed by autologous stem cell rescue, demonstrating a possible advantage for patients under 14 years of age [143, 147]. Whole lung radiotherapy is indicated in patients with pulmonary disease, and may prolong survival. However, firm data are lacking and a systematic review failed to confirm a survival advantage [160]. Radiation doses are given in Table 6.

A recent review of stereotactic body radiotherapy (SBRT) for metastatic and recurrent Ewing sarcoma and osteosarcoma reported on 14 patients with 27 osseous or pulmonary lesions. Estimated local control at 2 years in the lesions treated with curative intent was 85 %. However, there was significant toxicity especially if concurrent chemotherapy and re-irradiation were given [161].

The role of surgical resection of residual metastases is less well defined. Patients with bone or bone marrow metastases and patients with recurrent disease still fare poorly, with 5-year survival rates of between 10 and 45 % [24, 162, 163].

Guidance on the management of small suspicious lung nodules is available in trial protocols [108, 131].

Patients relapsing more than 2 years after diagnosis and without bone marrow or multiple bone involvement have a better outcome than others [126, 162, 164, 165].

Table 5 Radiotherapy dose and fractionation for ewing sarcoma

Setting	Dosage
Pre-operative radiotherapy	The total dose for preoperative irradiation is 50.4 Gy in 28 fractions in a single phase to the PTV. If there are concerns about organ tolerance or wound healing, then this dose can be reduced to 45 Gy in 25 Gy fractions
Post-operative radiotherapy	The total dose for postoperative radiotherapy is 54 Gy in 30 fractions, delivered as 45 Gy in 25 fractions to PTV1, and 9 Gy in 5 fractions to PTV2
Definitive radiotherapy	The total dose for definitive radiotherapy is 54 Gy in 1.8 Gy fractions, delivered as a single phase. A boost of 5.4 Gy in 3 fractions may be considered if desired, keeping within standard normal tissue dose constraints

Fractionation: conventionally fractionated radiotherapy (once daily fractions, five 1.8 Gy fractions per week) is the preferred fractionation schedule. In very young children, fractionation using 1.6 Gy fractions may be considered

Taken from: Euro–Ewing-2012 radiotherapy guidelines [158]

Table 6 Radiotherapy doses for whole lung radiotherapy

Whole lung radiotherapy	The dose for whole lung radiotherapy is 15 Gy in 10 fractions for patients <14 years, or 18 Gy in 12 fractions for patients ≥14 years. Dose may be specified to 100 % for an optimised plan, or to the mid plane dose (MPD) for simulated opposed fields. However, it should be noted that this will result in a dose of approximately 10 % higher in the lungs than that prescribed, and so optimisation of dosimetry is recommended if fields are simulated

Taken from: Euro–Ewing-2012 Radiotherapy Guidelines [158]

Doxorubicin therapy is usually not feasible after relapse because of previously administered cumulative doses. Chemotherapy regimens are not standardised and currently often comprise alkylating agents (cyclophosphamide, high-dose ifosfamide) in combination with topoisomerase inhibitors (etoposide, topotecan) or irinotecan with temozolomide [23, 133, 137, 138]. Given the poor outcomes after relapse, patients should be recruited to prospective clinical trials to investigate the role of second-line/experimental therapies wherever possible. At time of writing, an international trial, rEECur, is open to recruitment [151]. Radiotherapy may be helpful to palliate local symptoms.

Treatment evaluation

Change in the size of the soft tissue mass is easily evaluated on MRI, and is a reliable indicator of tumour response [166]. Dynamic MRI is not as reliable as in osteosarcoma, as remaining small tumour foci may not be detected. Sequential FDG PET evaluation and whole body MRI scanning is under evaluation [53, 112].

Disease progression during chemotherapy may mandate changes in treatment or earlier primary local control measures. A radiological increase in tumour size may be due to necrosis rather than tumour progression.

Key recommendations

- For Ewing sarcoma, systemic treatment with chemotherapy is standard. All new cases of Ewing's sarcoma of bone should be discussed at the National Ewing Multidisciplinary Team meeting.
- When treating the primary tumour with curative intent, all of the pre-chemotherapy volume should be treated with surgery, radiotherapy or both.
- If radiotherapy is indicated (e.g. the anatomical location of the tumour makes complete resection impossible or there has been an incomplete response to chemotherapy as identified radiologically), then preoperative radiotherapy may be advantageous.
- Patients with relapsed/progressive disease should be considered for clinical trials.

Chondrosarcoma

Assessing the grade of chondrosarcomas is difficult and variation in opinion is common, even between experts [28]. The diagnosis of chondrosarcoma requires discussion in a bone sarcoma MDT. Surgery is the treatment of choice.

Low grade cartilage tumours may recur locally but are unlikely to metastasise. Biopsy-confirmed low grade central chondrosarcomas in extremity long bones can be managed by complete curettage with or without adjuvant measures (e.g. phenol, cement, cryotherapy) with a high chance of success. Low grade peripheral chondrosarcomas (arising from osteochondromas) should be completely surgically removed, aiming to excise the tumour with a covering of normal tissue.

Higher grade chondrosarcomas (including clear cell chondrosarcoma) and all chondrosarcomas of the pelvis or axial skeleton should be surgically excised with wide margins [29, 30].

Mesenchymal chondrosarcoma may be responsive to chemotherapy and some patients may be considered for adjuvant or neoadjuvant therapy [114]. There is uncertainty about the chemotherapy sensitivity of dedifferentiated chondrosarcoma but it can be treated like osteosarcoma, although survival is poorer [31]. Survival after a diagnosis of dedifferentiated chondrosarcoma remains dismal. Complete excision is recommended if feasible, but there is a very high risk of local recurrence following pathological fracture. If wide margins cannot be reliably achieved with limb salvage, then amputation may maximize the chances of local control but there remains a high risk that metastases will develop.

Key recommendations

- Diagnosis of a chondrosarcoma requires discussion in a bone sarcoma MDT.
- Management of chondrosarcoma is surgical excision with wide margins for all but low grade central limb chondrosarcoma where curettage may be adequate.
- There are no data to support the routine use of chemotherapy.

Undifferentiated pleomorphic sarcomas.

Treatment strategies mimic those of osteosarcoma, with age-adjusted chemotherapy and complete *en-bloc* resection including any soft tissue component if possible.

Chordoma

Assessment in a specialist centre with expertise in managing chordomas is essential. To date, conventional therapy for chordoma has been complete surgical resection [167]. High dose radiotherapy using proton beams or carbon ions may be used post-operatively, and are promising alternatives to surgery for some patients, particularly those with high sacral tumours [74, 81, 82].

Surgical excision of tumours of the skull base or cervical spine should aim to remove as much tumour as possible, whilst preserving neurological function and therefore quality of life. R0 resection is rarely possible. Eight studies (summarized by Stacchiotti et al. [35]) have shown that surgery (R1 and R2 resections) followed by radiotherapy in selected patients produced 5-year estimated overall survival of 55–86 % in patients with chordoma of the skull base and/or cervical spine.

Metastases are rare but local recurrence is common and difficult to cure [168]. Treatment for local recurrence may include surgery and/or radiation therapy and/or systemic treatment (Table 7) [4, 35]. Molecular targeted agents may be effective [169, 170].

Other bone sarcomas

Prognosis and prognostic factors after a diagnosis of spindle cell sarcoma are similar to those of patients with osteosarcoma [41, 171, 172]. Treatment should be similar.

Adamantinoma is a malignant tumour occurring in the tibia. Most are low grade but higher grade areas in the primary tumour may require systemic therapy. Complete excision is the treatment of choice.

Giant cell tumours of bone

Giant cell tumours of bone require highly specialised treatment and all patients should be referred to a specialist bone sarcoma MDT for diagnosis and to coordinate treatment. Curettage alone is associated with a high risk of local recurrence (up to 50 %). Although there is no randomized controlled trial evidence, numerous case series suggest improved local control if adjuvants such as high speed burring and cement are used.

Denosumab is a novel RankL inhibitor which has been shown in clinical trials to suppress the formation and activity of osteoclasts. It is licensed for use by the European medicines agency from 2014. Denosumab is indicated in inoperable cases or those where the morbidity of surgery would be excessive. Denosumab is given as a monthly subcutaneous injection after three loading doses at weekly intervals. All patients require daily calcium and vitamin D supplements and females must avoid pregnancy. Significant side effects include hypocalcaemia, osteonecrosis of the jaw and atypical fractures [173, 174].

Emerging evidence suggests that whilst initial control is excellent (96 %), later recurrences can arise and most tumours recur if the drug is stopped (after around 9 months). Hence in inoperable cases life-long treatment may be required. The consequences of this, particularly in younger patients, are not known.

Using denosumab to reduce the size of a giant cell tumour prior to surgery may be advantageous but surgery should incorporate the extent of the original tumour to avoid recurrence. While clear guidance on the optimal duration of pre-operative treatment has yet to emerge, prolonged exposure to denosumab may make subsequent curettage more difficult. Treatment for up to 6 months before surgery is a reasonable pragmatic approach.

Follow-up

Follow-up after treatment aims to detect local recurrence, to detect metastatic disease for which treatment might be beneficial, to manage the long term toxicity of chemotherapy and radiotherapy and to look for long term complications of surgical treatment [4]. Local recurrences are often first detected by patients and therefore they should be given information about what to do if local recurrence is suspected.

The clinical follow-up of patients treated for high-grade tumours should include physical examination of the primary tumour site, and assessment of the functional outcome and possible complications of any reconstruction. Local and chest imaging should be included. Evidence for the optimum frequency of follow-up and the best imaging investigations is lacking although a recently reported randomised controlled trial showed no benefit of greater frequency of follow-up with regular cross sectional imaging over standard follow-up [178]. However, current protocols recommend follow-up at intervals of 2–4 months for the first 3 years after completion of therapy, every 6 months for year 4 and 5 and annually thereafter [24, 93].

For low grade bone sarcomas, the frequency of follow-up visits can be reduced to 4–6 monthly for 2 years and then annually. Late metastases as well as local

Table 7 Sarcoma advisory group guidelines—bone sarcomas

Sarcoma type	Category	1st line	2nd line	3rd line and other
Other high grade bone sarcomas including malignant fibrous histiocytoma, leiomyosarcoma, angiosarcoma, spindle cell sarcoma, dedifferentiated chondrosarcoma		Doxorubicin, cisplatin ± methotrexate [101]	Ifosfamide, etoposide ± methotrexate [102]	Gemcitabine and docetaxel [103]
Giant cell tumour	Locally advanced unresectable/metastatic	Denosumab [175]		
Chordoma	Locally advanced, unresectable or metastatic: non-dedifferentiated dedifferentiated	Imatinib [171] doxorubicin or doxorubicin and cisplatin [176]	Addition of sirolimus [170] or Sunitinib [177]	

Taken from London and South East Sarcoma Network (LSESN) guidelines [98]

recurrences and failure of reconstructions may occur more than 10 years after diagnosis in all tumours and there is no universally accepted stopping point for follow-up [4].

It is important to evaluate the long-term toxicity effect of chemotherapy and radiotherapy as well as immediate chemotherapy-related complications [64]. Monitoring for late effects should be undertaken, depending on the treatment given and in conjunction with late effect services when available [127, 179, 180].

Secondary cancers may arise in survivors of bone sarcomas, either related to or independent of irradiation. Secondary leukaemia, particularly acute myeloid leukaemia may rarely be observed following chemotherapy as early as 2–5 years after treatment [181, 182].

Key recommendations

- Standard follow-up for all sarcoma cases is currently chest X-ray and clinical review. The role of regular cross sectional imaging remains uncertain.
- At the end of treatment patients should receive information about the risk of local and systemic recurrence.
- Patients should have access to services for the late effects of treatment including chemotherapy, radiotherapy, surgery and psychsocial support.

Authors' contributions

All authors contributed to the content of the manuscript. All authors read and approved the final manuscript.

Author details

[1] Newcastle upon Tyne Hospitals NHS Foundation Trust, Freeman Hospital, Newcastle upon Tyne NE7 7DN, UK. [2] Nuffield Orthopaedic Centre, Oxford OX3 7LD, UK. [3] Royal Manchester Children's Hospital, Manchester M13 9WL, UK. [4] Royal Orthopaedic Hospital, Birmingham B31 2AP, UK. [5] The Royal Marsden, Sutton SM2 5PT, UK. [6] Birmingham Children's Hospital, Birmingham B4 6NH, UK. [7] Queen Elizabeth Hospital, Birmingham B15 2TH, UK. [8] University College Hospital, London NW1 2PG, UK.

Acknowledgements

We would like to thank the following people for reading and commenting on the final manuscript: Lindsay Campbell, Glasgow, Scotland; Rod Duncan, Glasgow, Scotland; John Barr, Belfast, Northern Ireland; CR Chandraseka, Liverpool, England; Dermot Murphy, Glasgow, Scotland; Angela Edgar, Edinburgh, Scotland; Lin Russell, Birmingham, England; Ivon Van Heugten, Changing Faces, London, England.

Competing interests

The authors declare that they have no competing interests.

References

1. National Health Service (NHS) Highly Specialised Commissioning Group. http://www.england.nhs.uk/commissioning/spec-services/npc-crg/group-b/b12/. Accessed 30 Jan 2014.
2. Grimer R, Athanasou N, Gerrand C, Judson I, Lewis I, Morland B, Peake D, Seddon B, Whelan J. UK guidelines for the management of bone sarcomas. Sarcoma. 2010;317462:14. doi:10.1155/2010/317462.
3. National Comprehensive Cancer Network. NCCN Clinical Practice Guidelines in Oncology. Bone Cancer, Version 1.2015. http://www.nccn.org/professionals/physician_gls/pdf/bone.pdf. Accessed 02 Sep 2015.
4. The ESMO/European Sarcoma Network Working Group. Bone sarcomas: ESMO clinical practice guidelines for diagnosis, treatment and follow-up. Ann Oncol. 2014;25(Suppl 3):113–23.
5. National Institute for Health and Care Excellence (NICE) Quality Standard QS78 Sarcoma; 2015. http://www.nice.org.uk/guidance/qs78. Accessed 02 Feb 2015.
6. National Institute for Health and Care Excellence (NICE) Suspected cancer: recognition and referral NICE guideline [NG12]; 2015. http://www.nice.org.uk/guidance/ng12. Accessed 21 Sep 2015.
7. National Cancer Intelligence Network (NCIN). Bone sarcoma incidence and survival. Tumours diagnosed between 1985 and 2009.Report R12/05 October 2012 www.ncin.org.uk/. Accessed 02 Feb 2015.
8. Grimer RJ, Briggs TR. Earlier diagnosis of bone and soft tissue tumours. J Bone Joint Surg Br. 2010;92(11):1489–92. doi:10.1302/0301-620X.92B11.24326.
9. Stiller CA, Craft AW, Corazziari I, EUROCARE Working Group. Survival of children with bone sarcoma in Europe since. Results from the EUROCARE study. Eur J Cancer. 1978;2001(37):760–6.
10. Kager L, Zoubek A, Dominikus M, Lang S, Bodmer N, Jundt G, Klingebiel T, Jürgens H, Gadner H, Bielack S. COSS study group. Osteosarcoma in very young children: experience of the cooperative osteosarcoma study group. Cancer. 2010;116(22):5316–24.
11. Malhas AM, Grimer RJ, Abudu A, Carter SR, Tillman RM, Jeys L. The final diagnosis in patients with a suspected primary malignancy of bone. J Bone Joint Surg Br. 2011;93:980–3.
12. Hauben EI, Hogendoorn PCW. Epidemiology of primary bone tumors and economical aspects of bone metastases. In: Heymann D, editor. Bone cancer: progression and therapeutic approaches. 1st ed. London: Academic Press; 2009. p. 3–8.
13. Whelan JS, Jinks RC, McTiernan A, Sydes MR, Hook JM, Trani L, Uscinska B, Bramwell V, Lewis IJ, Nooij MA, et al. Survival from high-grade localised extremity osteosarcoma: combined results and prognostic factors from three European Osteosarcoma Intergroup randomised trials. Ann Oncol. 2012;23:1607–16.
14. Fletcher CD, Bridge JA, Hogendoorn P, Mertens F, editors. WHO classification of tumours of soft tissue and bone. 4th ed. Lyon: France IARC Press; 2013.
15. Eyre R, Feltbower RG, Mubwandarikwa E, Eden TO, McNally RJ. Review: epidemiology of bone tumours in children and young adults. Pediat Blood Cancer. 2009;53:941–52.
16. Kalra S, Grimer RJ, Spooner D, Carter SR, Tillman RM, Abudu A. Radiation induced sarcomas of bone. Factors that affect outcome. J Bone Joint Surg Br. 2007;89B:808–13.
17. SEER. http://seer.cancer.gov/statfacts/html/bones.html. Accessed 29 May 2015.
18. Dorfman HD, Czerniak B. Bone Cancers. Cancer. 1995;75:203–10.
19. Mascarenhas L, Siegel S, Spector L, Arndt C, Femino D, Malogolowkin M. Malignant bone tumours. SEER AYA Monograph, Chapter 8. 2002. p. 97–109.
20. Fuchs B, Pritchard DJ. Etiology of osteosarcoma. Clinical Orthop Rel Res. 2002;397:40–52.
21. Hansen MF, Seton M, Merchant A. Osteosarcoma in Paget's disease of bone. J Bone Min Res. 2006;21(Suppl 2):58–63.
22. Specht K, Sung YS, Zhang L, Richter GHS, Fletcher CD, Antonescu CR. Distinct transcriptional signature and immunoprofile of *CIC-DUX4*-fusion positive round cell tumors compared to *EWSR1*-rearranged Ewing sarcomas– further evidence toward distinct pathological entities. Genes Chromosome Cancer. 2014;53(7):622–33.
23. Bernstein M, Kovar H, Paulussen M, Randall RL, Schuck A, Teot LA, Jüergens H. Ewing's sarcoma family of tumors: current management. Oncologist. 2006;11:503–19.
24. Paulussen M, Bielack S, Jürgens H, Casali PG, ESMO Guidelines Working Group. Ewing's sarcoma of the bone: ESMO clinical recommendations for diagnosis, treatment and follow-up. Ann Oncol. 2009;20(4):140–2.
25. Francis M, Dennis N, Charman J, Lawrence G, Grimer R. Bone and Soft Tissue Sarcomas UK Incidence and Survival: 1996 to 2010 November 2013 Version 2.0 NCIN. http://www.ncin.org.uk/publications/reports/. Accessed 29 May 2015.

26. Lai X, Chen S. Identification of novel biomarker candidates for immunohistochemical diagnosis to distinguish low-grade chondrosarcoma from echondroma. Proteonomic. 2015;15(13):2358–68. doi:10.1002/pmic.201400528 **(Epub 2015 Apr 24)**.
27. Verdegaal SH, Bovee JV, Pansuriya TC, Grimer RJ, Ozger H, Jutte PC, San Julian M, Biau DJ, van der Geest IC, Leithner A, et al. Incidence, predictive factors and prognosis of chondrosarcoma in patients with Ollier Disease and Maffucci Syndrome: an International Multicenter Study of 161 patients. Oncologist. 2011;16:1771–9.
28. Eefting D, Schrage YM, Geirnaerdt MJ, Le Cessie S, Taminiau AH, Bovée JV, Hogendoorn PC. EuroBoNeT consortium. Assessment of interobserver variability and histologic parameters to improve reliability in classification and grading of central cartilaginous tumors. Am J Surg Pathol. 2009;33:50–7.
29. Gelderblom H, Hogendoorn PCW, Dijkstra SD, van Rijswijk CS, Krol AD, Taminiau AH, Bovée JV. The clinical approach towards chondrosarcoma. Oncologist. 2008;13:320–9.
30. Riedel RF, Larrier N, Dodd L, Kirsch D, Martinez S, Brigman BE. The clinical management of chondrosarcoma. Curr Treat Options Oncol. 2009;10:94–106.
31. Grimer RJ, Gosheger G, Taminiau A, Biau D, Matejovsky Z, Kollender Y, San-Julian M, Gherlinzoni F, Ferrari C. Dedifferentiated chondrosarcoma: prognostic factors and outcome from a European group. Eur J Cancer. 2007;43:2060–5.
32. Romeo S, Bovee JV, Kroon HM, Tirabosco R, Natali C, Zanatta L, Sciot R, Mertens F, Athanasou N, Alberghini M, et al. Malignant fibrous histiocytoma and fibrosarcoma of bone: a reassessment in the light of currently employed morphological, immunochemical and molecular approaches. Virchows Arch. 2012;461:561–70.
33. Doyle LA. Sarcoma classification: an update based on the 2013 World Health Organization classification of tumors of soft tissue and bone. Cancer. 2014;120:1763–74.
34. Jeon DG, Song WS, Kong CB, Kim JR, Lee SY. MFH of bone and osteosarcoma show similar survival and chemosensitivity. Clin Orthop Rel Res. 2011;469:584–90.
35. Stacchiotti S. Sommer J on behalf of a chordoma global consensus group: a position paper from the medical and patient community. Lancet Oncol. 2015;16(2):e71–83.
36. Giannoulis DK, Gantsos A, Giotis D, Paschos NK, Vagionas A, Arnaoutoglou CM, Pentheroudakis G, Xenakis TA. Multiple recurrences and late metastasis of adamantinoma in the tibia: a case report. J Orthop Surg. 2014;22(3):420–2.
37. Roque P, Mankin HJ, Rosenberg A. Adamantinoma: an unusual bone tumour. Chir Organi Mov. 2008;92(3):149–54.
38. Viswanathan S, Jambhekar NA. Metastatic giant cell tumor of bone: are there associated factors and best treatment modalities? Clin Orthop Rel Res. 2010;468(3):827–33.
39. Bergovec M, Kubat O, Smerdelj M, Seiwerth S, Bonevski A, Orlic D. Epidemiology of musculoskeletal tumors in a national referral orthopedic department A study of 3482 cases. Cancer Epidemiol. 2015;39(3):298–302. doi:10.1016/j.canep.2015.01.015 **(Epub Feb 18 2015)**.
40. Campanacci M, Giunti A, Olmi R. Metaphyseal and diaphyseal localization of giant cell tumors. Chir Organi Mov. 1975;62(1):29–34.
41. Pakos EE, Grimer RJ, Peake D, Spooner D, Carter SR, Tillman RM, Abudu S, Jeys L. The other bone sarcomas: prognostic factors and outcomes for spindle cell sarcomas of bone. J Bone Joint Surg Br. 2011;93(9):1271–8.
42. Whelan JS, Pollock RC, Cassoni M, Windsor RE. Primary bone tumours. In: Price P, Sikora K, editors. Treatment of cancer. 6th ed. Boca Raton: CRC Press; 2014.
43. Grimer RJ, Sneath RS. Diagnosing malignant bone tumours. J Bone Joint Surg Br. 1990;72B:754–6.
44. Pizzo PA, Poplack DG. Osteosarcoma: principles and practice of pediatric oncology, 5th edn. 2006;35:1074–115.
45. Bielack SS, Machatschek JN, Flege S, Jürgens H. Delaying surgery with chemotherapy for osteosarcoma of the extremities. Exp Opin Pharmacother. 2004;5:1243–56.
46. Federman N, Bernthal N, Eilber FC, Tap WD. The multidisciplinary management of osteosarcoma. Curr Treat Opt Oncol. 2009;10:82–93.
47. National Institute for Health and Care Excellence (NICE). Guidance on cancer services—improving outcomes for people with sarcoma: the manual [needs assessment, evidence review, list of recommendations]; 2006. **(Developed by the National Collaborating Centre for Cancer)**.
48. National Institute for Health and Care Excellence (NICE) Quality Standard QS55 Young People with Cancer; 2014. http://www.nice.org.uk/guidance/qs55/resources/guidance-children-and-young-people-with-cancer-pdf. Accessed 10 Jan 2016.
49. Mankin HJ, Lange TA, Spanier SS. The hazards of biopsy in patients with malignant primary bone and soft-tissue tumors. J Bone Joint Surg Ser A. 1982;64(8):1121–7.
50. Andreou D, Bielack DD, Carrle D, Kevric M, Kotz R, Winkelmann W, Jundt G, Werner M, Fehlberg S, Kager L, et al. The influence of tumor- and treatment-related factors on the development of local recurrence in osteosarcoma after adequate surgery. An analysis of 1335 patients treated on neoadjuvant Cooperative Osteosarcoma Group protocols. Ann Oncol. 2011;22:1228–35.
51. Healthcare Improvement Scotland. http://www.healthcareimprovementscotland.org/our_work/cancer_care_improvement/programme_resources/scottish_referral_guidelines.aspx. Accessed 29 Feb 2016.
52. West of Scotland Cancer Network www.woscan.scot.nhs.uk. Accessed 29 Feb 2016.
53. Meyer JS, Nadel HR, Marina N, Womer RB, Brown KL, Eary JF, Gorlick R, Grier HE, Randall RL, Lawlor ER, et al. Imaging guidelines for children with Ewing sarcoma and osteosarcoma: a report from the Children's Oncology Group Bone Tumor Committee. Pediat Blood Cancer. 2008;51:163–70.
54. Picci P, Vanel D, Briccoli A, Talle K, Haakenaasen U, Malaguti C, Monti C, Ferrari C, Bacci G, Saeter G, et al. Computed tomography of pulmonary metastases from osteosarcoma: the less poor technique. A study of 51 patients with histological correlation. Ann Oncol. 2001;12:1601–4.
55. Wang S, Shi H, Yu Q. Osteosarcoma of the jaws: demographic and CT imaging features. Dentomaxillofacial Radiol. 2012;41:37–42.
56. Benz MR, Tchekmedyian N, Eilber FC, Federman N, Czernin J, Tap WD. Utilization of positron emission tomography in the management of patients with sarcoma. Curr Opin Oncol. 2009;21:345–51.
57. Newman EN, Jones RL, Hawkins DS. An evaluation of [F-18]-fluorodeoxy-D-glucose positron emission tomography, bone scan, and bone marrow aspiration/biopsy as staging investigations in Ewing sarcoma. Pediatr Blood Cancer. 2013;60(7):1113–7.
58. Quartuccio N, Fox J, Kuk D, Wexler LH, Baldari S, Cistaro A, Schöder H. Pediatric bone sarcoma: diagnostic performance of $^{(18)}$F-FDG PET/CT versus conventional imaging for initial staging and follow-up. Am J Roentgenol. 2015;204(1):153–60.
59. Bajpai J, Gamnagatti S, Kumar R, Sreenivas V, Sharma MC, Khan SA, Rastogi S, Malhotra A, Safaya R, Bakhshi S. Role of MRI in osteosarcoma for evaluation and prediction of chemotherapy response: correlation with histological necrosis. Pediatr Radiol. 2011;41:441–50.
60. Enneking WF, Spanier SS, Goodman MA. A system for the surgical staging of musculoskeletal sarcoma. Clin Orthop. 1980;53:106–20.
61. Edge SB, Byrd DR, Compton CC, Fritz AG, Greene FL, Trotti A (Eds.) AJCC Cancer Staging Manual, 7th edn. New York, NY: Springer 2010.
62. Bramer JA, van Linge JH, Grimer RJ, Scholten RJ. Prognostic factors in localized extremity osteosarcoma: a systematic review. Eur J Surg Oncol. 2009;35:1030–6.
63. Leavey PJ, Collier AB. Ewing sarcoma: prognostic criteria, outcomes and future treatment. Exp Rev Anticancer Ther. 2008;8:617–24.
64. Carrle D, Bielack SS. Current strategies of chemotherapy in osteosarcoma. Int Orthop. 2006;30:445–51.
65. Altuntas AO, Slavin J, Smith PJ, Schlict SM, Powell GJ, Ngan S, Toner G, Choong PF. Accuracy of computed tomography guided core needle biopsy of musculoskeletal tumours. ANZ J Surg. 2005;75:187–91.
66. Pramesh CS, Deshpande MS, Pardiwala DN, Agarwal MG, Puri A. Core needle biopsy for bone tumours. Eur J Surg Oncol. 2001;27:668–71.
67. Royal College of Pathologists Standards and datasets for reporting cancers: dataset for histopathology reports on primary bone tumours. February 2015. www.rcpath.org. Accessed 24 Feb 2015.
68. SNOMED CT. The language of the NHS Care Records Service www.connectingforhealth.nhs.uk/publications 3769 (revised November 07). Accessed 24/02/215.
69. Machado I, Noguera R, Pellin A, Lopez-Guerrero JA, Piqueras M, Navarro S, Llombart-Bosch A. Molecular diagnosis of Ewing sarcoma family of

tumors: a comparative analysis of 560 cases with FISH and RT-PCR. Diag Mol Pathol. 2009;18:189–99.
70. UK Clinical Research Network Study Portfolio. http://public.ukcrn.org.uk/search/. Accessed 29 Feb 2016.
71. National Cancer Research Institute Clinical Studies Groups. http://csg.ncri.org.uk/portfolio/portfolio-maps/ Accessed 29 Feb 2016.
72. Burgert EO, Nesbit ME, Garnsey LA, Gehan EA, Herrmann J, Vietti TJ, Cangir A, Tefft M, Evans R, Thomas P. Multimodal therapy for the management of nonpelvic, localized Ewing's sarcoma of bone: intergroup study IESS-II. J Clin Oncol. 1990;8:1514–24.
73. Anninga JK, Gelderblom H, Fiocco M, Kroep JR, Taminiau AH, Hogendoorn PC, Egeler RM. Chemotherapeutic adjuvant treatment for osteosarcoma: where do we stand? Eur J Cancer. 2011;16:2431–45.
74. Delaney T, Liebsch NJ, Pedlow FX, Adams J, Dean S, Yeap BY, McManus P, Rosenberg AE, Nielsen GP, Harmon DC, et al. Phase II study of high-dose photon/proton radiotherapy in the management of spine sarcomas. Int J Radiat Oncol Biol Phys. 2009;74(3):732–9.
75. Chen Y, Ciernik F, Niemierko A, Kobayashi, Y. Torunn, D. Ebb, D. Harmon, K. Raskin, and others. Treatment of unresectable osteosarcoma with proton therapy. Int J Radiat Oncol. 2009; 75(3).**(Abst 2770)**.
76. Blattmann C, Oertel S, Schulz-Ertner D, Rieken S, Haufe S, Ewerbeck V, Unterberg A, Karapanagiotou-Schenkel I, Combs SE, Nikoghosyan A, et al. Non-randomized therapy trial to determine the safety and efficacy of heavy ion radiotherapy in patients with non-resectable osteosarcoma. BMC Cancer. 2010;10:96. doi:10.1186/1471-2407-10-96.
77. Noël G, Feuvret L, Ferrand R, Boisserie G, Mazeron JJ, Habrand JL. Radiotherapeutic factors in the management of cervical-basal chordomas and chondrosarcomas. Neurosurgery. 2004;55:1252–60.
78. Ares C, Hug EB, Lomax AJ, Bolsi A, Timmermann B, Rutz HP, Schuller JC, Pedroni E, Goitein G. Effectiveness and safety of spot scanning proton radiation therapy for chordomas and chondrosarcomas of the skull base: first long-term result. Int J Radiat Oncol Biol Phys. 2009;75(4):1111–8.
79. Yasuda M, Bresson D, Chibbaro S, Cornelius JF, Polivka M, Feuvret L, Takayasu M, George B, et al. Chordomas of the skull base and cervical spine: clinical outcomes associated with a multimodal surgical resection combined with proton-beam radiation in 40 patients. Neurosurg Rev. 2012;35(2):171–82.
80. Ciernik IF, Niemierko A, Harmon DC, Kobayashi W, Chen YL, Yock TI, Ebb DH, Choy E, Raskin KA, Liebsch N, et al. Proton-based radiotherapy for unresectable or incompletely resected osteosarcoma. Cancer. 2011;117(19):4522–30.
81. Imai R, Kamada T, Sugahara S, Tsuji H, Tsujii H. Br J Radiol. 2011;84(1):48–54. doi:10.1259/bjr/13783281 **(Epub 2011 Mar 22)**.
82. Staab AI, Rutz HP, Ares C, Timmermann B, Schneider R, Bolsi A, Albertini F, Lomax A, Goitein G, Hug E. Spot-scanning-based proton therapy for extracranial chordoma. Int J Radiat Oncol Biol Phys. 2011;81(4):489–96. doi:10.1016/j.ijrobp.2011.02.018 **(Epub 15 Apr 2011)**.
83. NHS Commissioning website. http://www.england.nhs.uk/commissioning/spec-services/npc-crg/group-b/b01/. Accessed 29 Feb 2016.
84. Salunke AA, Chen Y, Tan JH, Chen X, Khin LW, Puhaindran ME. Does pathological fracture affect the prognosis in patients with osteosarcoma of the extremities? a systematic review and meta-analysis. Bone Joint J. 2014;96:1396–403.
85. Xie C, Guo W, Li Y, Sun X. Pathological fracture does not influence local recurrence and survival in high-grade extremity osteosarcoma with adequate surgical margins. J Surg Oncol. 2012;106(7):820–5.
86. Reddy KI, Wafa H, Gaston CL, Grimer RJ, Abudu AT, Jeys LM, Carter SR, Tillman RM. Does amputation offer any survival benefit over limb salvage in osteosarcoma patients with poor chemonecrosis and close margins? Bone Joint J. 2015;97(1):115–20.
87. Bramer JA, Abudu AA, Grimer RJ, Carter SR, Tillman RM. Do pathological fractures influence survival and local recurrence rate in bony sarcomas? Eur J Cancer. 2007;43(13):1944–51.
88. Carrle D, Bielack S. Osteosarcoma lung metastases detection and principles of multimodal therapy. In: Jaffe et al, editor. Pediatric and Adolescent Osteosarcoma: Cancer Treatment and Research, 152. DOI 10.1007/978-1-4419-0284-9_8. Springer Science+Business Media, LLC 2009.
89. Bacci G, Ferrari S, Bertoni F, Rimondini S, Longhi A, Bacchini P, Forni C, Manfrini M, Donati D, Picci P. Prognostic factors in nonmetastatic Ewing's sarcoma of bone treated with adjuvant chemotherapy: analysis of 359 patients at the Istituto Ortopedico Rizzoli. J Clin Oncol. 2000;18:4–11.
90. Altaf S, Enders F, Jeavons E, Krailo M, Barkauskas DA, Meyers P, Arndt C. High BMI at diagnosis is associated with inferior survival in patients with osteosarcoma: a report from the Children's Oncology Group. Pediatr Blood Cancer. 2013;60(12):2042–6.
91. Collins M, Wilhelm M, Conyers R, Herschtal A, Whelan J, Bielack S, Kager L, Kühne T, Sydes M, Gelderblom H, et al. Benefits and adverse events in younger versus older patients receiving neoadjuvant chemotherapy for osteosarcoma: findings from a meta-analysis. J Clin Oncol. 2013;31:2310–2.
92. Janeway KA, Barkauskas DA, Krailo MD, Meyers PA, Schwartz CL, Ebb DH, Seibel NL, Grier HE, Gorlick R, Marina N. Outcome for adolescent and young adult patients with osteosarcoma. Cancer. 2012;118(18):4579–605.
93. Bielack S, Carrle D, Casali PG. ESMO Guidelines Working Group. Osteosarcoma: ESMO clinical recommendations for diagnosis, treatment and follow-up. Ann Oncol. 2009;20(4):137–9.
94. Grimer RJ. Surgical options for children with osteosarcoma. Lancet Oncol. 2005;6(2):85–92.
95. Lewis IJ, Nooij MA, Whelan J, Sydes MR, Grimer R, Hogendoorn PC, Memon MA, Weeden S, Uscinska BM, van Glabbeke M, et al. The MRC BO06 and EORTC 80931 collaborators and European osteosarcoma intergroup: improvement in histologic response but not survival in osteosarcoma patients treated with intensified chemotherapy: a randomized phase III trial of the European osteosarcoma intergroup. J Natl Cancer Inst. 2007;99:112–28.
96. Grimer RJ, Cannon SR, Taminiau AM, Bielack S, Kempf-Bielack B, Windhager R, Dominkus M, Saeter G, Bauer H, Meller I, et al. Osteosarcoma over the age of forty. Eur J Cancer. 2003;39:157–63.
97. Goorin AM, Schwartzentruber DJ, Devidas M, Gebhardt MC, Ayala AG, Harris MB, Helman LJ, Grier HE, Link MP, Pediatric Oncology Group. Presurgical chemotherapy compared with immediate surgery and adjuvant chemotherapy for nonmetastatic osteosarcoma: Pediatric Oncology Group Study POG-8651. J Clin Oncol. 2003;21:1574–80.
98. London and South East Sarcoma Network. Sarcoma guidelines. http://www.lsesn.nhs.uk/guidelines.html. Accessed 31 Jan 2014.
99. Daw NC, Neel MD, Rao BN, Billups CA, Wu J, Jenkins JJ, Quintana J, Luchtman-Jones L, Villarroel M, Santana VM. Frontline treatment of localized osteosarcoma without methotrexate: results of the St Jude Children's Research Hospital OS99 trail. Cancer. 2011;117(12):2770–8.
100. Picci P, Sangiorgi L, Rougraff BT, Neff JR, Casadei R, Campanacci M. Relationship of chemotherapy-induced necrosis and surgical margins to local recurrence in osteosarcoma. J Clin Oncol. 1994;12:2699–705.
101. Meyers PA, Schwartz CL, Krailo MD, Healey JH, Bernstein ML, Betcher D, Ferguson WS, Gebhardt MC, Goorin AM, Harris M, et al. Children's Oncology Group. Osteosarcoma: the addition of muramyl tripeptide to chemotherapy improves overall survival—a report from the Children's Oncology Group. J Clin Oncol. 2008;26:633–8.
102. Goorin AM, Harris MB, Bernstein M, Ferguson W, Devidas M, Siegal GP, Gebhardt MC, Schwartz CL, Link M, Grier HE. Phase II/III trial of etoposide and high-dose ifosfamide in newly diagnosed metastatic osteosarcoma: a Pediatric Oncology Group trial. J Clin Oncol. 2002;20(2):426–33 **(Epub 2002/01/12)**.
103. Navid F, Willert JR, McCarville MB, Furman W, Watkins A, Roberts W, Daw NC. Combination of gemcitabine and docetaxel in the treatment of children and young adults with refractory bone sarcoma. Cancer. 2008;113(2):419–25.
104. Eiber F, Guiliano A, Eckhardt J, Patterson K, Moseley S, Goodnight J. Adjuvant chemotherapy for osteosarcoma: a randomized prospective trial. J Clin Oncol. 1987;5:21–6.
105. Bernthal NM, Federman N, Eilber FR, Nelson SD, Eckardt JJ, Eilber FC, Tap WD. Long-term results (>25 years) of a randomized, prospective clinical trial evaluating chemotherapy ion patients with high-grade, operable osteosarcoma. Cancer. 2012;118:5888–93.
106. van Dalen EC, van As JW, de Camargo B. Methotrexate for high-grade osteosarcoma in children and young adults Review. London: Wiley; 2009. http://onlinelibrary.wiley.com/doi/10.1002/14651858.CD006325.pub3/full. Accessed 20 Jan 2016.

107. Whelan J, Patterson D, Perisoglou M, Bielack S, Marina N, Smeland S, Bernstein M. The role of interferons in the treatment of osteosarcoma. Pediatr Blood Cancer. 2010;54(3):350–4. doi:10.1002/pbc.22136.
108. Whelan J, Bielack SS, Marina N, Smeland S, Jovic G, Hook JM, Krailo M, Anninga J, Butterfass-Bahloul T, Böhling T, et al. EURAMOS collaborators. EURAMOS-1, an international randomised study for osteosarcoma: results from pre-randomisation treatment. Ann Oncol. 2015;26:407–14.
109. Bielack SS, Smeland S, Whelan JS, Marina N, Jovic G, Hook JM, Krailo MD, Gebhardt M, Pápai Z, Meyer J, et al. EURAMOS-1 investigators. Methotrexate, doxorubicin, and cisplatin (MAP) plus maintenance pegylated interferon alfa-2b versus MAP alone in patients with resectable high-grade osteosarcoma and good histologic response to preoperative MAP: first results of the EURAMOS-1 Good Response Randomized Controlled Trial. J Clin Oncol. 2015;33(20):2279–87. doi:10.1200/JCO.2014.60.0734.
110. Bielack SS, Kempf-Bielack B, Delling G, Exner GU, Flege S, Helmke K, Kotz R, Salzer-Kuntschik M, Werner M, Winkelmann W, et al. For the cooperative German-Austrian-Swiss osteosarcoma group. Prognostic factors in high grade osteosarcoma of the extremities or trunk: an analysis of 1,702 patients treated on neoadjuvant cooperative osteosarcoma study group protocols. J Clin Oncol. 2002;20:776–90.
111. Byun BH, Kong CB, Lim I, Kim BI, Choi CW, Song WS, Cho WH, Jeon DG, Koh JS, Lee SY, et al. Early response monitoring to neoadjuvant chemotherapy in osteosarcoma using sequential 18 F-FDG PET/CT and MRI. Eur J Nucl Med Mol Imag. 2013;41:1553–62.
112. Wang CS, Du LJ, Si MJ, Yin QH, Chen L, Shu M, Yuan F, Fei XC, Ding XY. Noninvasive assessment of response to neoaduvant chemotherapy in osteosarcoma of long bones with diffusion-weighted imaging: an initial in vivo study. PLoS One. 2013;8(8):e72679.
113. National Institute for Health and Care Excellence (NICE) Neutropenic sepsis: prevention and management of neutropenic sepsis in cancer patients. NICE Guidelines [CG151]; 2012. http://www.nice.org.uk/guidance/cg151. Accessed 02 Feb 2015.
114. Frezza AM, Beale T, Bomanji J, Jay A, Kalavrezos N, Dileo P, Whelan J, Strauss SJ. Is [F-18]-fluorodeoxy-D-glucose positron emission tomography of value in the management of patients with craniofacial bone sarcomas undergoing neo-adjuvant treatment? BMC Cancer. 2014;14:23–9.
115. Kager L, Zoubek A, Potschger U, Kastner U, Flege S, Kempf-Bielack B, Branscheid D, Kotz R, Salzer-Kuntschik M, Winkelmann W, et al. Cooperative German-Austrian-Swiss Osteosarcoma Study Group. Primary metastatic osteosarcoma: presentation and outcome of patients treated on neoadjuvant Cooperative Osteosarcoma Study Group protocols. J Clin Oncol. 2003;21:2011–8.
116. Gelderblom H, Jinks RC, Sydes M, Bramwell VH, van Glabbeke M, Grimer RJ, Hogendoorn PC, McTiernan A, Lewis IJ, Nooij MA, et al. European Osteosarcoma Intergroup. Survival after recurrent osteosarcoma: data from 3 European Osteosarcoma Intergroup (EOI) randomized controlled trials. Eur J Cancer. 2011;47(6):895–902.
117. Garcia Franco CE. Torre W, Tamura A, Guillén-Grima F, San-Julian M, Martin-Algarra S, Pardo FJ. Long-term results after resection for bone sarcoma pulmonary metastases. Eur J Cardiothorac Surg. 2010;37:1205–8.
118. Ferrari S, Briccoli A, Mercuri M, Bertoni F, Picci P, Tienghi A, Del Prever AB, Fagioli F, Comandone A, Bacci G. Postrelapse survival in osteosarcoma of the extremities: prognostic factors for long-term survival. J Clin Oncol. 2003;21:710–5.
119. Kempf-Bielack B, Bielack SS, Juergens H, Branscheid D, Berdel WE, Exner GU, Göbel U, Helmke K, Jundt G, Kabisch H, et al. Osteosarcoma relapse after combined modality therapy: an analysis of unselected patients in the cooperative osteosarcoma study group (COSS). J Clin Oncol. 2005;23(3):559–68.
120. Berger M, Grignani G, Ferrari S, Biasin E. Brach del Prever A, Aliberti S, Saglio F, Aglietta M, Fagioli F. Phase 2 trial of two courses of cyclophosphamide and etoposide for relapsed high risk osteosarcoma patients. Cancer. 2009;115:2980–7.
121. Munoz A, Alfaro J, Pardo N, García-Miguel P, Quintero V, Gros L, Melero C, Antuña MJ, Ocete G, de Las Heras J, et al. Long-term results of the Spanish protocol SO-95 for the treatment of non-metastatic high-grade osteosarcoma of the extremeties in children. Clin Transl Oncol. 2009;11:387–92.
122. Anderson PM, Subbiah V, Rohren E. Bone-seeking radiopharmaceuticals as targeted agents of osteosarcoma: samarium-153-EDTMP and radium-223. Adv Exp Med Biol. 2014;804:291–304. doi:10.1007/978-3-319-04843-7_16.
123. Grignani G, Palmerini E, Ferraresi V, D'Ambrosio L, Bertulli R, Asaftei SD, Tamburini A, Pignochino Y, Sangiolo D, Marchesi E, et al. Italian Sarcoma Group. Sorafenib and everolimus for patients with unresectable high-grade osteosarcoma progressing after standard treatment: a non-randomised phase 2 clinical trial. Lancet Oncol. 2015;16(1):98–107.
124. Buddingh EP, Anninga JK, Versteegh MI, Taminiau AH, Egeler RM, van Rijswijk CS, Hogendoorn PC, Lankester AC, Gelderblom H. Prognostic factors in pulmonary metastasized high grade osteosarcoma. Paediat Blood Cancer. 2010;54:216–21.
125. He JP, Hao Y, Li M, Wang J, Guo FJ. Tumor-to-background ratio to predict response to chemotherapy of osteosarcoma better than standard uptake values. Orthop Surg. 2014;6(2):145–53.
126. Leavey PJ, Mascarenhas L, Marina N, Chen Z, Krailo M, Miser J, Brown K, Tarbell N, Bernstein ML, Granowetter L, et al. Children's Oncology Group. Prognostic factors for patients with Ewing sarcoma (EWS) at first recurrence following multi-modality therapy: a report from the Children's Oncology Group. Pediatr Blood Cancer. 2008;51:334–8.
127. Bacci G, Forni C, Longhi A, Ferrari S, Donati D, De Paolis M, Barbieri E, Pignotti E, Rosito P, Versari M. Long-term outcome for patients with non-metastatic Ewing's sarcoma treated with adjuvant and neoadjuvant chemotherapies. 402 patients treated at Rizzoli between 1972 and 1992. Eur J Cancer. 2004;40:73–83.
128. Paulussen M, Ahrens S, Craft AW, Dunst J, Fröhlich B, Jabar S, Rübe C, Winkelmann W, Wissing S, Zoubek A, Jürgens H. Ewing's tumors with primary lung metastases: survival analysis of 114 (European Intergroup) Cooperative Ewing's Sarcoma Studies patients. J Clin Oncol. 1998;16:3044–52.
129. Bacci G, Palmerini E, Staals EL, Longhi A, Barbieri E, Alberghini M, Ferrari S. Ewing's sarcoma family tumours of the humerus: outcome of patients treated with radiotherapy, surgery or surgery and adjuvant radiotherapy. Radiother Oncol. 2009;93:383–7.
130. Schuck A, Ahrens S, Paulussen M, Kuhlen M, Könemann S, Rübe C, Winkelmann W, Kotz R, Dunst J, Willich N, Jürgens H. Local therapy in localized Ewing tumors: results of 1058 patients treated in the CESS 81, CESS 86, and EICESS 92 trials. Int J Radiat Oncol Biol Phys. 2003;55:168–77.
131. EURO-E.W.I.N.G 99 treatment manual. http://www.cancer.gov/clinicaltrials/search/view?cdrid=68608&version=healthprofessional. Accessed 03 Feb 2015.
132. Nesbit ME, Gehan EA, Burgert EO Jr, Vietti TJ, Cangir A, Tefft M, Evans R, Thomas P, Askin FB, Kissane JM. Multimodal therapy for the management of primary, nonmetastatic Ewing's sarcoma of bone: a long-term follow-up of the first intergroup study. J Clin Oncol. 1990;8:1664–74.
133. Grier HE, Krailo MD, Tarbell NJ, Link MP, Fryer CJ, Pritchard DJ, Gebhardt MC, Dickman PS, Perlman EJ, Meyers PA, et al. Addition of ifosfamide and etoposide to standard chemotherapy for Ewing's sarcoma and primitive neuroectodermal tumor of bone. New Eng J Med. 2003;348:694–701.
134. Jürgens H, Exner U, Gadner H, Harms D, Michaelis J, Sauer R, Treuner J, Voûte T, Winkelmann W, Winkler K. Multidisciplinary treatment of primary Ewing's sarcoma of bone: a 6-year experience of a European cooperative trial. Cancer. 1988;61:23–32.
135. Paulussen M, Craft AW, Lewis I, Hackshaw A, Douglas C, Dunst J, Schuck A, Winkelmann W, Köhler G, Poremba C, et al. European Intergroup Cooperative Ewing's Sarcoma Study-92. Results of the EICESS-92 study: two randomized trials of Ewing's sarcoma treatment—cyclophosphamide compared with ifosfamide in standard-risk patients and assessment of benefit of etoposide added to standard treatment in high-risk patients. J Clin Oncol. 2008;26(27):4385–93.
136. Pinkerton CR, Bataillard A, Guillo S, Oberlin O, Fervers B, Philip T. Treatment strategies for metastatic Ewing's sarcoma. Eur J Cancer. 2001;37:1338–44.
137. Wagner LM, McAllister N, Goldsby RE, Rausen AR, McNall-Knapp RY, McCarville MB, Albritton K. Temozolomide and intravenous irinotecan for treatment of advanced Ewing sarcoma. Pediat Blood Cancer. 2007;48:132–9.
138. Burdach S, Meyer-Bahlburg A, Laws HJ, Haase R, van Kaik B, Metzner B, Wawer A, Finke R, Göbel U, Haerting J, et al. High-dose therapy for

patients with primary multifocal and early relapsed Ewing's tumors: results of two consecutive regimens assessing the role of total-body irradiation. J Clin Oncol. 2003;21:3072–8.

139. Le Deley M-C, Paulussen M, Lewis I, Brennan B, Ranft A, Whelan J, Le Teuff G, Michon J, Ladenstein R, Marec-Brard P, et al. Cyclophosphamide compared with ifosfamide in consolidation treatment of standard-risk Ewing sarcoma: results of the Randomized Noninferiority Euro-EWING99-R1 Trial. J Clin Oncol. 2014;32(23):2440–8.
140. Womer RB, West DC, Krailo MD, Dickman PS, Pawel BR, Grier HE, Marcus K, Sailer S, Healey JH, Dormans JP, et al. Randomized controlled trial of interval-compressed chemotherapy for the treatment of localized Ewing sarcoma: a report from the Children's Oncology Group. J Clin Oncol. 2012;30:4148–54.
141. Ferrari S, Sundby Hall K, Lutsch R, Tienghi A, Wiebe T, Fagioli F, Alvegard TA, Brach Del Prever A, Tamburini A, Alberghini M, et al. Nonmetastatic Ewing family tumours: high-dose chemotherapy with stem cell rescue on poor responder patients. Results of the Italian Sarcoma Group/Scandinavian Sarcoma Group III protocol. Ann Oncol. 2011;22(5):1221–7.
142. Juergens C, Weston C, Lewis I, Whelan J, Paulussen M, Oberlin O, Michon J, Zoubek A, Jürgens H, Craft A. Safety assessment of intensive induction with vincristine, ifosfamide, doxorubicin, and etoposide (VIDE) in the treatment of Ewing tumors in the EURO-E.W.I.N.G. 99 clinical trial. Pediat Blood Cancer. 2006;47(1):22–9.
143. Ladenstein R, Potschger U, Le Deley MC, Whelan J, Paulussen M, Oberlin O, van den Berg H, Dirksen U, Hjorth L, Michon J, et al. Primary disseminated multifocal Ewing sarcoma: results of the Euro-EWING 99 trial. J Clin Oncol. 2010;28:3284–91.
144. Ferrari S, del Prever AB, Palmerini E, Staals E, Berta M, Balladelli A, Picci P, Fagioli F, Bacci G, Vanel D. Response to high-dose ifosfamide in patients with advanced/recurrent Ewing sarcoma. Pediatr Blood Cancer. 2009;52(5):581–4.
145. Saylors RL 3rd, Stine KC, Sullivan J, Kepner JL, Wall DA, Bernstein ML, Harris MB, Hayashi R. Vietti TJ; Pediatric Oncology Group. Cyclophosphamide plus topotecan in children with recurrent or refractory solid tumors: a Pediatric Oncology Group phase II study. J Clin Oncol. 2001;19(15):3463–9.
146. Casey DA, Wexler LH, Merchant MS, Chou AJ, Merola PR, Price AP, Meyers PA. Irinotecan and temozolomide for Ewing sarcoma: the Memorial Sloan-Kettering experience. Pediatr Blood Cancer. 2009;53(6):1029–34.
147. McTiernan A, Driver D, Michelagnoli MP, Kilby AM, Whelan JS. High dose chemotherapy with bone marrow or peripheral stem cell rescue is an effective treatment option for patients with relapsed or progressive Ewing's sarcoma family of tumours. Ann Oncol. 2006;17:1301–5.
148. Fox E, Patel S, Wathen JK, Schuetze S, Chawla S, Harmon D, Reinke D, Chugh R, Benjamin RS, Helman LJ. Phase II Study of sequential gemcitabine followed by docetaxel for recurrent Ewing sarcoma, osteosarcoma, or unresectable or locally recurrent chondrosarcoma: results of sarcoma alliance for research through collaboration study 003. Oncol. 2012;17(3):321. doi:10.1634/theoncologist.2010-0265 **(Epub 23 Feb 2012)**.
149. Mora J, Cruz CO, Parareda A, de Torres C. Treatment of relapsed/refractory pediatric sarcomas with gemcitabine and docetaxel. J Pediatr Hematol Oncol. 2009;31(10):723–9.
150. Kebudi R, Gorgun O, Ayan I. Oral etoposide for recurrent/progressive sarcomas of childhood. Pediatr Blood Cancer. 2004;42(4):320–4.
151. Euro Ewing Consortium. http://www.euroewing.eu/clinical-trials/ee2012-trial. Accessed 29/2/2016.
152. Indelicato DJ, Keole SR, Shahlaee AH, Shi W, Morris CG, Marcus RB Jr. Definitive radiotherapy for Ewing tumors of extremities and pelvis: long-term disease control, limb function, and treatment toxicity. Int J Radiat Oncol Biol Phys. 2008;72(3):871–7.
153. DuBois SG, Krailo MD, Gebhardt MC, Donaldson SS, Marcus KJ, Dormans J, Shamberger RC, Sailer S, Nicholas RW, Healey JH, et al. Comparative evaluation of local control strategies in localized Ewing sarcoma of bone: a report from the Children's Oncology Group. Cancer. 2015;121(3):467–75.
154. Patel S, Delaney T. Advanced-technology radiation therapy for bone sarcomas. Cancer Control. 2008;15(1):21–37.
155. Sterzing F, Stoiber EM, Nill S, Bauer H, Huber P, Debus J, Münter MW. Intensity modulated radiotherapy (IMRT) in the treatment of children and adolescents–a single institution's experience and a review of the literature. Radiat Oncol. 2009;4:37. doi:10.1186/1748-717X-4-37.
156. Mounessi FS, Lehrich P, Haverkamp U, Willich N, Bolling T, Eich HT. Pelvic Ewing sarcomas. Three-dimensional conformal vs. intensity-modulated radiotherapy. Strahlenther Onkol. 2013;189(4):308–14. doi:10.1007/s00066-012-0304-z **(Epub 2013 Feb 28)**.
157. Pérez-Muñoz I, Grimer RJ, Spooner D, Carter S, Tillman RRR, Abudu A, Jeys L. Use of tissue expander in pelvic Ewing's sarcoma treated with radiotherapy. Eur J Surg Oncol. 2014;40(2):197–201. doi:10.1016/j.ejso.2013.09.001.
158. Euro-Ewing Radiotherapy Guidelines, Chapter XVII. In: EUROpean Ewing tumour Working Initiative of National Groups Ewing Tumour Studies 1999. EE 99 Amended Version 14th February 2006. https://www.skion.nl/workspace/uploads/ee99_amended_treo__2006_02_14.pdf. Accessed 20 Jan 2016.
159. Bernstein ML, Devidas M, Lafreniere D, Souid AK, Meyers PA, Gebhardt M, Stine K, Nicholas R, Perlman EJ, Dubowy R, Pediatric Oncology Group, Children's Cancer Group Phase II Study 9457, Children's Oncology Group, et al. Intensive therapy with growth factor support for patients with Ewing tumor metastatic at diagnosis: Pediatric Oncology Group/Children's Cancer Group Phase II Study 9457—a report from the Children's Oncology Group. J Clin Oncol. 2006;24:152–9.
160. Whelan JS, Burcombe RJ, Janinis J, Baldelli AM, Cassoni AM. A systematic review of the role of pulmonary irradiation in the management of primary bone tumours. Ann Oncol. 2002;13:23–30.
161. Brown LC, Lester RA, Grams MP, Haddock MG, Olivier KR, Arndt CA, Rose PS, Laack NN. Stereotactic radiotherapy for metastatic and recurrent Ewing sarcoma and osteosarcoma. Sarcoma. 2014;418270:9. doi:10.1155/2014/418270.
162. Cotterill SJ, Ahrens S, Paulussen M, Jürgens HF, Voûte PA, Gadner H, Craft AW. Prognostic factors in Ewing's tumor of bone: analysis of 975 patients from the European Intergroup Cooperative Ewing's Sarcoma Study Group. J Clin Oncol. 2000;18:3108–14.
163. Cangir A, Vietti TJ, Gehan EA, Burgert EO Jr, Thomas P, Tefft M, Nesbit ME, Kissane J, Pritchard D. Ewing's sarcoma metastatic at diagnosis. Results and comparisons of two intergroup Ewing's sarcoma studies. Cancer. 1990;66:887–93.
164. McTiernan AM, Cassoni AM, Driver D, Michelagnoli MP, Kilby AM, Whelan JS. Improving outcomes after relapse in Ewing's Sarcoma: analysis of 114 patients from a single institution. Sarcoma. 2006;2006:1–8.
165. Stahl M, Ranft A, Paulussen M, Bölling T, Vieth V, Bielack S, Görtitz I, Braun-Munzinger G, Hardes J, Jürgens H, et al. Risk of recurrence and survival after relapse in patients with Ewing sarcoma. Pediatr Blood Cancer. 2011;57(4):549–53.
166. Abudu A, Davies AM, Pynsent PB, Mangham DC, Tillman RM, Carter SR, Grimer RJ. Tumour volume as a predictor of necrosis after chemotherapy in Ewing's sarcoma. J Bone Joint Surg Br. 1999;81(2):317–22.
167. Boriani S, Bandiera S, Biagini R, Bacchini P, Boriani L, Cappuccio M, Chevalley F, Gasbarrini A, Picci P, Weinstein JN. Chordoma of the mobile spine: 50 years of experience. Spine. 2006;31:493–503.
168. Xie L, Whalley N, Adasonia K, Grimer R, Jeys L. Can local recurrence of a sacral chordoma be treated by further surgery? Bone Joint J. 2015;97(5):711–5.
169. Stacchiotti S, Marrari A, Tamborini E, Palassini E, Virdis E, Messina A, Crippa F, Morosi C, Gronchi A, Pilotti S, et al. Response to imatinib plus sirolimus in advanced chordoma. Ann Oncol. 2009;20:1886–94.
170. Stacchiotti S, Longhi A, Ferraresi V, Grignani G, Comandone A, Stupp R, Bertuzzi A, Tamborini E, Pilotti S, Messina A, et al. Phase II study of imatinib in advanced chordoma. J Clin Oncol. 2012;30(9):914–20.
171. Brewer P, Sumathi V, Grimer RJ, Carter SR, Tillman RM, Abudu A, Jeys L. Primary leiomyosarcoma of bone: analysis of prognosis. Sarcoma. 2012;636849:4. doi:10.1155/2012/636849.
172. National Cancer Institute (NCI). General information about osteosarcoma and malignant fibrous histiosarcoma (MFH) of bone. http://www.cancer.gov/cancertopics/types/bone. Accessed 02 Feb 2015.
173. Chawla S, Henshaw R, Seeger L, Choy E, Blay JY, Ferrari S, Kroep J, Grimer R, Reichardt P, Rutkowski P, et al. Safety and efficacy of denosumab for adults and skeletally mature adolescents with giant cell tumour of bone: interim analysis of an open-label, parallel-group, phase 2 study. Lancet Oncol. 2013;14(9):901–8.

174. Rutkowski P, Ferrari S, Grimer RJ, Stalley PD, Dijkstra SP, Pienkowski A, Vaz G, Wunder JS, Seeger LL, Feng A, et al. Surgical downstaging in an open-label phase II trial of denosumab in patients with giant cell tumor of bone. Ann Surg Oncol. 2015;22(9):2860–8. doi:10.1245/s10434-015-4634-9.
175. Thomas D, Henshaw R, Skubitz K, Chawla S, Staddon A, Blay JY, Roudier M, Smith J, Ye Z, Sohn W, et al. Denosumab in patients with giant-cell tumour of bone: an open-label, phase 2 study. Lancet Oncology. 2010;11(3):275–80.
176. Fleming GF, Heimann PS, Stephens JK, Simon MA, Ferguson MK, Benjamin RS, Samuels BL. Dedifferentiated chordoma. Response to aggressive chemotherapy in two cases. Cancer. 1993;72(3):714–8 **(Epub 1993/08/01)**.
177. George S, Merriam P, Maki RG, Van den Abbeele AD, Yap JT, Akhurst T, Harmon DC, Bhuchar G, O'Mara MM, D'Adamo DR, et al. Multicenter phase II trial of sunitinib in the treatment of nongastrointestinal stromal tumor sarcomas. J Clin Oncol. 2009;27(19):3154–60.
178. Puri A, Gulia A, Hawaldar R, Ranganathan P, Badwe RA. Does intensity of surveillance affect survival after surgery for sarcomas? results of a randomized noninferiority trial. Clin Orthop Rel Res. 2014;472(5):1568–75.
179. Aksnes LH, Bauer HC, Dahl AA, Fosså SD, Hjorth L, Jebsen N, Lernedal H, Hall KS. Health status at long-term follow up in patients treated for extremity localized Ewing sarcoma or osteosarcoma: a Scandinavian sarcoma group study. Pediatr Blood Cancer. 2009;53:84–9.
180. Langer T, Stöhr W, Paulides M, Kremers A, Dörr HG, Göbel U, Beck JD. Prospective multicenter registration of major late sequelae in sarcoma patients using the late effects surveillance system (LESS). Klinische Pädiatrie. 2005;217:176–81.
181. Bassal M, Mertens AC, Taylor L, Neglia JP, Greffe BS, Hammond S, Ronckers CM, Friedman DL, Stovall M, Yasui YY, et al. Risk of selected subsequent carcinomas in survivors of childhood cancer: a report from the childhood cancer survivor study. Clin Oncol. 2006;24(3):476–83.
182. Rodriguez-Galindo C, Poquette C, Marina NM, Head DR, Cain A, Meyer WH, Santana VM, Pappo AS. Hematologic abnormalities and acute myeloid leukemia in children and adolescents administered intensified chemotherapy for the Ewing sarcoma family of tumours. J Pediat Oncol. 2000;22(4):321–9.

14

Cytotoxic and targeted therapy for treatment of pseudomyogenic hemangioendothelioma

Jason Joseph[1], Wei-lien Wang[2], Madhavi Patnana[3], Naveen Ramesh[1], Robert Benjamin[1], Shreyaskumar Patel[1] and Vinod Ravi[1*]

Abstract

Pseudomyogenic hemangioendothelioma (PMH) is a recently described, indolent vascular tumor that usually presents in the distal extremities. PMH typically has a multi-focal presentation and can involve several tissue planes including the dermis, subcutis, muscle, and bone. This soft tissue tumor predominantly affects men between 20 and 50 years of age. PMH tumors typically are resected but frequently recur locally; thus, more efficacious treatment options are needed. Herein, we report two cases of patients with PMH who were treated with systemic therapy. To the best of our knowledge, our report is the first to describe a response of PMH either to gemcitabine/taxane cytotoxic chemotherapy or to a mammalian target of rapamycin inhibitor. In the first case, a 45-year-old man with PMH of the right ilium was treated with gemcitabine plus docetaxel. Although chemotherapy was ultimately halted owing to gemcitabine-induced pulmonary toxicity, positron emission tomography-computer tomography scans taken after three cycles of gemcitabine plus docetaxel illustrated a noticeable response to the regimen. In the second case, a 22-year-old man with PMH of the right distal femur and metastases in the left ilium showed no response to gemcitabine plus docetaxel therapy, but underwent surgical resection after cisplatin and doxorubicin resulted in stable disease. DNA sequencing of his tumor revealed the presence of a tuberous sclerosis 1 (TSC1) mutation, so daily everolimus, which inhibits mammalian target of rapamycin, was started. Two months after beginning everolimus, the patient underwent magnetic resonance imaging of the pelvis, which revealed mild shrinkage of PMH metastases in the left iliac bone. Despite the apparent heterogeneity of response to gemcitabine/taxane chemotherapy in our two patients, these two cases indicate that gemcitabine/taxane and mammalian target of rapamycin inhibitor may serve as systemic treatment options for PMH and warrant further investigation.

Keywords: Pseudomyogenic, Hemangioendothelioma, Soft tissue tumor, Sarcoma, mTOR inhibitor

Background

Pseudomyogenic hemangioendothelioma (PMH) is a rare indolent vascular tumor that typically presents in the distal extremities and may present in multiple tissue planes, including the dermis, subcutis, muscle, and bone [1, 2]. Over the last three decades, PMH has been determined to be the same pathological entity as epithelioid sarcoma-like hemangioendothelioma and fibroma-like variant of epithelioid sarcoma [2–5]. The tumor has a 4.6:1 male predominance and typically occurs in men between 20 and 50 years of age. Histopathologically, PMH resembles a myogenic neoplasm with a striking rhabdomyoblast appearance and spindle cell morphology. However, PMH lacks true muscle markers such as desmin and has an immunophenotype and highly membranous pattern in line with endothelial differentiation [2, 5]. PMH has recently been characterized molecularly to have a balanced t(7;19) translocation resulting in a SERPINE1-FOSB fusion [6]. PMH does not typically

*Correspondence: vravi@mdanderson.org
[1] Department of Sarcoma Medical Oncology, Unit 0450, The University of Texas MD Anderson Cancer Center, 1515 Holcombe Blvd., Houston, TX 77030, USA

transform into high-grade disease or metastasize. However, PMH frequently recurs locally after excision [2].

While much has been published concerning the characterization of PMH, much remains to be learned about the natural history of the disease and efficacy of treatment. In the majority of PMH cases, excision is the management modality of choice, but over a third of patients experience local recurrence or new nodules in adjacent soft tissue during follow up [2]. Previous accounts demonstrate an indolent course of disease and most studies have shown that the disease does not progress before or after therapy. In a large case series (n = 50), only one patient died of PMH. Nevertheless, since PMH presents as multifocal tumors in 70 % of patients, systemic therapy options are acutely needed [2].

To the best of our knowledge, only two published reports [5, 7] in the literature discuss a response by PMH to therapeutic options other than excision.

Here, we report two cases of patients who had PMH that responded to systemic therapy: one patient exhibited a noticeable response to gemcitabine plus docetaxel and one patient demonstrated a response to everolimus, a mammalian target of rapamycin (mTOR) inhibitor.

Case presentation

Case 1

In October 2010, a 45-year-old man presented to his local physician with pain in his right groin, which the patient attributed to a muscle strain from playing soccer. As his pain worsened, the patient went to an orthopedic surgeon who obtained a magnetic resonance imaging (MRI) study that showed a mass within the right anterior ilium. In December 2010, the patient was examined by physicians in the Department of Orthopaedic Oncology at The University of Texas MD Anderson Cancer Center, and a biopsy of the right ilium mass revealed a malignant epithelioid and spindle cell neoplasm most consistent with PMH. The patient was treated with two cycles of intra-arterial cisplatin (120 mg/m^2) administered every 3 weeks. Due to hearing loss, administration was modified to intravenously with a slow infusion rate over 24 h for the next two cycles. Restaging positron emission tomography-computed tomography (PET-CT) studies revealed a minor tumor response to cisplatin.

Because the patient's hearing loss worsened, therapy was switched to a combination of gemcitabine (900 mg/m^2) and docetaxel (100 mg/m^2) administered in 3 week cycles, beginning 3 weeks after cessation of cisplatin. Restaging PET-CT studies performed after completion of the third cycle revealed that the PMH had significantly responded to gemcitabine plus docetaxel (Fig. 1). Unfortunately, despite this significant improvement, there was evidence of gemcitabine-induced pulmonary toxicity. Therefore, cytotoxic chemotherapy was halted, and a tapering dose of steroids was given to the patient to treat the pulmonary toxicity. The patient's edema was managed with furosemide and amiloride.

During a follow-up visit 3 months after cessation of gemcitabine and docetaxel, the patient's PET-CT scans showed mild progression of disease in the right iliac bone with enlarging lucencies. This finding suggested that the PMH progressed in the absence of gemcitabine and docetaxel treatment. Therapy with weekly paclitaxel (80 mg/m^2) was therefore started. However, after 4 months of paclitaxel, therapy was discontinued because the patient experienced hearing loss, rhinitis, and neuropathy characterized by tingling of the hands and feet. Restaging studies performed 16 months following cessation of cytotoxic chemotherapy revealed stable disease.

The tumor response to the combination of gemcitabine and a taxane was clearly demonstrated on the PET-CT scans. PMH progressed once chemotherapy was stopped, and taxane treatment led to disease stability, suggesting that gemcitabine plus taxane could be an effective treatment for PMH.

Case 2

In June 2011, a 22-year-old man presented to his local physician with a painless, dime-shaped nodule in his right lateral thigh. Approximately 1 year later, the mass began to enlarge and induce pain, and the patient saw a dermatologist who performed a punch biopsy that was inconclusive. In September 2012, an excisional biopsy was performed at MD Anderson Cancer Center, and the pathologist concluded that the mass was consistent with PMH originating from the right femur. Baseline imaging included MRI of the right thigh which showed multiple enhancing lesions in the distal right femur and lateral soft tissues, extending for a length of 6.8 cm and centered approximately 7 cm proximal to the articular surface of the lateral femoral condyle. A baseline PET-CT study revealed a hypermetabolic mass in the right distal femur (standardized uptake value, maximum of 15.2) and a 1.3 cm left acetabular lytic lesion (standardized uptake value, maximum of 7.9), suspicious for metastatic disease (Fig. 2). After the patient was evaluated by physicians in the Department of Sarcoma Medical Oncology at MD Anderson, therapy with gemcitabine (900 mg/m^2) and docetaxel (75 mg/m^2) was started and given in 3 week cycles. The cytotoxic chemotherapy was well tolerated. However, imaging showed no evidence of tumor response after two cycles, and treatment was halted.

Therapy was then changed to doxorubicin (90 mg/m^2 as a continuous infusion over 72 h) and cisplatin (120 mg/m^2 as an intravenous infusion over 4 h), but the patient had mucositis, tinnitus, neutropenic fever,

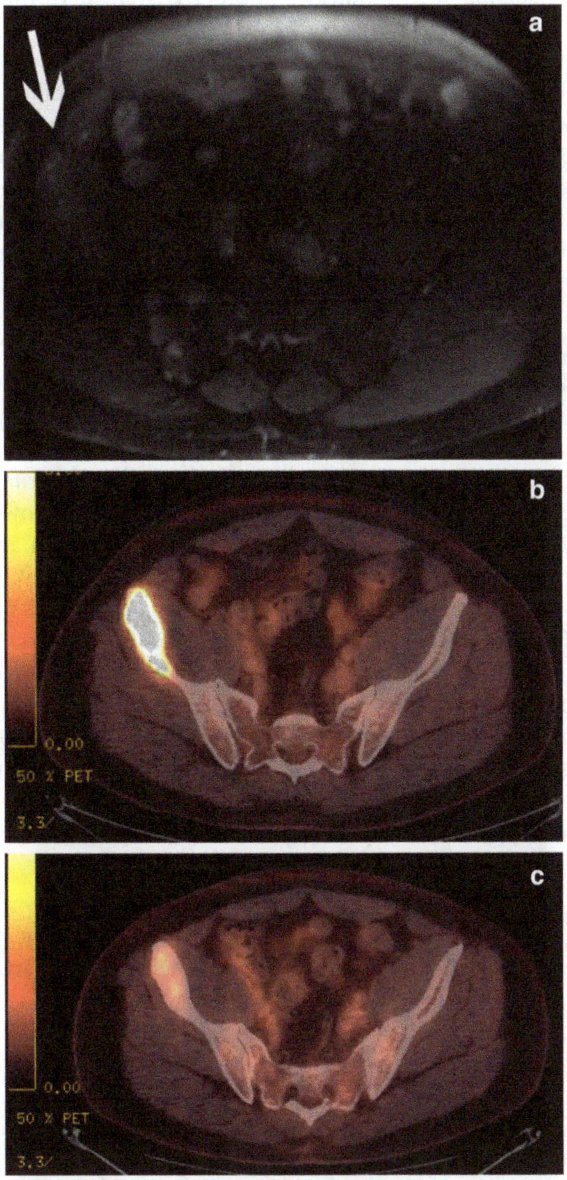

Fig. 1 Imaging studies for 45-year-old patient ("Case 1") with pseudomyogenic hemangioendothelioma. **a** Baseline fat saturated T1-weighted axial magnetic resonance image with intravenous contrast enhancement of the pelvis demonstrates multiple enhancing tumor foci in the right iliac bone (*white arrow*). **b** Positron emission tomography-computed tomography (PET-CT) fusion image through the pelvis demonstrates diffuse metabolic activity in the right anterior iliac bone (disease in the right posterior iliac bone at the level of the sacroiliac joint was also present but is not shown). This image was obtained 1 month before the patient began gemcitabine/docetaxel. **c** PET-CT fusion image through the pelvis after three cycles of gemcitabine/docetaxel demonstrates a significant metabolic response

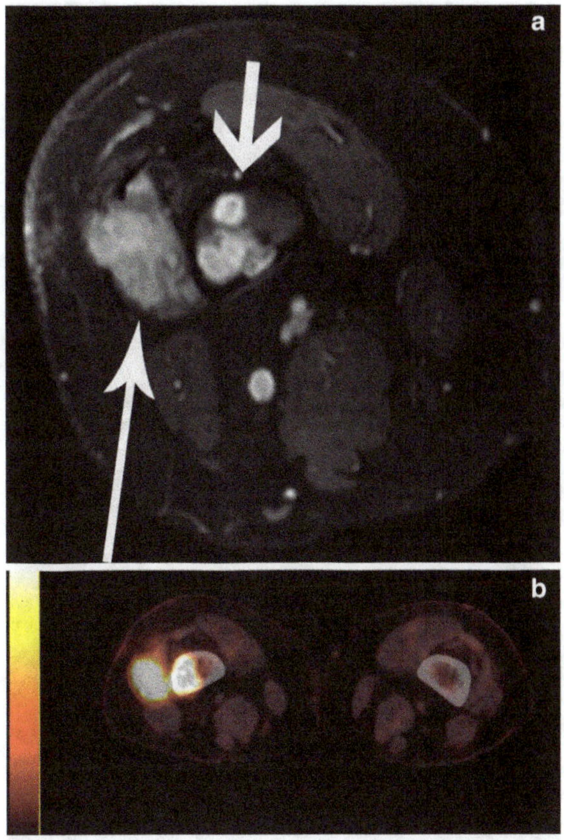

Fig. 2 Baseline magnetic resonance imaging (MRI) and positron emission tomography-computed tomography (PET-CT) studies for a 22-year-old man ("Case 2") with pseudomyogenic hemangioendothelioma. **a** Baseline contrast-enhanced, fat-saturated T1-weighted axial MR image of the right thigh demonstrates multifocal enhancing lesions in the distal femoral metadiaphysis (*short white arrow*) and vastus intermedius muscle and subcutaneous fat. **b** PET-CT fusion image through the distal femurs demonstrates corresponding hypermetabolic activity. Restaging examinations after two cycles of gemcitabine and docetaxel (not shown) did not demonstrate any significant response

and ototoxicity during the first cycle. The cisplatin dose was reduced to 100 mg/m^2 as a slow infusion over 24 h to prevent ototoxicity and doxorubicin was changed to bolus doxorubicin with dexrazoxane (90 mg/m^2) in a 3 week cycle to reduce mucositis caused by continuous intravenous infusion of doxorubicin. The patient tolerated the regimen better during the second cycle, and the PMH remained stable.

In July 2013, the patient underwent surgical resection to remove the right distal femoral lesion. DNA sequencing of the tumor revealed the presence of a tuberous sclerosis 1 (TSC1):c.1760A >Gp.K587R mutation. Owing to the TSC1 mutation, therapy with everolimus (10 mg/day) was started. Two months later, the patient underwent MRI of the pelvis, which revealed mild interval healing of the small intramedullary metastases in the supra-acetabular region of the left iliac bone (Fig. 3).

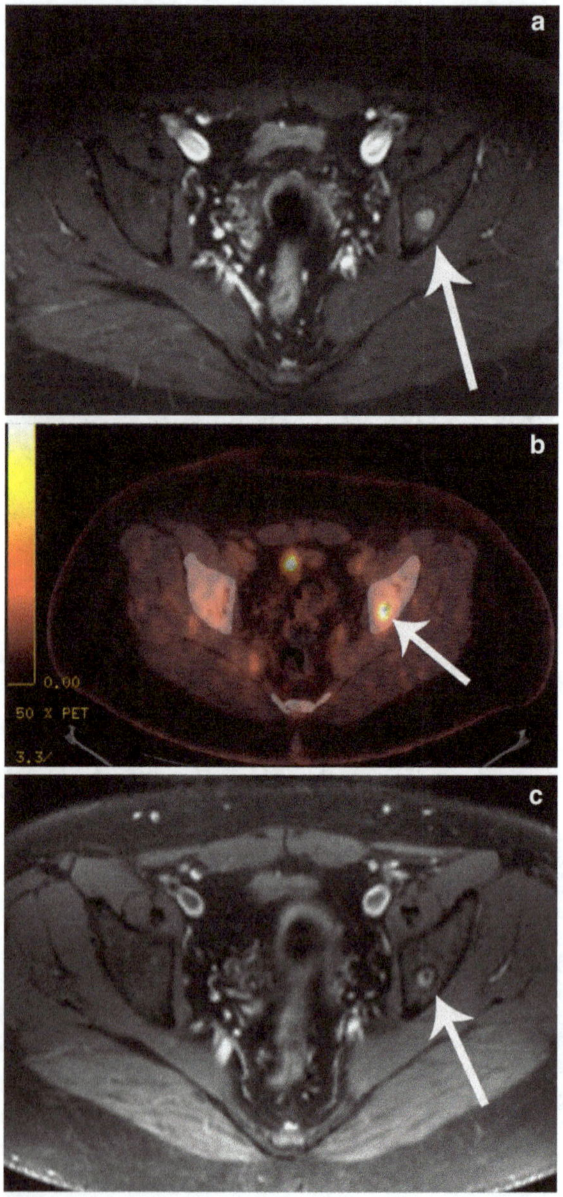

Fig. 3 Imaging studies obtained during treatment for a 22-year-old man ("Case 2") with pseudomyogenic hemangioendothelioma. **a** Fat-saturated T1-weighted axial magnetic resonance image with intravenous contrast enhancement of the pelvis demonstrates a solitary enhancing tumor focus in the supra-acetabular region of the left iliac bone (*white arrow*), before everolimus treatment. **b** Positron emission tomography-computed tomography fusion image through the pelvis demonstrates corresponding metabolic activity. This image was obtained before the patient began everolimus treatment. **c** Fat-saturated T1-weighted axial MR image with intravenous contrast enhancement of the pelvis obtained after 2 months of everolimus demonstrates partial response of the solitary enhancing tumor focus in the supra-acetabular region of the left iliac bone

Restaging MRI studies of the pelvis were performed 5 months after the start of everolimus treatment and revealed generally stable disease and no evidence of recurrent disease in the thigh. Owing to the stability of the disease, the patient decided to cease everolimus therapy and pursue cryotherapy. Overall, the mTOR inhibitor provided a noticeable response in the tumor, which had not responded to doxorubicin and cisplatin. Thus, targeted therapy could serve as a viable treatment option for PMH.

Discussion

To the best of our knowledge, only two previous descriptions of outcomes from PMH therapy other than resection have been published [5, 7]. The first report described a 36-year-old man with multiple lesions in his right lower leg treated with isolated limb perfusion (melphalan and tumor necrosis factor alpha) followed by four cycles of ifosfamide and doxorubicin. The treatment did not elicit significant shrinkage of the tumor, but the lesion remained stable after 9 months of follow-up [5]. The second study reported a response of PMH to metronomic oral cyclophosphamide and prednisolone. The patient's lesion decreased in size after 10 months of therapy before the patient became non-compliant; however, the report did not include any quantifiable data or imaging concerning lesion size and progression [7].

A review of all published literature on pseudomyogenic hemangioendothelioma was performed to summarize major findings of this newly characterized soft tissue tumor. Of the 63 total reported cases, 78 % of patients were males. PMH presented in the extremities in 79 % of cases and was multifocal at diagnosis in over two-thirds of patients. 90 % of cases utilized excision as the treatment modality of choice (Table 1).

In the first of our cases, the patient exhibited a noticeable treatment response to gemcitabine plus docetaxel. As the 3 month follow-up PET-CT scans clearly indicate, a significant tumor response was achieved following therapy (Fig. 1). The progression of the tumor 3 months after cessation of chemotherapy suggests that the tumor response directly resulted from the gemcitabine and docetaxel therapy. Furthermore, the resumption of a taxane led to disease stability, suggesting that gemcitabine plus a taxane could be an effective treatment for PMH.

Unlike patient 1, patient 2's tumor did not respond to gemcitabine plus docetaxel but ultimately showed stability following treatment with cisplatin and doxorubicin. The differing outcomes following gemcitabine plus

Table 1 Reported cases of pseudomyogenic hemangioendothelioma

References	Cases (N)	Sex	Tumor location	Multifocality at diagnosis	Management
Sheng [1]	1	Male: 100 % (1of 1) Female: 0 % (0 of 1)	Extremity: 100 % (1 of 1)	100 % (1 of 1)	Excision: 100 % (1 of 1)
Hornick and Fletcher [2]	50	Male: 82 % (41 of 50) Female: 18 % (9 of 50)	Extremity: 78 % (39 of 50) Trunk: 18 % (9 of 50) Head and neck: 4 % (2 of 50)	66 % (33 of 50)	Excision: 92 % (46 of 50) Post-operative radiation: 16 % (8 of 50) Chemotherapy: 12 % (6 of 50)
Amary et al. [5]	5 (1 case included in Hornick was excluded)[a]	Male: 50 % (2 of 4) Female: 50 % (2 of 4)	Extremity: 100 % (4 of 4)	75 % (3 of 4)	Excision: 75 % (3of 4) Chemotherapy: 25 % (1 of 4)
Stuart et al. [7]	1	Male: 100 % (1 of 1) Female: 0 % (0 of 1)	Extremity: 100 % (1 of 1)	100 % (1 of 1)	Chemotherapy: 100 % (1 of 1)
Sheng and Wang [9]	1	Male: 0 % (0 of 1) Female: 100 % (1 of 1)	Extremity: 100 % (1 of 1)	100 % (1 of 1)	Excision: 100 % (1 of 1)
Requena et al. [10]	2	Male: 50 % (1 of 2) Female: 50 % (1 of 2)	Extremity: 50 % (1 of 2) Head and neck: 50 % (1 of 2)	100 % (2 of 2)	Excision: 100 % (2 of 2)
Righi [11]	2	Male: 50 % (1 of 2) Female: 50 % (1 of 2)	Extremity: 100 % (2 of 2)	100 % (2 of 2)	Excision: 100 % (2 of 2)
Karakasli et al. [12]	1	Male: 100 % (1 of 1)	Extremity: 100 % (1 of 1)	0 % (0 of 1)	Excision: 100 % (1 of 1)
McGinity [13]	1	Male: 100 % (1 of 1) Female: 0 % (0 of 1)	Extremity: 0 % (0 of 1) Trunk: 100 % (1 of 1)	0 % (0 of 1)	Excision: 100 % (1 of 1)
Total	63	Male: 78 % (49 of 63) Female: 22 % (14 of 63)	Extremity: 79 % (50 of 63) Trunk: 16 % (10 of 63) Head and neck: 5 % (3 of 63)	Multifocality at diagnosis: 68 % (43 of 63)	Excision: 90 % (57 of 63) Post-op radiation: 13 % (8 of 63) Chemotherapy: 13 % (8 of 63)

[a] Patient 5 of this report was already accounted for in the series by Hornick et al. [2]

docetaxel treatment in the two cases reflect PMH's heterogeneity of response to cytotoxic chemotherapy. The discovery of a TSC1 mutation in patient 2's tumor prompted the use of an mTOR inhibitor. An mTOR inhibitor was selected due to its potential to inhibit aberrant mTOR signaling in perivascular epithelioid cell tumors with similar TSC1 mutations [8]. The mTOR inhibitor used in case 2 provided a noticeable response in the PMH metastases in the supra-acetabular region of the left iliac bone. Thus, systemic therapy targeted to the mutations detected by DNA sequencing could be a promising option for PMH that warrants further investigation.

Conclusion

To the best of our knowledge, our report is the first to describe a response of PMH either to gemcitabine/taxane chemotherapy or to an mTOR inhibitor. These observations are especially noteworthy because previous treatment options have typically dealt with local excision and a high rate of recurrence or chemotherapeutic approaches which lack a significant response. There is much to be learned about systemic treatment of pseudomyogenic hemagioendothelioma, but these two cases demonstrate two distinct treatment approaches that warrant further investigation.

Abbreviations

MRI: magnetic resonance imaging; mTOR: mammalian target of rapamycin; PET-CT: positron emission tomography-computed tomography; PMH: pseudomyogenic hemangioendothelioma; TSC1: tuberous sclerosis 1.

Authors' contributions

JJ compiled all patient data, completed a literature review and wrote the manuscript, VR conceived of the study, participated in its design and coordination, and helped draft the manuscript, RB helped conceive of the study and gave valuable insight while drafting the manuscript, MP aided in choosing and interpreting all PET/CT and MRI images, NR aided in analyzing and interpreting data used in the manuscript, SP helped conceive of the study and gave valuable insight while drafting the manuscript, WW confirmed histopathological diagnosis for both cases. All authors read and approved the final manuscript.

Author details

[1] Department of Sarcoma Medical Oncology, Unit 0450, The University of Texas MD Anderson Cancer Center, 1515 Holcombe Blvd., Houston, TX 77030, USA. [2] Department of Pathology, The University of Texas MD Anderson Cancer Center, Houston, TX, USA. [3] Department of Diagnostic Radiology, The University of Texas MD Anderson Cancer Center, Houston, TX, USA.

Competing interests

The authors declare that they have no competing interests.

References

1. Sheng WQ, Wang J. Primary pseudomyogenic haemangioendothelioma of bone. Histopathology. 2012;61(6):1219–24.
2. Hornick JL, Fletcher CD. Pseudomyogenic hemangioendothelioma: a distinctive, often multicentric tumor with indolent behavior. Am J Surg Pathol. 2011;35(2):190–201.
3. Billings SD, Folpe AL, Weiss SW. Epithelioid sarcoma-like hemangioendothelioma. Am J Surg Pathol. 2003;27(1):48–57.
4. Mirra JM, Kessler S, Bhuta S, Eckardt J. The fibroma-like variant of epithelioid sarcoma. A fibrohistiocytic/myoid cell lesion often confused with benign and malignant spindle cell tumors. Cancer. 1992;69(6):1382–95.
5. Amary MF, O'Donnell P, Berisha F, Tirabosco R, Briggs T, Pollock R, et al. Pseudomyogenic (epithelioid sarcoma-like) hemangioendothelioma: characterization of five cases. Skelet Radiol. 2013;42(7):947–57.
6. Walther C, Tayebwa J, Lilljebjörn H, Magnusson L, Nilsson J, von Steyern FV, Øra I, Domanski HA, Fioretos T, Nord KH, Fletcher CD, Mertens F. A novel SERPINE1-FOSB fusion gene results in transcriptional up-regulation of FOSB in pseudomyogenic haemangioendothelioma. J Pathol. 2014;232(5):534–40.
7. Stuart LN, Gardner JM, Lauer SR, Monson DK, Parker DC, Edgar MA. Epithelioid sarcoma-like (pseudomyogenic) hemangioendothelioma, clinically mimicking dermatofibroma, diagnosed by skin biopsy in a 30-year-old man. J Cutan Pathol. 2013;40(10):909–13.
8. Wagner AJ, Malinowska-Kolodziej I, Morgan JA, Qin W, Fletcher CD, Vena N, Ligon AH, Antonescu CR, Ramaiya NH, Demetri GD, Kwiatkowski DJ, Maki RG. Clinical activity of mTOR inhibition with sirolimus in malignant perivascular epithelioid cell tumors: targeting the pathogenic activation of mTORC1 in tumors. J Clin Oncol. 2010;28(5):835–40.
9. Sheng W, Pan Y, Wang J. Pseudomyogenic hemangioendothelioma: report of an additional case with aggressive clinical course. Am J Dermatopathol. 2013;35(5):597–600.
10. Requena L, Santonja C, Martinez-Amo JL, Saus C, Kutzner H. Cutaneous epithelioid sarcomalike (pseudomyogenic) hemangioendothelioma: a little-known low-grade cutaneous vascular neoplasm. JAMA Dermatol. 2013;149(4):459–65.
11. Righi A, Gambarotti M, Picci P, Dei Tos AP, Vanel D. Primary pseudomyogenic haemangioendothelioma of bone: report of two cases. Skelet Radiol. 2014;44(5):727–31.
12. Karakasli A, Karaaslan A, Erduran M, Capkin S, Tuna EB, Havitcioglu H. Pseudomyogenic (epithelioid sarcoma-like) hemangioendothelioma with bone invasion. J Orthop. 2014;11(4):197–9.
13. McGinity M, Bartanusz V, Dengler B, Birnbaum L, Henry J. Pseudomyogenic hemangioendothelioma (epithelioid sarcoma-like hemangioendothelioma, fibroma-like variant of epithelioid sarcoma) of the thoracic spine. Eur Spine J. 2013;22(Suppl 3):S506–11.

15

Metastatic meningioma presenting as a malignant soft tissue tumour

Catherine McCarthy[1], Monika Hofer[2], Marianna Vlychou[3], Robar Khundkar[4], Paul Critchley[4], Simon Cudlip[5], Olaf Ansorge[2] and Nick A. Athanasou[3*]

Abstract

Background: Extracranial metastasis of malignant meningioma to soft tissues is extremely rare and its clinical, radiological and pathological features are not well-characterised.

Case presentation: We report a case of a 58 year old man who presented with a mobile mass within the left trapezius muscle. The patient had previously undergone surgery for a right frontal lobe high grade anaplastic meningioma. Histology of the soft tissue lesion showed metastatic anaplastic meningioma with clumps of pleomorphic tumour cells which expressed epithelial membrane antigen, cytokeratin and P63 but were negative for other epithelial and mesenchymal markers. A PET-CT scan revealed additional metastatic lesions in the left pleura, liver and iliac bone.

Conclusions: Metastatic malignant meningioma can very rarely present as a high grade pleomorphic malignant soft tissue tumour and needs to be distinguished from soft tissue sarcomas and metastatic carcinomas that express epithelial antigens.

Keywords: Meningioma anaplastic, Metastasis, Soft tissue, Tumour

Background

Meningiomas are relatively common primary intracranial tumours that arise within the leptomeninges or dura mater; these tumours exhibit morphological and immunophenotypic evidence of origin from meningothelial cells which are present in the arachnoid membrane and arachnoid villi associated with the intradural venous sinuses and their tributaries [1]. The majority of meningiomas arise within the cranial cavity and are supratentorial dura-based lesions that develop most commonly in the vicinity of the superior sagittal sinus, over the cerebral convexities or in contact with the falx cerebri. Approximately 12% arise in the spine.

Meningiomas show considerable morphologic variation and are most commonly benign tumours (Grade I) [2, 3]. Atypical (Grade II) and anaplastic (Grade III) meningiomas, which have aggressive/malignant potential, are distinguished on the basis of mitotic activity and a number of other features (e.g. pleomorphism, cellularity, necrosis). Anaplastic meningiomas commonly recur and very rarely have been known to metastasise to extracranial tissues and organs [3–5]. The true prevalence of metastatic malignant meningioma is unknown as many reported cases and case series include cases of "benign metastasising meningioma", as well as tumours that were in the past incorrectly classified as meningiomas (e.g. angioblastic meningioma which is now known to be a solitary fibrous tumour).

The most frequently reported sites of extracranial metastasis of malignant meningioma are lung, spine and liver [3–13]. There are very few reports of malignant meningioma metastasising to deep soft tissues [4, 14–16]. We report a case of a metastatic anaplastic meningioma which presented as a growing soft tissue tumour in the trapezius muscle and review the literature regarding soft tissue involvement by metastatic meningioma.

*Correspondence: nick.athanasou@ndorms.ox.ac.uk
[3] Nuffield Department of Orthopaedics, Rheumatology and Musculoskeletal Sciences, Nuffield Orthopaedic Centre, University of Oxford, Windmill Road, Oxford OX3 7HE, UK

Case presentation

A 55 year old man was admitted to hospital with a head injury that resulted in hearing loss on the left side with pulsatile tinnitus and a vague feeling of disorientation. A CT scan showed an irregular extra-axial solitary lesion lying adjacent to the falx on the right of the midline measuring 3 × 4 × 6 cm with significant mass-effect and peritumoral oedema involving most of the right frontal lobe. There was evidence of underlying bone remodelling with vascular dural supply and heterogeneous enhancement after contrast administration with a deep cystic component. There were fringes of tumour interdigitating with the brain substance indicating probable brain invasion (Fig. 1). The findings were consistent with an aggressive frontal meningioma. Partial surgical removal of the lesion in the right frontal lobe was undertaken. On histological examination, the lesion was classified as an atypical (WHO Grade II) meningotheliomatous meningioma.

A year later, the patient experienced an episode of seizures and a CT scan revealed three new lesions at the site of the previously excised meningioma with extensive perilesional oedema. An MRI confirmed the CT findings indicative of tumour and also detected invasion and occlusion of the anterior part of the superior sagittal sinus (Fig. 2). Partial resection of the recurrent mass was again undertaken. Histology of the tumour specimen showed features of an anaplastic (WHO Grade III) meningotheliomatous meningioma with lobules of tumour containing cells with round or oval vesicular nuclei. Focally, there were cells which showed more prominent nuclear pleomorphism. There was increased mitotic activity and extensive tumour necrosis was noted (Fig. 3). Post-operative follow-up revealed residual tumour in the anterior part of the superior sagittal sinus, along the falx and the right frontal convexity. Follow-up imaging also confirmed interval progression of the residual meningioma.

The patient completed a course of radiotherapy and, nine months later, a mobile soft tissue lump on his back was noted. A thoracic CT scan revealed a soft tissue lesion superficially located in the inferior portion of the left trapezius muscle. The lesion was lobulated, had a low attenuation centre, showed peripheral enhancement and did not exhibit evidence of matrix calcification (Fig. 4). The lesion increased in size and a subsequent MRI scan performed 6 months later confirmed the presence of a solid soft tissue mass up to 5 cm in diameter in the medial left trapezius muscle. The lesion indented the underlying paravertebral muscles but remained well-defined and did not invade the deeper musculature. The lesion returned isointense T1-W signal relative to skeletal muscle and heterogeneous high T2-W signal. There was no internal calcification, haemorrhage or cystic degeneration. Peripheral feeding vessels were present (Fig. 5). A PET-CT scan demonstrated that the intramuscular lesion was extremely FDG avid with an SUVmax of 22.1 (Fig. 6). PET-CT also revealed disseminated, markedly FDG avid metastases in liver, bone and pleura and residual meningioma in the right frontal lobe.

The lesion was biopsied and showed a largely lobulated tumour containing collections of tumour cells, many of which showed similar features to those seen in the

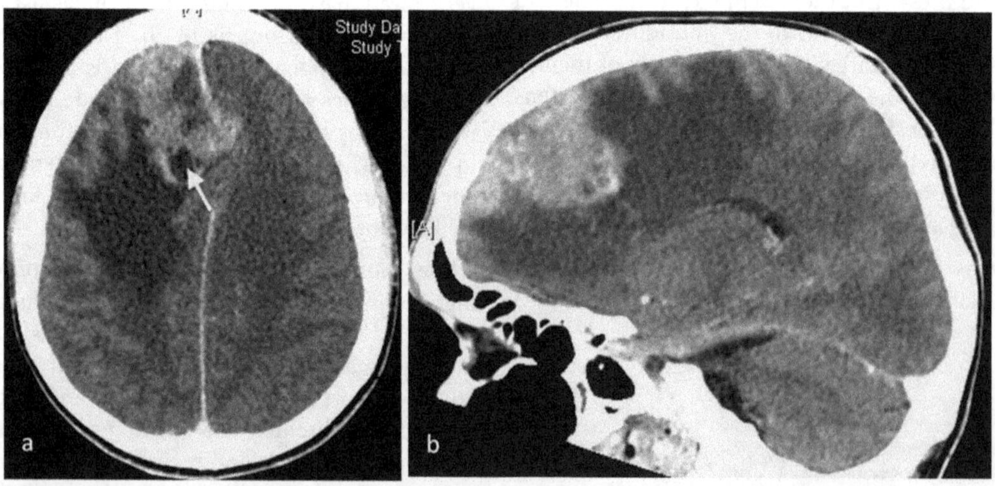

Fig. 1 Axial CT post contrast image (**a**) and sagittal reconstruction (**b**) shows an irregular extra-axial solid mass with heterogeneous enhancement and deep cystic change (*arrow*) adjacent to the falx extending into the right frontal lobe. There is significant peritumoral oedema and mass effect involving the right frontal lobe with displacement of the midline. These findings, together with tumour interdigitating with the brain substance, are consistent with an aggressive frontal meningioma

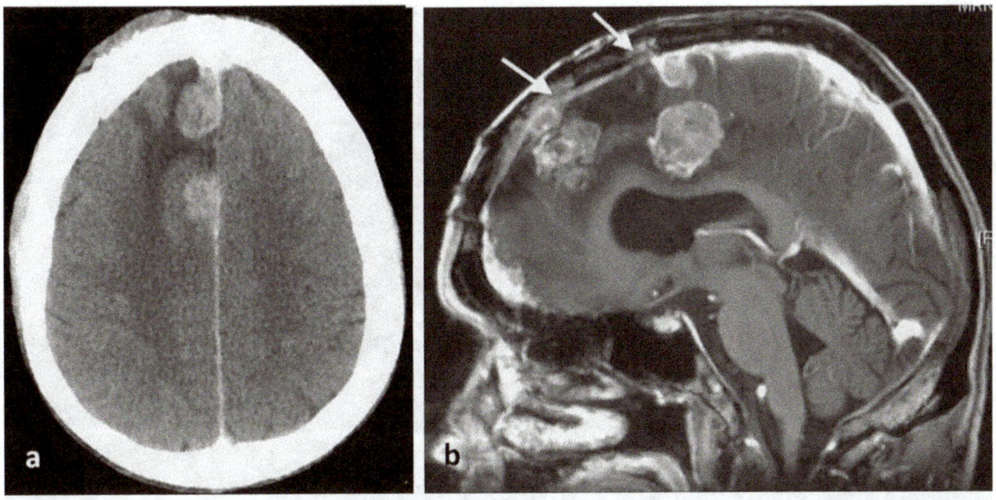

Fig. 2 Axial CT post contrast image showing: **a** nodular enhancing masses and perilesional oedema in the right frontal lobe, indicative of local recurrence of the meningioma. **b** A sagittal T1-weighted MR image post contrast confirming the presence of three lesions and invasion of the superior sagittal sinus (*arrows*)

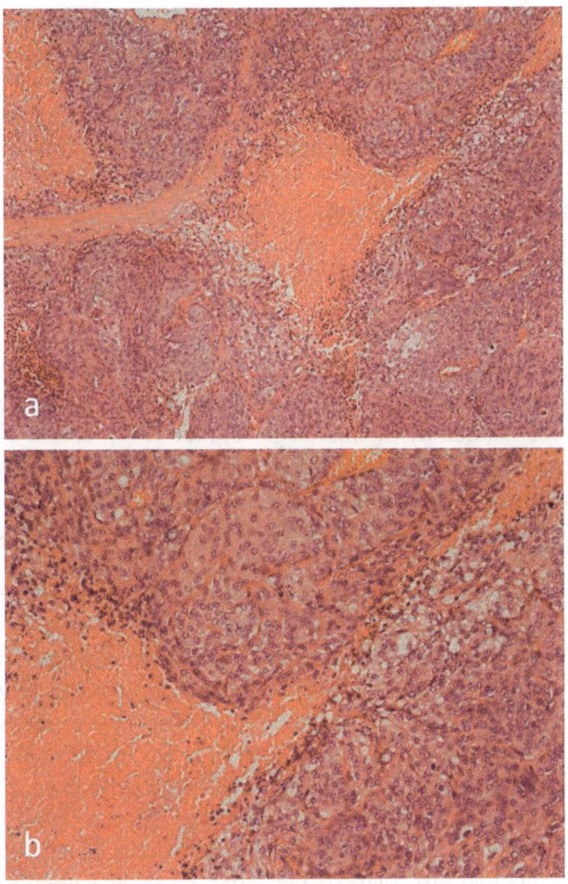

Fig. 3 Histology of the anaplastic (Grade III) meningioma of the frontal lobe showing; **a** lobules of meningotheliomatous tumour containing cells with round vesicular nuclei, **b** areas of focal tumour necrosis containing more pleomorphic tumour cells

frontal lobe tumour. There were a few whorled collections of tumour cells with round or oval vesicular nuclei (Fig. 7). There was prominent nuclear pleomorphism, a high mitotic rate and focal tumour necrosis. Focally there were solid areas of proliferation of pleomorphic tumour cells, some of which had vacuolated cytoplasm. Immunohistochemistry showed strong expression of epithelial membrane antigen (EMA) and P63; there was also focal expression of cytokeratin (CK7+, CK20−), nuclear staining for IN-1, and a high Ki-67 fraction. There was no expression of desmin, S100, CD10, CD30, CD68, myogenin, smooth muscle actin, estrogen receptor, progesterone receptor, chromogranin, carcinoembryonic antigen or TTF1. There was initially some difficulty in establishing the pathological diagnosis as the previous history of recurrent atypical/anaplastic meningioma was not provided to the reporting pathologist whose initial differential diagnosis included a soft tissue metastasis of carcinoma and a primary soft tissue sarcoma expressing the epithelial markers. However, once the history of meningioma and the radiological findings were taken into account, it was clear that the soft tissue mass represented a metastasis of the previously diagnosed anaplastic meningotheliomatous meningioma.

A wide local excision of the lesion, which measured 5 × 3 × 2 cm, was performed; this included a cuff of normal muscle around the lesion and a 1 cm margin of skin around the previous biopsy scar. Histological findings in the resection specimen were similar to those of the biopsy. Further follow up of the patient by CT scan showed no recurrence of the soft tissue lesion but progression of disease in the brain.

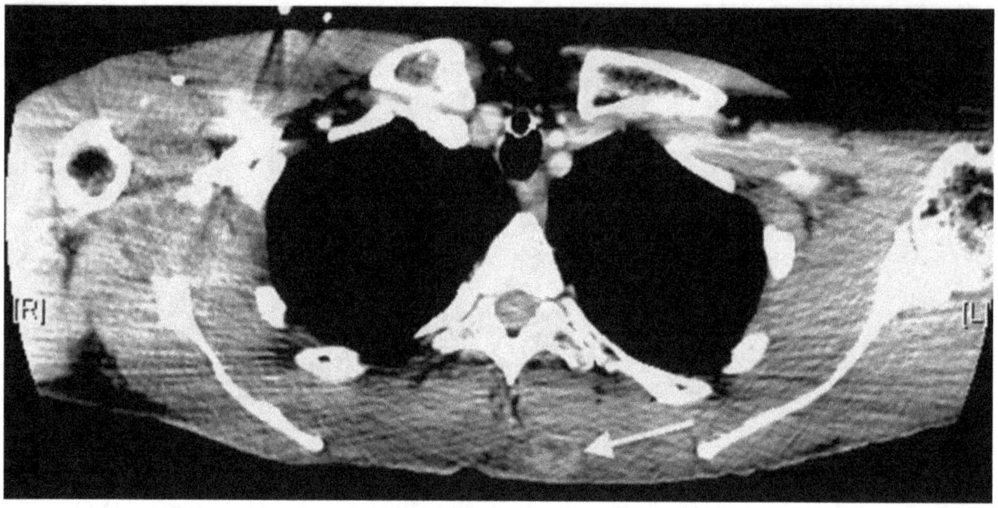

Fig. 4 Axial thorax CT post contrast image showing an ill-defined soft tissue mass (*arrow*) superficially located in the left trapezius muscle with peripheral enhancement and low signal in the centre

Discussion

Extracranial metastasis of meningioma occurs rarely with only a few case reports documenting deep soft tissue as a site of metastasis [4, 14–17]; it is not clear from many of these reports whether, as in our case, the metastasis involved soft tissue alone or whether other contiguous structures, such as lymph nodes and bone, were also involved. Doxtader et al. [14] described an aggressive meningioma in an 8 year old patient with metastasis to cervical soft tissue and lymph nodes. There is also a report of an isolated "chest wall" metastasis and of a bone/soft tissue metastasis from an atypical primary meningioma of the nasal septum that clinically simulated a soft tissue sarcoma [15, 16]. In a review of the literature between 1886 and 1958, Karasick et al. [5] reported 56 patients who developed extracranial meningioma metastasis, none of which were in soft tissue. In the database review of Enam et al. [9], the incidence of meningioma metastasis was 0.76% with no soft tissue metastasis being noted. Forest et al. [3] also carried out a database review totalling 1291 meningiomas and identified only four cases of metastatic meningioma, none of which was in soft tissues.

A recent review of the literature on all reports of distant metastasis of intracranial meningiomas found that in 115 patients with 164 metastatic lesions, 83.9% were Grade I (benign), 20.0% were Grade II (atypical) and 40% Grade III (anaplastic) meningiomas [4]. This analysis excluded pathological entities such as "angioblastic meningioma", meningeal carcinomas and sarcomas, all of which were formerly considered to represent subtypes of meningioma. In this review, 6% of cases developed in cervical soft tissue, 2.4% in skin and subcutaneous tissue and 1.8% in muscle. Haematogenous spread of meningiomas through the paravertebral and jugular venous systems, which also drain thoracic tissues, has been postulated and could account for the relatively high frequency of the neck and upper trunk as a site of soft tissue and lymph node metastasis. Although anaplastic and atypical meningiomas were most commonly associated with metastatic lesions, comprising 31.3 and 19.1% of cases respectively, it was noted that Grade I meningiomas can also give rise to metastatic lesions. It was also noted that in 93% of cases the intracranial meningioma was diagnosed and resected before the distant metastasis appeared. The prognosis of intracranial meningioma is determined by the histological grade [1, 2], and in our case progression of the intracranial tumour to a higher histological grade was noted.

Radiological features of the chest wall tumour in our case were not specific; the diagnosis of a metastatic tumour was supported radiologically by the interval increase in the size of the lesion, as well as high FDG uptake and the finding of lesions at other sites on the PET-CT scan. Multiple deposits were also observed in other extracranial sites in previous reports of soft tissue metastasis from malignant meningioma [3, 4]. The tumour in the frontal lobe showed several radiological findings that have been described as potential markers of atypical or malignant meningiomas including indistinct or irregular tumour margins, marked peritumoral oedema, inhomogeneous enhancement post-contrast, intrinsic cyst-like areas, disruption of the arachnoid at the brain-tumour interface and adjacent bone destruction [18–24].

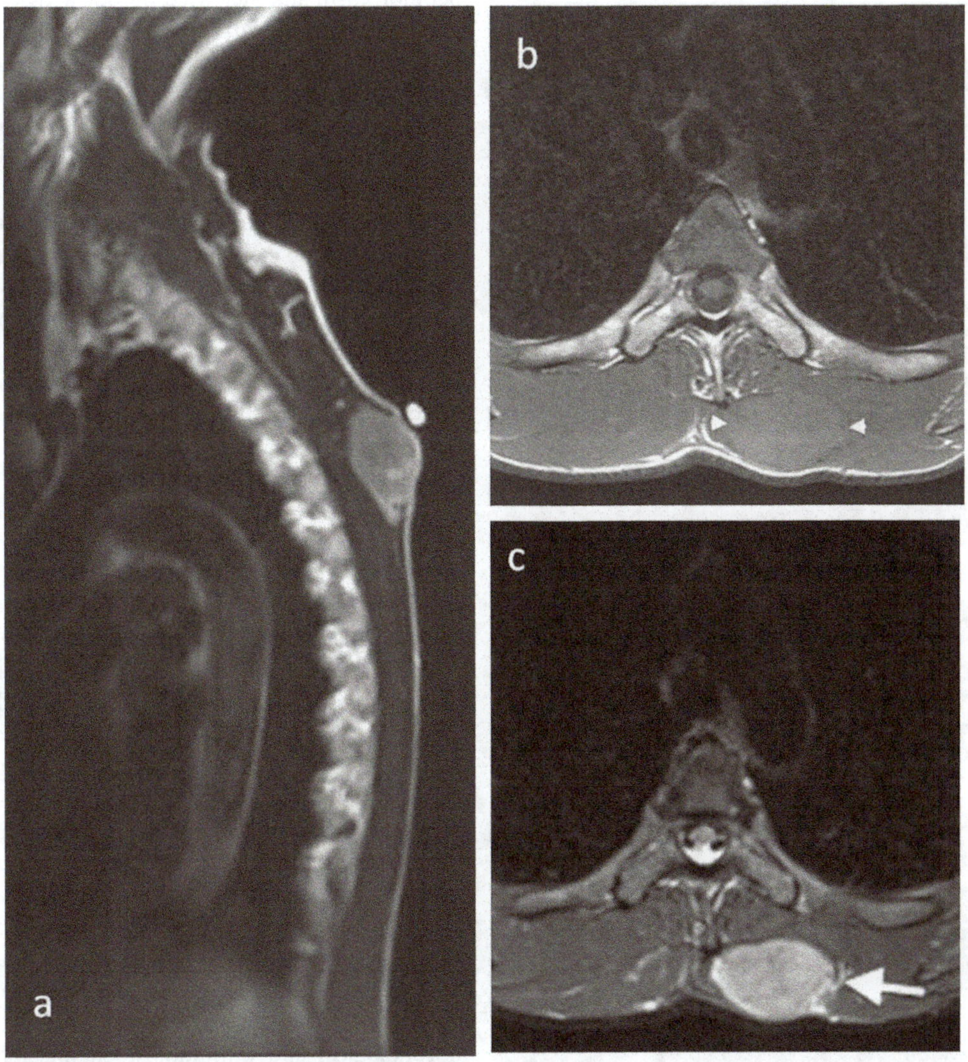

Fig. 5 Sagittal T2 (**a**), axial T1 (**b**) and axial T2 fat saturated (**c**) MR images demonstrate a solid well defined soft tissue mass in the medial left trapezius muscle which returns isointense T1-W (between *arrow heads*) and heterogeneous predominantly high T2-W signal relative to skeletal muscle. There is mass effect on the deeper paravertebral muscles and peripheral feeding vessels along the lateral aspect of the lesion (*arrow*)

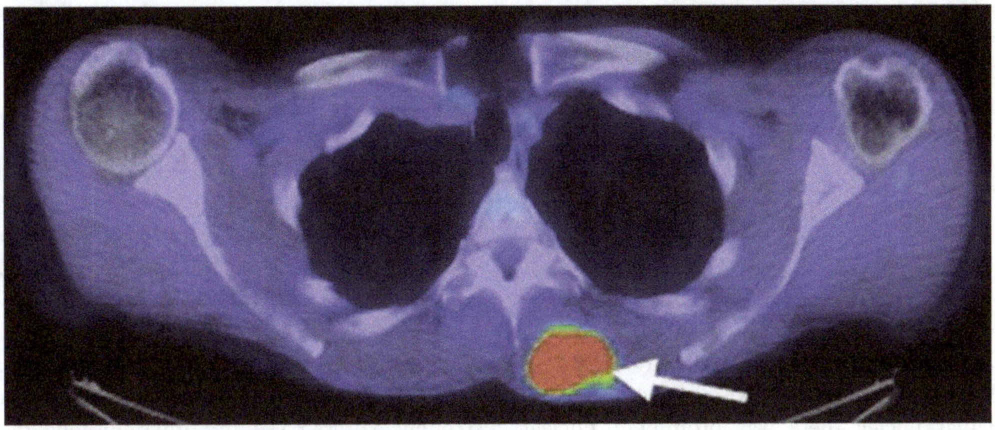

Fig. 6 PET-CT confirms the presence of an FDG avid soft tissue mass in the left trapezius muscle

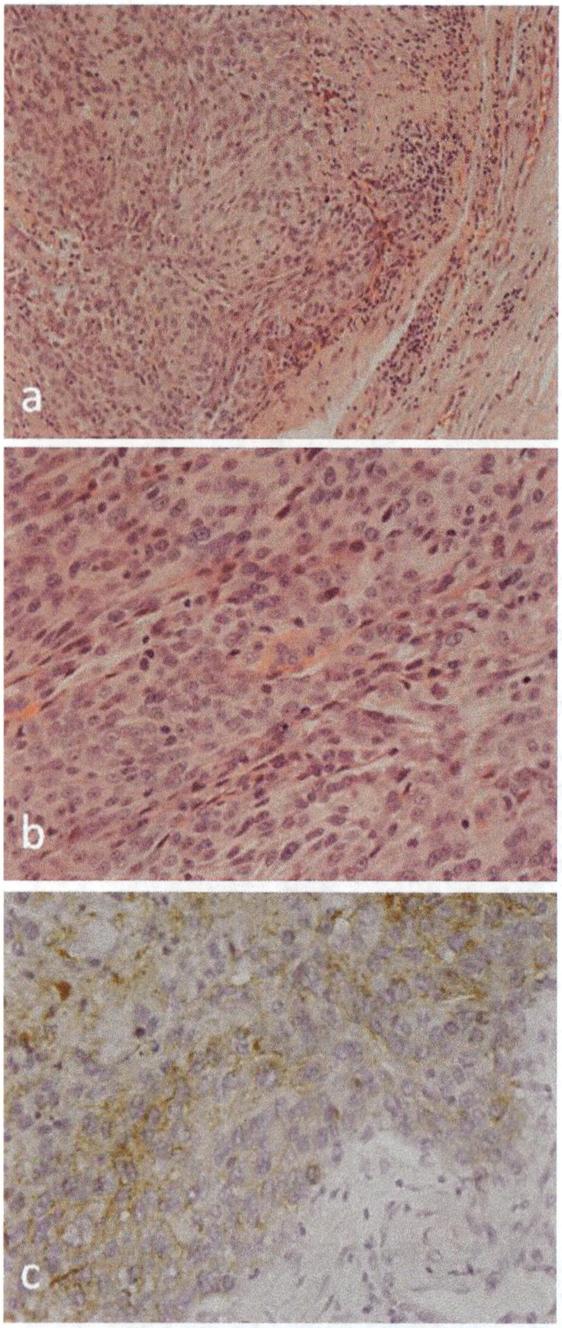

Fig. 7 Histology of the metastatic meningioma in soft tissues showing: **a** lobules of tumour showing features of meningotheliomatous meningioma similar to the primary brain tumour **b** areas where tumour cells exhibit marked nuclear pleomorphism and contain prominent nucleoli. **c** Expression of EMA by tumour cells

Histological features of the chest wall tumour showed that it was focally necrotic and contained collections of tumour cells with elongated cytoplasm and round or oval vesicular nuclei; there was prominent nuclear pleomorphism and increased mitotic activity. Morphologically, the differential diagnosis was wide and included sarcoma, lymphoma, metastatic melanoma and carcinoma. Immunohistochemistry showed expression of epithelial markers on tumour cells with diffuse, strong staining for EMA and focal staining for cytokeratin. In the absence of any previous history, and taking into account other immunohistochemical findings, these features were thought to favour metastatic carcinoma or a sarcoma expressing epithelial markers. Several sarcomas are known to express epithelial markers, including synovial sarcoma, epithelioid sarcoma, epithelioid malignant peripheral nerve sheath tumour, myoepithelioma and leiomyosarcoma [25] Morphological and immunophenotypic features were not typical of any of these specific tumour types. Soft tissue metastasis of carcinoma is well recognised with autopsy series reporting that this occurs in 0.75–9% of patients who die of metastatic carcinoma [26–29]. Lung is the most common primary carcinoma that results in soft tissue metastasis with a mean prevalence of 2.3% being reported [30], and the cytokeratin profile in our case was consistent with a metastatic lung carcinoma; it was not typical for metastatic renal or colon carcinoma, both which have also been reported to produce soft tissue metastasis with relative frequency. Although metastatic malignant meningioma is much less common than metastatic carcinoma, the prevalence of metastatic meningioma in skin, subcutaneous tissue and muscle is, at least in one case series [4], comparable to that of metastatic carcinoma. In our case the diagnosis of metastatic meningioma became clear when the full past history of the patient was recognised. It could be argued that the possibility of malignant meningioma should have been suspected earlier given that the morphological and immunohistochemical findings were so typical of this tumour with focal, occasionally whorled collections of strongly EMA+ tumour cells being typical of a meningotheliomatous meningioma [1, 2]. It should be noted that in more diagnostically challenging cases certain genetic/cytogenetic abnormalities such as inactivating mutations of NF2, monosomy 22, as well as specific alterations in gene expression, may also be useful in establishing the diagnosis of metastatic meningioma [31].

Conclusion

Knowledge of the clinical and radiological information was essential to establish the diagnosis of metastatic malignant meningioma in our case, particularly the previous history of anaplastic meningioma and the radiological identification of FDG avid lesions at several sites. Although very rare, the possibility of metastatic meningioma should be considered in the differential diagnosis of a malignant soft tissue tumour, where tumour cells strongly express EMA and other epithelial markers.

Abbreviations

PET: positron-emission tomography; FDG: fludeoxyglucose; EMA: epithelial membrane antigen; WHO: World Health Organization; CT: computed tomography; MRI: magnetic resonance imaging; CK: cytokeratin.

Authors' contributions

MV, CM, RK and NAA were the major contributors in writing the manuscript. NAA made the final editing of the manuscript. PC, RK and SC cared for the patient during her time in the hospital and provided details of surgical treatment. MV, CM, MH, OA assisted in the radiological and pathological data collection and the preparation of the manuscript. All authors read and approved the final manuscript.

Author details

[1] Department of Radiology, Nuffield Orthopaedic Centre, Windmill Road, Oxford OX3 7HE, UK. [2] Department of Neuropathology, Oxford University Hospitals Oxford, Oxford OX3 9DU, UK. [3] Nuffield Department of Orthopaedics, Rheumatology and Musculoskeletal Sciences, Nuffield Orthopaedic Centre, University of Oxford, Windmill Road, Oxford OX3 7HE, UK. [4] Sarcoma Service, Nuffield Orthopedic Centre, Windmill Road, Oxford OX3 7HE, UK. [5] Department of Neurosurgery, Oxford University Hospitals, Oxford OX3 9DU, UK.

Acknowledgements

We thanks Mrs. Sarah Turton for typing the manuscript.

Competing interests

The authors declare that they have no competing interests.

Funding

MV was an EU-funded visitor on the Erasmus + program.

References

1. Lamszus K. Menigioma pathology, genetics and biology. J Neuropathol Exp Neurol. 2004;63:275–86.
2. Louis DN, Perry A, Reifenberger G, von Deimling A, Figaella-Branger D, Cavenee WK, Ohgaki H, Wiestler OD, Kleihues P, Ellison DW. The 2016 World Health Organisation classification of tumours of the central nervous system: a summary. Acta Neuropathol. 2016;131:803–20.
3. Forest F, Berremila SA, Gyenes C, Ginguene C, Kassir R, et al. Metastatic meningiomas; an unusual clinical and pathological diagnosis with highly variable outcome. J Neurooncol. 2014;120:411–21.
4. Surov A, Gottschling S, Bolz J, Kornhuber M, Alfieri A, Holzhausen HJ, et al. Distant metastases in meningioma: an underestimated problem. J Neurooncol. 2013;112:323–7.
5. Karasick JL, Mullan SF. A survey of metastatic meningiomas. J Neurosurg. 1974;40:206–12.
6. Chuang HC, Lee HC, Cho DY. Intracranial malignant meningioma with multiple spinal metastases—a case report and literature review: case report. Spine. 2006;31:E1006–10.
7. Fabi A, Nuzzo C, Vidiri A, Ciccarese M, Felici A, Cattani F, Cognetti F. Bone and lung metastases from intracranial meningioma. Anticancer Res. 2006;26:3835–7.
8. Cabada T, Bermejo R, Bacaicoa C, Martínez-Peñuela A. Metastatic meningioma: the role of whole-body diffusion-weighted imaging. Oncol Lett. 2011;2:931–3.
9. Enam SA, Abdulraf S, Mehta B, Malik GM, Mahmood A. Metastasis in meningioma. Acta Neurochir (Wien). 1996;138:1172.
10. Younis GA, Sawaya R, DeMonte F, Hess KR, Albrecht S, Bruner JM. Aggressive meningeal tumours: a review of a series. J Neurosurg. 1995;82:17–27.
11. Couldwell WT, Fankhauser H, de Tribolet N. Osseous metastases from benign interventricular meningioma. Case report. Acta Neurochir. 1992;117:195–9.
12. Slavin ML. Metastatic malignant meningioma. J Clin Neuroopthamol. 1989;9:55–9.
13. Adlakha A, Rao K, Adlakha H, Perry A, Crotty TB, Scheithauer BW, et al. Meningioma metastatic to the lung. Mayo Clin Proc. 1999;74(11):1129–33.
14. Doxtader EE, Butts SC, Holsapple JW, Fuller CE. Aggressive pediatric meningioma with soft tissue and lymph node metastases: a case report. Pediatr Dev Pathol. 2009;12(3):244–8.
15. Williamson BE, Stanton CA, Levine EA. Chest wall metastasis from recurrent meningioma. Am Surg. 2001;67:966–8.
16. Baek BJ, Shin JM, Lee CK, Lee JH, Lee KH. Atypical primary meningioma in the nasal septum with malignant transformation and distant metastasis. BMC Cancer. 2012;12:275.
17. Lee GC, Choi SW, Kim SH, Kwon HJ. Multiple extracranial metastases of atypical menigiomas. J Korean Neurosurg Soc. 2009;45:107–11.
18. New PF, Hesselink JR, O'Corroll CP, Kleinman GM. Malignant meningiomas: CT and histologic criteria, including a new CT sign. Am J Neuroradiol. 1982;3:267–76.
19. Liu Y, Chotai S, Chen M, Jin S, Qi ST, Pan J. Preoperative radiologic classification of convexity meningioma to predict the survival and aggressive meningioma behaviour. PLoS ONE. 2015;10:e0118908.
20. Hsu CC, Pai CY, Kao HW, Hsueh CJ, Hsu WL, Lo CP. Do aggressive imaging features correlate with advanced histopathological grade in meningiomas? J Clin Neurosci. 2010;17:584–7.
21. Nagar VA, Ye JR, Ng WH, et al. Diffusion-weighted MR imaging: diagnosing atypical or malignant meningiomas and detecting tumour dedifferentiation. Am J Neuroradiol. 2008;29:1147–52.
22. Hakyemez B, Yildirim N, Gokalp G, Erdogan C, Parlak M. The contribution of diffusion-weighted MR imaging to distinguishing typical from atypical meningiomas. Neuroradiology. 2006;48:513–20.
23. Yin B, Liu L, Zhang BY, Li YX, Li Y, Geng DY. Correlating apparent diffusion coefficients with histopathologic findings on meningiomas. Eur J Radiol. 2012;81:4050–6.
24. Surov A, Gottschling S, Mawrin C, et al. Diffusion-weighted imaging in meningioma: prediction of tumour grade and association with histopathological parameters. Transl Oncol. 2015;8:517–23.
25. Miettinen M. Immunohistochemistry of soft tissue tumours: modern soft tissue pathology: tumours and non-neoplastic conditions. Cambridge: Cambridge University press; 2010. p. 44–104.
26. Spencer PS, Helm TNL. Skin metastasis in cancer patients. Cutis. 1987;39:119–21.
27. Lookingbill DP, Spangler N, Sexton FM. Skin involvement as the presenting sign of internal carcinoma. A retrospective study of 7316 cancer patients. J Am Acad Dermatol. 1990;22:19–26.
28. Hidaka T, Ischii Y, Kitamura S. Clinical features of skin metastasis from lung cancer. Intern Med. 1996;35:459–62.
29. Nguyen NC, Chaar BT, Osman MM. Prevalence and patterns of soft tissue metastasis; detection with true whole-body F-18 FG PET/CT. BMC Med Imaging. 2007;12(7):8.
30. Perisano C, Spinelli MS, Graci C, et al. Soft tissue metastasis in lung cancer: a review of the literature. Eur Rev Med Pharmacol Sci. 2012;16:1908–14.
31. Yuzawa S, Nishihara H, Tanaka S. Genetic landscape of meningioma. Brain Tumour Pathol. 2016;33:237–47.

16

Tumor volume is a better predictor of post-operative wound complications compared to tumor size in soft tissue sarcomas of the proximal lower extremity

Michael Ziegele[1], David M. King[1] and Manpreet Bedi[2*]

Abstract

Background: Wide local excision with or without radiation therapy (RT) and chemotherapy is widely accepted as appropriate management for soft tissue sarcomas (STS) of the extremity. Although survival and local control rates are comparable to amputation, post-operative wound complications (WC) following limb salvage can result in significant morbidity for the patient. Certain risk factors such as location, pre-operative RT, and age have been shown to increase the risk of WCs. Somewhat surprisingly, size has not consistently been shown to impact WC rates. The goal of this study is to assess whether tumor volume, as opposed to the traditional measurement of the largest dimension in one plane, correlates with the development of post-operative WCs.

Methods: Between 2000 and 2013, 81 patients with STS of the proximal lower extremity, buttock and pelvis were retrospectively identified from our prospective database. We reviewed the impact of patient, tumor, and treatment variables on postoperative WC. Predictors for WC were evaluated using the Fisher exact test for univariate analysis and logistic regression for multivariate analysis. Tumor volume was determined using the medical image merge (MIM) ® software program (version 6.5.4, MIM Software, Cleveland, OH). Tumor size (diameter) was determined the historical way of measuring the widest dimension on the sagittal, coronal, and axial planes from the MRI scan at midplane.

Results: The overall WC rate within 6 months of tumor resection was 32 %. WC were more likely to occur with larger tumor volumes ($p = 0.015$), although not with tumor diameters ≥ 10 cm ($p = 0.55$). Neither volume of subcutaneous fat ($p = 0.34$) or depth of the subcutaneous fat layer ($p = 0.82$) significantly impacted WC rates. Tumor proximity to skin surface also did not significantly impact WC risk ($p = 0.73$).

Conclusions: Increase in tumor volume led to a higher risk of post-operative WCs. Assessing tumor volume may allow clinicians to better counsel patients on their risk of post-operative WCs. Tumor volume, as opposed to size alone, should be considered in future sarcoma outcome studies.

Background

Approximately 12,000 patients in the United States each year are diagnosed with soft tissue sarcomas (STS), representing roughly 1 % of all adult malignancies [1]. In the past, due to concern for high local recurrence rates with local excision, amputation was routinely performed. However, there has been a transition in the management of STS of the extremity towards limb salvage resection in combination with radiation therapy (RT) with or without chemotherapy. This treatment approach has resulted in excellent local control rates [2, 3].

Despite advances in the treatment of STS, post-operative wound complications (WC) following surgical resection of the tumor remain an important source of morbidity for patients. WC have been reported in 16–56 % of surgical cases [4, 5], and can include

*Correspondence: mbedi@mcw.edu
[2] Department of Radiation Oncology, Medical College of Wisconsin, 9200 West Wisconsin Ave, Milwaukee, WI 53226, USA

complications such as seromas, hematomas, wound necrosis, wound dehiscence, cellulitis, and abscess formation.

Considerable research has been dedicated towards investigating risk factors for WC follow surgical resection of STS. Risk factors include, but are not limited to, location of disease, tumor size and proximity to skin, and timing of radiation. Tumor location is a strong predictive factor, with tumors located in the lower extremity (LE) experiencing higher rates of WC following surgery [6–10]. Korah et al. demonstrated that tumor location was the single most important risk factor for WC, and also reports a wound reoperation rate of 29 % for LE tumors vs. 4 % in upper extremity (UE) tumors [7].

Although location of the primary tumor has been consistently shown to impact the development of post-operative WCs, this has not been the case for tumor size. Moreover, most studies that evaluate size as a risk factor take into consideration the maximal dimension of the primary tumor. While the maximal measurement in one dimension gives an idea of tumor size, the overall size, or volume, difference between a 3 × 10 cm tumor and a 9 × 10 cm tumor is notable. There has been little information on the volume of the tumor and correlation to post-operative WCs.

Similar to tumor size, body mass index (BMI) and the amount of subcutaneous fat has not repeatedly been shown to influence WCs. This lack of consistency perhaps demonstrates that more than one measurement variable effects this outcome.

The objective of this study was to investigate additional variables that might impact post-operative WCs following surgical resection of STS. Specifically, utilizing a combination of volumetric and linear data gathered from preoperative MRIs, we determined if tumor volume and the ratio of subcutaneous (SC) fat, muscle and tumor impacted WC risk. To our knowledge the impact of SC fat on WC rates has never been investigated in STS, although high levels of SC fat have been linked with increased WC rates in other surgical procedures [11–13]. Additionally, the ability of tumor diameter to predict WC risk in comparison to tumor volume has never been investigated.

Methods

This research was reviewed and approved by the Institutional Review Board (IRB) and all investigators completed training in both human research and patient privacy.

Patient population

All patients with localized primary STS of the proximal LE, buttock, and pelvis who underwent wide surgical resection, with or without radiation, and/or chemotherapy between 2000 and 2013 were reviewed. Pelvic tumors in this study included sarcomas in the pelvis and buttock that were extra-peritoneal. No retroperitoneal or peritoneal tumors were included in this study. Additional exclusion criteria included metastatic disease on initial presentation, age <18 years old, STS of locations other than the proximal LE, buttock, or pelvis, recurrent or non-oncologic resection of sarcomas at first presentation to our sarcoma center, and small subcutaneous tumors. All patients underwent resection. Patients who had radiation (preoperative or post-operative) or no radiation were included in the study. Patients who did not have complete medical records including treatment information and a pathology report, and follow-up of less than 6 months were also excluded. Histopathologic types demonstrating rhabdomyosarcoma, extraosseous primitive neuroectodermal tumor, Kaposi's sarcoma, angiosarcoma, and desmoid fibromatosis were also excluded.

Eighty-one patients were identified in our database who met the inclusion criteria. Patients were staged according to the 2009 American Joint Committee on Cancer (AJCC) system seventh edition.

Treatment

All patients were discussed at a multidisciplinary tumor board consisting of surgical and musculoskeletal oncologists, medical and radiation oncologists, radiologists and pathologists. Treatment recommendations from this tumor board were presented to the patient.

Radiotherapy and chemotherapy

Patients included in this study had either preoperative, post-operative or no RT. Those that had preoperative RT received a median dose of 50 Gy using 3D-conformal radiation or intensity-modulated radiotherapy (IMRT). Patients who received post-operative RT received a median dose of 60 Gy.

Chemotherapy was recommended and administered in patients who were typically <70 years of age, with large (>5 cm), deep, and high-grade lesions. Chemotherapy was a doxorubicin-ifosfamide based regimen given for 1–3 cycles based on clinical response and tolerance.

Surgery

Limb-sparing resection was performed in all patients. Wide surgical resection was performed by fellowship trained musculoskeletal oncologists grossly through normal tissue planes with sacrifice of arteries or veins that were involved by tumor. Preservation of neurovascular structures was performed when possible. The goal of surgery was to achieve negative margins (R0). Vascular or reconstructive plastic surgeons were involved in cases that required vascular reconstruction, difficult wound closures and free flap reconstructions.

Data collection

Pre-operative MRIs were downloaded into the medical image merge (MIM) ® software program (version 6.5.4, MIM Software, Cleveland, OH). MRI's were acquired within 1 month prior to limb-sparing resection. Post-operative MRI's were also identified for linear measurements from the incision to the deep fascia. Using axial views, tumors were identified and contoured from proximal to distal tip, generating data on maximal tumor diameter and tumor volume. Volumes of subcutaneous fat and lean mass (including muscle, bone, and blood vessels) were gathered in a similar manner by contouring the structures from the proximal to distal boundaries of the tumor (Fig. 1). Tumor proximity to skin surface was measured from the point of maximal tumor diameter on the axial view to the future incision site determined from the patient's post-operative MRI. Maximal subcutaneous fat layer depth was also measured in this manner, along the length of the tumor and directly adjacent to the future incision site.

Patient data, including age, sex, BMI, diabetic and smoking status, presence of cardiovascular disease, KPS score, tumor histology and stage/grade, use of flap reconstruction, and treatment with chemotherapy were gathered from the existing orthopedic oncology database of STS patients.

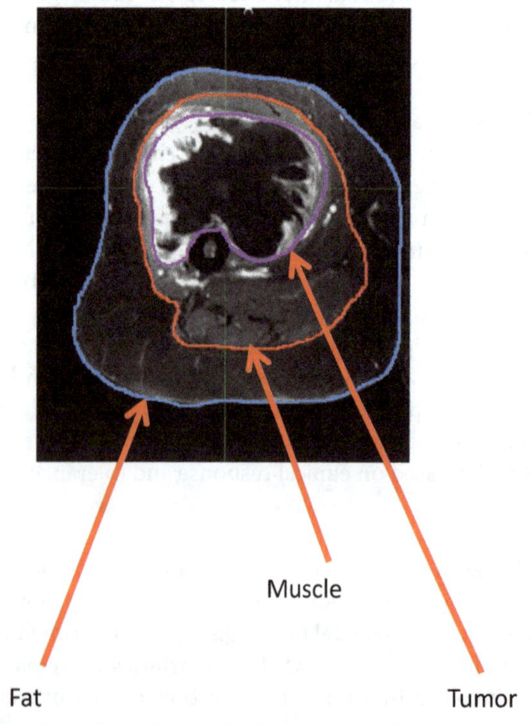

Fig. 1 Forty-eight year old with a high grade myxofibrosarcoma of the proximal thigh. Axial (*A*), coronal (*B*) and sagittal (*C*) views with contours of fat (*blue*), muscle (*red*) and tumor (*purple*)

Outcomes

Post-operative WCs were defined as by the Canadian Multicenter Trial and were recorded if they occurred within 6 months following limb-salvage surgery (Table 1). In general, patients who required re-operation, prolonged wound care or antibiotics after resection were considered WC [10].

Statistical analysis

Statistical software MedCalc (Version 15.6; MedCalc Software bvba, Ostend, Belgium) was used for all data analysis. Clinical, pathologic and treatment characteristics for WC were assessed and summarized in Table 2. Wound outcome was a dichotomous variable. The fisher exact test was used for univariate analysis (UVA). If a variable had a p value of less than 0.25, then it was used in the multivariate model. A logistic regression analysis was used for multivariate analysis (MVA). For all analysis, type I error was maintained at 0.05 and all tests were two-sided.

A receiver operative characteristic (ROC) curve was constructed and used to examine whether the volumetric data could differentiate between tumors that were predisposed to post-operative WCs versus those that were not predisposed to post-operative WCs.

Results

Eighty-one patients with stage I–III STS of the LE and buttock underwent treatment at this institution and were eligible for the study. Sixty-nine (85 %) patients had tumors located in the proximal LE, eight (10 %) had tumors in the buttock, and four (5 %) had tumors located in the pelvic region. An overview of patient, tumor, and treatment characteristics can be found in Table 2. Median age at diagnosis was 57 (range: 26–84), and median follow-up was 1.7 years. All 81 patients underwent limb-salvage resection; no patient underwent an amputation at the time of definitive resection.

The overall WC rate within 6 months of tumor resection and as defined by the Canadian Multicenter Trial [10], was 32 % (26 of 81 patients). Of these, ten (38 %) patients developed wound dehiscence and necrotic wounds, ten (38 %) patients developed infection, five (20 %) patients had delayed wound healing, and one (4 %) patient developed a post-operative hematoma. Fifty-four (67 %) patients had high grade tumors, four (5 %) intermediate grade, and 23 (28 %) low grade. There was no significant difference in WC rates in patients with

Table 1 Canadian multicenter wound complication definition

Wound complication category	Definition
Surgical complications	Secondary operations required for wound treatment (debridement, secondary closure procedures such as rotationplasty, free flaps, or skin grafts) Invasive procedure required for wound care (drainage of hematoma, seroma, or infected wound collection) Deep wound packing required at any time (deep packing defined as packing deep to dermis in an area of dehisced wound) to an area of the wound measuring ≥2 cm in length
Non-surgical complications	Readmission to hospital for wound care Prolonged dressing changes, including packing of the wound for >6 weeks from wound break down Failure of epithelialization of skin graft by 4 weeks after surgery

high grade (29.7 %) vs. low/intermediate grade (37.0 %) tumors (p = 0.61).

Median BMI of patients in our study was 28.8. WC occurred in 15 patients (37.5 %) with a BMI >28.8, and in eleven patients (28.2 %) with a BMI <28.8; this difference was not significant on UVA (p = 0.47) or MVA (p = 0.18). Similarly, when BMI was analyzed as a continuous variable, it did not significantly impact WC rates (OR 1.0448, 95 % CI 0.9746–1.1201, p = 0.22).

Forty-three patients had a tumor diameter of ≥10 cm. The WC rate was 39.5 % with tumors that were >10 cm compared to 23.6 % when the primary tumor measured <10 cm. This failed to reach statistical significance (p = 0.15). Increasing tumor volume, however, was associated with higher WC rates. The median tumor volume of patients in this study was 228.1 mL. WC occurred in 17/41 (41.5 %) patients with a tumor volume ≥228.1 mL, and in 9/40 (22.5 %) patients with a tumor volume <228.13 mL; p = 0.015). Increasing tumor volume was also significant when assessing this measure as a continuous variable (p = 0.015, OR 1.0010, 95 % CI 1.0001–1.0018). This finding held on MVA (p = 0.03, OR 1.0010, 95 % CI 1.0001–1.0018). A scatter plot depicting tumor size versus volume is located in Fig. 1.

The volume of subcutaneous fat did not significantly impact WC rates in this study (p = 0.34, OR 1.0002, CI 0.9998–1.0005). In addition, ratios comparing volumes of lean mass to subcutaneous fat (p = 0.69, OR 0.8683, 95 % CI 0.4306–1.7507) and volumes of subcutaneous fat to tumor (p = 0.55, OR 0.9822, 95 % CI 0.9257–1.0421) failed to reveal a significant relationship to WC on logistic regression. Depth of the subcutaneous fat layer at the incision site likewise did not impact WC rates.

Seventy (86 %) patients underwent preoperative RT, three (4 %) patients underwent postoperative RT, and eight (10 %) patients received both pre- and postoperative RT. There were no significant differences in WC rates between these groups. Fifty-six (69 %) patients received neoadjuvant chemotherapy, which had no significant impact on WC rates upon UVA (35.7 vs. 31.6 %, p = 0.44). No patient included in our study received adjuvant chemotherapy.

Primary closure was utilized for 50 (62 %) patients, while 31 (38 %) patients were selected for a vascularized flap closure with plastic surgery. Use of the flap closure was associated with higher WC rates (45 %) than primary closure (26 %), a difference which was significant on MVA (OR 3.6969, 95 % CI 1.2432–10.9938, p = 0.02). No other variables were significant on UVA or MVA (Table 3).

Local control in this cohort was 100 % and the distant metastasis rate was 30.8 %. Median survival was not met, but 2-year overall survival was 93.4 %. Median and 2-year progression-free survival was 66 months and 65 %, respectively. Similarly, median and 2-year distant metastasis-free survival was 66 months and 65 %, respectively.

Discussion

While pre-operative RT combined with wide surgical resection of STS improves disease free survival and has become the standard in limb salvage care at many institutions, post-operative WCs remain a considerable source of morbidity for patients. Several studies have investigated variables that influence post-operative WCs, which include, but are not limited to tumor size and location, proximity to skin surface, radiation field size, and timing of radiation [4, 14–16].

Location of the primary tumor has consistently been shown to impact post-operative WCs. Moore et al. reports a 23 % difference in WC rate for proximal LE tumors and proximal UE tumors [6]. Tumors in the adductor compartment of the proximal thigh are particularly prone to WC, a trend likely explained by disruption of the lymphatic network of the LE which occurs during surgery [6]. For this study, we wanted to eliminate the

Table 2 Clinical, pathologic, and treatment characteristics

Age (years)	
Mean	58.2
Median	57
Range	26–84
Gender	
F	30 (37 %)
M	51 (63 %)
Performance status (KPS)	
81–100	71(88 %)
≤80	10 (12 %)
Cardiovascular disease	
No	74 (91 %)
Yes	7 (9 %)
Diabetes	
No	72 (89 %)
Yes	9 (11 %)
Smoking history	
No	57 (70 %)
Yes	24 (30 %)
Stage	
I	20 (25 %)
II	10 (12 %)
III	51 (63 %)
Size	
<10 cm	38 (47 %)
≥10 cm	43 (53 %)
Location	
Proximal lower extremity	69 (85 %)
Buttock	8 (10 %)
Hip/pelvis	4 (5 %)
Grade	
Low	23 (28 %)
Intermediate	4 (5 %)
High	54 (67 %)
Histology	
Undifferentiated	10 (12 %)
Liposarcoma/leiomyosarcoma	31 (38 %)
Myxofibrosarcoma	11 (14 %)
Synovial	4 (5 %)
Spindle cell	13 (16 %)
Other	12(15 %)
Neoadjuvant chemotherapy	
No	25 (31 %)
Yes	56 (69 %)
Timing of RT	
No RT	8 (10 %)
Preoperative RT	70 (86 %)
Post-operative RT	3 (4 %)
Flap reconstruction	
No	50 (62 %)
Yes	31(38 %)

Table 3 UVA of WC variables

Variable	p value
BMI (>28/<28)	0.474
Neoadjuvant chemo (Y/N)	0.440
Cardiovascular disease (Y/N)	0.675
Diabetes (Y/N)	0.458
Smoking (Y/N)	0.798
Grade (high grade/non-high grade)	0.615
KPS score (>80/≤80)	0.278
Sex (M/F)	0.474
Tumor size (≥10 cm/<10 cm)	0.156
Flap closure (Y/N)	0.055

confounding influence of tumor location on WC risk. Therefore, our cohort only included patients with tumors in the proximal LE, buttock, or pelvic area.

Tumor size is a strong predictor of WC risk, a relationship which is demonstrated by multiple studies [4, 6, 7, 10, 17]. Tumors greater than 10 cm [4, 6, 10], 8 cm [7], and even 5 cm in diameter [18] have all been shown to be associated with higher WC risk. A probable explanation for the impact of tumor size on WC rates is that larger tumors generate a greater dead-space in the soft tissue following resection, predisposing the patient to seromas, hematomas, and infection. Our study did not demonstrate that tumors greater than 10 cm in diameter were associated with a statistically significant higher risk of WCs. We did however find a statistically significant relationship between tumor volume and WC rate, establishing that increasing tumor volume predicts a greater risk of postoperative WC. This finding first corroborates prior research on the importance of tumor size as a risk factor for postoperative WC. More notably however, it also suggests that tumor volume, rather than tumor diameter or cross-sectional area, is a more powerful predictor of postoperative WC risk. Moreover, as conveyed in Fig. 2,

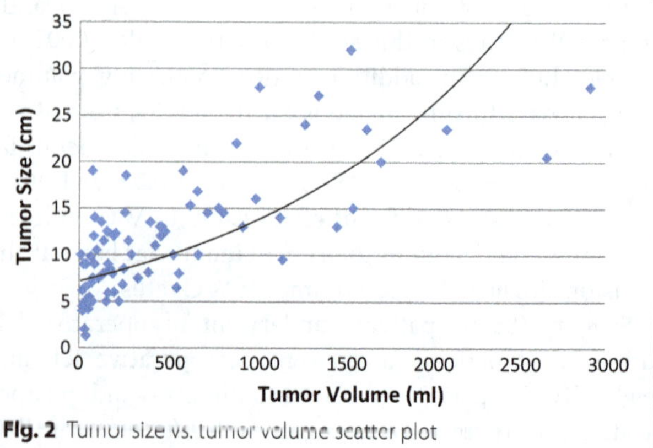

Fig. 2 Tumor size vs. tumor volume scatter plot

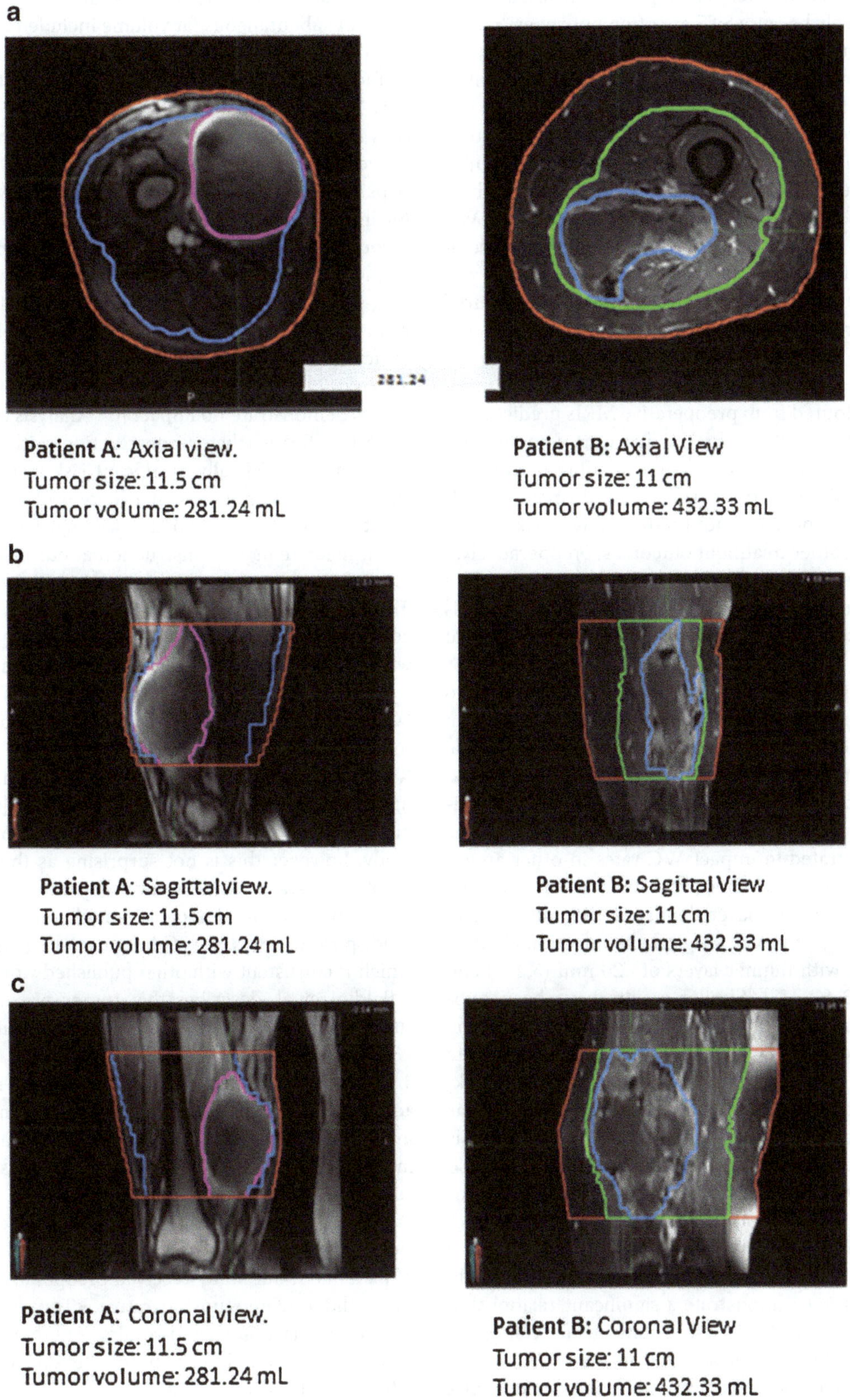

Fig. 3 **a** Patient A and B's Tumor size and corresponding volume on axial view. **b** Patient A and B's tumor size and corresponding volume on sagittal view. **c** Patient A and B's tumor size and corresponding volume on coronal view

there seems to be little relationship between size and volume, most likely because STS are often not spherical, but have an irregular shape. Thus, as mentioned above, maximal dimension may only provide one component influencing WC, and it is truly the volume that impacts this outcome. By measuring a 3-dimensional tumor in only one plane it is easy to over or under estimate true tumor burden, thereby misjudging the soft-tissue defect which will be left post-resection along with the associated WC risk (Fig. 3a–c). Work by Geller et al. has previously demonstrated that tumor volume is associated with WC risk [5]. In this study however, tumor volume was measured from final gross pathology specimens and was also not compared to tumor diameter or cross sectional area. To our knowledge, our study is the first to assess if tumor volumes contoured from preoperative MRIs predict postoperative WC risk. It also for the first time demonstrates that volumetric measurements may be more representative of tumor size than measuring tumor diameter, a finding which has implications for predicting WC risk, as well as potentially other treatment outcomes, preoperatively.

With the expanding obesity epidemic in the United States, the impact of subcutaneous fat on WC risk is a crucial area of investigation in STS. BMI has failed to demonstrate a significant association with WCs in prior studies [6], as well as our own. However, BMI fails to take into account factors such as gender differences in adipose tissue distribution and also levels of lean muscle mass which may weaken any association with WC risk. Levels of subcutaneous fat tissue surrounding the incision site has yet to be investigated in STS, although it has been demonstrated to impact WC rates in other arenas of surgery. In one study of cervical spine fusions, patients with subcutaneous fat layer depths of >40 mm were at significantly higher risk of surgical site infection (18.2 %) than patients with thinner layers of <20 mm (5.2 %) and <10 mm (2.3 %) [17]. Similar results have been published in gynecologic and general surgery, indicating that the thickness of SC fat surrounding the incision site impacts WC risk [11–13, 19, 20]. Increased SC fat thickness necessitates a longer surgical incision, as well as increased retraction which may lead to tissue necrosis at the operative site. A thicker subcutaneous layer also increases wound tension at closure, placing the patient at increased risk for wound dehiscence and also reducing tissue microperfusion and oxygen availability to the wound [21]. In contrast to the aforementioned research, our study did not demonstrate a significant relationship between WC risk and either subcutaneous fat volume or depth of the adipose layer adjacent to the incision. One limitation to our study which may have impacted results is that a nine of the preoperative MRIs had small sections of peripheral tissue cut off, not allowing us to fully contour fat and muscle layers. Additionally, our measurement of subcutaneous fat volume included adipose tissue from the entire circumference of the leg, not just surrounding the incision site. An avenue for future research may be measurement of the SC fat volume surrounding only the leg compartment specific to the tumors location.

Reconstruction of surgical wounds with vascularized flaps is utilized as an alternative to primary closure following resection of STS. It is intended to lower WC risk through minimizing residual dead space and also substituting previously irradiated soft tissues with healthy and well-vascularized tissue from a donor site. The literature returns mixed results on the impact of plastic reconstruction on WC risk; some studies conclude that it lowers risk [22], others find that it increases it [4], while yet others demonstrate no impact [6]. Analysis of our patient cohort indicates that reconstruction with vascularized flaps was a statistically significant risk factor for WC. It should be noted however that there is likely a strong element of selection bias in this finding. Patients selected for immediate flap reconstruction at our institution were often those felt to be at higher risk for postoperative WC. These included patients with greater tumor volumes, vascular involvement of their tumor, and host comorbidities which may have increased their risk for WCs.

The association between preoperative RT and increased WC risk has been well established. O'Sullivan et al. reported an 18 % increase in WC rate with preoperative RT in comparison to postoperative RT, a finding which has been replicated by additional studies [6, 23]. Timing of RT was not a significant risk factor for WC in our study; however this is not surprising as the vast majority of our patients underwent preoperative RT. Similarly, the administration of neoadjuvant chemotherapy did not predispose patients to WC in our study. This is a finding which is consistent with other published work.

Baldini et al. describes that tumor proximity to skin surface impacts WC risk, reporting that tumors located <3 mm from the skin surface increase risk for WC (OR 3.9) [4]. This finding however has not been replicated in additional research [6], and is also not shown in our findings. Timing of radiotherapy in our study may be a factor in this negative result. Baldini et al. suggests that preoperative RT of superficial tumors delivers an unavoidably high radiation dose to the surgical flaps used in wound closure, increasing the risk for WC. While the majority of patients in our study received preoperative RT (86 %), some did undergo postoperative RT or no RT at all, which may have impacted results. Another possibility is that our small sample size limited our ability to find a significant relationship.

One weakness of our study was our small sample size. STS are exceedingly rare cancers, and by restricting our study population to only patients with tumors in the proximal LE, buttock, or pelvis, we limited our sample size. This could potentially explain why some of our results did not reach the level of statistical significance. For instance, prior research has demonstrated diabetes to be powerful risk factor for WC following resection of STS [4, 6]. In our study there were large differences in WC risk for patients with diabetes (44.4 vs. 30.6 %). This difference was not significant however, which may be due to our analysis being underpowered. Additional limitations to our study include the retrospective nature of the study and the inherent biases which come with this design, as well as the limited field of view on nine of the preoperative MRIs which limited our ability to accurately contour structures. Another limitation of the study is the potential error in the volume measurements. Contouring structures on MRI scans is a very operator dependent process, and results may vary from person to person based on contouring technique. We attempted to limit the potential impact of this by having all measurements acquired by a single researcher. Although all data was generated by a single researcher in our study, the intra and inter-observer variability associated with the volume measurement technique is unknown and attempts to replicate this research in the future may be prone to this bias.

Conclusions

In this study, it was tumor volume, more than size that impacted the development of post-operative WCs. Our study demonstrates that gathering data on tumor volume, rather than diameter, may be a more accurate means of predicting WC risk. Tumor volume measurements could allow clinicians to more accurately counsel patients regarding their risk of WCs and also arrange for more aggressive follow-up and prophylactic regimens to combat the risk of WC. Further investigations on the relationship between volumetric parameters and treatment outcomes are warranted.

Abbreviations

BMI: body mass index; CI: confidence interval; Gy: gray; MIM: medical image merge; MVA: multivariate analysis; STS: soft tissue sarcomas; UVA: univariate analysis; WC: wound complication.

Authors' contributions

MZ: conducted a literature search, analysis and drafted the manuscript. MB: assisted with the literature search, formulated project design, performed data analysis, and assisted in manuscript construction and editing. DK: formulated project design and supervised the study. DK also assisted in manuscript construction and editing. All authors read and approved the final manuscript.

Author details

[1] Department of Orthopaedic Surgery, Medical College of Wisconsin, 9200 West Wisconsin Ave, Milwaukee, WI 53226, USA. [2] Department of Radiation Oncology, Medical College of Wisconsin, 9200 West Wisconsin Ave, Milwaukee, WI 53226, USA.

Competing interests

The authors declare that they have no competing interests.

Funding source

There were no funding sources available for this project.

References

1. Jemal A, Murray T, Ward E, Samuels A, Tiwari RC, Ghafoor A, Feuer EJ, Thun MJ. Cancer statistics, 2005. CA Cancer J Clin. 2005;55(1):10–30 **(Erratum in: CA Cancer J Clin. 2005 Jul-Aug;55(4):259. PubMed PMID: 15661684)**.
2. Suit HD, Spiro I. Role of radiation in the management of adult patients with sarcoma of soft tissue. Semin Surg Oncol. 1994;10(5):347–56.
3. Yang JC, Chang AE, Baker AR, Sindelar WF, Danforth DN, Topalian SL, DeLaney T, Glatstein E, Steinberg SM, Merino MJ, Rosenberg SA. Randomized prospective study of the benefit of adjuvant radiation therapy in the treatment of soft tissue sarcomas of the extremity. J Clin Oncol. 1998;16(1):197–203.
4. Baldini EH, Lapidus MR, Wang Q, Manola J, Orgill DP, Pomahac B, Marcus KJ, Bertagnolli MM, Devlin PM, George S, Abraham J, Ferrone ML, Ready JE, Raut CP. Predictors for major wound complications following preoperative radiotherapy and surgery for soft-tissue sarcoma of the extremities and trunk: importance of tumor proximity to skin surface. Ann Surg Oncol. 2013;20(5):1494–9. doi:10.1245/s10434-012-2797-1 **(Epub 2012 Dec 15)**.
5. Geller DS, Hornicek FJ, Mankin HJ, Raskin KA. Soft tissue sarcoma resection volume associated with wound-healing complications. Clin Orthop Relat Res. 2007;459:182–5.
6. Moore J, Isler M, Barry J, Mottard S. Major wound complication risk factors following soft tissue sarcoma resection. Eur J Surg Oncol. 2014;40(12):1671–6. doi:10.1016/j.ejso.2014.10.045.
7. Korah MP, Deyrup AT, Monson DK, Oskouei SV, Weiss SW, Landry J, Godette KD. Anatomic tumor location influences the success of contemporary limb-sparing surgery and radiation among adults with soft tissue sarcomas of the extremities. Int J Radiat Oncol Biol Phys. 2012;82(2):933–9. doi:10.1016/j.ijrobp.2010.11.020 **(Epub 2011 Feb 6)**.
8. Prendergast B, Fiveash JB, Gibbs CP, Scarborough MT, Indelicato DJ. Radiotherapy for soft tissue sarcoma of the proximal lower extremity. Sarcoma. 2010;2010:829498. doi:10.1155/2010/829498 **(Epub 2010 Oct 14)**.
9. Schwartz A, Rebecca A, Smith A, Casey W, Ashman J, Gunderson L, Curtis K, Chang YH, Beauchamp C. Risk factors for significant wound complications following wide resection of extremity soft tissue sarcomas. Clin Orthop Relat Res. 2013;471(11):3612–7. doi:10.1007/s11999-013-3130-4 **(Epub 2013 Jun 28)**.
10. O'Sullivan B, Davis AM, Turcotte R, Bell R, Catton C, Chabot P, Wunder J, Kandel R, Goddard K, Sadura A, Pater J, Zee B. Preoperative versus postoperative radiotherapy in soft-tissue sarcoma of the limbs: a randomised trial. Lancet. 2002;359(9325):2235–41.
11. Tsukada K, Miyazaki T, Kato H, Masuda N, Fukuchi M, Fukai Y, Nakajima M, Ishizaki M, Motegi M, Mogi A, Sohda M, Moteki T, Sekine T, Kuwano H. Body fat accumulation and postoperative complications after abdominal surgery. Am Surg. 2004;70(4):347–51.
12. Yamada T, Okabayashi K, Hasegawa H, Tsuruta M, Abe Y, Ishida T, Matsui S, Kitagawa Y. Age, preoperative subcutaneous fat area, and open laparotomy are risk factors for incisional hernia following colorectal cancer surgery. Ann Surg Oncol. 2015;23(Suppl 2):236–41.
13. Soper DE, Bump RC, Hurt WG. Wound infection after abdominal hysterectomy: effect of the depth of subcutaneous tissue. Am J Obstet Gynecol. 1995;173(2):465–9 **(discussion 469-71)**.
14. Cannon CP, Ballo MT, Zagars GK, Mirza AN, Lin PP, Lewis VO, et al. Complications of combined modality treatment of primary lower extremity soft tissue sarcomas. Cancer. 2006;107:2455–61.

15. Arbeit JM, Hilaris BS, Brennan MF. Wound complications in the multimodality treatment of extremity and superficial truncal sarcomas. J Clin Oncol. 1987;5:480–8.
16. Kunisada T, Ngan SY, Powell G, Choong PFM. Wound complications following pre-operative radiotherapy for soft tissue sarcoma. EJSO. 2002;28:75–9.
17. Mehta AI, Babu R, Sharma R, Karikari IO, Grunch BH, Owens TR, Agarwal VJ, Sampson JH, Lad SP, Friedman AH, Kuchibhatla M, Bagley CA, Gottfried ON. Thickness of subcutaneous fat as a risk factor for infection in cervical spine fusion surgery. J Bone Joint Surg Am. 2013;95(4):323–8. doi:10.2106/JBJS.L.00225.
18. Cannon CP, Ballo MT, Zagars GK, Mirza AN, Lin PP, Lewis VO, Yasko AW, Benjamin RS, Pisters PW. Complications of combined modality treatment of primary lower extremity soft-tissue sarcomas. Cancer. 2006;107(10):2455–61.
19. Fujii T, Tsutsumi S, Matsumoto A, Fukasawa T, Tabe Y, Yajima R, Asao T, Kuwano H. Thickness of subcutaneous fat as a strong risk factor for wound infections in elective colorectal surgery: impact of prediction using preoperative CT. Dig Surg. 2010;27(4):331–5. doi:10.1159/000297521 **(Epub 2010 Aug 3)**.
20. Sugisawa N, Tokunaga M, Tanizawa Y, Bando E, Kawamura T, Terashima M. Intra-abdominal infectious complications following gastrectomy in patients with excessive visceral fat. Gastric Cancer. 2012;15:206–12.
21. Guo S, Dipietro LA. Factors affecting wound healing. J Dent Res. 2010;89(3):219–29. doi:10.1177/0022034509359125 **(Epub 2010 Feb 5. Review)**.
22. Griffin AM, Dickie CI, Catton CN, Chung PW, Ferguson PC, Wunder JS, O'Sullivan B. The influence of time interval between preoperative radiation and surgical resection on the development of wound healing complications in extremity soft tissue sarcoma. Ann Surg Oncol. 2015;22:2824–30.
23. Peat BG, Bell RS, Davis A, O'Sullivan B, Mahoney J, Manktelow RT, Bowen V, Catton C, Fornasier VL, Langer F. Wound-healing complications after soft-tissue sarcoma surgery. Plast Reconstr Surg. 1994;93(5):980–7.

17

Antiangiogenic effects in patients with progressive desmoplastic small round cell tumor: data from the French national registry dedicated to the use of off-labeled targeted therapy in sarcoma (OUTC's)

Sarah Bétrian[1*], Christophe Bergeron[2], Jean-Yves Blay[3], Emmanuelle Bompas[4], Philippe A. Cassier[3], Laure Chevallier[5], Jérome Fayette[3], Magali Girodet[5], Cécile Guillemet[6], Axel Le Cesne[7], Perrine Marec-Berard[2], Isabelle Ray-Coquard[3] and Christine Chevreau[1]

Abstract

Background: Desmoplastic small round cell tumor (DSRCT) is a very rare mesenchymal tumor that mainly affects teenagers and young adults with a mean age at diagnosis around 20–25 years. Although initial management still needs standardization, many centers will use multimodal treatment including intensive chemotherapy, extensive surgical resection followed by radiotherapy. Despite this, prognosis remains very poor and the median overall survival is 25 months. Recurrent disease is mainly treated by chemotherapy. Recently, due to the unmet medical need for recurrent disease, targeted therapies were explored for DSRCT.

Methods: In this study, we assessed the response rate and progression free survival in nine cases of progressive DSRCT included in the OUTC's registry and treated with antiangiogenics targeted agents (sunitinib, sorafenib and bevacizumab). OUTC's, a French national registry, collects data about the use of off-label targeted therapy in sarcoma.

Results: Eight males and one woman were included, with median age at diagnosis of 27.3 years (range from 9 to 48 years). They received a mean 3 lines (2–5) of treatment before antiangiogenic agent initiation. Six patients received sunitinib, two received sorafenib and one bevacizumab. Median progression free survival was 3.1 months (range 2–5.5 months) and best response observed was 5.5 months stable disease. Most patients had manageable low-grade toxicities, mainly fatigue, abdominal pain and skin toxicity.

Conclusions: Despite very limited activity of antiangiogenics in our study, prospective collection of cases of these rare tumors together with molecular data should guide therapeutic decision and enhance outcome.

Keywords: Desmoplastic small round cell tumor, Antiangiogenic, Chemotherapy treatment, Sunitinib

Background

Desmoplastic small round cell tumor (DSRCT) was first described in 1989 by Gerald and Rosai [1], as a tumor made of small round blue cells separated by abundant desmoplastic stroma. Fewer than 800 cases have been reported in the literature. DSRCT is therefore rare. DSRCT is an aggressive tumor, which mainly affects teenagers and young adults, predominantly males (sex ratio 4:1 to 9:1) with a peak incidence in the third decade of life.

On histological examination, tumor cells may display epithelial, mesenchymal and neuronal markers [2].

*Correspondence: Betrian.sarah@iuct-oncopole.fr
[1] Departments of Oncology and Clinical Research, Institut Claudius Regaud, Institut Universitaire du Cancer, Toulouse Oncopole, 1 avenue Irène Joliot-Curie, 31059 Toulouse Cedex, France

DSRCT is associated with a unique translocation t(11:22) (p13, q12) resulting in a fusion of the EWSR1 and the Wilm's tumor WT1 genes. The chimeric product acts as an aberrant transcriptional factor and several transcriptional oncogenic targets have been identified including platelet derived growth factor A (PDGFA), insulin like growth factor 1 (IGF1) and WT-1 [3]. However, this has not yet been translated in efficient targeted therapy in this disease.

DRSCT typically involves the abdominal and peritoneal cavity, but extra-peritoneal organs may be affected [4–6]. Retroperitoneal lymph nodes, liver or lung metastases occur up to 50% cases at diagnosis [7]. There is no validated disease staging system, although the peritoneal cancer index (PCI) may be used for peritoneal disease [8] and Hayes-Jordan et al. have proposed a staging system specific to DSRCT [9].

With only one large case series described, the best therapeutic strategy remains unclear. DSRCT has a poor prognosis with a median OS of 25 months [7] and a 29 and 18% 3 and 5-years survival rate [10, 11]. A few small series suggest that intensive chemotherapy followed by extensive debulking surgery and abdominal radiation may improve the outcome of patients with operable disease [7, 12, 13]. Polychemotherapy schedule using alkylating agents and anthracyclins such as P6 protocol (cyclophosphamide, doxorubicin, vincristine, ifosfamide, etoposide, irinotecan and platinum alternating schedule) is associated with better outcome. A few centers have advocated the use of hyperthermic intraperitoneal chemotherapy (HIPEC) but, in the absence of randomized study, it is difficult to decipher the actual treatment effect from a selection bias in these series [14, 15]. Whole abdominal pelvic radiation therapy (WAP RT) and increasing development of intensity modulated radiation therapy were also described as a part of the adjuvant treatment [16, 17].

Overall, despite multimodal strategy, long term survivor rate remains low, with fewer than 20% of patients achieving 5-year survival [12]. Tumor recurrence and progression is the rule. After first line treatment, several cytotoxic agents have been studied, alone or in combination, including vinorelbine and cyclophosphamide [18], irinotecan [19], trabectedin [20, 21]. However, response rates are low and only partial responses are described and response duration remains short, range from 3 to 9 months.

Recently, there has been interest in the potential role of antiangiogenic tyrosine kinase inhibitors. Indeed, expression of EWS-WT1 induces PDGFA, a potent mitogen for fibroblast and endothelial cells. Particularly, PDGFA blockade may be interesting in DSRCT because of a profuse stromal reaction and neoangiogenesis surrounding tumor cells [3]. Thus, tyrosine kinase PDGFA receptor (PDGFRA) inhibitors such as imatinib and multikinase inhibitors, sunitinib and pazopanib, have been tested in DSRCT [22–24]. Our study reports nine cases of progressive DSRCT treated with antiangiogenic targeted agents, and registered in the national registry "OUTC's" dedicated to the use of off-labeled targeted therapy in sarcoma.

Patients and methods

Registry

OUTC's registry (Observatoire de l'Utilisation des Thérapies Ciblées dans le Sarcome) aims to collect, in a prospective manner, all medical data regarding the use of off-label targeted therapies in sarcoma to assess their efficacy and toxicity profile [25]. Off-label prescription is authorized in France for rare disease under control of experts, based on published data reporting potential activity.

Patients

Patients with confirmed progressive DSRCT, not amendable to curative treatment, were included. As our study was not interventional, written consent was not required. However, patients were informed and gave oral consent for data collection and use of clinical data for research purposes. All patients received a detailed information letter and had the opportunity to withdraw their consent at any time. Children could be included with their parent's consent. Progressive DSRCT was confirmed, in seven of our nine cases, by a systematic pathological review as part of two databases dedicated to collection and management of cases of soft tissue and visceral sarcomas (REePS: https://rreps.sarcomabcb.org/; and European Conticabase: https://conticabase.sarcomabcb.org/). All data were collected by the coordination center (Centre Léon Bérard, Lyon) after approval of the Centre Léon Bérard Clinical Trial Review Committee and two French data protection authorities (CCTIRS: Additional file 1; and CNIL: Additional file 2). Five university hospitals (all members of the GSF-GETO) participated and included all consecutive patients. Once a patient was registered, follow-up was established every 2 months by the coordination center.

Study endpoints

The primary objective was to describe the efficacy of antiangiogenics agents in advanced DSRCT. Efficacy endpoints included response rate [i.e. partial and complete response (PR, CR)], according to RECIST criteria, disease control rate (i.e. rate of CR, PR and stable disease (SD) as best overall response) and progression free survival (PFS) under treatment. Secondary objective included characterization of safety profile.

Statistical methods

Descriptive analysis was done using median values and range. PFS was defined as the time from start of AAT until progressive disease according to RECIST, or death. Safety evaluation was based on the frequency and severity of toxicities, graded according to the common terminology criteria for adverse events.

Results

Patient characteristics

From July 2002 to July 2013, 9 patients in 5 institutions were registered and received antiangiogenics targeted therapies (AAT) for advanced desmoplastic tumors. Patient and tumor characteristics, tumor staging and treatment are summarized in Table 1. There were 8 males. The median age at diagnosis was 27.3 years (range 9–48 years) and two patients were under the age of 18 years at diagnosis. Most patients had metastatic disease at diagnosis and have received multimodal treatment. Seven patients had surgical debulking of the primary tumor. First-line chemotherapy was generally based on anthracycline, ifosfamide and methotrexate. Three patients received radiotherapy as part of first line treatment. Median PFS after first line treatment was 19.5 months (range 6–47 months). Relapsed and progressive disease was treated with various chemotherapy regimens containing platinum, gemcitabine, irinotecan, temozolomide or trabectedine. Overall, for relapsed disease, complete response was observed for 2 first relapsed patients, with HIPEC and FOLFIRI regimen for one and etoposide, carboplatine, thiotepa and busulfan for the other one (PFS 17 and 12 months respectively). For the other patients short disease stabilization was the best response obtained with these second line regimens. Overall, second line treatment was associated with a median PFS of 10.5 months (range 2–17 months).

The median time from diagnosis to AAT was 3.6 years (range 10–78 months). Two patients received others targeted therapies, in 3rd line treatment, as part of a clinical trial (Ridaforolimus, mTOR inhibitor/SUCCEED trial *NCT00538239*, Dalotuzumab, IGFR1 inhibitor/DALORI trial) before they both received sunitinib. The median number of previous chemotherapy treatments before AAT was 3 (range 2–5). All patients had confirmed progressive disease at the time of initiation of AAT. In seven cases the decision to use off-label AAT was made after discussion in a multidisciplinary meeting. Six patients received sunitinib, two patients received sorafenib and one received bevacizumab. All treatments are summarized in Table 2.

Table 1 Patient and disease characteristics

	Total (n = 9)
Sex	
Male	8
Female	1
Age at histological diagnosis (years)	
Mean (SD)	27,3
Range (years)	9–48
Tumor localization	
Abdomen	7
Head and neck	1
Pelvis	1
Histological subtype	
DSRCT	4
Desmoplastic medulloblastoma	1
Desmoplastic tumor with multiple differentiation	2
Unclassified desmoplastic tumor	2
Tumor stage (AJCC/IUCC)	
Unknown	2
IV_B	7
Metastases at diagnosis	
Yes	6
Liver	4
Peritoneum	2
Other	1
Surgery of primary tumor	
Yes	7
Resection quality	
R_0	0
R_1	3
R_2	2
Unknown	2

SD standard deviation, *AJCC* American Joint Committee on Cancer, *IUCC* Union for International Cancer Control

AAT efficacy

Efficacy data were collected every 2 months. Individual responses to previous treatments and AAT are detailed in Table 2. The median PFS was 3.1 months for patients who received sunitinib. Overall, for the nine patients treated with AAT, the disease control rate at 2 months was 66.7% and PFS was also 3.1 months. The patient treated with bevacizumab died from progressive disease at 2 months and the patients treated with sorafenib had progressive disease at 4 months. Overall, for these nine patients, the best response had been stable disease.

AAT safety

The main toxicities are presented in Table 3. Among the six patients treated with sunitinib, gastro-intestinal toxicity and fatigue were the most common adverse events

Table 2 Treatment response and duration

Patient	First treatment	Surgery resection quality	Radiotherapy	PFS 1	Relapses treatments/*PFS*	Lines of treatment before TT	TT type	PFS with TT (months)
1	MAID[a]-ASCT[b]	R2	_	12 months	Gemcitabine-cisplatine/2,5 months	2	Sunitinib	2
2	LV5Fu-Ciplatine	_	_	8 months	HIPEC[c]-FOLFIRI[d]/17 months FOLFIRI/3 months Holoxan-etoposide/3 months Adriamycine-cyclophosphamide/*2 months*	*5*	Sorafenib	3.5
3	MAI[e]	R1	Yes	39 months	Gemcitabine-docetaxel/4 months Adriamycine-holoxan/3 months Cisplatine-irinotecan/6 months Trabectedine/9 months	5	Sorafenib	4
4	Adriamycine-etposide-Cisplatine-Cyclophosphamide + VAI[f]	R2	_	44 months	Carboplatine-etoposide/13 months	2	Sunitinib	5.5
5	Cyclophosphamide-etoposide-carboplatine	R1	Yes	47 months	Etoposide-carboplatine-busulfan-thiotepa/12 months Temozolamide/5 months TEMIRI[g]/*4 months*	4	Bevacizumab	2
6	MAI	_	_	6 months	VAC[h]/6 months	2	Ridaforolimus *PFS* 23 months Sunitinib	4 OS 38 months
7[j]	Bevacizumab-IVADo[i]	R1	Yes	7 months	Navelbine-cyclophosphamide/10 months	2	Dalotuzumab *PFS* 2 months Sunitinib	3
8	Adriamycine-ifosfamide-etoposide	_	_	6 months	Cyclophosphamide/3 months Trabectedine/4 months	3	Sunitinib	2 OS 19 months
9	MAI	_	_	7 months	VAC/3 months	2	Sunitinib	2

[a] Mesna-Adriblastine-Ifosfamide-Dacarbazine

[b] Autologous stem cell transplantation

[c] Hyperthermic intraperitoneal chemotherapy

[d] 5 Fluorouracile-Oxaliplatine-Irinotecan

[e] Mesna-Adriblastine-Ifosfamide

[f] Vincristine-Actinomycine D-Ifosfamide

[g] Temozolamide-Irinotecan

[h] Vincristine-Actinomycine D-Cyclophosphamide

[i] Ifosfamide-Vincristine-Actinomycine D-Doxorubicine

[j] This patient had TT bevacizumab in first line treatment as part of BERNIE study in combination with IVADo polychemotherapy. The second relapse was treated with dalotuzumab, he received temodal-irinotecan for third relapse (PFS 8 months) and he finally had sunitinib for the fourth relapse

(AEs) (n = 4). One patient had grade 3 hepatitis, but otherwise, most AEs were low grade and none required interruption of sunitinib. One patient treated with sorafenib had grade 1 skin toxicity and grade 2 cough. The other patient treated with sorafenib had grade 3 abdominal pain that required cessation of treatment. Overall, the toxicity profile seen with these agents was similar to that observed in others studies [26]. There were no grade IV adverse events and no toxic deaths occurred during follow-up.

Discussion

Relapsed and refractory DSRCT remains associated with very poor prognosis. As noted above, multimodal therapy that combines polychemotherapy, debulking surgery

Table 3 TT toxicities

Sunitinib (n = 6)	Total N	Grade 1 N	Grade 2 N	Grade 3 N
Skin toxicity	1	1	0	0
Fatigue	3	2	0	1
Nausea	1	1	0	0
Diarrhea	1	1	0	0
Abdominal pain	1	1	0	0
Hepatic cytolysis	1	0	0	1
Dyspnoea	1	0	0	1
Hematoxicity	2	1 *(anemia)*	0	1 *(lymphopenia)*
Sorafenib (n = 2)				
Skin toxicity	1	1	0	0
Abdominal pain	1	0	0	1
Cough	1	0	1	0

and radiotherapy is associated with better outcome than less comprehensive treatment [7, 12].

In our case series, clinical patients characteristics are comparable to those of previous series. Seven of our nine patients had debulking surgery even in presence of metastatic disease at diagnosis. First-line chemotherapy was based on anthracyclines, ifosfamide and etoposide using regimens adapted from the P6 protocol. These approaches are similar than those used in the most studies reported to date and are considered as standard care. The median PFS following first-line treatment was 19.5 months, which is comparable with PFS reported in the literature [11, 27].

There is no standard approach beyond first line, and patients received in most cases chemotherapy and salvage surgery when feasible. Gemcitabine, temozolamide, irinotecan and trabectedine were the main cytotoxic agents used. Overall, second line treatment was associated with a median PFS of 10.5 months (range 2–17 months). The only one patient who was treated with sunitinib monotherapy had a PFS of only 2 months. These data suggest that, if performance status allows, treatment for relapsed disease should again be based on combination chemotherapy.

Recent data suggest the interest of novel targeted therapy, against several biological processes involved in DSRCT pathogenesis, to treat recurrent diseases. Based on Ewing sarcoma model and EWS-Fli translocation, leading to dysregulation of insulin growth factor 1 (IGF1) receptor and dependence on IGF1 [28, 29], humanized monoclonal antagonist IGF1 receptor (IGF1R) antibodies have been developed [30, 31]. As part of clinical trial, one of our patients received the IGF1R antibody dalotuzumab, with a low PFS.

The modest efficacy of these signaling inhibitors and the development of resistance provide a rationale for the use of antiangiogenic multi-targeted kinase inhibitors. Only a few AATs have been tested in patients with relapsed and refractory DSRCT. Imatinib was used in a phase II study for two patients with DSRCT expressing KIT and/or PDGFRα with very limited response [22]. This may be explained by the fact that KIT expression probably leads to tumorigenicity as a spectrum, with more reliance on other kinase pathways, and may be targeted by other tyrosine kinase small molecules inhibitors [22]. Sunitinib is a multi-targeted agent that potently inhibits PDGFR, KIT, FLT3, CSF-1 and RET, as well as vascular endothelial growth factor (VEGF) receptor tyrosine kinases. It targets multiple signaling pathways in tumor, stromal, and endothelial compartments that are relevant to DSRCT [32]. Six of our patients received sunitinib as AAT for progressive disease with a median PFS of 3.1 months. Thus, sunitinib activity seems to be comparable to recent eight cases reported by Italiano et al. with median PFS of 2.6 months [23].

Overall, our results are similar to those described in the other retrospective analyses of monochemotherapy and most AAT for progressive DSRCT (Table 4). Efficacy was modest and the best response obtained was stable disease. However, a retrospective study of pazopanib in nine DSRCT cases reported promising results with a 9.2 months PFS [24]. Such as sunitinib, pazopanib is an orally available inhibitor of the tyrosine kinases of several factors including the vascular endothelial growth factor receptors (VEGFR) 1–3, c-KIT, and the platelet-derived growth factor receptors (PDGFR) alpha and beta, and has been approved for advanced soft tissue sarcoma.

This cohort, although small and retrospective, confirms the safety of AATs. AEs were mostly low grade and manageable, similar to those previously reported in other series.

Moreover, recent data on olaratumab, a recombinant human IgG1 monoclonal antibody that specifically binds PDGFRA and receptor activation, and its FDA approval, may significantly improve outcome of patients with soft tissue sarcoma. In this study, only one patient had an undifferentiated round cell sarcoma negative for EWS in olaratumab treatment arm [34].

Conclusions

OUTC'S program allows the collection of data on the off-label use of TTs in rare tumors such as DSRCT. This is especially useful since such patients are generally ineligible for clinical trials. Moreover new treatment development in DSRCT remains poor. Despite negative results, this study suggests that AAT with sunitinb, sorafenib or bevacizumab monotherapy doesn't seem to be the best

Table 4 Literature data of chemotherapy agents and TT for advanced TT

Chemotherapy agent	Patients number	Best response	PFS	References
Vinorelbine-Cyclophosphamide	2	2 PR	4 and 15 months	Ferrari et al. [18]
Irinotecan	8	4 SD, 4 PD	Unknown	Bisogno et al. [19]
Trabectedine	2	2 SD	4 months	Frezza et al. [21]
TT agent				
Imatinib	7	1 PR, 4 PD, 2 NA	1 month	Chao et al. [22]
Sunitinib	8	2 PR, 3 SD, 3 PD	2.6 months	Italiano et al. [23]
Pazopanib[c]	9	2 PR, 5 SD, 2 PD, CBR[a] 78%	9.2 months	Frezza et al. [24]
Temsirolimus	1	SD	10 months	Thijs et al. [33]
Ganitumab	16	1 PR, 10 SD, 4 PD, CBR[b] 25%	19 months	Tap et al. [30]

PR partial response, *SD* stable disease, *PD* progressive disease, *NA* non assessable, *CBR* clinical benefit rate (PR + SD >12 weeks[a], 24 weeks[b])

[c] Retrospective analysis from data comprising three DSRCT patients treated within the EORTC phase II study 62043, three in the EORTC phase III study 62072 (PALETTE), along with three patients treated in the UK on the subsequent pazopanib named patient program

approach to treat progressive DSRCT. Identification of molecular pathways and specific mutations involved in DSRCT pathogenesis may allow the development of new targeted and combination treatments to improve response rate and survival in relapsed and progressive DSRCT. Thus, IGFR1 inhibitors and multi-targeted kinase inhibitors may be another treatment strategy, probably in combination with chemotherapy. Prospective collection of cases of these rare tumors treated with targeted therapies together with increased molecular data understanding should improve therapeutic decision and enhance outcome.

Additional files

Additional file 1. CCTIRS (Comité Consultatif sur le traitement de l'information en matière de recherché dans le domaine de la santé) approved the relevance of the personal name specific data with regard to the objective of the research.

Additional file 2. CNIL (Comité National d'Information et Libertés) French committee in charge of watching that the computing is in the service of the citizen and that it strikes a blow neither at the human identity, nor at the human rights, nor at the private life, nor at the personal or public freedoms.

Abbreviations

DSRCT: desmoplastic small round cell tumor; PDGFA: platelet derived growth factor A; PDGFRA: platelet derived growth factor receptor A; IGF1: insulin like growth factor 1; WAP RT: whole abdominal pelvic radiation therapy; HIPEC: hyperthermic intraperitoneal chemotherapy; AAT: anti-angiogenic targeted therapy.

Authors' contributions

Study conception and design: JYB, IRC. Acquisition of data: CB, JYB, EP, PC, JF, CG, ALC, PMB, IRC, CC. Data management: LC, MG. Analysis and interpretation of data: SB, CC IRC. Drafting and revision of the manuscript: SB, CC, IRC, PMB. Obtained funding: IRC. Administrative, technical and material support: IRC. Study supervision: CC, IRC. All authors read and approved the final manuscript.

Author details

[1] Departments of Oncology and Clinical Research, Institut Claudius Regaud, Institut Universitaire du Cancer, Toulouse Oncopole, 1 avenue Irène Joliot-Curie, 31059 Toulouse Cedex, France. [2] Departments of Oncology and Clinical Research, Centre Léon Berard and Institut d'Hématologie et d'Oncologie Pédiatrique, Lyon, France. [3] Departments of Oncology and Clinical Research, Centre Léon Berard, Lyon, France. [4] Departments of Oncology and Clinical Research, Institut de Cancérologie de l'Ouest, Rene Gauducheau, St Herblain, France. [5] Clinical Research Department, CRA, Centre Léon Berard, Lyon, France. [6] Departments of Oncology and Clinical Research, Centre Henri Becquerel, Rouen, France. [7] Departments of Oncology and Clinical Research, Institut Gustave Roussy, Paris, France.

Acknowledgements

The authors would like to acknowledge the DAM's association and the Ain department's league for financial support, Laure Chevallier and Muriel Rogasick for OUTC's data management.

Competing interests

Dr. LE CESNE declares honoraria from Pharmamar, Novartis-GSK, Lilly and Pfizer. All remaining authors declare that they have no competing interests. Dr. MAREC-BERARD reported receiving travel stipends from Novartis, Pharmamar SARL, ROCHE. All remaining authors declare that they have no competing interests.

Ethics approval and consent to participate

The study was approved by the two committees: CNIL (Commission Nationale d'Information et Libertés: French national agency regulating data protection) and CCTIRS (Comité Consultatif sur le traitement de l'information en matière de recherche dans le domaine de la santé) (Additional file 1). The study had to be approved by the Multidisciplinary Sarcoma Board (MSB) of all participating centers according to the French Cancer Plan recommendations. As the study was not interventional, formal written consent was not required by French law. However, patients were informed and gave oral consent for data collection and use of clinical data for research purposes. Children could be included with their parents' consent. All patients received a detailed information letter and had the opportunity to withdraw their consent at any time.

Funding

This study was financially supported by Dam's (Détecter Alerter Mobiliser sarcomes) patients advocacy group and the Ain department league.

References

1. Gerald WL, Rosai J. Case 2 desmoplastic small cell tumor with divergent differentiation. Pediatr Pathol. 1989;9:177–83.
2. Zhang J, Dalton J, Fuller C. Epithelial marker-negative desmoplastic small round cell tumor with atypical morphology: definitive classification by fluorescence in situ hybridization. Arch Pathol Lab Med. 2007;131:646–9.
3. Gerald WL, Haber DA. The EWS-WT1 gene fusion in desmoplastic small round cell tumor. Semin Cancer Biol. 2005;15:197–205.
4. Tison V, Cerasoli S, Morigi F, Ladanyi M, Gerald WL, Rosai J. Intracranial desmoplastic small-cell tumor: report of a case. Am J Surg Pathol. 1996;20:112–7.
5. Yue X, Wang JZ, Tian Y, Wang KJ. Paratesticular desmoplastic small round cell tumor with metastasis: a report of two cases. Kaohsiung J Med Sci. 2014;30:104–5.
6. Nakayama J, Nassau S, Atkins K, Modesitt SC. Desmoplastic small round cell tumor of the ovary: a rare but devastating disease in young women. Gynecol Oncol Case Rep. 2014;7:16–8.
7. Honoré C, Amroun K, Vilcot L, Mir O, Domont J, Terrier P, Le Cesne A, Le Péchoux C, Bonvalot S. Abdominal desmoplastic small round cell tumor: multimodal treatment combining chemotherapy, surgery, and radiotherapy is the best option. Ann Surg Oncol. 2015;22:1073–9.
8. Dufresne A, Cassier P, Couraud L, Marec-Bérard P, Meeus P, Alberti L, Blay JY. Desmoplastic small round cell tumor: current management and recent findings. Sarcoma. 2012;2012:714986.
9. Hayes-Jordan A, Green H, Fitzgerald N, Xiao L, Anderson P. Novel treatment for desmoplastic small round cell tumor: hyperthermic intraperitoneal perfusion. J Pediatr Surg. 2010;45:1000–6.
10. Mingo L, Seguel F, Rollán V. Intraabdominal desmoplastic small round cell tumour. Pediatr Surg Int. 2005;21:279–81.
11. Kushner BH, LaQuaglia MP, Wollner N, Meyers PA, Lindsley KL, Ghavimi F, Merchant TE, Boulad F, Cheung NK, Bonilla MA, et al. Desmoplastic small round-cell tumor: prolonged progression-free survival with aggressive multimodality therapy. J Clin Oncol. 1996;14:1526–31.
12. Lal DR, Su WT, Wolden SL, Loh KC, Modak S, La Quaglia MP. Results of multimodal treatment for desmoplastic small round cell tumors. J Pediatr Surg. 2005;40:251–5.
13. Shoushtari AG. MM. Predictors of overall survival in patients diagnosed with desmoplastic small round cell tumor (DSRCT). J Clin Oncol. 2014;32(5):2014.
14. Hayes-Jordan A, Green HL, Lin H, Owusu-Agyemang P, Fitzgerald N, Arunkumar R, Mejia R, Okhuysen-Cawley R, Mauricio R, Fournier K, et al. Complete cytoreduction and HIPEC improves survival in desmoplastic small round cell tumor. Ann Surg Oncol. 2014;21:220–4.
15. Bakrin N, Bereder JM, Decullier E, Classe JM, Msika S, Lorimier G, Abboud K, Meeus P, Ferron G, Quenet F, et al. Peritoneal carcinomatosis treated with cytoreductive surgery and hyperthermic intraperitoneal chemotherapy (HIPEC) for advanced ovarian carcinoma: a French multicentre retrospective cohort study of 566 patients. Eur J Surg Oncol. 2013;39:1435–43.
16. Pinnix CC, Fontanilla HP, Hayes-Jordan A, Subbiah V, Bilton SD, Chang EL, Grosshans DR, McAleer MF, Sulman EP, Woo SY, et al. Whole abdominopelvic intensity-modulated radiation therapy for desmoplastic small round cell tumor after surgery. Int J Radiat Oncol Biol Phys. 2012;83:317–26.
17. Desai NB, Stein NF, LaQuaglia MP, Alektiar KM, Kushner BH, Modak S, Magnan HM, Goodman K, Wolden SL. Reduced toxicity with intensity modulated radiation therapy (IMRT) for desmoplastic small round cell tumor (DSRCT): an update on the whole abdominopelvic radiation therapy (WAP-RT) experience. Int J Radiat Oncol Biol Phys. 2013;85:e67–72.
18. Ferrari A, Grosso F, Stacchiotti S, Meazza C, Zaffignani E, Marchianò A, Casanova M. Response to vinorelbine and low-dose cyclophosphamide chemotherapy in two patients with desmoplastic small round cell tumor. Pediatr Blood Cancer. 2007;49:864–6.
19. Bisogno G, Riccardi R, Scagnellato A, Arcamone G, Miglionico L, Carli M. No effect of irinotecan in patients with resistant desmoplastic small round cell tumor. Pediatr Blood Cancer. 2010;54:182–3.
20. López-González A, Cantos B, Tejerina E, Provencio M. Activity of trabectidin in desmoplastic small round cell tumor. Med Oncol. 2011;28(Suppl 1):S644–6.
21. Frezza AM, Whelan JS, Dileo P. Trabectedin for desmoplastic small round cell tumours: a possible treatment option? Clin Sarcoma Res. 2014;4:3.
22. Chao J, Budd GT, Chu P, Frankel P, Garcia D, Junqueira M, Loera S, Somlo G, Sato J, Chow WA. Phase II clinical trial of imatinib mesylate in therapy of KIT and/or PDGFRalpha-expressing Ewing sarcoma family of tumors and desmoplastic small round cell tumors. Anticancer Res. 2010;30:547–52.
23. Italiano A, Kind M, Cioffi A, Maki RG, Bui B. Clinical activity of sunitinib in patients with advanced desmoplastic round cell tumor: a case series. Target Oncol. 2013;8:211–3.
24. Frezza AM, Benson C, Judson IR, Litiere S, Marreaud S, Sleijfer S, Blay JY, Dewji R, Fisher C, van der Graaf W, Hayward L. Pazopanib in advanced desmoplastic small round cell tumours: a multi-institutional experience. Clin Sarcoma Res. 2014;4:7.
25. Eberst L, Cropet C, Le Cesne A, Pautier P, Penel N, Adenis A, Chevreau C, Bay JO, Collard O, Cupissol D, et al. The off-label use of targeted therapies in sarcomas: the OUTC'S program. BMC Cancer. 2014;14:870.
26. Ravaud A, Motzer RJ, Pandha HS, George DJ, Pantuck AJ, Patel A, Chang YH, Escudier B, Donskov F, Magheli A, et al. Adjuvant sunitinib in high-risk renal-cell carcinoma after nephrectomy. N Engl J Med. 2016;375:2246–54.
27. Whelan J, Khan A, Sharma A, Rothermundt C, Dileo P, Michelagnoli M, Seddon B, Strausss S. Interval compressed vincristine, doxorubicin, cyclophosphamide alternating with ifosfamide, etoposide in patients with advanced Ewing's and other small round cell sarcomas. Clin Sarcoma Res. 2012;2:12.
28. Karnieli E, Werner H, Rauscher FJ, Benjamin LE, LeRoith D. The IGF-I receptor gene promoter is a molecular target for the Ewing's sarcoma-Wilms' tumor 1 fusion protein. J Biol Chem. 1996;271:19304–9.
29. Finkeltov I, Kuhn S, Glaser T, Idelman G, Wright JJ, Roberts CT, Werner H. Transcriptional regulation of IGF-I receptor gene expression by novel isoforms of the EWS-WT1 fusion protein. Oncogene. 2002;21:1890–8.
30. Tap WD, Demetri G, Barnette P, Desai J, Kavan P, Tozer R, Benedetto PW, Friberg G, Deng H, McCaffery I, et al. Phase II study of ganitumab, a fully human anti-type-1 insulin-like growth factor receptor antibody, in patients with metastatic Ewing family tumors or desmoplastic small round cell tumors. J Clin Oncol. 2012;30:1849–56.
31. Naing A, LoRusso P, Fu S, Hong DS, Anderson P, Benjamin RS, Ludwig J, Chen HX, Doyle LA, Kurzrock R. Insulin growth factor-receptor (IGF-1R) antibody cixutumumab combined with the mTOR inhibitor temsirolimus in patients with refractory Ewing's sarcoma family tumors. Clin Cancer Res. 2012;18:2625–31.
32. Chow LQ, Eckhardt SG. Sunitinib: from rational design to clinical efficacy. J Clin Oncol. 2007;25:884–96.
33. Thijs AM, van der Graaf WTA, van Herpen CML. Temsirolimus for metastatic desmoplastic small round cell tumor. Pediatr Blood Cancer 2010;55(7):1431–2.
34. Tap WD, Jones RL, Van Tine BA, Chmielowski B, Elias AD, Adkins D, Agulnik M, Cooney MM, Livingston MB, Pennock G, et al. Olaratumab and doxorubicin versus doxorubicin alone for treatment of soft-tissue sarcoma: an open-label phase 1b and randomised phase 2 trial. Lancet. 2016;388:488–97.

Regional chemotherapy by isolated limb perfusion prior to surgery compared with surgery and post-operative radiotherapy for primary, locally advanced extremity sarcoma

Jens Jakob[1†], Henry G. Smith[2†], Michelle J. Wilkinson[2], Tim Pencavel[2], Aisha B. Miah[2], Joseph M. Thomas[2], Per-Ulf Tunn[3], Lothar R. Pilz[4], Dirk C. Strauss[2], Peter Hohenberger[5] and Andrew J. Hayes[2*]

Abstract

Background: Induction chemotherapy by isolated limb perfusion (ILP) with melphalan and tumour necrosis factor-α is an effective strategy to facilitate limb-conserving surgery in locally advanced extremity sarcoma. In a comparison of cohorts matched for grade, size and surgical resectability, we compared the outcome of patients undergoing induction ILP prior to limb-conserving surgery and selective post-operative radiotherapy with patients undergoing limb-conserving surgery and routine post-operative radiotherapy.

Methods: Patients with primary, grade 2/3 sarcomas of the lower limbs over 10 cm in size were identified from prospectively maintained databases at 3 centres. Patients treated at a UK centre underwent limb-conserving surgery and post-operative radiotherapy (Standard cohort). Patients at two German centres underwent induction ILP, limb-conserving surgery and selective post-operative radiotherapy (ILP cohort).

Results: The Standard cohort comprised 80 patients and the ILP cohort 44 patients. Both cohorts were closely matched in terms of tumour size, grade, histological subtype and surgical resectability. The median age was greater in the Standard vs the ILP cohort (60.5 years vs 56 years, $p = 0.033$). The median size was 13 cm in both cohorts. 5-year local-recurrence (ILP 12.2%, Standard 20.1%, $p = 0.375$) and distant metastases-free survival rates (ILP 49.6%, Standard 46.0% $p = 0.821$) did not differ significantly between cohorts. Fewer patients received post-operative radiotherapy in the ILP cohort compared with the Standard cohort (27% vs 82%, $p < 0.001$).

Conclusion: In comparative cohorts, the outcomes of patients undergoing induction ILP prior to surgery did not differ from those undergoing standard management, although induction ILP was associated with a reduced need for adjuvant radiation.

Keywords: Soft tissue sarcoma, Isolated limb perfusion, Adjuvant radiotherapy, Postoperative complications

*Correspondence: andrew.hayes@rmh.nhs.uk
†Jens Jakob and Henry George Smith contributed equally to this work
[2] Sarcoma Unit, Department of Academic Surgery, Royal Marsden Hospital NHS Foundation Trust, Fulham Road, London SW3 6JJ, UK
Full list of author information is available at the end of the article

Background

Extremity soft tissue sarcomas (ESTS) are rare tumours comprising over 50 different histological subtypes [1, 2]. Optimal management of locally advanced ESTS requires multimodal therapy and the precise role of isolated limb perfusion (ILP) in the overall treatment strategy remains to be fully defined. For small or superficial ESTS, treatment usually involves surgery alone, gaining wide surgical margins while preserving function. Adjuvant radiotherapy is reserved for high-grade tumours greater than 5 cm or small tumours that focally involve margins adjacent to a critical structure [3]. When sarcomas attain even greater dimensions, such as over 10 cm, it becomes increasingly difficult to achieve negative margins without recourse to amputation or function-limiting surgery. While amputation for ESTS does not improve survival for sarcoma over limb-conserving surgery, it may still be considered for large sarcomas when the risk for local recurrence is viewed as significant [4–6].

Induction chemotherapy by ILP using melphalan with recombinant human tumour necrosis factor alpha (TNFα) prior to a limb-conserving surgical resection was introduced as a strategy for locally advanced sarcomas considered irresectable other than by an amputation [7]. TNFα is a multifunctional cytokine, which causes increased vascular permeability, associated with increased extravasation of cytotoxic agents and selective destruction of tumour-associated vessels by endothelial apoptosis and inflammation [8–10]. A multi-institutional case series of patients with locally advanced sarcomas, considered to be irresectable with limb-conserving surgery and adjuvant radiotherapy, which were treated using ILP with TNFα reported a limb salvage rate of 84% [7]. In light of these results, TNFα has been licensed for this indication since 2006.

ILP is now used more widely in large, high-grade tumours that are compatible with limb-conserving surgery but risk positive resection margins. Such patients would undergo an induction ILP prior to a wide resection of the primary tumour, with the aim of gaining as wide a margin as is compatible with preserving limb function. Post-operative radiotherapy is then typically only offered if the pathology specimen demonstrates viable tumour at a compromised margin. The alternative, which might be considered the standard management, would be a function-preserving wide resection with adjuvant radiotherapy to compromised margins. It is known that with adjuvant radiotherapy, planned microscopic positive margins over a critical structure are fully compatible with long-term local control [11].

In a retrospective cohort analysis, we sought to determine whether the peri-operative morbidity and oncological outcomes differed between these alternative multi-modality approaches to large high-grade sarcoma of the lower limb.

Patients and methods

Patient selection

Patients were identified from 1996 to 2010 using prospectively maintained databases at the Royal Marsden Hospital London, UK (defined as the Standard cohort) and the Sarcoma Center Berlin-Brandenburg and the University Medical Center Mannheim, Germany (defined as the ILP cohort). In the ILP cohort, all patients with a primary, unifocal, intermediate or high-grade (G2 and G3) ESTS of the lower limb with a maximum dimension of over 10 cm who underwent an induction ILP prior to a surgical resection were included. In the Standard cohort, all patients with the same characteristics but who had undergone limb-conserving surgery were included. Patients with disseminated disease at diagnosis or who had received pre-operative systemic chemotherapy were excluded.

Grading was according to the FNCLCC system [12]. Each tumour was staged as T2b N0 MO G2 or G3, corresponding to stage IIb or III in the AJCC system [13]. Size was defined by pre-operative cross sectional imaging (CT or MRI) and confirmed after pathological analysis. The administration of adjuvant radiotherapy in either cohort was not an inclusion criterion and all decisions relating to radiotherapy were made on an individual patient basis.

Treatment

The ILP cohort underwent induction ILP with TNFα (Beromun™, Boehringer Ingelheim, Germany) and melphalan followed by a wide or compartmental resection of the tumour 6–10 weeks later. Adjuvant radiation was not given routinely but considered in case of R1 resections or where the rate of necrosis post-ILP was considered suboptimal. The Standard cohort underwent a wide or compartmental resection, with radiotherapy offered at 6–12 weeks post-operatively [14].

Isolated limb perfusion

ILP has been described in detail before [7]. The procedure was performed under general anaesthesia. The perfusions were hyperthermic, with a target temperature of 38–39.5 °C. TNFα was administered after a stable limb circuit without leakage had been established, at a dose of 2–4 mg. Melphalan was applied 15 min later, at a dose of 10 mg/L of perfused limb volume. Total perfusion time was 90 min. The extremity was then rinsed with hydroxyl ethyl starch.

Surgical resection

The surgical approach in both cohorts was to achieve negative surgical histopathological margins where possible in the context of a limb-conserving operation. En-bloc resections with wide margins (1–2 cm of uninvolved tissue or an intact adjacent fascial layer) were performed whenever possible. When the tumour abutted major vessels or motor nerves, the adventitia or epineurium was taken as the margin of resection. When vessels were encased, they were resected and reconstructed. When the tumour abutted the bone, the periosteum was taken en-bloc with the tumour. Soft tissue reconstruction with pedicled or free-flaps was performed whenever necessary.

Adjuvant radiotherapy

Post-operative radiotherapy was administered 6–10 weeks post-surgery. In the Standard cohort, post-operative radiotherapy was considered for all cases. However, the final decision was made by a multi-disciplinary team in light of post-operative histology, the surgical margins and the patient's age and co-morbidities. In the ILP cohort, radiotherapy was administered in selected cases when there was a suboptimal histopathological response (less than 90% necrosis or viable tumour present at a surgical margin).

Histopathological analysis

Histopathologic analysis included assessment of resection margins and pathological response. A macroscopically positive margin was defined as R2 resection. If the tumour extended into the resection margin (<1 mm) on microscopic examination, the margin was defined as R1 resection and margins without actual involvement of the resection margin (>1 mm or an intact fascial plane) were considered microscopically negative (R0).

Follow-up

Patients were followed up every 3–4 month intervals for the first 3 years, then twice a year for up to 5 years, and annually thereafter.

Cohort comparison for resectability

To ensure that the tumours in both cohorts were equivalent in terms of resectability, three independent sarcoma surgeons working at major European sarcoma centres reviewed anonymised MRI's from patients within each cohort and scored the compatibility of the tumours with limb-conserving surgery and adjuvant radiotherapy alone. Twenty patients were randomly selected from each cohort. The anonymised images, together with basic patient details (gender, age, histopathology and tumour size), were then distributed to the assessors who ranked the images based on resectability from 1 to 10, with 1 being easily resectable by limb-conserving surgery and 10 indicating that limb conservation was impossible and amputation was required (Fig. 1).

Statistical analysis

To identify risk factors for local recurrence, metastasis and death from disease, stepwise Cox proportional-hazards regression analyses were performed using SPSS version 20. The influence of age (<65 vs. ≥ 65 years), tumour size, tumour grade (2 vs. 3), resection margin (R0 vs. R1), post-operative irradiation (yes vs. no), and local recurrence were assessed. Overall survival, systemic and local recurrences were calculated using Kaplan–Meier method and compared using the logrank test (Graphpad Prism, Version 6.0).

Results

Patient characteristics

Details of patient demographics are shown in Table 1. 80 patients were identified in the Standard cohort and compared to 44 patients in the ILP cohort (Fig. 2). The median age of patients in the Standard cohort was 60.5 years (range 18–92), which was significantly older than the ILP cohort with a median age of 56 years (range 17–82), (Mann–Whitney test $p=0.033$). There was no difference in tumour size between the two cohorts with both having a median tumour size of 13 cm (Standard range 10–29, ILP range 10–34), ($p=0.915$ Mann–Whitney test). The proportion of grade 2 and 3 tumours was also similar with the Standard cohort having 52 (65%) of patients with grade 3 tumours and the ILP cohort 31 patients (70.5%) ($p=0.840$ Fisher's exact test). No significant difference was found in the score of resectability between the two groups (Standard Cohort vs ILP median 4.45 vs 5.05 $p=0.314$, mean 5.12 vs 4.23 $p=0.112$) although the ILP cohort had slightly higher absolute scores (Additional file 1: Figure S1).

Treatment

Details of operative characteristics, complications, resection margins, final tumour histology and follow-up are shown in Table 2. Patients in the ILP cohort were significantly more likely to undergo vascular reconstruction. The use of flaps was also more common in this cohort. No significant difference in significant complications, defined as wound infections or collections requiring surgical or radiological intervention, was noted between the two cohorts. Two patients (5%) in the ILP cohort required an amputation. One amputation was performed in the peri-operative period due to procedure-related complications. The other amputation was performed 18 months after surgery due to chronic ulceration following a

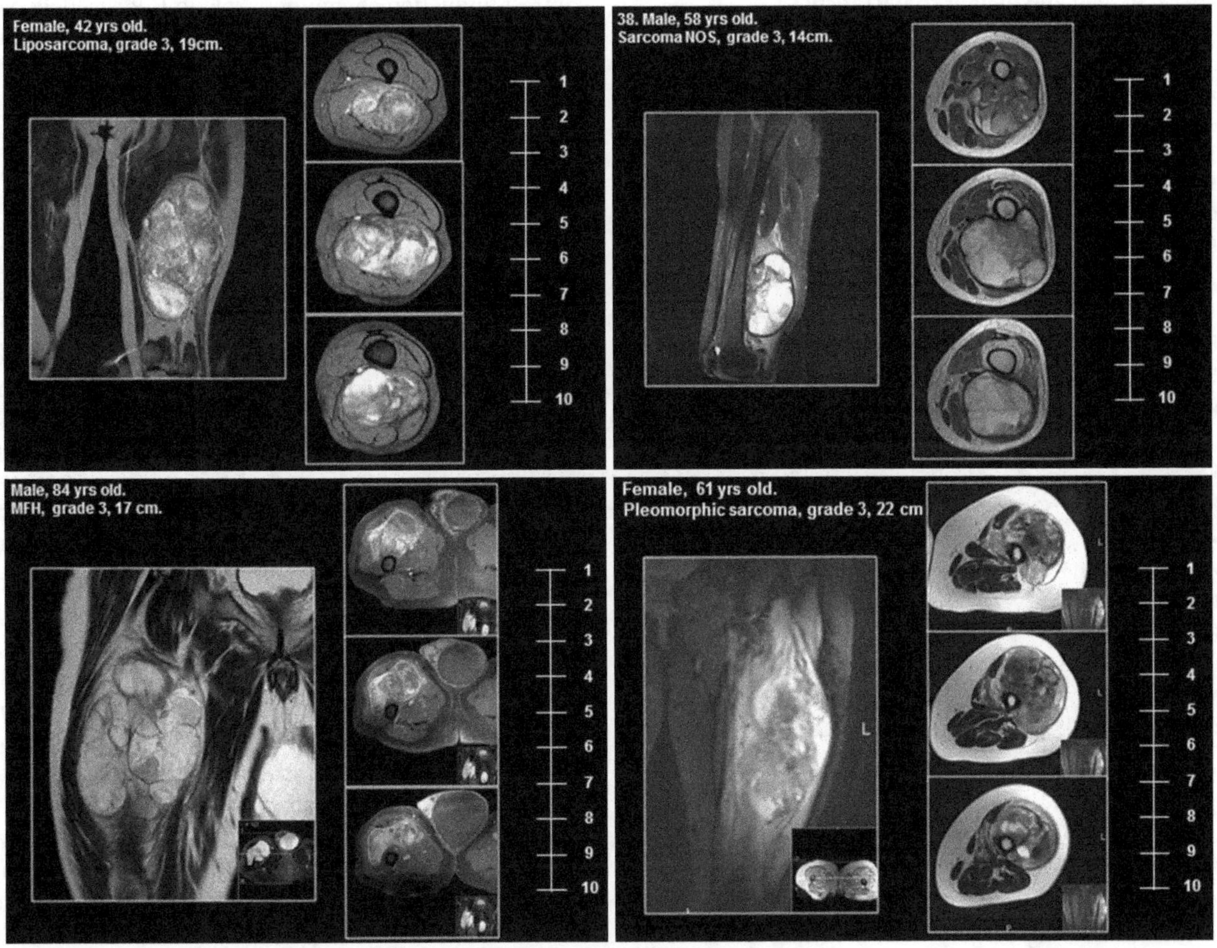

Fig. 1 Examples of MRI imaging of patients used for comparison of tumour resectability in cohorts

wound infection. No patients in the Standard cohort required amputation. In the Standard cohort 66 (82%) of patients received adjuvant radiotherapy compared to 12 (27%) patients in the ILP cohort ($p<0.001$, Chi square). The reasons for omitting radiotherapy in the Standard cohort were age and associated performance status (4 patients, median age 87.3 years), a compartmental resection achieving negative margins in all planes (6 patients, median age 57.7 years) or the rapid development of pulmonary metastases in the early post-operative period (4 patients). In the ILP cohort, the local recurrence rate in patients not receiving adjuvant radiotherapy was not significantly different to those who did (12.5% vs 8%, $p=1.0$ unpaired t-test).

Oncological Outcomes

The median follow-up for the Standard and ILP cohorts was 31 (4–194) months and 36 (8–163) months, respectively. The 5-year local recurrence-free (ILP cohort 12.2%, Standard cohort 20.1%, $p=0.375$ log-rank test) and distant metastases-free survival (ILP cohort 49.6%, Standard cohort 46.0%, $p=0.821$ log-rank test) did not significantly differ between cohorts (Fig. 3). Furthermore, at the time of writing, the local failure rate (i.e. patients developing local recurrence or requiring amputation) for both treatment arms was identical at 16%. Treatment strategy was not predictive of local or distant recurrence, with the only factors found to increase the risk of local recurrence on multivariate analysis being age and a positive (R1) resection margin (Table 3). The 5-year overall survival was worse in the Standard cohort compared to the ILP cohort (46.8% vs 63.8%, $p=0.020$ log-rank test). However, in a Cox proportional hazard model, when the differences in age between the two cohorts were accounted for, the overall survival on multivariate analysis between the ILP and Standard cohorts was virtually identical (HR 1.02, 95% CI 1.00–1.04, $p=0.043$).

Table 1 Patient and tumour characteristics

	Standard cohort	ILP cohort	Overall
Number of patients	80	44	124
Age at operation (median), years	60.5	56	57.5
Gender			
Male	46 (57.5%)	24 (54.5%)	70 (56.5%)
Female	34 (42.5%)	20 (45.5%)	54 (43.5%)
Tumour site			
Thigh	74 (92.5%)	30 (68.2%)	104 (83.9%)
Popliteal fossa	1 (1.3%)	5 (11.4%)	6 (4.8%)
Leg	5 (6.3%)	9 (20.5%)	14 (11.3%)
Median tumour size (cm)	13	13	13
Tumour grade			
II	28 (35.0%)	13 (29.5%)	41 (33.1%)
III	52 (65.0%)	31 (70.5%)	83 (66.9%)
Histology			
Pleomorphic	35 (43.8%)	20 (45.5%)	55 (44.4%)
Liposarcoma	13 (16.3%)	10 (22.7%)	23 (18.5%)
Leiomyosarcoma	9 (11.3%)	5 (11.4%)	14 (11.3%)
Solitary fibrous tumour	3 (3.8%)	1 (2.3%)	4 (3.2%)
MPNST	2 (2.5%)	2 (4.5%)	4 (3.2%)
Other	18 (23.8%)	6 (13.6%)	24 (19.4%)

MPNST malignant peripheral nerve sheath tumour

Discussion

Standard treatment for locally advanced ESTS consists of limb-conserving surgery with adjuvant radiotherapy that may be delivered pre or post-operatively [15]. The role of (neo)adjuvant chemotherapy outside of specific chemo-sensitive subtypes in ESTS is controversial. In the EORTC 62931 study, Woll et al. randomised patients with localised, grade II or III extremity sarcoma to receive adjuvant cheomotherapy in the form of doxorubicin, ifosfamide and lenogastrim in addition to surgery, radiotherapy and, if appropriate, ILP [16]. No benefit in terms of relapse-free or overall survival with this adjuvant regime compared to the control cohort were identified (5-year OS 66.5% vs 67.8%). More recently, in the ISG-STS 1001 study, Gronchi et al. randomised patients with localised, high-grade extremity sarcoma of 5 specified subtypes to receive neoadjuvant standard chemotherapy, in the form of epirubicin and ifosfamide, or histotype-tailored regimes [17]. This trial closed early after an interim analysis demonstrated no benefit in the histotype-tailored regimes. However, at 48 months, overall suvrival in the standard cohort was 89%, which suggests a potential benefit to neoadjuvant standard chemotherapy in these histological subtypes. As of yet, there is consensus regarding the role of (neo)adjuvant chemotherapy and its use is not considered standard in the most recent guidelines [18]. In contrast, induction chemotherapy with ILP is widely recognised to produce markedly better response rates than systemic chemotherapy and has a well-established role in facilitating function-preserving resections in locally advanced ESTS that would otherwise require amputation [7, 19–24].

With induction ILP increasingly used for ESTS that may be amenable to standard surgical management, the question as to which strategy, if either, is superior has arisen. Previous case series have clearly shown that induction ILP prior to surgery is an effective approach to deal with compromised surgical margins, as wide surgical resections were not possible. Similarly adjuvant radiotherapy has been shown to be effective in preventing local relapse after positive surgical margins [25]. The ability to directly compare these treatment strategies is hampered by the rarity of locally advanced non-metastatic primary ESTS and the scarcity of specialist centres performing ILP. As such, a randomized study comparing these strategies is not feasible [26]. Although subject to the limitations of any retrospective study, this comparison of matched cohorts provides valuable evidence to compare these two approaches.

The present study has found that the peri-operative and oncological outcomes of patients undergoing induction ILP prior to surgical resection are very similar to those undergoing standard surgical management. No significant difference was found in the rate of peri-operative complications between cohorts. Although two patients in the ILP cohort required amputations, only one was due to procedure-related complications. Similarly, no significant difference was found in the rates of local recurrence between these treatment arms, despite the use of adjuvant radiotherapy being significantly less frequent in the ILP cohort. There are no clear guidelines regarding the use of radiotherapy following ILP, although it is typically considered following an inadequate response on histological assessment of the specimen. However, following a microscopically complete resection with over 50% necrosis in the specimen, adjuvant radiotherapy is unlikely to be of additional benefit [27].

As a retrospective study, this series is subject to the bias inherent with this methodology. However, analysis of the tumour characteristics in terms of grade, size and histological subtype showed that the cohorts were well matched and this is reflected in the identical rate of metastatic spread. Similarly the assessment of the tumours "resectability" by independent experts indicated that the technical difficulty of surgery appeared to be similar in both cohorts. Although the cohorts were reasonably well matched, they were not randomized and we identified some important differences. There was a higher proportion of popliteal fossa and leg tumours in the ILP cohort. It is generally accepted that achieving local control for

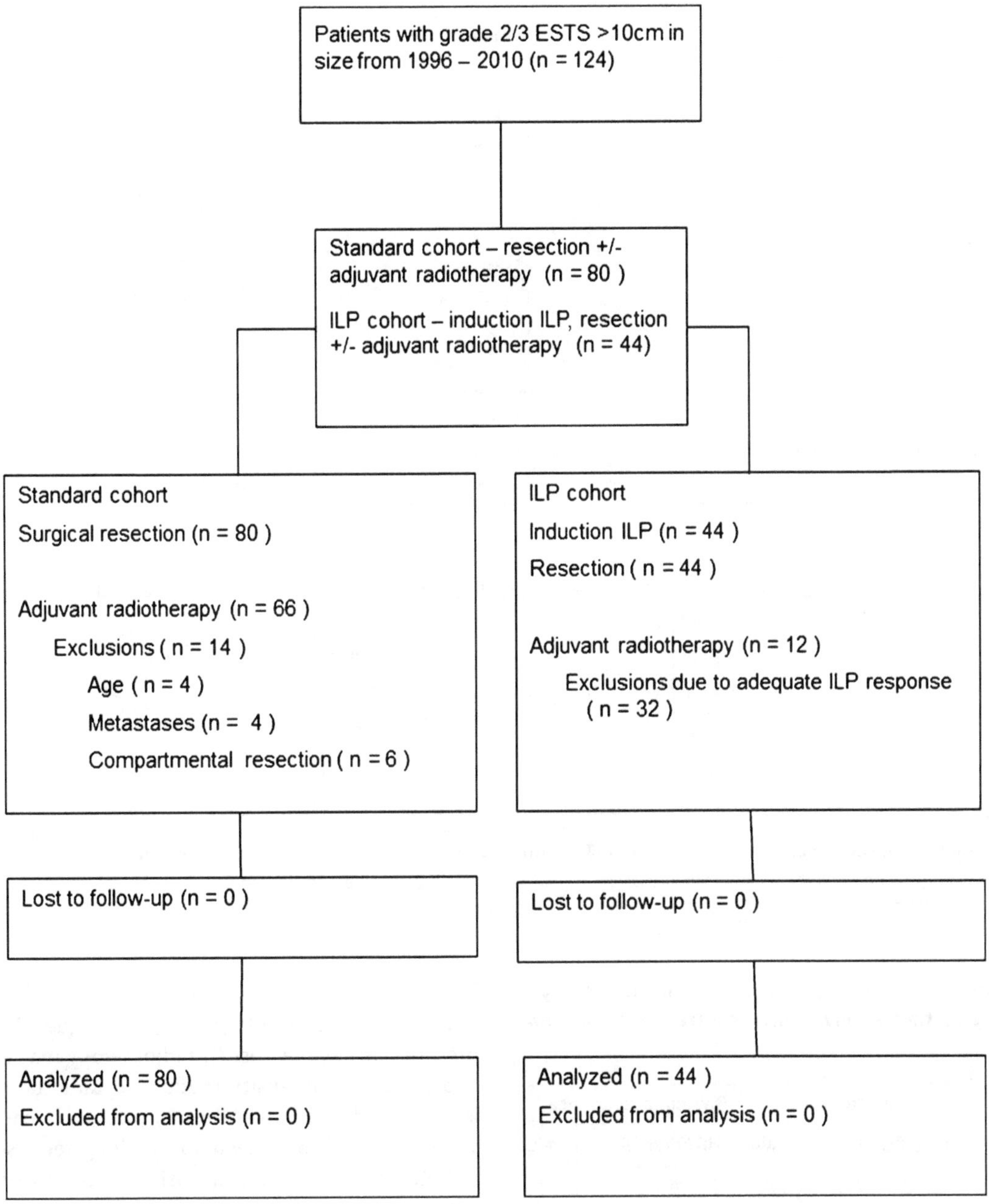

Fig. 2 CONSORT diagram of the Standard and ILP cohorts

sarcomas is more challenging in the distal than the proximal extremity. Therefore, this may represent a bias towards patients with more challenging tumours being referred to specialist centres providing ILP. A further limitation to this study is the inability to comment on the post-operative limb-function in each cohort, an additional important factor that may influence the choice of treatment strategy in these patients.

In the absence of any significant difference in outcomes between these treatment strategies, the morbidity associated with their use becomes increasingly important. Induction ILP carries the risks associated with an additional operation and short term toxicity associated with regional chemotherapy. That being said, the peri-operative morbidity associated with ILP is generally very low. Severe regional toxicity following ILP is rare occurring in 2–15% and the need for amputation even more so with rates of 0–2% [28]. The long-term complications from external beam radiotherapy, the technique used in the majority of patients in this study, are well documented

Table 2 Post-operative outcomes in standard and ILP cohorts

	Standard N=80	ILP N=44	p value
Complications			
All	25 (31%)	17 (39%)	0.43
Wound infection	12 (15%)	7 (16%)	1.0
Collection	13 (16%)	8 (18%)	0.81
Amputation	0 (0%)	2 (5%)	0.12
Resection margin			
R0	65 (81%)	39 (89%)	0.32
R1	15 (19%)	5 (11%)	
Follow-up, months			
Median	31	36	0.3373
(Range)	(4–194)	(8–163)	
Local recurrence	13 (16%)	5 (11%)	0.597
Local recurrence OR post-operative amputation	13 (16%)	7 (16%)	1
Systemic recurrence	43 (54%)	23 (52%)	1

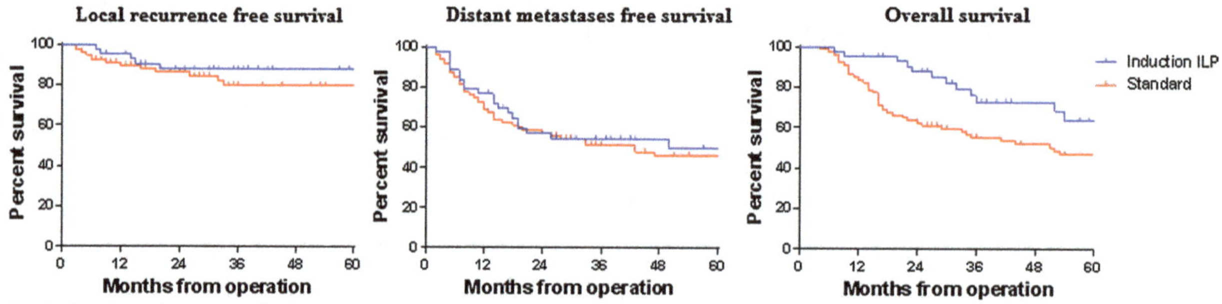

Fig. 3 Oncological outcomes for the ILP and Standard cohorts (logrank test was used to assess comparison)

Table 3 Multivariate cox proportional hazard analysis of factors effecting survival and recurrence of tumours by cohort

	Local recurrence		Systemic recurrence	
	HR (95% CI)	p value	HR (95% CI)	p value
Standard	1.66 (0.64–4.27)	0.295	1.04 (0.63–1.73)	0.867
ILP	1		1	
Increasing Age	1.04 (1.01–1.08)	0.02	1.02 (0.99–1.03)	0.78
			1	
Increasing size	0.951 (0.84–1.08)	0.44	1.04 (0.99–1.09)	0.98
			1	
R1	3.63 (1.36–9.69)	0.01	1.56 (0.85–2.89)	0.153
R0	1		1	
Grade 3	1.74 (0.56–5.35)	0.33	0.91 (0.55–1.51)	0.704
Grade 2	1		1	

[29]. However, during the period of this study, advances have been made in radiotherapy techniques. When given pre-operatively, the dose of radiotherapy may be reduced and the use of intensity-modulated radiotherapy, which is associated with lower toxicity rates, is becoming more widespread [15, 30]. Even so, the long-term sequelae of radiotherapy, including the risk of second malignancies, remain significant and are of particular importance in young patients [31].

Conclusion

Induction ILP followed by a wide resection provides an alternative treatment to standard therapy in the management of locally advanced ESTS. Consideration should be given to induction ILP in young patients with large, high-grade extremity sarcomas who would benefit most from avoiding radiotherapy.

Authors' contributions

Study concept and design: JJ, AJH, JMT, PH, DS. Acquisition, analysis and interpretation of data: HGS, MJW, TP, JJ, PUT, PH, AJH, DCS. Drafting manuscript: HGS, MJW, JJ, AJH. All authors read and approved the final manuscript.

Author details

[1] Department of Surgery, Division of Surgical Oncology, University Hospital Mannheim, University of Heidelberg, Mannheim, Germany. [2] Sarcoma Unit, Department of Academic Surgery, Royal Marsden Hospital NHS Foundation Trust, Fulham Road, London SW3 6JJ, UK. [3] Department of Orthopedic Oncology, Helios Klinikum Berlin-Buch, Sarcoma Center Berlin-Brandenburg, Berlin, Germany. [4] Medical Faculty Mannheim, University of Heidelberg, Mannheim, Germany. [5] Department of Surgery, Division of Surgical Oncology and Thoracic Surgery, University Hospital Mannheim, University of Heidelberg, Mannheim, Germany.

Acknowledgements

JJ was granted a research fellowship by the Royal Marsden NHS foundation trust. The authors acknowledge financial support by Deutsche Forschungsgemeinschaft and Ruprecht-Karls-Universität Heidelberg within the funding programme. No other funding was received for this study.

Competing interests

Peter Hohenberger and Jens Jakob received honoraria from Boehringer Ingelheim.

References

1. Grimer R, Judson I, Peake D, Seddon B. Guidelines for the management of soft tissue sarcomas. Sarcoma. 2010;2010:506182.
2. Rastrelli M, Tropea S, Basso U, Roma A, Maruzzo M, Rossi CR. Soft tissue limb and trunk sarcomas: diagnosis, treatment and follow-up. Anticancer Res. 2014;34(10):5251–62.
3. Casali PG, Blay JY. experts ECECPo: soft tissue sarcomas: ESMO clinical practice guidelines for diagnosis, treatment and follow-up. Ann Oncol. 2010;21(Suppl 5):v198–203.
4. Alamanda VK, Crosby SN, Archer KR, Song Y, Schwartz HS, Holt GE. Amputation for extremity soft tissue sarcoma does not increase overall survival: a retrospective cohort study. Eur J Surg Oncol. 2012;38(12):1178–83.
5. Rosenberg SA, Tepper J, Glatstein E, Costa J, Baker A, Brennan M, DeMoss EV, Seipp C, Sindelar WF, Sugarbaker P, et al. The treatment of soft-tissue sarcomas of the extremities: prospective randomized evaluations of (1) limb-sparing surgery plus radiation therapy compared with amputation and (2) the role of adjuvant chemotherapy. Ann Surg. 1982;196(3):305–15.
6. Williard WC, Hajdu SI, Casper ES, Brennan MF. Comparison of amputation with limb-sparing operations for adult soft tissue sarcoma of the extremity. Ann Surg. 1992;215(3):269–75.
7. Eggermont AM, Schraffordt Koops H, Klausner JM, Kroon BB, Schlag PM, Lienard D, van Geel AN, Hoekstra HJ, Meller I, Nieweg OE, et al. Isolated limb perfusion with tumor necrosis factor and melphalan for limb salvage in 186 patients with locally advanced soft tissue extremity sarcomas. The cumulative multicenter European experience. Ann Surg. 1996;224(6):756–64 **(discussion 764-755)**.
8. Bazzoni F, Beutler B. The tumor necrosis factor ligand and receptor families. N Engl J Med. 1996;334(26):1717–25.
9. Locksley RM, Killeen N, Lenardo MJ. The TNF and TNF receptor superfamilies: integrating mammalian biology. Cell. 2001;104(4):487–501.
10. ten Hagen TL, Eggermont AM. Changing the pathophysiology of solid tumours: the potential of TNF and other vasoactive agents. Int J Hyperthermia. 2006;22(3):241–6.
11. O'Donnell PW, Griffin AM, Eward WC, Sternheim A, Catton CN, Chung PW, O'Sullivan B, Ferguson PC, Wunder JS. The effect of the setting of a positive surgical margin in soft tissue sarcoma. Cancer. 2014;120(18):2866–75.
12. Coindre JM. Grading of soft tissue sarcomas: review and update. Arch Pathol Lab Med. 2006;130(10):1448–53.
13. Edge SB, Compton CC. The American Joint Committee on Cancer: the 7th edition of the AJCC cancer staging manual and the future of TNM. Ann Surg Oncol. 2010;17(6):1471–4.
14. Pitcher ME, Thomas JM. Functional compartmental resection for soft tissue sarcomas. Eur J Surg Oncol. 1994;20(4):441–5.
15. O'Sullivan B, Davis AM, Turcotte R, Bell R, Catton C, Chabot P, Wunder J, Kandel R, Goddard K, Sadura A, et al. Preoperative versus postoperative radiotherapy in soft-tissue sarcoma of the limbs: a randomised trial. Lancet. 2002;359(9325):2235–41.
16. Woll PJ, Reichardt P, Le Cesne A, Bonvalot S, Azzarelli A, Hoekstra HJ, Leahy M, Van Coevorden F, Verweij J, Hogendoorn PC, et al. Adjuvant chemotherapy with doxorubicin, ifosfamide, and lenograstim for resected soft-tissue sarcoma (EORTC 62931): a multicentre randomised controlled trial. Lancet Oncol. 2012;13(10):1045–54.
17. Gronchi A, Ferrari S, Quagliuolo V, Broto JM, Pousa AL, Grignani G, Basso U, Blay JY, Tendero O, Beveridge RD, et al. Histotype-tailored neoadjuvant chemotherapy versus standard chemotherapy in patients with high-risk soft-tissue sarcomas (ISG-STS 1001): an international, open-label, randomised, controlled, phase 3, multicentre trial. Lancet Oncol. 2017;18(6):812–22.
18. Group ESESNW. Soft tissue and visceral sarcomas: ESMO clinical practice guidelines for diagnosis, treatment and follow-up. Ann Oncol. 2014;25(Suppl 3):102–12.
19. Bonvalot S, Laplanche A, Lejeune F, Stoeckle E, Le Pechoux C, Vanel D, Terrier P, Lumbroso J, Ricard M, Antoni G, et al. Limb salvage with isolated perfusion for soft tissue sarcoma: could less TNF-alpha be better? Ann Oncol. 2005;16(7):1061–8.
20. Cherix S, Speiser M, Matter M, Raffoul W, Lienard D, Theumann N, Mouhsine E, Mirimanoff RO, Leyvraz S, Lejeune FJ, et al. Isolated limb perfusion with tumor necrosis factor and melphalan for non-resectable soft tissue sarcomas: long-term results on efficacy and limb salvage in a selected group of patients. J Surg Oncol. 2008;98(3):148–55.
21. Deroose JP, Eggermont AM, van Geel AN, Burger JW, den Bakker MA, de Wilt JH, Verhoef C. Long-term results of tumor necrosis factor alpha- and melphalan-based isolated limb perfusion in locally advanced extremity soft tissue sarcomas. J Clin Oncol. 2011;29(30):4036–44.
22. Gutman M, Inbar M, Lev-Shlush D, Abu-Abid S, Mozes M, Chaitchik S, Meller I, Klausner JM. High dose tumor necrosis factor-alpha and melphalan administered via isolated limb perfusion for advanced limb soft tissue sarcoma results in a > 90% response rate and limb preservation. Cancer. 1997;79(6):1129–37.
23. Pennacchioli E, Deraco M, Mariani L, Fiore M, Mussi C, Collini P, Olmi P, Casali PG, Santinami M, Gronchi A. Advanced extremity soft tissue sarcoma: prognostic effect of isolated limb perfusion in a series of 88 patients treated at a single institution. Ann Surg Oncol. 2007;14(2):553–9.
24. Jakob J, Tunn PU, Hayes AJ, Pilz LR, Nowak K, Hohenberger P. Oncological outcome of primary non-metastatic soft tissue sarcoma treated by neoadjuvant isolated limb perfusion and tumor resection. J Surg Oncol. 2014;109(8):786–90.
25. Yang JC, Chang AE, Baker AR, Sindelar WF, Danforth DN, Topalian SL, DeLaney T, Glatstein E, Steinberg SM, Merino MJ, et al. Randomized prospective study of the benefit of adjuvant radiation therapy in the treatment of soft tissue sarcomas of the extremity. J Clin Oncol. 1998;16(1):197–203.
26. Bonvalot S, Gronchi A. ILP and RT: the study that will never be. Ann Surg Oncol. 2011;18(2):303–5.
27. Deroose JP, Burger JW, van Geel AN, den Bakker MA, de Jong JS, Eggermont AM, Verhoef C. Radiotherapy for soft tissue sarcomas after isolated limb perfusion and surgical resection: essential for local control in all patients? Ann Surg Oncol. 2011;18(2):321–7.
28. Smith HG, Hayes AJ. The role of regional chemotherapy in the management of extremity soft tissue malignancies. Eur J Surg Oncol. 2016;42(1):7–17.
29. Davis AM, O'Sullivan B, Turcotte R, Bell R, Catton C, Chabot P, Wunder J, Hammond A, Benk V, Kandel R, et al. Late radiation morbidity following randomization to preoperative versus postoperative radiotherapy in extremity soft tissue sarcoma. Radiother Oncol. 2005;75(1):48–53.
30. Folkert MR, Singer S, Brennan MF, Kuk D, Qin LX, Kobayashi WK, Crago AM, Alektiar KM. Comparison of local recurrence with conventional and intensity-modulated radiation therapy for primary soft-tissue sarcomas of the extremity. J Clin Oncol. 2014;32(29):3236–41.
31. Hall EJ, Wuu CS. Radiation-induced second cancers: the impact of 3D-CRT and IMRT. Int J Radiat Oncol Biol Phys. 2003;56(1):83–8.

19

Intraosseous papillary intralymphatic angioendothelioma (PILA)

Marco Gambarotti[1], Alberto Righi[1,5*], Marta Sbaraglia[2], Giuseppe Bianchi[3], Piero Picci[1], Daniel Vanel[1] and Angelo Paolo Dei Tos[1,2,4]

Abstract

Background: Papillary intralymphatic angioendothelioma (PILA) is a locally aggressive, rarely metastasizing vascular tumor, generally occurring in the soft tissues, with less than 40 cases described in the literature and only three cases reported in bone.

Case presentation: We describe the case of a 51-year-old male with an intraosseous PILA of the proximal edge of his left clavicle and two other lesions evident on imaging. The patient was treated with marginal resection of the clavicle lesion but was lost to follow-up 1 month after surgery.

Conclusions: PILA can also occur in bone, albeit very rarely, and has to be considered in the differential diagnosis of vascular bone tumors.

Keywords: Papillary intralymphatic angioendothelioma, Dabska tumor, Bone

Background

Papillary intralymphatic angioendothelioma (PILA) is a rare vascular tumor defined in the latest edition of the WHO tumor classification [1] as a "rarely metastasizing lymphatic vascular neoplasm". It was initially considered a malignant tumor due to the fact that two patients had lymph node metastases [2]. The tumor was subsequently renamed PILA in 1998 by Fanburg-Smith et al. [3], considering its borderline behavior and prominent lymphatic phenotype. To the best of our knowledge, less than 40 cases of PILA have been described in the literature [2–17]. The majority of these cases occur in soft tissues, with only three cases reported in bone [2, 13, 15]. Due to its rarity, multifocality and morphological features, the diagnosis of PILA often represents a challenge for the pathologist.

The aim of the present study is to report a new case of PILA occurring in bone, describing the clinical, radiological, and histological features.

*Correspondence: alberto.righi@ior.it
[5] Istituto Ortopedico Rizzoli, Via di Barbiano 1/10, 40136 Bologna, Italy

Case presentation

Only one patient with intraosseous PILA was referred to and treated at our center between 1901 and 2016. This patient was a 51-year-old male with a painful lesion of the proximal edge of his left clavicle, which had been present for 2 months.

Imaging studies (Fig. 1A) revealed a lytic lesion in the medial end of the left clavicle with cortical destruction and soft tissue invasion. The signal was isointense on T1-weighted (Fig. 1B) and heterogeneously hyperintense on fat-saturated T2-weighted MRI (Fig. 1C) and after contrast medium injection (Fig. 1D).

Two other lesions were radiologically evident in the right clavicle and left distal femur.

The patient underwent a needle biopsy. Histologically, a vascular lesion was evident, with hypercellular areas and the neoplastic cells had a focal epithelioid appearance. A final diagnosis of low-grade hemangioendothelioma was made.

Partial resection of the clavicle was performed. Grossly, a gray-reddish lesion was present in the clavicle, with infiltration of the soft tissues (Fig. 2A). The tumor

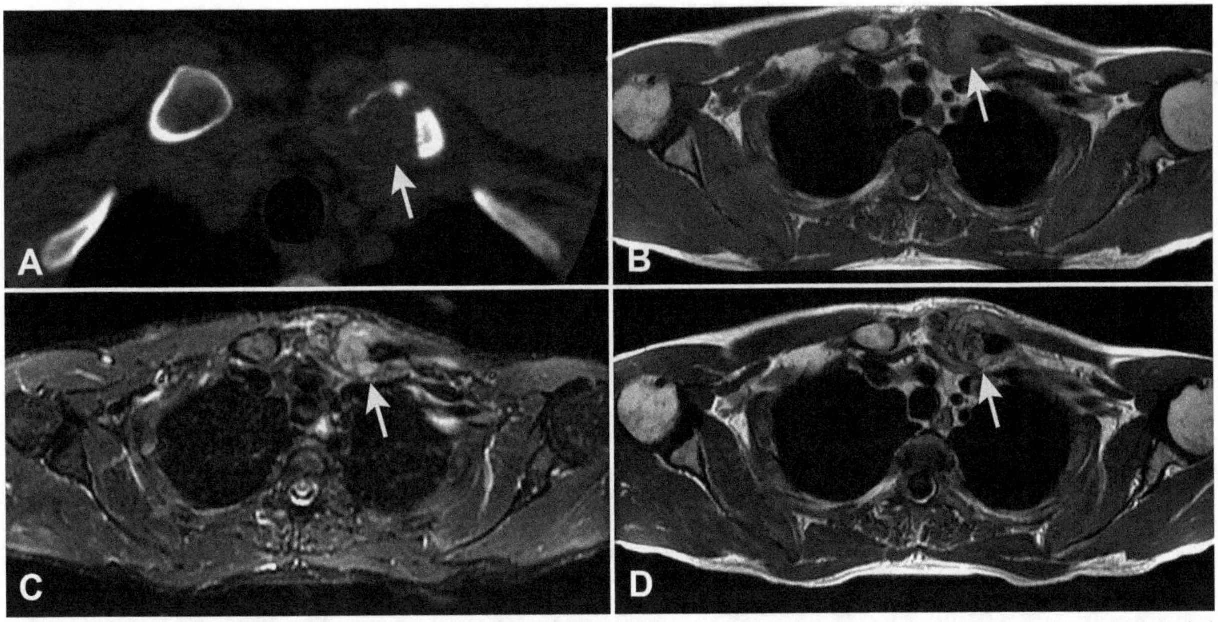

Fig. 1 On CT **A** the lesion (see arrows) involves the medial end of the clavicle and is purely lytic; the cortex is destroyed and soft tissues are invaded. On axial MRI the signal is isointense on T1-weighted (**B**), and heterogeneously hyperintense on fat-saturated T2-weighted (**C**) and after contrast medium injection (**D**)

measured 8 × 4 × 3 cm. Histologically, the tumor was composed of multiple vascular channels, with some areas appearing as glomerulus-like structures (Fig. 2B), with papillary projections into the lumen (Fig. 2C–E). Papillae were covered by plump endothelial cells, some with a hobnail appearance. Immunohistochemically, the neoplastic cells were positive for podoplanin (D2-40), a lymphatic vessel marker (Fig. 2F), and for endothelial markers (CD31 and ERG). Surgical margins were focally marginal.

The patient was lost to follow-up 1 month after surgery.

Discussion and conclusions

PILA is a rarely metastasizing lymphatic vascular neoplasm first described in 1969 by Dabska et al. [4]. To date less than 40 cases have been described in the literature [2–17].

Clinically, this extremely rare tumor more commonly occurs in infants, children and young adults [2, 13, 15], although it can also occur in the elderly [15] without sex predilection [15]. It is generally localized in the dermis and subcutaneous tissue of the extremities [3] and less commonly in the trunk, head and neck [2, 13]. Few cases have been reported in deeper locations, including the spleen [16], tongue [14], and testis [11, 17].

Only three cases have been reported in bone [2, 13, 15], as summarized in Table 1. The case reported by Li et al. [15] was characterized by multiple bone lesions in the facial bones. Our case was also characterized by multifocality on MR imaging. In the case described by McCarthy et al. [2], radiographs revealed periosteal reaction on the medial aspect of the distal femoral metaphysis and faint intraosseous radiolucency in the epiphysis. Almost identical features were described by Nakayama et al. [13]. In the case described by Bin et al. [15], CT-scan showed multifocal osteolytic lesions with soft tissue mass. On MRI the lesion showed low intensity on T1-weighted images and high intensity on T2-weighted images [2, 13].

The pain and radiological features of the tumor are consistent with a well-circumscribed radiolucent lesion, generally with sclerotic margins on CT-scan, and are suggestive of osteoid osteoma [2, 13]. Langerhans cell histiocytosis also has to be considered in the differential diagnosis [15].

Histologically, PILA is composed of a proliferation of spindle- to polygonal-shaped, slightly atypical cells forming numerous interconnecting capillary and cavernous vascular cavities [2, 13, 15], with papillary projections into the lumen. The papillae consist of a fibrovascular core covered by slightly atypical plump cuboidal endothelial cells, with a hobnail or "match-head" appearance [2, 13, 15]. Solid areas and glomerulus-like structures may be present [15]. Mitoses are rare and necrosis is absent [15]. Immunohistochemically, the expression of podoplanin (D2-40) is consistent with its lymphatic phenotype [1].

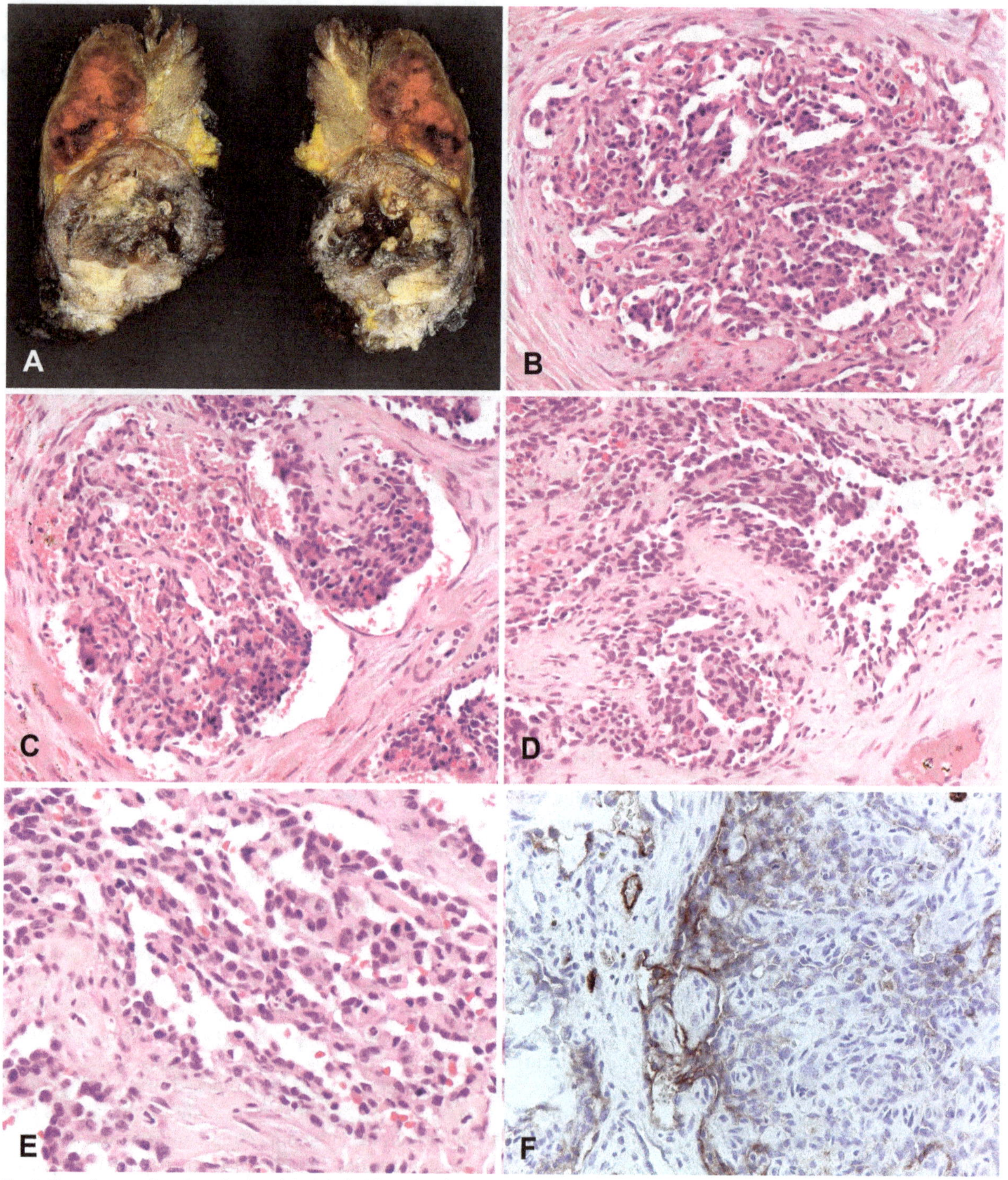

Fig. 2 Gross features **A** an 8 cm. Lesion of the left clavicle, with soft tissue invasion. Histological features of the lesion, composed of glomerulus-like structures (**B**), with papillary structures projecting into the lumen, covered by plump "hobnail" endothelial cells (**C–E**). Immunohistochemical positivity for podoplanin (D2-40) in the neoplastic cells (**F**)

Two vascular lesions, retiform hemangioendothelioma and papillary endothelial hyperplasia (Masson's hemangioma), may be confused with PILA due to the presence of "hobnail" cells and papillary projections [2, 15]. However, the former is a locally aggressive, rarely metastasizing vascular tumor characterized by distinctive branching of

Table 1 Clinicopathological features of papillary intralymphatic angioendotheliomas reported in literature

No	Age	Sex	Site	Treatment	Follow-up (months)	References
1	45	F	Distal femur (epiphysis)	Complete curettage	NED 12	[2]
2	39	F	Distal femur (metaphysis)	Curettage and wide re-excision	NED 500	[13]
3	1	M	Facial bones (multiple lesions)	Complete curettage	NED 24	[15]
4	51	M	Left clavicle (multiple lesions)	Marginal resection	Lost to follow-up	Current case

arborizing blood vessels, imparting a pattern reminiscent of rete testis [2, 15]. The latter is a reactive endothelial proliferation with vascular thrombosis, characterized by papillary projections with hyaline or fibrin cores associated with thrombotic material, and often free-floating in the vascular lumens [2, 15].

"Hobnail" cells and papillary projections associated with podoplanin immunohistochemical expression are also helpful in distinguishing PILA from epithelioid hemangioma and lymphangioma-like Kaposi sarcoma [15].

PILA can be locally invasive with the potential to metastasize. Lymph node metastases have been reported [7] and a case of angiosarcoma arising within a PILA has been described [9]. In 2000 Dabska performed a 30-year review of the six patients originally reported in 1969: one patient died of widespread pulmonary metastases [18]. Accordingly, long-term follow-up should be performed in soft tissue PILA, although more recent series demonstrate no local recurrences or metastases [3] and an excellent prognosis with complete excision [2].

Due to the low numbers of intraosseous PILA reported in the literature, the difference between intraosseous and soft tissue PILA in tumor prognosis is unknown; similarly, no consensus has been reached as to the proper treatment of intraosseous PILA [13], although complete curettage seems sufficient to avoid recurrences [2].

In conclusion, we describe a new case of PILA of bone, with multifocal presentation on imaging. This very rare vascular tumor generally occurs in soft tissues, but can also be present in bone, thus extending the spectrum of vascular bone tumors.

Authors' contributions

All authors were involved in clinical data acquisition. AR and MG drafted the manuscript. DV and PP conceived the study. GB, MS and APDT revised the article critically for important intellectual content. All authors read and approved the final manuscript.

Author details

[1] Department of Pathology, Rizzoli Institute, Bologna, Italy. [2] Department of Pathology, Treviso Regional Hospital, Treviso, Italy. [3] Orthopaedic Oncology Department, Rizzoli Institute, Bologna, Italy. [4] University of Padua School of Medicine, Padua, Italy. [5] Istituto Ortopedico Rizzoli, Via di Barbiano 1/10, 40136 Bologna, Italy.

Acknowledgements

None.

Competing interests

Prof. Angelo Paolo Dei Tos is Editor-in-Chief of Clinical Sarcoma Research.

Funding

None.

References

1. Fanburg-Smith JC. Papillary intralymphatic angioendothelioma. In: Fletcher CDM, Bridge JA, Hogendoorn PCW, Mertens F, editors. World Health Organization classification of tumors of soft tissue and bone. Lyon: IARC Press; 2013. p. 148–9.
2. McCarthy EF, Lietman S, Argani P, Frassica FJ. Endovascular papillary angioendothelioma (Dabska tumor) of bone. Skeletal Radiol. 1999;28:100–3.
3. Fanburg-Smith JC, Michal M, Partanen TA, Alitalo K, Miettinen M. Papillary intralymphatic angioendothelioma (PILA): a report of twelve cases of a distinctive vascular tumor with phenotypic features of lymphatic vessels. Am J Surg Pathol. 1999;23:1004–10.
4. Dabska M. Malignant endovascular papillary angioendothelioma of the skin in childhood. Clinicopathologic study of 6 cases. Cancer. 1969;24:503–10.
5. Bernić A, Novosel I, Krizanac S. An unusual mole: an adult case of Dabska tumor. Coll Antropol. 2012;36:171–2.
6. Rumana M, Khursheed N, Ramzan A. Congenital occipital encephalocele with Dabska tumor: report of an unusual case. Pediatr Neurosurg. 2012;48:48–50.
7. de Saint-Maur PP, Audouin J, Cazier A, Le Tourneau A, Molina T, Diebold J. Nodal intralymphatic papillary endothelial tumor with Dabska-like features: report of a case in two mesenteric lymph nodes. Histopathology. 2011;59:1027–9.
8. Neves RI, Stevenson J, Hancey MJ, Vangelisti G, Miraliakbari R, Mackay D, Clarke L. Endovascular papillary angioendothelioma (Dabska tumor): underrecognized malignant tumor in childhood. J Pediatr Surg. 2011;46:e25–8.
9. Antosz Z, Zaniewski M, Kostecki J, Poreba R. Angiosarcoma arising within a malignant endovascular papillary angioendothelioma (Dabska tumor). Neuro Endocrinol Lett. 2010;31:454–6.
10. Ward KA, Ecker PM, White RR, Melnik TE, Gulbahce EH, Wilke MS, Sangueza OP. Papillary intralymphatic angioendothelioma of the thigh: a case report and review of the literature. Dermatol Online J. 2010;16:4.
11. Bhatia A, Nada R, Kumar Y, Menon P. Dabska tumor (endovascular papillary angioendothelioma) of testis: a case report with brief review of literature. Diagn Pathol. 2006;1:12.
12. Ide F. Oral endovascular papillary angioendothelioma (Dabska tumor). J Oral Pathol Med. 2004;33:249.
13. Nakayama T, Nishino M, Takasu K, Hayakawa K, Toguchida J, Tanaka C. Endovascular papillary angioendothelioma (Dabska tumor) of bone. Orthopedics. 2004;27:327–8.
14. Takaoka K, Sakurai K, Noguchi K, Hashitani S, Urade M. Endovascular papillary angioendothelioma (Dabska tumor) of the tongue: report of a case. J Oral Pathol Med. 2003;32:492–5.
15. Li B, Li Y, Tian XY, Li Z. Unusual multifocal intraosseous papillary intralymphatic angioendothelioma (Dabska tumor) of facial bones: a case report and review of literature. Diagn Pathol. 2013;8:160.
16. Katz JA, Mahoney DH, Shukla LW, Smith CW, Gresik MV, Hawkins HK. Endovascular papillary angioendothelioma in the spleen. Pediatr Pathol. 1988;8:185–93.
17. Schultheis AM, Sandmann M, Steurer S. Strong ERG positivity in papillary intralymphatic angioendothelioma of the testis of a 24-year-old male: a case report. Case Rep Pathol. 2013;2013:531479.

20

The use of whole exome sequencing and murine patient derived xenografts as a method of chemosensitivity testing in sarcoma

Nicholas Calvert[1*], Jiansha Wu[3], Sophie Sneddon[3], Jennifer Woodhouse[4], Richard Carey-Smith[1], David Wood[1] and Evan Ingley[2,3]

Abstract

Background: Soft tissue and bone sarcoma represent a broad spectrum of different pathology and genetic variance. Current chemotherapy regimens are derived from randomised trials and represent empirical treatment. Chemosensitivity testing and whole exome sequencing (WES) may offer personalized chemotherapy treatment based on genetic mutations.

Methods: A pilot, prospective, non-randomised control experimental study was conducted. Twelve patients with metastatic bone or soft tissue sarcoma that had failed first line chemotherapy treatment were enrolled for this study. Human tissue taken at surgical biopsy under general anaesthetic was divided between two arms of the trial. Subsections of the tumour were used for WES and the remainder was implanted subcutaneously in immunodeficient mice (PDX). Results of WES were analysed using a bioinformatics pipeline to identify mutations conferring susceptibility to kinase inhibitors and common chemotherapeutic agents. PDX models exhibiting successful growth underwent WES of the tumour and subsequent chemosensitivity testing.

Results: WES was successful in all 12 patients, with successful establishment PDX tumours models in seven patients. WES identified potential actionable therapeutics in all patients. Significant variation in predicted therapeutics was demonstrated between three PDX samples and their matched tumour samples.

Conclusion: Analysis of WES of fresh tumour specimens via a bioinformatics pipeline may identify potential actionable chemotherapy agents. Further research into this field may lead to the development of personalized cancer therapy for sarcoma.

Keywords: Sarcoma, Chemosensitivity, Whole exome sequencing

Background

The mainstay of systemic cancer therapies has been empirically derived cytotoxic combination protocols based on histological appearance, organ of origin, and tumour staging. This approach has proven effective in lymphomas and other germ cell tumours, but their efficacy has been less in bone and soft-tissue sarcoma due to their heterogeneity [1]. For patients with chemotherapy resistant sarcoma, the significant toxicity of these agents result in morbidity and mortality without therapeutic benefit. This has led to an interest in developing ex vivo chemosensitivity testing to predict drug response prior to patient administration.

Recent advances have been made in the utilization of genomic data to facilitate development of targeted therapeutic agents. An example of this is the identification of key genes and signaling pathways in gastrointestinal stromal tumours (GIST). Identification of oncogene mutations in *KIT*, *PDGRFα* and *BRAF* have led to the development of selective kinase inhibitors to target them [2–4].

The whole human genome contains approximately 3×10^9 base pairs, containing coding (exons) and

*Correspondence: Nicholas.calvert@health.wa.gov.au

[1] Department of Orthopaedic Surgery, Sir Charles Gairdner Hospital, Nedlands, WA 6009, Australia

non-coding (introns) regions [5]. Less than ~ 10% of the genome is characterized and the clinical implications of mutations throughout the genome are poorly understood [6]. It is estimated that 85% of disease-causing mutations are found in the coding region of the genome, the exome [7, 8]. As such, limiting the analysis to exome sequencing rather than whole genome sequencing provides the most cost-effective method and the greatest possibility of identifying clinically relevant mutations.

The implantation of patient derived tumours into immunodeficient mice is a recently developed technique to provide a more representative microenvironment for measuring tumour response to chemotherapy agents. Reliable mouse models that recapitulate the biological profiles of sarcomas have been developed as a research tool in sarcomas [9] and indeed one such model led to the description of a possible cell of origin of synovial sarcoma [10]. These xenografts provide a more complete model of the biological behaviour and metastatic potential of tumours than cell line studies [11, 12].

Tyrosine kinases play an important role in the modulation of cell signalling pathways. Their role in oncogenesis of several forms of cancer was recently discovered and arises from genetic mutation that causes dysregulation of these pathways to stimulate a variety of biologic pathways, including angiogenesis and cell growth. Tyrosine kinase inhibitors competitively inhibit ATP binding or impede activation/activity of these kinases, thus leading to pathway deactivation [13].

The use of these drugs in sarcoma has been limited in comparison to other malignancies. In a recent review [14], it was shown that the response rate of soft tissue sarcomas to a variety of kinase inhibitors in phase 2 and phase 3 trials remained well below 10%. However, it should be noted that these trials tended to group together different tumour types. As previously mentioned, sarcoma has a high tendency for heterogeneity between types and subtypes, hence these broad studies may not provide a representative view on the efficacy of this drug class. By identifying gene mutations targetable by tyrosine kinase inhibitors in individual sarcoma samples it may be possible to tailor therapies and improve response rates.

Herein, we describe a comparison of whole exome analysis of germline, tumour, and murine patient derived xenografts (PDX), with implementation of a bioinformatics pipeline for chemosensitivity prediction in 12 patients with bone and soft tissue sarcoma.

Methods

A prospective case series study was conducted from March 2016 to March 2017. Institutional approval to conduct the trial was obtained from the Human Ethics Committee. Twelve adult patients with bone or soft tissue sarcoma who had failed to respond to standard chemotherapy, or newly diagnosed local recurrence of bone or soft tissue sarcoma following chemotherapy, were enrolled in the trial. Under-age patients, or those with a cognitive impairment preventing them from providing informed consent were excluded from the trial. Informed consent was obtained by an investigator.

Following informed consent, samples of the tumour were taken at the time of surgical biopsy under general or local anaesthesia.

Generation of patient-derived xenografts (PDX)

Subsections of the tumour sample were divided between whole exome sequencing (WES) and implantation subcutaneously in immunodeficient mice. Patient blood samples were sent for WES for germline exome identification. DNA was extracted from tumour and blood using a Blood and Cell Culture DNA mini kit according the manufacturer's instructions (Qiagen, Hilden, Germany). DNA was quantitated using a NanoDrop (ThermoFisher Scientific, Waltham, MA) and integrity checked by agarose electrophoresis and ethidium bromide staining. Tumour tissue was sliced into approximately 2 mm^3 fragments, mixed with extracellular matrix (Matrigel, at 1 mg/mL) (Corning, Tewksbury, MA) and implanted subcutaneously via an 18G needle on the right flank of 6–10 week-old female NSG (NOD.Cg-$Prkdc^{scid}$ $IL2R\gamma^{tm1Wjl}$/SzJ) mice (Jackson Laboratory, Bar Harbor, ME). PDX models with successful establishment of tumours were subsequently biopsied with sections of the tumour sent for WES. All PDX tumour biopsies performed for exome sequencing were performed from zero passage mice to minimise the amount of model acquired mutations, which have been demonstrated to increase with each passage [15].

Exome sequencing and data processing

Samples for WES were prepared using an Agilent SureSelect Target Enrichment Kit and libraries were sequenced via 100 bp PE using an Illumina HiSeq 4000 sequencer (Macrogen, Seoul, Republic of Korea). With 100× read depth for germline DNA, and 200× read depth for primary tumour and PDX DNA.

Application of the IMPACT pipeline

Sequence data were then analysed using a modified version of the Integrating Molecular Profiles with Actionable Therapeutics (IMPACT) pipeline developed at the University of Colorado [16]. All analysis parameters were as per those outlined by Hintzsche et al. [16].

Further functional analysis of the gene mutations identified as a potential kinase inhibitor target was performed to investigate whether targeting these kinases had known effects on tumour biology. Known molecular pathways were explored using WebGestalt [17] and identification of the site of these mutations on the kinase proteins were explored using the UniProt Knowledge Database [18].

The actionable therapeutics identified for each PDX sample was compared with it's matched list of tumour derived actionable therapeutics using Fisher's exact test of independence for assessment of statistical significance.

Results

Establishment of tumours in PDX models was successful in seven patients. Patient demographics are outlined in Table 1. Figure 1 lists identified single nucleotides variants that were predicted to be deleterious by six algorithms (SIFT, Polyphen2, MutationTaster, FATHMM, CADD, GERP) [19–24] or by two algorithms if the variant is listed in COSMIC [25].

Sequencing metrics

Sequencing metrics are outlined in Table 2. Whole exome sequencing was performed to a median depth of 142. A median of 122,945,876 reads were generated for each sample. A median of 475 somatic mutations per sample were identified for the tumour samples, with a median of 34,442 for the PDX.

Direct tumour analysis

Potential kinase inhibitor targets were identified in six of the twelve samples. These samples were of osteosarcoma, Ewing's sarcoma, undifferentiated pleomorphic sarcoma, alveolar rhabdomyosarcoma, and leiomyosarcoma. The results of this analysis are outlined in Table 3.

Analysis using the bioinformatics pipeline successfully identified potential actionable therapeutics in all the twelve samples. An example of the generated list of potential actionable therapeutics is outlined in Table 4. The results for all patients are listed in Additional file 1.

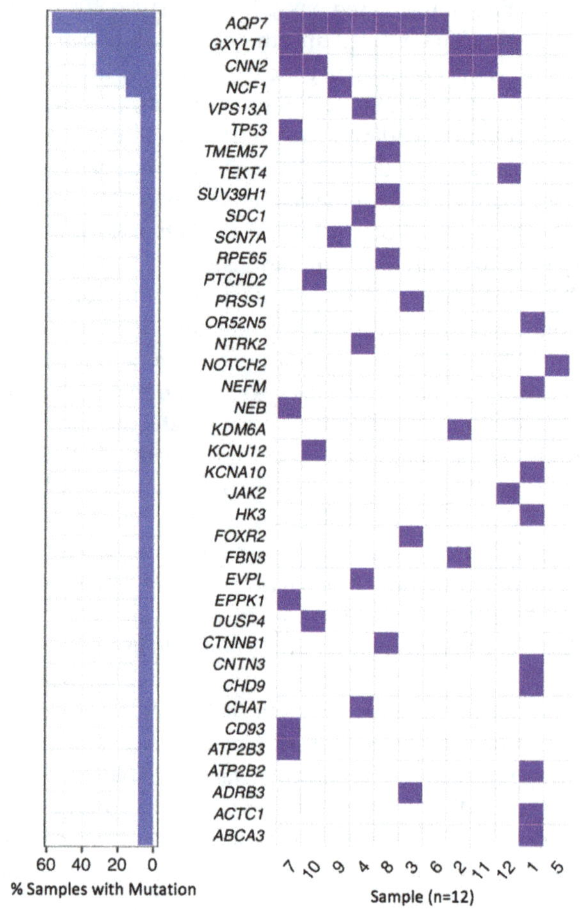

Fig. 1 Waterfall plot of single nucleotide variants predicted to be deleterious or likely deleterious

One sample of osteosarcoma demonstrated a mutation of the KIT gene. This gene is a proto-oncogene responsible for the encoding of c-kit, and plays a role in cell survival and proliferation. The mutation identified (E142Q) lies in the extracellular domain and may alter the structure of the receptor. The same mutation of the ALK gene (C928fs) was demonstrated in a sample of Ewing's sarcoma and leiomyosarcoma. The exact action of this ALK mutation on oncogenesis is still unclear, however it has been implicated in numerous malignancies including non-small cell lung cancer [26]. The identified frameshift mutation is located extracellularly before the kinase domain, and may result in a decoy receptor being produced. A mutation of ABL2 was demonstrated in a patient with undifferentiated pleomorphic sarcoma. This gene has been implicated in numerous solid organ tumours [27] and plays a role in cell growth and survival. The identified frameshift (I471fs) lies within the protein

Table 1 Patient demographics

Patients (n)	12
Male	6
Female	6
Median age (range)	49 (23–68)
Type of sarcoma (n)	
Osteosarcoma	2
Undifferentiated pleomorphic sarcoma	2
Leiomyosarcoma	2
Synovial sarcoma	1
Ewing's sarcoma	1
Alveolar rhabdomyosarcoma	1
Chordoma	1
Metastatic angiosarcoma	1
Dedifferentiated liposarcoma	1

Table 2 Sequencing metrics

Diagnosis	Depth	Reads (M)	% on-target reads	Somatic mutations	Synonymous	Non-synonymous	INDEL	Frame-shift	Stop gain/loss
Osteosarcoma									
Germline	88.1	75	89.1						
Tumour	153.2	134	81.5	479	144	290	12	24	9
PDX	282.7	141	53.9	96,393	79,080	15,354	440	1334	139
Dedifferentiated liposarcoma									
Germline	74.7	71	89.8						
Tumour	148.5	123	79.4	458	154	250	14	28	12
Leiomyosarcoma									
Germline	94.9	778	79.0						
Tumour	145.7	116	81.1	384	118	218	15	26	7
Osteosarcoma									
Germline	72.1	613	74.7						
Tumour	175.2	148	79.0	575	179	331	18	30	17
PDX	142.1	123	80.2	288,522	232,825	48,320	1496	5307	477
Synovial sarcoma									
Germline	71.5	784	58.3						
Tumour	159.6	134	79.5	471	169	245	13	32	12
Ewing's sarcoma									
Germline	65.8	730	58.4						
Tumour	122.7	128	61.0	529	191	262	21	45	10
PDX	141.7	125	75.5	7089	3399	3416	115	105	53
Undifferentiated pleomorphic sarcoma									
Germline	77.1	677	75.4						
Tumour	139.6	132	72.5	522	202	271	15	26	7
PDX	168	137	79.4	118,641	97,602	18,574	568	1651	207
Alveolar rhabdo-myosarcoma									
Germline	83.1	727	86.6						
Tumour	152.6	132	86.3	591	187	325	25	39	12
PDX	187.3	159	76.7	24,851	12,266	10,617	121	331	117
Leiomyosarcoma									
Germline	98.8	880	76.7						
Tumour	166	147	80.2	368	112	220	5	20	11
PDX	159.8	134	77.9	34,442	28,019	5701	183	470	67
Chordoma									
Germline	70.7	617	77.5						
Tumour	145.8	141	78.9	440	147	247	7	31	8
Metastatic angiosarcoma									
Germline	72	632	76.1						
Tumour	202.2	176	78.2	489	177	249	17	36	10
PDX	147	121	77.7	10,376	7892	2238	42	148	52
Undifferentiated pleomorphic sarcoma									
Germline	78.6	692	82.4						
Tumour	146	119	82.6	405	147	210	16	25	7

kinase domain, and may alter receptor function. A second patient with the same tumour demonstrated a JAK2 mutation, a kinase with important roles in cell growth and development. The observed mutation (S593F) was present in the second protein kinase domain, which is thought to be responsible for catalytic activity. Finally, a mutation of NTRK1 was identified in a sample of alveolar rhabdomyosarcoma. Gene fusions with this gene are

Table 3 Predicted kinase inhibitors

Patient	Diagnosis	Database	Gene	Variant	Therapeutic
Pt1	Osteosarcoma	NCI match clinical trials	KIT	E142Q	Sunitinib
		DSigDB FDA approved kinase inhibitors	KIT	E142Q	Imatinib, Sorafenib, Dasatanib, Sunitinib, Nilotinib, Pazopanib, Axitinib, Cabozantinib
Pt6	Ewing's sarcoma	DSigDB FDA approved kinase inhibitors	ALK	C928fs	Crizotinib, Ceritinib
Pt7	Undifferentiated pleomorphic sarcoma	DSigDB FDA approved kinase inhibitors	ABL2	I471fs	Dasatinib
Pt8	Alveolar rhabdomyosarcoma	DSigDB FDA approved kinase inhibitors	NTRK1	G18E	Imatinib
Pt9	Leiomyosarcoma	DSigDB FDA approved kinase inhibitors	ALK	C928fs, F921L	Crizotinib, Ceritinib
Pt12	Undifferentiated pleomorphic sarcoma	DSigDB FDA approved kinase inhibitors	JAK2	S593F	Ruxolitinib

Table 4 Predicted actionable therapeutics for patient 1

Drug	Targets hit	Potential targets	*P* value (hypergeometric test)
Letrozole	1	5	< 0.001
Fludarabine	1	6	0.001
Sunitinib	1	9	0.001
Gemcitabine	1	11	0.002
Imatinib	1	10	0.002
Clofarabine	1	12	0.002
Regorafenib	1	18	0.005
Cytarabine	1	18	0.005
Doxorubicin	1	104	0.133
Cisplatin	–	–	–
Methotrexate	–	–	–
Ifosfamide	–	–	–

Diagnosis was of osteosarcoma. Therapeutics that the patient had received are highlighted in italics

potentially oncogenic via up regulation of the TRKA protein. The mutation demonstrated (G18E) lies outside of the functional domains and as such selective inhibition would be not appear to be beneficial.

In four patients, actionable therapeutics were identified that are already in use as treatment for the corresponding sarcoma: Methotrexate was identified for an osteosarcoma patient as well as a synovial sarcoma patient; Doxorubicin was identified for an Ewing's sarcoma patient and Vincristine was identified for an alveolar rhabdomysarcoma patient.

PDX actionable therapeutics comparison

Establishment of PDX tumour lineages was successful for seven patients. Failure of tumour establishment was defined as lack of observable tumour growth within 24 weeks.

All seven PDX tumours underwent WES from which potential actionable therapeutics were identified. Samples from three patients were assessed to be statistically significant different in terms of actionable therapeutics identified in direct tumour and PDX analysis (Table 5). The primary tumours for these three samples were osteosarcoma, undifferentiated pleomorphic sarcoma, and leiomyosarcoma.

Discussion

This study outlines a method for the use of WES in combination with the IMPACT bioinformatics pipeline to generate a list of potentially actionable chemotherapeutics in bone and soft tissue sarcoma.

Analysis of the WES data with the bioinformatics pipeline found tyrosine kinase inhibitor targets for half of the patients. Kinase targets found in the analysis were for osteosarcoma (*KIT*), Ewing's sarcoma (*ALK*), undifferentiated pleomorphic sarcoma (*JAK2, ABL2*), alveolar rhabdomyosarcoma (*NTRK1*), and leiomyosarcoma (*ALK*). Of these targets, two have been described previously in the literature for their respective malignancy. Two separate studies [28, 29] have described the presence of *ALK* mutations in Ewing's sarcoma and have hypothesized that this mutation may be targetable with Crizotinib. Over expression of the KIT gene and resultant increased levels, has previously been identified as a potential therapeutic target in paediatric osteosarcoma [30].

As this is a non-validated method this trial did not aim to alter patient drug treatment. Indeed, due to advance stage of disease in which the biopsies were performed, the majority of patients were deceased at the time of results becoming available. Of note, one patient with osteosarcoma elected to undergo treatment with the predicted tyrosine kinase inhibitor whilst in the terminal

Table 5 Comparison of potential actionable therapeutics between direct tumour analysis and PDX analysis

Diagnosis	PDX-therapeutics identified (n)	Novel in comparison to tumour (n)	Tumour-therapeutics identified (n)	P-value
Osteosarcoma	6	6	9	1.000
Osteosarcoma	24	22	11	*0.019*
Ewing's sarcoma	16	15	13	0.161
Undifferentiated pleomorphic sarcoma	19	11	29	*< 0.001*
Alveolar rhabdomyosarcoma	6	5	3	0.219
Leiomyosarcoma	9	4	6	*0.025*
Metastatic angiosarcoma	11	11	10	1.000

Each of the seven PDX samples are listed with their primary diagnosis. P-values were calculated using Fisher's exact test of independence

Italic values indicate significance of P-value ($p < 0.05$)

stages of their disease. A temporary clinical response was demonstrated with a reduction in size of his recurrent tumour. Whist this is far from conclusive, such a result provides some promise that guided treatment may be feasible.

A list of potentially actionable therapeutics was generated for all twelve fresh tumour specimens. Four patients had received chemotherapy agents that were predicted to be actionable, and in none of these were more than one of their current agents predicted to be actionable. The interpretation of this result is difficult, as enrolled patients had already undergone chemotherapy treatment. Darwinian selection pressure in response to chemotherapy exposure may have resulted in the tumours already developing resistance to previous chemotherapy agents. Identifying whether these predicted agents truly are effective is difficult. As this method of drug prediction is not validated we were unable to utilise these results in chemotherapeutic selection. Due to the heterogeneity of sarcoma the data on non-traditional chemotherapy regimes is scarce. Therefore, a larger trial is required with biopsy performed prior to commencement of chemotherapy, and subsequent tracking of chemotherapy response. This would clarify whether there is correlation between predicted drugs and clinical course.

Of the genes predicted to be deleterious four were present in more than one sample. A mutation of AQP7 was present seven samples. This gene encodes for Aquaporin 7, and there is some early evidence that it may play a role in tumour cell function [31]. Four demonstrated mutations in GXYLT1 and four had mutations in CNN2. GXYLT1 is involved in the Notch protein pathway, it's potential role in these malignancies is unclear. CNN2 is known to play a role in smooth muscle contraction and cell adhesion. A sample of alveolar rhabdomyosarcoma and a sample of undifferentiated pleomorphic sarcoma both demonstrated a mutation in NCF1, mutation of which can be associated with chronic granulomatous disease.

Results of pipeline analysis of PDX samples to identify tyrosine kinase inhibitors indicated varied results in comparison to fresh tumour samples. Of the seven PDX models, five had targetable mutations identified in fresh tumour samples with only three of these remaining present in the PDX analysis. Analysis of all seven PDX samples demonstrated the presence of novel targetable gene mutations in comparison to fresh tumour. The most marked of this was the osteosarcoma sample from patient 4, which demonstrated no actionable kinase inhibitor targets in the tumour WES and 35 novel actionable kinase targets with 227 novel variants in the PDX WES.

Actionable chemotherapeutics were successfully predicted in all seven PDX samples. Pipeline analysis identified novel chemotherapeutics in all samples in comparison to fresh tumour results. Samples from three patients were found to be significantly different statistically in terms of actionable therapeutics identified in direct tumour and PDX analysis. These three samples were for osteosarcoma, undifferentiated pleomorphic sarcoma, and leiomyosarcoma.

Of the twelve patients enrolled in this trial two had osteosarcoma, two had leiomyosarcoma, and two had undifferentiated pleomorphic sarcoma. The two osteosarcomas demonstrated different mutation, kinase inhibitor, and actionable therapeutic profiles. The leiomyosarcoma samples had different drug profiles but both demonstrated a mutation in AQP7. Likewise, the undifferentiated pleomorphic sarcomas had different drug profiles but a mutation of the gene GXYLT1 was present in both.

The results obtained in this study raise several interesting questions. Despite poor earlier evidence for the use of tyrosine kinase inhibitors in sarcoma, the results of the pipeline analysis may suggest that they could play a role if selected individually for patients. It is possible that the genetic mutations that confer a susceptibility to these agents occurs sporadically throughout the sarcoma subtypes. Therefore, careful selection may provide a response in a subset of patients. Secondly, it is interesting to note that very few of the patient's received chemotherapeutics that were predicted to be actionable by pipeline analysis. An intriguing finding is that pipeline analysis of a chordoma sample indicated the presence of 17 potential actionable therapeutics. Except in rare cases of aggressive chordoma, this sarcoma has traditionally been regarded as having a poor response to chemotherapy [32].

Several limitations are inherent in the design of this study. As this is a pilot investigation, the small number and heterogeneity of the population studied prevents any definitive conclusions to be made. As such, this study is intended to generate hypotheses for further studies and establish a protocol for a larger trial. In comparison to Stebbing et al. [9] a lower rate of successful graft incorporation in the PDX models was seen, 58% in comparison to 75%. The reason for this is unclear, as the patient population and technique were similar, and may relate to the smaller sample size in this trial. Although a list of potentially actionable therapeutics was generated for each patient, due to the small sample size it is not possible to meaningfully compare the predicted therapeutics to the observed clinical response of the tumour to the received chemotherapeutics. A larger patient population would be required to establish any significant correlation between the results. Lastly, the heterogeneity of the patient tumour type acts as a limitation in this study, a limitation that can be noticed in a significant proportion of the sarcoma literature. However, it could be argued that due to the rarity and vast heterogeneity of these tumours amongst type and subtype, which is becoming increasingly apparent with genetic analysis, it may not be possible to apply the traditional study design to this malignancy successfully. Therefore, the use of "n of 1" trial designs and similar methods may have a significant role to play.

It should be noted that this is a pilot study and further research into this area is required. This is especially important when considering cost and infrastructure required for large scale multi-centre trials. Continued research into the use of WES and drug prediction using bioinformatics pipelines, such as IMPACT, for sarcoma are strongly encouraged. Larger numbers are required to permit meaningful correlation of predicted drug responses and observed clinical response. As this technique is not clinically validated, such a trial would provide support for the development of a multi-centre prospective trial in which chemotherapy selection is guided by chemosensitivity pipeline results.

Conclusion

This study provides support for the development of a large-scale trial utilising WES and the IMPACT bioinformatics pipeline to determine potential actionable chemotherapy agents and tyrosine kinase inhibitors. With further advances it is possible that drug prediction via WES may provide clinicians with the ability to deliver personalized therapy to patients with sarcoma and other malignancies.

Authors' contributions

NC was involved in conceptualisation, data curation, investigation, formal analysis, methodology, software, writing. DW was involved in conceptualisation, funding acquisition, investigation, supervision, methodology. RC-S was involved in conceptualisation, funding acquisition, investigation, supervision, methodology. EI and JW were involved in conceptualisation, investigation, methodology. JW was involved in patient recruitment data curation, project administration. All authors read and approved the final manuscript.

Author details

[1] Department of Orthopaedic Surgery, Sir Charles Gairdner Hospital, Nedlands, WA 6009, Australia. [2] Murdoch University, Murdoch, WA 6150, Australia. [3] Harry Perkins Institute of Medical Research, The University of Western Australia, 6 Verdun Street, Nedlands, WA 6009, Australia. [4] Hollywood Functional Rehabilitation Centre, 117 Stirling Hwy, Nedlands, WA 6009, Australia.

Competing interests

The authors declare that they have no competing interests.

Funding

A financial Grant from the Abbie Basson Sarcoma Foundation Ltd charity was received for the conduct of this trial.

References

1. Nielsen TO, West RB. Translating gene expression into clinical care: sarcomas as a paradigm. J Clin Oncol. 2010;28:1796–805.
2. Taylor BS, Barretina J, Maki RG, Antonescu CR, Singer S, Ladanyi M. Advances in sarcoma genomics and new therapeutic agents. Nat Rev Cancer. 2011;11(8):541–57.
3. Agaram NP, Wong GC, Guo T, Maki RG, Singer S, DeMatteo RP, Besmer P, Antonescu CR. Novel V600E BRAF mutations in imatinib-naive and imatinib-resistant gastrointestinal stromal tumors. Genes Chromosomes Cancer. 2008;47:853–9.
4. Heinrich MC, Corless CL, Duensing A, McCreevey L, Chen C-J, Joseph N, Singer S, Griffith DJ, Haley A, Town A, Demetri GD, Fletcher CD, Fletcher JA. PDGFRA activating mutations in gastrointestinal stromal tumors. Science. 2003;299(5607):708–10.
5. Rabbani B, Tekin M, Mahdieh N. The promise of whole-exome sequencing in medical genetics. J Hum Genet. 2014;59(1):5–15.
6. Rizzo JM, Buck MJ. Key principles and clinical applications of "next-generation" DNA sequencing. Cancer Prev Res. 2012;5:887–900.
7. Botstein D, Risch N. Discovering genotypes underlying human phenotypes: past successes for mendelian disease, future approaches for complex disease. Nat Genet. 2003;33:228–37.
8. Majewski J, Schwartzentruber J, Lalonde E, Montpetit A, Jabado N. What can exome sequencing do for you? J Med Genet. 2011;48:580–9.
9. Stebbing J, Paz K, Schwartz GK, Wexler LH, Maki R, Pollock RE, Morris R, Cohen R, Shankar A, Blackman G, Harding V, Vasquez D, Krell J, Zacharoulis S, Ciznadija D, Katz A, Sidransky D. Patient-derived xenografts for individualized care in advanced sarcoma. Cancer. 2014;120:2006–15.
10. Haldar M, Hancock JD, Coffin CM, Lessnick SL, Capecchi MR. A conditional mouse model of synovial sarcoma: insights into a myogenic origin. Cancer Cell. 2007;11:375–88.
11. Neve RM, Chin K, Fridlyand J, Yeh J, Baehner FL, Fevr T, Clark L, Bayani N, Coppe JP, Tong F, Speed T, Spellman PT, DeVries S, Lapuk A, Wang NJ, Kuo WL, Stilwell JL, Pinkel D, Albertson DG, Waldman FM, McCormick F, Dickson RB, Johnson MD, Lippman M, Ethier S, Gazdar A, Gray JW. A collection of breast cancer cell lines for the study of functionally distinct cancer subtypes. Cancer Cell. 2006;10:515–27.

12. Kao J, Salari K, Bocanegra M, Choi YL, Girard L, Gandhi J, Kwei KA, Hernandez-Boussard T, Wang P, Gazdar AF, Minna JD, Pollack JR. Molecular profiling of breast cancer cell lines defines relevant tumor models and provides a resource for cancer gene discovery. PLoS ONE. 2009;4:e6146.
13. Arora A, Scholar E. Role of tyrosine kinase inhibitors in cancer therapy. J Pharmacol Exp Ther. 2005;315(3):971–9.
14. Frezza A, Stacchiotti S, Gronchi A. Systemic treatment in advanced soft tissue sarcoma: what is standard, what is new. BMC Med. 2017;15:109.
15. Ben-David U, Ha G, Tseng YT, Greenwald NF, Oh C, Shih J, McFarland JM, Wong B, Boehm JS, Beroukhim R, Golub TR. Patient-derived xenografts undergo mouse-specific tumor evolution. Nat Genet. 2017;49(11):1567–75.
16. Hintzsche J, Kim J, Yadav V, Amato C, Robinson SE, Seelenfreund E, Shellman Y, Wisell J, Applegate A, McCarter M, Box N, Tentler J, De S, Robinson WA, Tan AC. IMPACT: a whole-exome sequencing analysis pipeline for integrating molecular profiles with actionable therapeutics in clinical samples. J Am Med Inform Assoc. 2016;23:721–30.
17. Wang J, Vasaikar S, Shi Z, Greer M, Zhang B. WebGestalt 2017: a more comprehensive, powerful, flexible and interactive gene set enrichment analysis toolkit. Nucleic Acids Res. 2017;45(W1):W130–7.
18. The UniProt Consortium. UniProt: the universal protein knowledgebase. Nucleic Acids Res. 2017;45:D158–69.
19. Kumar P, Henikoff S, Ng PC. Predicting the effects of coding non-synonymous variants on protein function using the SIFT algorithm. Nat Protoc. 2009;4:1073–81.
20. Adzhubei IA, Schmidt S, Peshkin L, Ramensky VE, Gerasimova A, Bork P, Kondrashov AS, Sunyaev SR. A method and server for predicting damaging missense mutations. Nat Methods. 2010;7:248–9.
21. Shihab HA, Gough J, Cooper DN, Stenson PD, Barker GL, Edwards KJ, Day IN, Gaunt TR. Predicting the functional, molecular, and phenotypic consequences of amino acid substitutions using hidden Markov models. Hum Mutat. 2013;34:57–65.
22. Kircher M, Witten DM, Jain P, O'Roak BJ, Cooper GM. A general framework for estimating the relative pathogenicity of human genetic variants. Nat Genet. 2014;46:310–5.
23. Cooper GM, Stone EA, Asimenos G, NISC Comparative Sequencing Program, Green ED, Batzoglou S, Sidow A. Distribution and intensity of constraint in mammalian genomic sequence. Genome Res. 2005;15:901–13.
24. Schwarz JM, Rödelsperger C, Schuelke M, Seelow D. MutationTaster evaluates disease-causing potential of sequence alterations. Nat Methods. 2010;7:575–6.
25. Forbes SA, Beare D, Boutselakis H, Bamford S, Bindal N, Tate J, Cole CG, Ward S, Dawson E, Ponting L, Stefancsik R, Harsha B, Kok CY, Jia M, Jubb H, Sondka Z, Thompson S, De T, Campbell PJ. COSMIC: somatic cancer genetics at high-resolution. Nucleic Acids Res. 2017;45(D1):D777–83.
26. Hallberg B, Palmer RH. The role of the ALK receptor in cancer biology. Ann Oncol. 2016;27(S3):iii4–15.
27. Wang J, Pendergast AM. The emerging role of ABL kinases in solid tumors. Trends Cancer. 2015;1(2):110–23.
28. Murga-Zamalloa C, Lim M. ALK-driven tumors and targeted therapy: focus on crizotinib. Pharmgenom Pers Med. 2014;7:87–94.
29. Fleuren ED, Roeffen MH, Leenders WP, Flucke UE, Vlenterie M, Schreuder HW, Boerman OC, van der Graaf WT, Versleijen-Jonkers YM. Expression and clinical relevance of MET and ALK in Ewing sarcomas. Int J Cancer. 2013;133(2):427–36.
30. Entz-Werle N, Gaub MP, Lavaux T, Marcellin L, Metzger N, Marec-Berard P, Schmitt C, Brugiere L, Kalifa C, Tabone MD, Pacquement H, Gentet P, Lutz P, Oudet P, Babin A. KIT gene in pediatric osteosarcomas: could it be a new therapeutic target? Int J Cancer. 2007;120(11):2510–6.
31. Papadopoulos MC, Saadoun S. Key roles of aquaporins in tumor biology. Biochim Biophys Acta. 2015;1848(10 Pt B):2576–83.
32. Chugh R, Tawbi H, Lucas D. Chordoma: the nonsarcoma primary bone tumor. Oncol. 2007;12(11):1344–50.

21

Non-canonical WNT6/WNT10A signal factor expression in EBV+ post-transplant smooth muscle tumors

Kristin Teiken[1*†], Mark Kuehnel[1†], Jan Rehkaemper[2], Hans Kreipe[1], Florian Laenger[1], Kais Hussein[1] and Danny Jonigk[1]

Abstract

Post-transplant smooth muscle tumors (PTSMTs) are rare mesenchymal neoplasms which occur after solid organ or haematopoietic stem cell transplantation. PTSMT typically consist of Epstein–Barr-virus (EBV)+ smooth muscle-like cells and show an intermediate malignancy. Their main occurrences are visceral organs, especially the liver, but intracranial appearances are described and associated with a poor prognosis. EBV drives the growth of PTSMT; however, the underlying molecular mechanisms still remain unclear. Gene expression analysis of a set of morphologically similar tumors (leiomyomas, leiomyosarcomas, angioleiomyomas and endothelial haemangiomas) from patients without immunosuppression or EBV-association was performed. Our findings indicate that PTSMT's growth is driven by two factors of the wingless-type protein family: WNT6 and WNT10A. We are first to report that in PTSMTs, a non-canonical activation of WNT, independent of beta-catenin, drives tumor cell proliferation via MTOR/AKT1, MYC and Cyclin D2.

Keywords: PTSMT, Post-transplant smooth muscle tumors, Angioleiomyomas, EBV, WNT

Background

Tumors with predominant or partial smooth muscle differentiation make up a broad spectrum of mesenchymal neoplasms. Most of these tumors are based on spontaneous mutations of a mesenchymal stem cell. A rare and virus-associated entity are the post-transplant smooth muscle tumors (PTSMT) [1, 2]. These tumors are typically positive for the Epstein–Barr virus (EBV) and can manifest themselves at any time and in any organ after transplantation [1]. Similar neoplasms can also occur in any other immunosuppressive condition, in particular after infection with human immunodeficiency virus (HIV; HIV-SMT) or congenital immune defects (CI-SMT) [1, 3, 4].

Post-transplant smooth muscle tumors are rare in regard to the total population (<1% of transplanted patients [5]) but represent an important clinical and radiological differential diagnosis in immune-compromised patients, particularly to post-transplant lymphoproliferative diseases (PTLD). In PTSMT, the site of manifestation determines the patients' outcome [2]. In particular, cerebral PTSMT has a poor prognosis, while histological features (mitotic rate, cellular atypia, and necrosis) have no prognostic impact [1].

Epstein–Barr virus is specialized to infect B cells and almost all adults harbor a small population of EBV+ non-neoplastic B cells, which are controlled by T cell homeostasis. It is not known how EBV enters non-B cell tissues, such as mesenchymal cells. It is thought that the PTSMT cell of origin is derived from a perivascular non-endothelial mesenchymal smooth muscle stem cell. EBV+ PTSMT have a type III-like latency with expression of EBV protein EBNA (Epstein–Barr nuclear antigen) but often lack EBV latent membrane protein 1 (LMP1) expression [6]. The tumorigenic role of EBV in smooth muscle neoplasms is not clear because particularly HIV-SMT can be EBV negative, indicating that the virus is not

*Correspondence: Teiken.Kristin@mh-hannover.de
†Kristin Teiken and Mark Kuehnel contributed equally to this work
[1] Institute of Pathology, Hannover Medical School (MHH), Carl-Neuberg-Str. 1, 30625 Hannover, Germany

absolutely necessary for aberrant smooth muscle proliferation [1].

In our previous works, we found a molecular microenvironment which is not related to EBV infection, but rather to smooth muscle differentiation [5]. In addition, EBV is able to induce neoangiogenesis, but we found only minor changes on the transcriptional level, including increased levels of angiopoietin 2 (ANGPT2) [7]. Defining driver mutations in PTSMT are still not known. However, we and others found up-regulation of MYC proto-oncogene transcripts, protein expression of phosphorylated mechanistic target of rapamycin kinase (MTOR) and phosphorylated AKT serine/threonine kinase 1 (AKT1) signaling factors [2, 6].

In the present analyses we wanted to asses if and which transcript profile of mesenchymal stem cell and signaling factors differ between PTSMT and other neoplasms with smooth muscle differentiation.

Methods

Tumor samples

EBV+ PTSMTs comprised six tumors from five patients; one patient had a tumor in the spleen and another in a cerebral sinus. We previously reported the clinical and histopathological characteristics of four of these patients [2]. The fifth patient was a female (age: 61 years) who developed a PTSMT in the liver 5 years after kidney transplantation (tumor diameter 3.1 cm, 10% Ki67, positive for EBV in situ hybridization (EBER), smooth muscle actin, caldesmon and desmin).

For control purposes, the following tumors were analyzed (Table 1, Fig. 1): (i) smooth muscle tumors (nine visceral leiomyomas and four central venous G1–2 leiomyosarcomas) and (ii) mixed smooth muscle and vascular tumors (28 with different histological subtypes of angioleiomyomas). Additionally, we added (iii) a vascular tumor control group (five endothelial haemangiomas), as the actual origin of PTSMT is still uncertain and aberrant myogenous venous wall cells are still under discussion as the cells of origin [2, 8]. Before performing molecular analysis, the angioleiomyomas were histologically sub grouped according to the old but current standard of Morimoto [9] (13/28 capillary solid, 7/28 venous, 5/28 cavernous, 3/28 mixed capillary-cavernous). All samples of formalin fixed and paraffin-embedded (FFPE) tumors were selected from the archive of the Institutes of Pathology in Muenster (12/28 angioleiomyomas) and Hannover (all other samples).

Transcript expression analysis

Samples contained >80% tumor tissue and RNA was extracted and purified with our established mineral oil method and RNeasy Mini Kit (Qiagen, Hilden, Germany) via Maxwell® system (Promega cooperation, Mannheim, Germany). RNA was quantified by Qubit® 2.0 fluorometer (Life Technologies/Thermo Fisher Scientific, Waltham, MA, USA). Transcript expression analysis was performed via NanoString nCounter™ system. NanoString uses digital fluorescent reporters for gene detection and enables analysis of small amount of RNA while minimizing background signals. We used the prefabricated stem cell panel (includes 193 target genes and six endogenous control genes) as described in the manufacturer's protocol (NanoString Technologies, Seattle, WA, USA). Endogenous control genes were glucuronidase beta (GUSB), glyceraldehyde-3-phosphate dehydrogenase (GAPDH), clathrin heavy chain (CLTC), hypoxanthine phosphoribosyltransferase 1 (HPRT1), phosphoglycerate kinase 1 (PGK1) and tubulin beta class I (TUBB).

Immunohistochemistry

Deparaffinized and rehydrated FFPE tissue sections (1–2 μm) were processed in an automated staining system (Benchmark ULTRA, Ventana Medical Systems, Inc.,

Table 1 Sample set and clinical data

Entities	PTSMT	Leiomyoma (LM)	Leiomyosarcoma (LMS)	Angioleiomyoma (ALM)	Endothelial haemangioma (EHA)
Number of tumors	n=6 (5 patients)	n=9	n=4	n=28	n=5
Age (median, range)	11.5 (6–61)	60 (29–71)	63 (45–71)	60 (23–79)	48 (32–58)
Gender	♀ 100% ♂ 0%	♀ 89% ♂ 11%	♀ 75% ♂ 25%	♀ 64% ♂ 36%	♀ 60% ♂ 40%
Tumor localisation	Kidney (n=2) Lung (n=1) Colon (n=1) Spleen (n=1) Confluens sinuum (n=1)	Stomach (n=3) Kidney (n=2) Skin (n=2) Esophagus (n=1) Mesenterium (n=1)	Pulmonary artery (n=2) Right atrium (n=1) Adrenal gland vein (n=1)	Lower extremities (n=13) Upper extremities (n=2) Head–Neck (n=3) Genital ♀ (n=2) Skin/soft tissue (n=8)	Lower extremities (n=3) Head–Neck (n=1) Mediastinal (n=1)

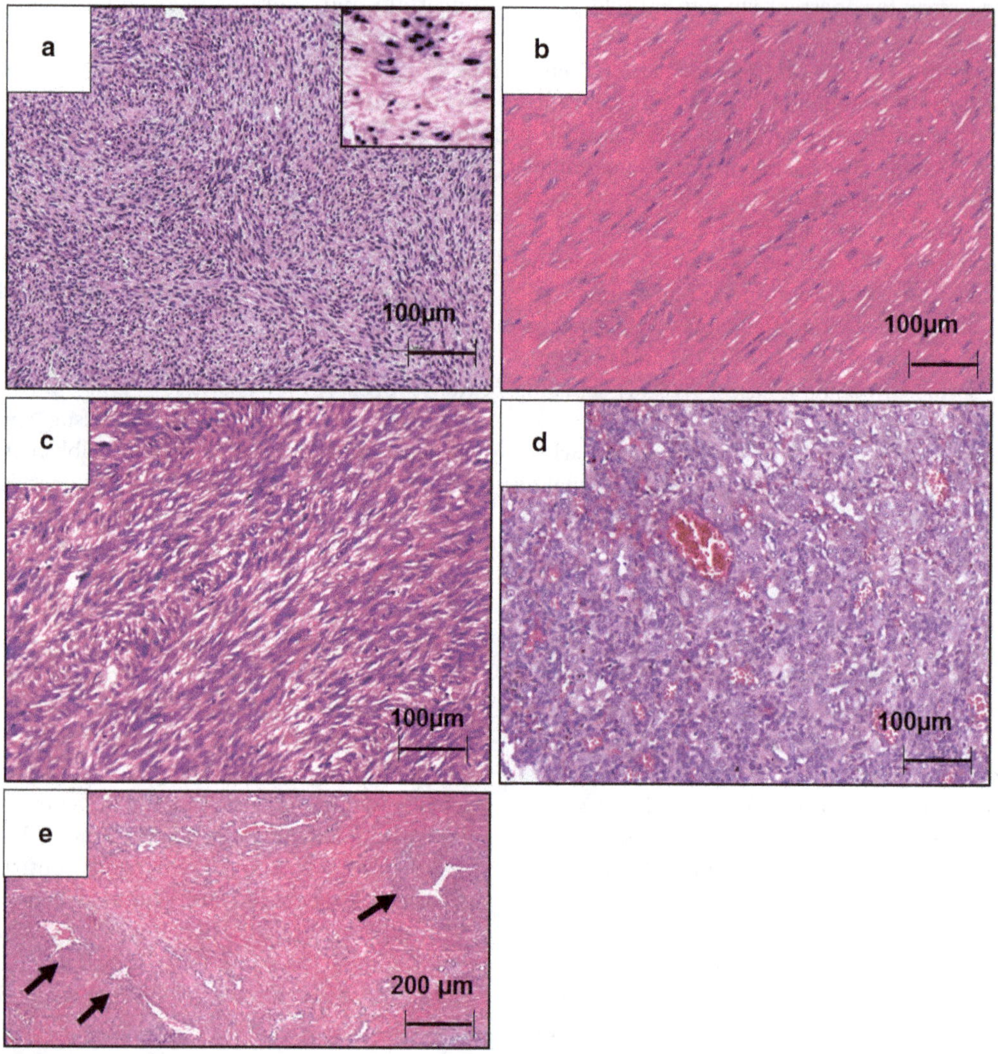

Fig. 1 Histological appearance of the five different entities. **a** Post transplant smooth muscle tumor (haematoxylin–eosin stain (HE stain, 100×) with inserted positive EBV-in situ hybridization (EBER), **b** visceral leiomyoma (HE stain, 100×), **c** visceral leiomyosarcoma of the central venous tract (right atrium, HE stain, 100×) with prominent atypia and increased level of mitosis figures, **d** endothelial haemangioma (HE stain, 100×) with prominent vessels, **e** angioleiomyoma (HE stain, 50×), in particular venous subtype with prominently walled vessels (arrows)

Tucson, AZ, USA). A monoclonal anti-beta-catenin antibody was used.

Data analysis

Raw data of transcript target gene expression were analyzed by nSolver™ software (NanoString Technologies) and set in relation to the average of endogenous control genes (geometric mean of controls as level of relative gene expression: reference gene index). Further statistical analysis for comparison of different tumor groups was performed with Prism 5.0 (Graph Pad Software, San Diego, CA, USA) by using the non-parametric Mann–Whitney test for two group comparison and the Krustal–Wallis test and post hoc Dunn-test for multiple comparisons. P values <0.05 were considered as statistically significant. Heatmaps were generated using R.

Results

Increased WNT6/WNT10A levels in PTSMT

Transcript analysis showed significant differential expression of several genes among the different types of smooth muscle tumors (Table 2, Additional file 1: Figure S1). Several factors were increased in only one type of tumor. PTSMT showed increased Wnt family member 6 (WNT6) and WNT10A levels while all other types of tumors showed no different expression or low levels of these two WNT factors (Fig. 2, Table 2). WNT6 and WNT10A are encoded as a gene cluster on chromosomal

Table 2 Significant differentially regulated genes in PTSMTs and leiomyosarcomas

Regulation	Gene	Median PTSMT	Median ALM	Median LM	Median LMS	Median EHA
Upregulated in PTSMT	WNT6	0.39301	0.00961	0.00439	0.01074	0.01285
	WNT10A	0.12282	0.00545	0.00482	0.00670	0.03415
	MYC	0.48877	0.13366	0.11219	0.24502	0.50480
	Cyclin D2	2.89498	0.54088	1.02805	0.44413	0.32572
Downregulated in PTSMT	WNT9B	0.00192	0.00416	0.00193	0.00951	0.01138
	GAS1	0.02407	0.05434	0.19764	0.28556	0.30450
	PRKD1	0.07241	0.21601	0.22282	0.15769	0.12693
	FGFR1	0.36842	0.80905	1.72532	0.93143	0.48040
	Beta-catenin	1.57460	2.09349	2.49687	2.23053	1.47197
Upregulated in leiomyosarcomas compared to PTSMT	WNT9B	0.00192	0.00416	0.00193	0.00951	0.01138
	GAS1	0.02407	0.05434	0.19764	0.28556	0.30450
	DHH	0.00297	0.01077	0.00831	0.00259	0.04553
	LFNG	0.23836	0.77146	0.22185	0.76354	2.24482
	MFNG	0.05390	0.07672	0.05256	0.05478	0.50480
	PRKACA	0.85552	1.53877	1.51137	1.44838	1.70591
	IGF	0.04295	0.12047	0.11971	0.16677	0.67152

segment 2q35. In individual PTSMT cases, both WNT factors were co-expressed at similar levels.

In addition to WNT6/WNT10A, cell cycle G1/S transition regulator Cyclin D2 (CCND2) was increased. As could be expected from our previous results on uterine leiomyomas and PTSMT [2], MYC proto-oncogene, bHLH transcription factor (MYC) transcripts were significantly higher in PTSMT than in non-uterine visceral leiomyomas (Fig. 2). These three factors are not encoded on 2q35 or any other chromosome 2 segment, but on chromosome 8 (MYC: 8q24) and chromosome 12 (CCND2: 12p13).

WNT9B (17q21.32), S phase entry blocker growth arrest specific 1 (GAS1) and serine/threonine protein kinase D1 (PRKD1) were expressed at low levels in PTSMT while the other analyzed tumor types showed higher levels, in particular, leiomyosarcomas. Similar to our previous results [7], fibroblast growth factor receptor 1 (FGFR1) levels are lower in PTSMT as compared to leiomyomas.

WNT signaling-related transcript levels of catenin beta 1 (CTNNB1) were not increased in PTSMT (Fig. 2, Table 2). Beta-catenin protein expression was evaluated by immunohistochemistry in PTSMT. All of them showed no nuclear beta-catenin protein localisation. Compared to the other tumor types, several other canonical and non-canonical WNT signaling pathway factors were not significantly deregulated in PTSMT, in particular, frizzled class receptors (FZD), WNT1-8, WNT9A, WNT10B, WNT11 and WNT16, beta-catenin-related transcription factor 7 (TCF7), WNT signaling pathway regulator adenomatous-polyposis-coli gen (APC), glycogen synthase kinase 3 beta (GSK-3beta), Cyclin D1 (CCND1) as well as the two small GTPase ROH family members ras homolog family member A (ROHA) and cell division cycle 42 (CDC42). These findings indicate that other canonical and non-canonical WNT pathways are not activated and affirm our theory. Therefore, the downstream effectors of the elevated WNT6/WNT10A levels remain unclear.

Different gene expression profiles in PTSMT and leiomyosarcomas

There were significant differences between visceral leiomyomas, angioleiomyomas and haemangiomas (Additional file 1: Figure S1).

In comparison to all other tumors, leiomyosarcomas showed several increased gene expression levels (Table 2). The following expression levels were significantly higher in leiomyosarcomas than in PTSMT (Table 2): WNT9B, GAS1, signaling factor desert hedgehog (DHH), the two Notch signaling pathway factors LFNG O-fucosylpeptide 3-beta-N-acetylglucosaminyltransferase provided (LFNG) and MFNG O-fucosylpeptide 3-beta-N-acetylglucosaminyltransferase (MFNG), protein kinase cAMP-activated catalytic subunit alpha (PRKACA) and insulin-like growth factor 1 (IGF1). Roland et al. [10] showed that leiomyosarcomas also express the IGF receptor which indicates paracrine activation.

Histopathological subgroups of angioleiomyomas show no molecularpathological correlation

There are three distinct histopathological subtypes of angioleiomyomas which were originally described on

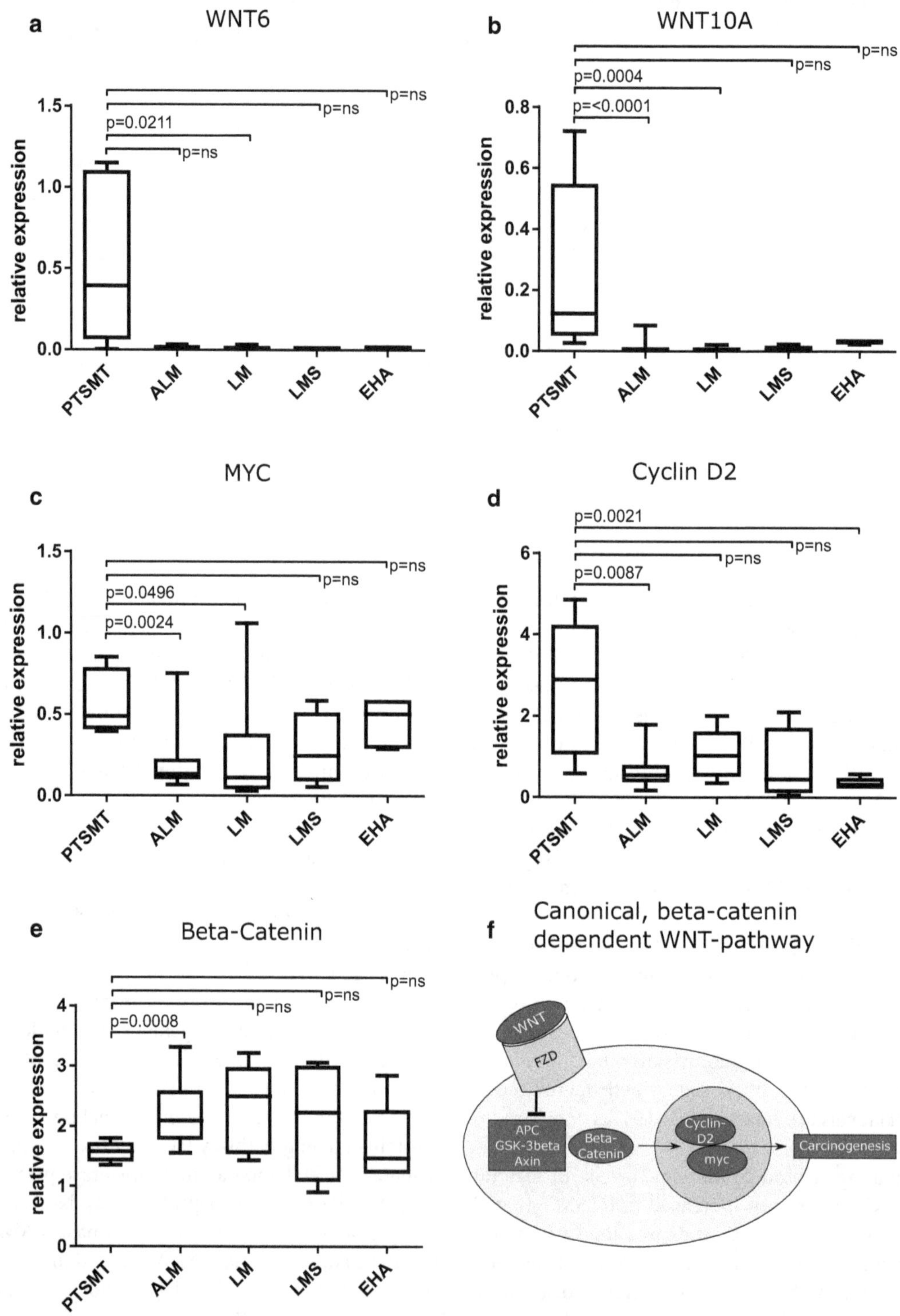

Fig. 2 **a–e** Significant upregulated gene members of the WNT signaling pathway in PTSMT. Note that non-significant (p = ns) differences between PTSMT and other tumors regarding WNT6 and WNT10A expression are related to non-detactable transcripts in several ALM, LMS and EHA (**a**, **b**). **f** Beta-catenin is bound and inactivated in a complex formation containing adenomatous polyposis coli gene (APC), glycogen synthase kinase 3 beta (GSK-3beta) and axin-1 (Axin). In the classical, beta-catenin-dependent WNT signaling pathway, members of WNT family bind to the frizzled class receptors (FZD) whereas beta-catenin is set free and initiates carcinogenesis via activation of MYC and Cyclin D2

the basis of histopathological features by Morimoto in 1973 [9]. Regarding the genes under investigation, manly these subgroups showed the same molecularpathological characteristics. Only six genes show significant differences between the angioleiomyoma types (ISL1, NCSTN, TCF7, WNT10A, WNT11, WNT7A) but their relative expression levels were very low, which indicates no biological relevance (< 0.4 compared to standardized reference gene index).

Discussion

Post-transplant smooth muscle tumor share morphological similarities with leiomyomas and low-grade leiomyosarcomas and only show rarely high-grade atypia. One of the main differences is the EBV association. Our previous molecular analysis showed no clear relationship between EBV infection of tumor cells and (de)regulation of gene expression. One reason could be that PTSMT usually do not express LMP1, a viral protein which is associated with manipulation of the host cell cycle and cytokine expression. In one of the very first analyses which addressed the question of specific signaling pathway deregulation in PTSMT, Ong et al. [6] demonstrated that these tumors express phosphorylated MTOR and phosphorylated AKT1 proteins and that Ras association domain family member 1 (RASSF1) was hypermethylated. Activated MTOR/AKT1 signaling, RASSF1 hypermethylation and MYC expression can also be found in a subset of leiomyosarcomas [6, 11, 12]. We could confirm our previous result that PTSMT have higher expression levels of MYC than uterine and non-uterine leiomyomas. In our current analysis we found that this difference regarding MYC was not significant in comparison to leiomyosarcomas. Remarkably, for the very first time, we could show that PTSMT are characterized by WNT6/WNT10A regulation while all other tumor entities under investigation showed almost no expression of these two factors. There are no reports on a particular WNT6 or WNT10A expression in EBV infected cells [13, 14]. Therefore, it is unlikely that EBV is the main cause of this WNT6/WNT10A expression. The only other known tumor entity characterized by WNT6/WNT10A overexpression are colorectal carcinomas and it is assumed that their mode of proliferation is linked to differential beta-catenin expression—as opposed to PTSMTs [15].

Both genes are encoded as a cluster on segment 2q35. Co-expression of these two factors indicates a co-regulation of the respective promotors. The fact that many canonical WNT signaling factors were not increased and that we found no nuclear beta-catenin indicates activation of the non-canonical WNT pathway. Similar to PTSMT, leiomyosarcomas usually show no aberrant nuclear beta-catenin expression [10, 16]. Non-canonical WNT signaling is often characterized by alternative signaling without cytoplasmic stabilization of soluble beta-catenin [17–19]. These include the WNT/calcium pathway and the planar cell polarity (PCP). In those alternative pathways, other WNT factors than WNT6 and WNT10A are usually involved [17–19]. In contrast to PTSMT, it has been shown in renal cell carcinoma that WNT10A is involved in canonical WNT/beta-catenin signaling [20]. In the murine kidney, Wnt6 is also related to canonical Wnt/beta-catenin signaling [21]. In mesenchymal cells expression of WNT6, WNT10A and WNT10B can be associated with osteoblastogenesis and inhibition of adipogenesis but not with smooth muscle differentiation [22]. WNT6 is involved in differentiation of non-smooth muscle myogenic cells, e.g. in the heart, and proliferation of stromal cells in the placenta [23–26]. There are reports which imply a special relationship between WNT/beta catenin signaling and CCND2 in glioma cells [27] but not in smooth muscle cells. At least in cardiomyocytes, there are evidences of a MYC-dependent activation of CCND2 [28]. In insulin sensitive pancreatic beta cells, activated MTOR leads to CCND2-associated proliferation [29, 30]. Therefore, these signaling factors could also be linked in PTSMT. Based on the finding that MTOR signaling is activated, Sirolimus has been used for targeted therapy in PTSMT [31].

Conclusions

In summary, we are the first to report that PTSMT cells may harbor a unique variant of a non-canonical WNT pathway, which is based on WNT6/WNT10A, and which may induce cell proliferation and differentiation via MTOR/AKT1, MYC and CCND2.

Additional file

Additional file 1: Figure S1. Heatmap of all investigated stem cell genes shows differences between the five entities. PTSMT: post-transplant smooth muscle tumors, ALM: angioleiomyomas and their histomorphological subtypes, LM: leiomyomas, EHA: endothelial haemangiomas and LMS: leiomyosarcomas of the central venous tract. Colors encode significance level of pairwise group comparison. The abbreviations of the five entities stand for the corresponding significantly different regulated group. ns: $p > 0.05$, *: $p \leq 0.05$, **: ≤ 0.01, ***: ≤ 0.001.

Abbreviations

AKT1: serin/threonin kinase 1; ANGPT2: angiopoietin 2; APS: adenomatous-polyposis-coli gen; CCND1: Cyclin-D1; CCND2: Cyclin-D2; CDC42: cell division cycle 42; CI-SMT: congenital immune defects-smooth muscle tumors; CLTC: clathrin heavy chain; CTNNB1: beta-catenin 1; DHH: desert hedgehog; EBER: Epstein–Barr virus; EBNA: Epstein–Barr nuclear antigen; EBV: Epstein–Barr virus-encoded small RNA; FFPE: formalin fixed and paraffin-embedded; FGFR1: fibroblast growth factor receptor 1; FZD: frizzled class receptor; GAPDH: glyceraldehyde-3-phosphate dehydrogenase; GAS1: S phase entry blocker growth arrest specific 1; GSK-3beta: glycogen synthase kinase 3 beta; GUSB: glucuronidase beta; HE: hematoxylin and eosin; HIV: human immunodeficiency virus; HIV-SMT: human immunodeficiency virus smooth muscle tumors;

HPRT1: hypoxanthine phosphoribosyltransferase 1; IGF: insulin like growth factor 1; ISL1: insulin gene enhancer protein; LFNG: LFNG *O*-fucosylpeptide 3-beta-*N*-acetylglucosaminyltransferase provided; LMP1: latent membrane protein 1; MFNG: MFNG *O*-fucosylpeptide 3-beta-*N*-acetylglucosaminyltransferase; MTOR: rapamycin kinase; NCSTN: nicastrin; PCP: planar cell polarity; PGK1: phosphoglycerate kinase 1; PRKACA: protein kinase cAMP-activated catalytic subunit alpha; PRKD1: serine/threonine protein kinase D1; PTLD: post-transplant lymphoproliferative disease; PTSMT: post-transplant smooth muscle tumor; RASSF1: Ras associated domain family member 1; ROHA: GTPase ROH family members ras homolog family member A; TCF7: beta-catenin-related transcription factor 7; TUBB: tubulin beta class 1; WNT6: WNT family gene member 6; WNT10A: WNT family gene member 10A.

Authors' contributions

Histomorphology (KT, DJ, KH, FL, JR, HK), molecular analysis (KT, MK, DJ), data collection, analysis of data and manuscript preparation (MK, KT, DJ, KH). All authors read and approved the final manuscript.

Author details

[1] Institute of Pathology, Hannover Medical School (MHH), Carl-Neuberg-Str. 1, 30625 Hannover, Germany. [2] Institute of Pathology, University of Muenster, Domagkstraße 17, 48149 Muenster, Germany.

Acknowledgements

This work was supported by the Collaborative Research Centre 738 (CRC 738), in particular Danny Jonigk and Florian Laenger. The authors would like to thank A. Hori for patiently translating the original angioleiomyoma paper by Morimoto form Japanese to German. Furthermore, the authors thank Annette Mueller-Brechlin, Regina Engelhardt and Christina Fiedler for their excellent technical support, Helge Stark for his statistical advice and Jan Lukas Robertus and Kara Diemer for editing the text.

Competing interests

The authors have no commercial associations relevant for this study and

Funding

The project was funded by the German Research Foundation as part of Collaborative Research Centre 738 (CRC738, Danny Jonigk, Florian Laenger).

References

1. Hussein K, Rath B, Ludewig B, Kreipe H, Jonigk D. Clinico-pathological characteristics of different types of immunodeficiency-associated smooth muscle tumours. Eur J Cancer. 2014;50(14):2417–24.
2. Jonigk D, Laenger F, Maegel L, Izykowski N, Rische J, Tiede C, Klein C, Maecker-Kolhoff B, Kreipe H, Hussein K. Molecular and clinicopathological analysis of Epstein–Barr virus-associated posttransplant smooth muscle tumors. Am J Transplant. 2012;12(7):1908–17.
3. Issarachaikul R, Shuangshoti S, Suankratay C. Epstein–Barr virus-associated smooth muscle tumors in AIDS patients: a largest case (series). Intern Med. 2014;53(20):2391–6.
4. Schober T, Magg T, Laschinger M, Rohlfs M, Linhares ND, Puchalka J, Weisser T, Fehlner K, Mautner J, Walz C, Hussein K, Jaeger G, Kammer B, Schmid I, Bahia M, Pena SD, Behrends U, Belohradsky BH, Klein C, Hauck F. A human immunodeficiency syndrome caused by mutations in CARMIL2. Nat Commun. 2017;8:14209.
5. Jonigk D, Izykowski N, Maegel L, Schormann E, Maecker-Kolhoff B, Laenger F, Kreipe H, Hussein K. MicroRNA expression in Epstein–Barr virus-associated post-transplant smooth muscle tumours is related to leiomyomatous phenotype. Clin Sarcoma Res. 2013;3(1):9.
6. Ong KW, Teo M, Lee V, Ong D, Lee A, Tan CS, Vathsala A, Toh HC. Expression of EBV latent antigens, mammalian target of rapamycin, and tumor suppression genes in EBV-positive smooth muscle tumors: clinical and therapeutic implications. Clin Cancer Res. 2009;15(17):5350–8.
7. Jonigk D, Izykowski N, Maegel L, Schormann E, Ludewig B, Kreipe H, Hussein K. Tumour angiogenesis in Epstein–Barr virus-associated post-transplant smooth muscle tumours. Clin Sarcoma Res. 2014;4(1):1.
8. Chaves NJ, Kotsimbos TC, Warren MA, et al. Cranial leiomyosarcoma in an Epstein–Barr virus (EBV)-mismatched lung transplant recipient. J Heart Lung Transplant. 2007;26:753–5.
9. Morimoto N. Angiomyoma (vascular leiomyoma): a clinicopathological study. Med J Kagoshima Univ. 1973;24:663–83.
10. Roland CL, Boland GM, Demicco EG, Lusby K, Ingram D, May CD, Kivlin CM, Watson K, Al Sannaa GA, Wang WL, Ravi V, Pollock RE, Lev D, Cormier JN, Hunt KK, Feig BW, Lazar AJ, Torres KE. Clinical observations and molecular variables of primary vascular leiomyosarcoma. JAMA Surg. 2016;151(4):347–54.
11. Setsu N, Yamamoto H, Kohashi K, Endo M, Matsuda S, Yokoyama R, Nishiyama K, Iwamoto Y, Dobashi Y, Oda Y. The Akt/mammalian target of rapamycin pathway is activated and associated with adverse prognosis in soft tissue leiomyosarcomas. Cancer. 2012;118(6):1637–48.
12. Tsiatis AC, Herceg ME, Keedy VL, Halpern JL, Holt GE, Schwartz HS, Cates JM. Prognostic significance of c-Myc expression in soft tissue leiomyosarcoma. Mod Pathol. 2009;22(11):1432–8.
13. Chou J, Lin YC, Kim J, You L, Xu Z, He B, Jablons DM. Nasopharyngeal carcinoma—review of the molecular mechanisms of tumorigenesis. Head Neck. 2008;30(7):946–63.
14. Pang MF, Lin KW, Peh SC. The signaling pathways of Epstein–Barr virus-encoded latent membrane protein 2A (LMP2A) in latency and cancer. Cell Mol Biol Lett. 2009;14(2):222–47.
15. Kirikoshi H, Sekihara H, Katoh M. WNT10A and WNT6, clustered in human chromosome 2q35 region with head-to-tail manner, are strongly coexpressed in SW480. Biochem Biophys Res Commun. 2001;283(4):798–805.
16. Gogou PN, Batistatou A, Pakos EE, Apostolikas N, Stefanou D, Tsekeris PG. Expression of E-cadherin, beta-catenin and topoisomerase II alpha in leiomyosarcomas. Clin Transl Oncol. 2009;11(8):548–51.
17. Cuppens T, Tuyaerts S, Amant F. Potential therapeutic targets in uterine sarcomas. Sarcoma. 2015;2015:243298.
18. Kim JH, Park SY, Jun Y, Kim JY, Nam JS. Roles of Wnt target genes in the journey of cancer stem cells. Int J Mol Sci. 2017;18(8):1604. https://doi.org/10.3390/ijms18081604.
19. Sedgwick AE, D'Souza-Schorey C. Wnt signaling in cell motility and invasion: drawing parallels between development and cancer. Cancers (Basel). 2016;8(9):80. https://doi.org/10.3390/cancers8090080.
20. Hsu RJ, Ho JY, Cha TL, Yu DS, Wu CL, Huang WP, Chu P, Chen YH, Chen JT, Yu CP. WNT10A plays an oncogenic role in renal cell carcinoma by activating WNT/beta-catenin pathway. PLoS ONE. 2012;7(10):e47649.
21. Beaton H, Andrews D, Parsons M, Murphy M, Gaffney A, Kavanagh D, McKay GJ, Maxwell AP, Taylor CT, Cummins EP, Godson C, Higgins DF, Murphy P, Crean J. Wnt6 regulates epithelial cell differentiation and is dysregulated in renal fibrosis. Am J Physiol Renal Physiol. 2016;311(1):F35–45.
22. Cawthorn WP, Bree AJ, Yao Y, Du B, Hemati N, Martinez-Santibanez G, MacDougald OA. Wnt6, Wnt10a and Wnt10b inhibit adipogenesis and stimulate osteoblastogenesis through a beta-catenin-dependent mechanism. Bone. 2012;50(2):477–89.
23. Hitchins L, Fletcher F, Allen S, Dhoot GK. Role of Sulf1A in Wnt1- and Wnt6-induced growth regulation and myoblast hyper-elongation. FEBS Open Bio. 2012;3:30–4.
24. Lavery DL, Martin J, Turnbull YD, Hoppler S. Wnt6 signaling regulates heart muscle development during organogenesis. Dev Biol. 2008;323(2):177–88.
25. Schmeckpeper J, Verma A, Yin L, Beigi F, Zhang L, Payne A, Zhang Z, Pratt RE, Dzau VJ, Mirotsou M. Inhibition of Wnt6 by Sfrp2 regulates adult cardiac progenitor cell differentiation by differential modulation of Wnt pathways. J Mol Cell Cardiol. 2015;85:215–25.
26. Wang Q, Lu J, Zhang S, Wang S, Wang W, Wang B, Wang F, Chen Q, Duan E, Leitges M, Kispert A, Wang H. Wnt6 is essential for stromal cell proliferation during decidualization in mice. Biol Reprod. 2013;88(1):5.
27. Zhang H, Wei DL, Wan L, Yan SF, Sun YH. Highly expressed lncRNA CCND2-AS1 promotes glioma cell proliferation through Wnt/beta-catenin signaling. Biochem Biophys Res Commun. 2017;482(4):1219–25.
28. Murray TV, Smyrnias I, Schnelle M, Mistry RK, Zhang M, Beretta M, Martin D, Anilkumar N, de Silva SM, Shah AM, Brewer AC. Redox regulation of cardiomyocyte cell cycling via an ERK1/2 and c-Myc-dependent activation of Cyclin D2 transcription. J Mol Cell Cardiol. 2015;79:54–68.
29. Lakshmipathi J, Alvarez-Perez JC, Rosselot C, Casinelli GP, Stamateris RE, Rausell-Palamos F, O'Donnell CP, Vasavada RC, Scott DK, Alonso LC, Garcia-Ocana A. PKCzeta is essential for pancreatic beta-cell replication during insulin resistance by regulating mTOR and Cyclin-D2. Diabetes. 2016;65(5):1283–96.

Giant cell tumour of the distal radius/ulna: response to pre-operative treatment with short-term denosumab

Catherine L. McCarthy*, Christopher L. M. H. Gibbons, Kevin M. Bradley, A. Bass Hassan, Henk Giele and Nicholas A. Athanasou

Abstract

Background: Treatment of giant cell tumour of bone (GCTB) of the distal radius/ulna poses a surgical challenge, as complex reconstructive surgery may be required. This study evaluates the clinical, radiological and pathological findings in five cases of GCTB of the distal forearm where a 3 month course of denosumab was given prior to surgery.

Methods: Patients with biopsy proven distal forearm GCTB, treated for 3 months with denosumab, followed by salvage surgery (curettage and cementation) were included. Wrist pain and function were assessed using the modified Mayo Wrist Score (MMWS). Plain radiographs, MRI and PET/CT were performed pre-treatment and 2 months after initiation of denosumab therapy. Histological comparison was made between the original biopsy and surgical curettage specimens.

Results: Five patients with an average age of 25 years were included in the study. Improvement in wrist pain and function was seen in all patients with the average MMWS increasing from 30 pre-treatment to 85 at 3 months. Plain radiographs demonstrated marginal sclerosis in all cases with reconstitution of cortical and subarticular bone by 2 months; internal matrix sclerosis and osseous consolidation was more variable. Increased tumour heterogeneity and low signal were observed on T2-weighted MR images. PET/CT revealed a decrease in average SUV from 14.8 pre-treatment to 4.7 at 2 months. Histology showed disappearance of osteoclasts and increased fibro-osseous tissue. Denosumab treatment has the potential to facilitate salvage surgery, thus avoiding bone resection and graft reconstruction. A good outcome was achieved apart from local recurrence in one case. Follow up ranged from 17 to 54 months.

Conclusion: Distal forearm GCTB responds clinically, radiologically and histologically to a short course of pre-operative denosumab therapy, which has the potential to facilitate salvage surgery.

Keywords: Giant cell tumour of bone, Distal forearm, Denosumab

Background

Giant cell tumour of bone (GCTB) is a benign but locally aggressive neoplasm, accounting for approximately 5% of primary bone tumours [1–3]; it commonly develops in the mature skeleton involving the epiphyseal region of long bones. The three most common locations where GCTB develops are the distal femur, proximal tibia and distal radius respectively.

In GCTB there is a proliferation of mononuclear stromal cells which highly express receptor activator of nuclear factor kappa-B ligand (RANKL), and an infiltrate of mononuclear macrophage-like cells and scattered multinucleated osteoclastic giant cells, both of which express RANK [1, 2, 4, 5]. In the presence of macrophage-colony stimulating factor, RANK + macrophages interact with RANKL + stromal cells to induce osteoclast formation. The numerous osteoclastic giant cells in GCTB are responsible for the extensive osteolysis that attends GCTB tumour growth. Denosumab is a human monoclonal antibody that targets and binds with high affinity and

*Correspondence: catherinemccarthy@doctors.org.uk
Nuffield Orthopaedic Centre, Windmill Road, Headington, Oxford OX3 7HE, UK

specificity to RANKL; it competitively inhibits RANK–RANKL binding, decreasing the formation, activity and survival of osteoclastic giant cells in GCTB, resulting in reduced bone resorption [5–8].

Traditionally, GCTB has been treated surgically by local curettage, with or without packing of the defect with polymethylmethacrylate (PMMA) cement or bone graft, and internal fixation when needed [9–12]. The aim of this approach is to remove the tumour whilst preserving normal anatomy and wrist function. The reported recurrence rate of GCTB following this treatment is, however, relatively high with more frequent recurrence noted in the distal radius and ulna [2, 3, 12–16]. Previous studies have shown that pre-operative denosumab therapy makes subsequent surgery more feasible and may result in surgical down-staging to a less morbid surgical salvage procedure [17, 18] allowing for improved patient function. There are currently no specific guidelines on the optimal duration of pre-operative denosumab therapy and recognising the imaging features of a positive tumoral response to denosumab is important for therapeutic decision making.

This study evaluates the clinical, radiological and pathological findings in five cases of GCTB of the distal forearm that received a planned short 3 month course of denosumab prior to surgery.

Methods

A retrospective review of patients presenting between 2012 and 2015 with GCTB of the distal upper extremity was conducted at our institution. Patients with biopsy proven (Campanacci grade 2/3) GCTB of the distal ulna or radius treated for 3 months with denosumab followed by surgical curettage and cementation, and with more than 12 months follow up, were included in the study. Excluded patients were those that lacked a pre-treatment biopsy and/or had received prior treatment for their GCTB, including denosumab treatment for more than 3 months, and/or had > 12 months follow-up.

Denosumab was administered by subcutaneous injection of 120 mg every 4 weeks with additional loading doses of 120 mg on days 8 and 15 of the first month. Daily supplements of calcium 500 mg and vitamin D 400 IU were taken and serum electrolytes were checked every 4 weeks. This was performed for a total of three cycles.

Clinical data collected included age, sex, location of tumour, length of follow-up and complications post-surgery. Patient wrist pain and function were assessed by the medical oncologist administering denosumab at the commencement of treatment and at 4 weekly intervals for the 3 month treatment using the modified Mayo Wrist Score (MMWS). Each assessment totaled 100 points divided among wrist pain (25 points), range of motion as a percentage of the opposite side (25 points), grip strength as a percentage of the opposite side (25 points), and the ability to return to regular employment or activities (25 points).

All patients were initially assessed with plain radiographs, magnetic resonance imaging, with and without gadolinium contrast (MRI), and positron emission tomography with fluorodeoxyglucose integrated with computed tomography (PET/CT). These studies were repeated 2 months after the commencement of denosumab therapy. All patients had post-operative and follow-up plain radiographs. All imaging studies were repeated if there was clinical or radiographic suspicion of recurrence.

Following 3 months denosumab treatment, surgical management consisted of careful and thorough curettage of all clinically visible disease, including bony septa and the neo-sclerotic intra-osseous margin, then painting the cavity with methylene blue and high speed burring of the sclerotic internal margins of the tumour. PMMA cement was used to fill the small defects created in the bone. No other adjuvants such as phenol or cryotherapy were used. The same sarcoma surgeon, with over 30 years experience, treated and followed up all cases.

In assessing the histological response to denosumab, comparison was made between the original biopsy specimen and surgical curettage specimens. The presence or absence of osteoclasts, the number of mononuclear stromal cells and the extent of fibrous matrix/bone formation was noted.

Results

Between May 2012 and July 2015, five patients fulfilling the inclusion criteria were referred to our unit with GCTB of the distal forearm. There were four females and one male with an average age of 25 years.

Pre-denosumab treatment findings

Clinical

The patients presented with increasing wrist pain (n = 5), wrist swelling (n = 4), reduced wrist grip (n = 3), reduced wrist movement and function (n = 5). The average MMWS score prior to treatment was 30. Table 1 presents demographic, clinical and radiological data on the cases in this study.

Radiological

Initial plain radiographs demonstrated in all cases a solitary, expansile, lytic lesion involving the epiphysis and extending up to the articular surface of the distal radius (n = 4) or ulna (n = 1). The physis was fused in all patients. Four lesions were graded as Campanacci grade 2 (active). These showed eccentric expansion of

Table 1 Demographic, clinical and radiological patient data

Patient #	Age	Sex	Site	Campanacci grade	Marginal sclerosis after denosumab	Intralesional matrix sclerosis after denosumab	Pre/post SUV on PET/CT	Time between denosumab and surgery (days)	Follow-up (months)	Local recurrence (time in months)
1	19	Male	Right radius	2	Yes	Moderate	19.5/8.8	23	47	No
2	21	Female	Right radius	2	Yes	Mild	7.2/3.2	18	17	No
3	39	Female	Right ulna	2	Yes	Mild	10.6/2.0	36	54	No
4	27	Female	Left radius	2	Yes	Moderate-marked	17/4.8	25	35	No
5	22	Female	Right radius	3	Yes	Moderate-marked	19.5/4.5	39	32	Yes (2)

bone with associated cortical thinning but no cortical destruction or pathologic fracture (Figs. 1a, 2a, 3a, 4a). One lesion was graded as Campanacci grade 3 (aggressive) with cortical breach of the radial styloid articular surface (Fig. 5a). MRI showed expansile subarticular lesions returning low to isointense signal relative to surrounding muscle on T1-weighted imaging (Fig. 3c) and heterogeneous predominantly high STIR and T2-weighted signal intensity (Figs. 3b, 4b). Gadolinium was administered in three cases and demonstrated diffuse enhancement in all cases. There were fluid–fluid levels in one patient indicative of secondary aneurysmal bone cyst change (Fig. 2b). There was a focal breach of the radial styloid articular surface with a small amount of soft-tissue extending into the radial aspect of the carpal joint in the Campanacci grade 3 lesion. In the remaining cases, the articular surface appeared intact. PET/CT revealed lytic, expansile lesions without a sclerotic rim and marked cortical thinning with an increased standardized uptake value (SUV) in all cases (Figs. 4c, 5b). The average pre-treatment SUV was 14.8 (Table 1). There were no distant lesions and the lungs were clear in all patients.

Histological

The diagnosis of GCTB was histologically confirmed pre-treatment in all cases. Histology showed a proliferation of mononuclear stromal cells, numerous macrophages and frequent scattered osteoclast-like giant cells, some of which were very large and contained a large number of nuclei (Fig. 6a).

Post-denosumab treatment findings

Clinical

Denosumab treatment was administrated for 3 months pre-surgery; it was generally well tolerated and the patients had no serious treatment-related adverse events. In all patients a decrease in wrist pain and improved wrist function was noted within 2 months of commencing denosumab therapy, with the average MMWS increasing to 75. The MMWS increased further to 85 at 3 months.

Radiological

Two months following the commencement of denosumab treatment, plain radiographs showed well-defined marginal sclerosis with reconstitution and mineralization of cortical bone in all cases. Varying degrees of internal matrix sclerosis and osseous consolidation resulted in increased radiopacity of the lesions (Figs. 1b, 2c, 3d, 5c). Cortical sclerosis resulted in mild cortical irregularity and modeling deformity involving the articular surface in two cases (Figs. 1b, 3d). The Campanacci grade 2 lesions showed no significant change in tumour size. The Campanacci grade 3 lesion showed a 15% increase in tumour volume in addition to considerable marginal and

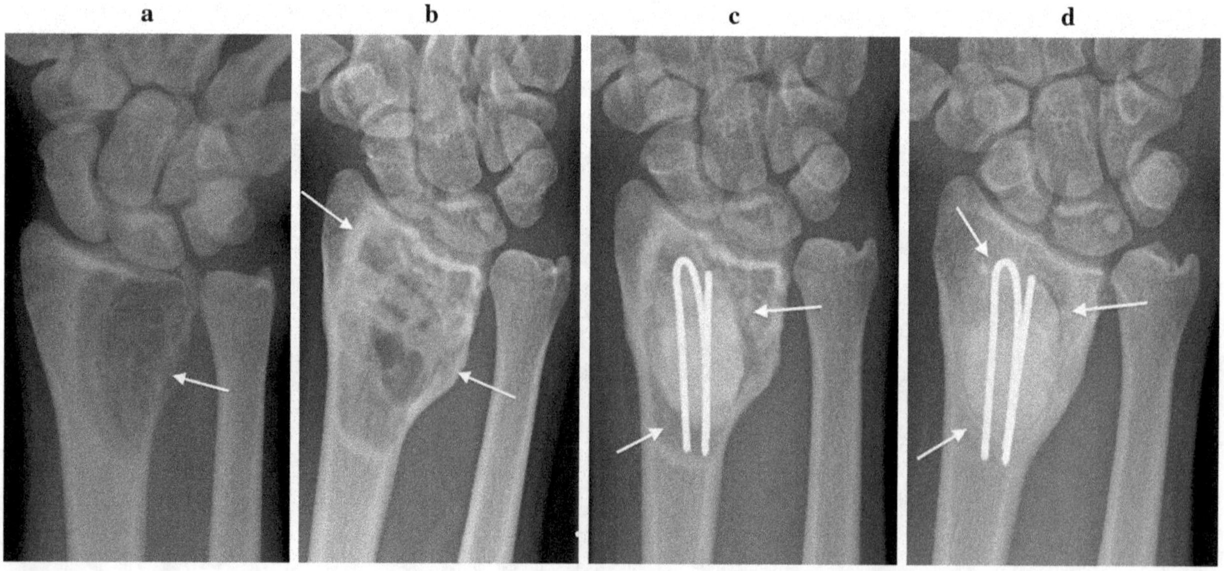

Fig. 1 Patient 1: pre denosumab, **a** frontal plain radiograph shows a lytic Campanacci grade 2 distal radial GCTB with mild expansion and cortical thinning (arrow). Post denosumab at 2 months, **b** frontal plain radiograph demonstrates sclerosis of the tumour margin (arrows) and radial articular surface. There is mild modeling deformity of the radial articular surface and moderate internal matrix osteosclerosis. Post surgical, **c** frontal plain radiograph 1 week post surgical curettage, cementoplasty and internal fixation shows lucency of the peripheral tumour cavity (arrows) and **d** 2 years post surgery with progressive infilling of the lesion with osteosclerosis around the cement despite no post operative denosumab therapy (arrows)

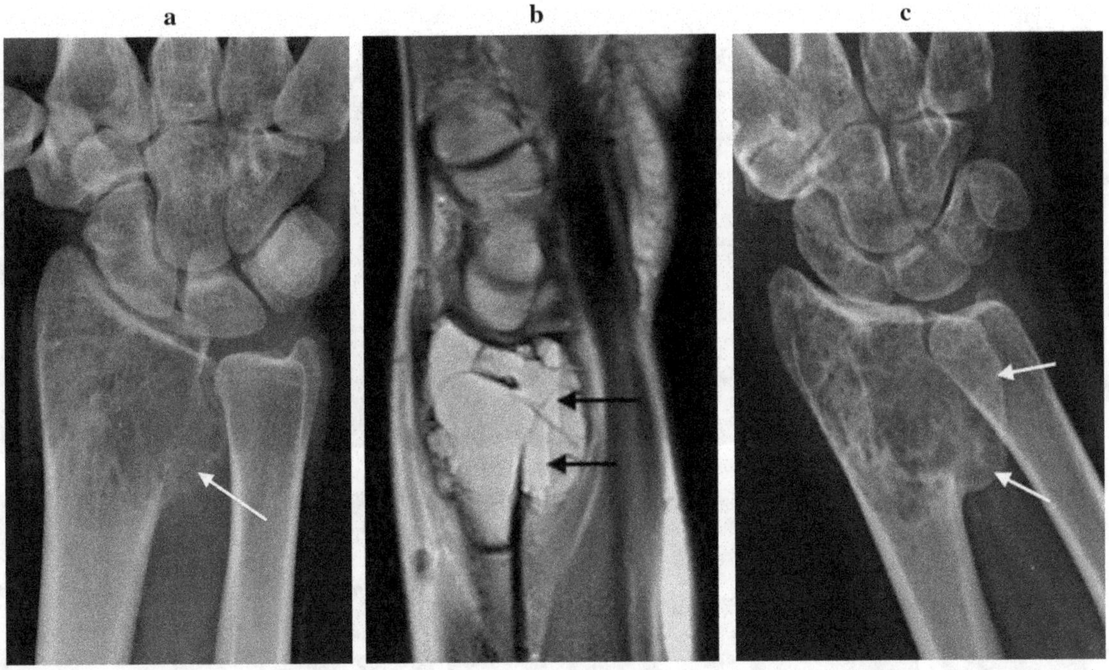

Fig. 2 Patient 2: pre denosumab, **a** frontal plain radiograph shows a lytic Campanacci grade 2 distal radial GCTB with medial expansion and cortical thinning (arrow). **b** Sagittal T2-weighted MR image demonstrates volar expansion and fluid fluid levels (arrows) indicating secondary aneurysmal bone cyst. Post denosumab at 2 months, **c** frontal plain radiograph demonstrates more clearly defined sclerotic tumour margins particularly along the expansile medial aspect of the lesion (arrows) and mild matrix osteosclerosis

matrix sclerosis after 2 months of denosumab treatment (Fig. 5c). MRI showed increased low signal marginal sclerosis with clearer definition of cortical margins (Fig. 3e, f). The articular surface appeared intact in all cases with no soft tissue mass. There was no significant change in T1 weighted signal (Fig. 3f). T2 weighted signal appeared more heterogeneous post-treatment with new areas of internal low T2 signal along with multiple central non-enhancing areas post-gadolinium (Figs. 3e, 4d). PET/CT confirmed radiologic evidence of bone repair with marginal and intralesional osteosclerosis in all patients. The average SUV at 2 months after commencing denosumab decreased to 4.7 (Figs. 4e, 5d; Table 1).

Histological

Histopathological examination of the treated GCTBs showed an absence of osteoclasts and an increase in well-vascularized cellular fibrous and fibrosseous tissue with focal areas of osteoid and woven bone formation (Fig. 6b); these were of variable thickness and shape and covered partly by bone lining cells. There were scattered macrophage-like cells but no giant cells were observed. There was no mitotic activity or nuclear pleomorphism of stromal cells, which appeared reduced in number within cellular fibrous tissue. The lesions were surrounded by organised reactive bone.

Outcome following denosumab treatment and salvage surgery

Curettage of the GCTB with insertion of PMMA cement was performed an average of 28 days after cessation of denosumab treatment. Internal fixation was used in one case due to bone destruction that necessitated support of the distal radial joint surface (Fig. 1c). There were no intraoperative complications.

Average follow-up was 37 months (Table 1). Four patients had a good clinical and functional outcome with no post-surgery complications or evidence of recurrence. One of these patients demonstrated progressive infilling of the tumour with osteosclerosis around the cement on plain radiographs over 2 years (Fig. 1d) despite no further denosumab therapy; this did not result in increased symptoms. One patient with the Campanacci grade 3 lesion had local tumor recurrence 2 months post-surgery; this was evident from radiographic imaging which showed progressive bone destruction with involvement of the radio-carpal joint (Fig. 5e). Resection of the distal radius with a vascularized free fibular graft (VFFG) and joint reconstruction was performed 7 months after initial surgery in this case. Twenty-three months after this intervention there has been no evidence of recurrence.

None of the patients has shown evidence of distal disease.

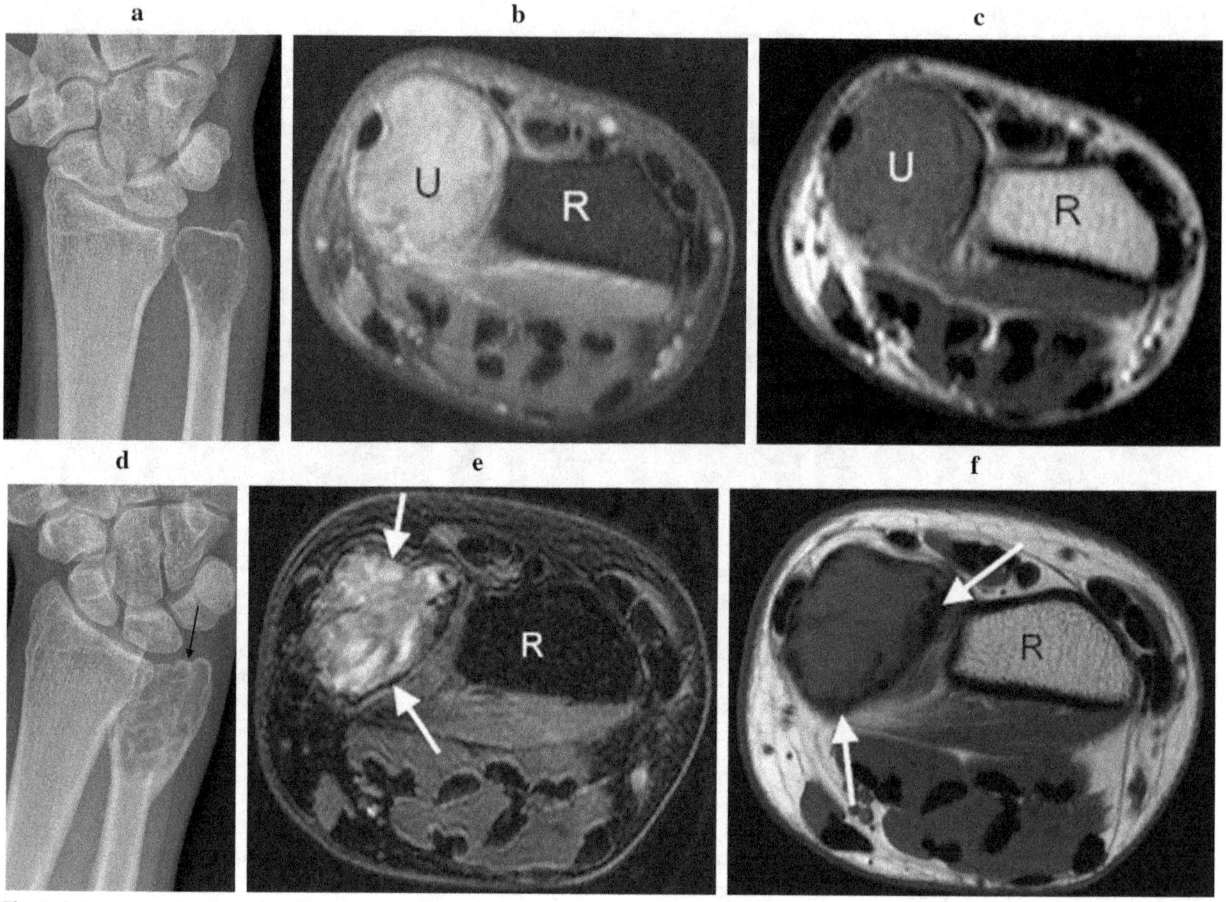

Fig. 3 Patient 3: pre denosumab, **a** frontal plain radiograph demonstrates a Campanacci grade 2 distal ulnar GCTB with mild expansion and cortical thinning. **b** Axial T2-weighted fat saturated and **c** axial T1-weighted MR images confirm an expansile heterogeneous predominantly high T2- and low to isointense T1-weighted distal ulnar lesion (*U* ulnar, *R* radius). Post denosumab at 2 months, **d** frontal plain radiograph shows marginal sclerosis and internal matrix sclerosis, with mild modeling deformity of the ulnar articular surface (black arrow). **e** Axial T2-weighted fat saturated and **f** axial T1-weighted MR images show definition of cortical margins with the formation of marginal sclerosis seen as peripheral low T1 and T2-W signal (white arrows). The tumour matrix is more heterogeneous with areas of low T2-W signal reflecting internal matrix consolidation (*R* radius)

Discussion

GCTB is a benign but locally aggressive tumour that occurs most commonly in a relatively young patient population. The distal radius is the third most common location where GCTB develops and, as in other sites, curettage of the tumour and cementation is often employed as first-line treatment [12, 16, 19–21]. However, distal radius/ulna GCTBs frequently recur following this treatment, usually within the first 2 years [22] and complex reconstructive surgery is often required, not only to limit local recurrence but also to preserve functional anatomy [12, 23].

There are a few previous case reports describing the effect of denosumab treatment on GCTB of the distal radius. A beneficial effect of denosumab was noted on a GCTB of the distal radius [24] and a locally aggressive giant cell-containing lesion of the radius diagnosed as aneurysmal bone cyst, a lesion which is also known to contain stromal cells that express RANKL [25, 26]. Matcuk et al. [27] noted rapid recurrence and aggressive growth of a GCTB after the cessation of long-term denosumab therapy, indicating that surgery is important in managing these tumours. This is the first case series examining the effect of a pre-operative short course of denosumab treatment on GCTB in bones of the distal forearm. As such, there are no guidelines on patient selection or optimal treatment in terms of dose and duration of denosumab administration; our denosumab schedule was based on previous phase 2 studies [6, 18, 28]. Denosumab was well tolerated in our cases, none of whom reported any of the known side effects of this drug [7, 8, 18].

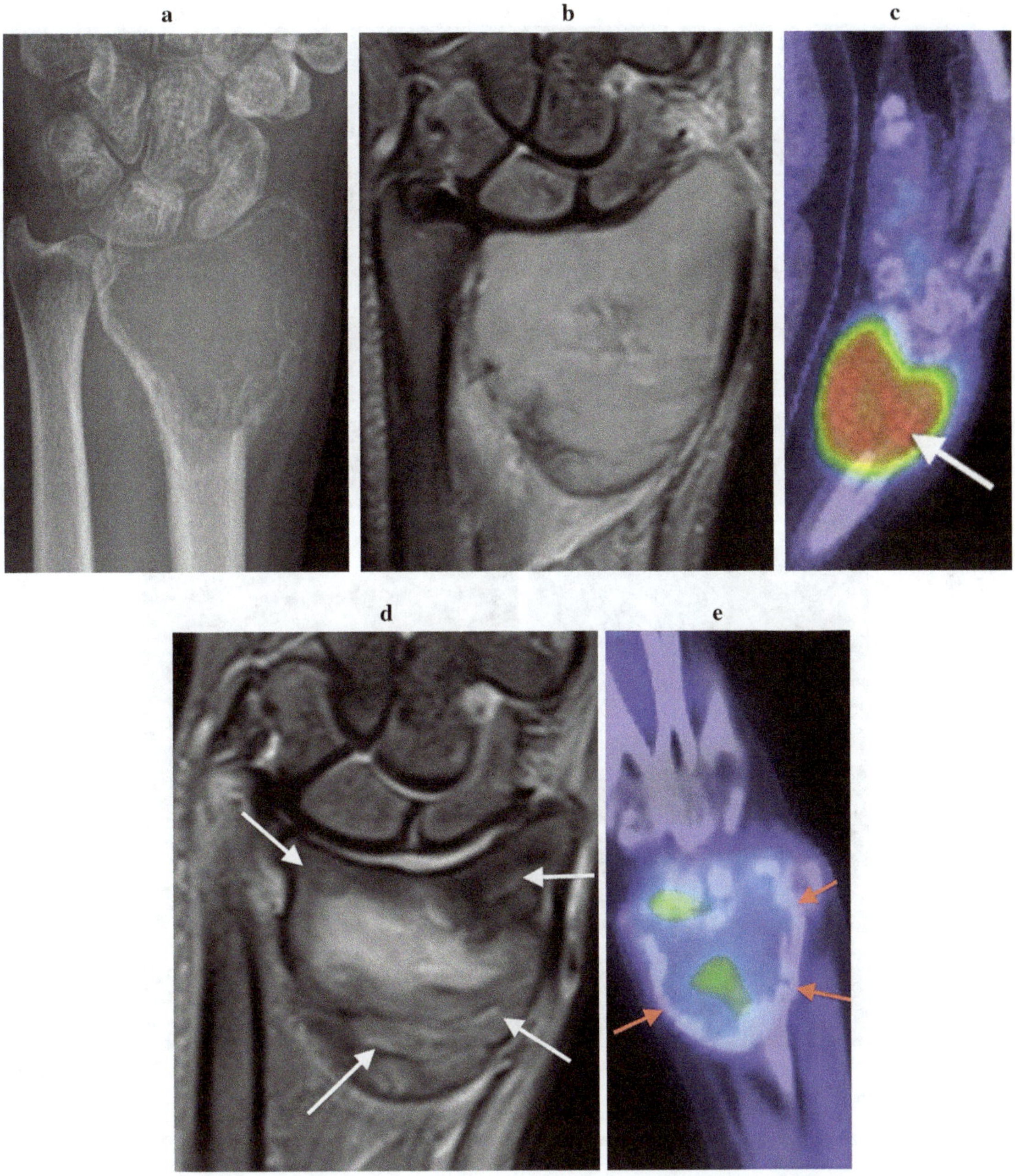

Fig. 4 Patient 4: pre denosumab, **a** frontal plain radiograph demonstrates a lytic expansile Campanacci grade 2 distal radial GCTB with cortical thinning. **b** Coronal STIR MR image shows the lesion returns heterogeneous predominantly high STIR MR signal. **c** Fused PET/CT image illustrates marked FDG uptake with a standardized uptake value (SUV) of 17 (arrow). Post denosumab at 2 months, **d** coronal STIR MR image shows increased heterogeneity of MR signal with areas of low STIR signal reflecting matrix osteosclerosis (white arrows). **e** Fused PET/CT image confirms a significant decrease in FDG uptake with an SUV of 4.8 and the formation of marginal sclerosis (red arrows)

The origin of pain in GCTB is multifactorial including mechanical stress from tumour related pressure, tumour growth with expansion of the periosteum, the loss of structurally significant bone and mechanical failure. The production of prostaglandins, endothelins and other noxious factors by the tumour cells are also known to result in pain [28]. Clinically, all five patients showed a significant decrease in wrist pain within 8 weeks of commencing denosumab therapy. This is in keeping with previous studies, which reported a clinically relevant decrease in pain with low or no analgesic use in most patients within 2 months of commencing denosumab therapy [6, 18, 28].

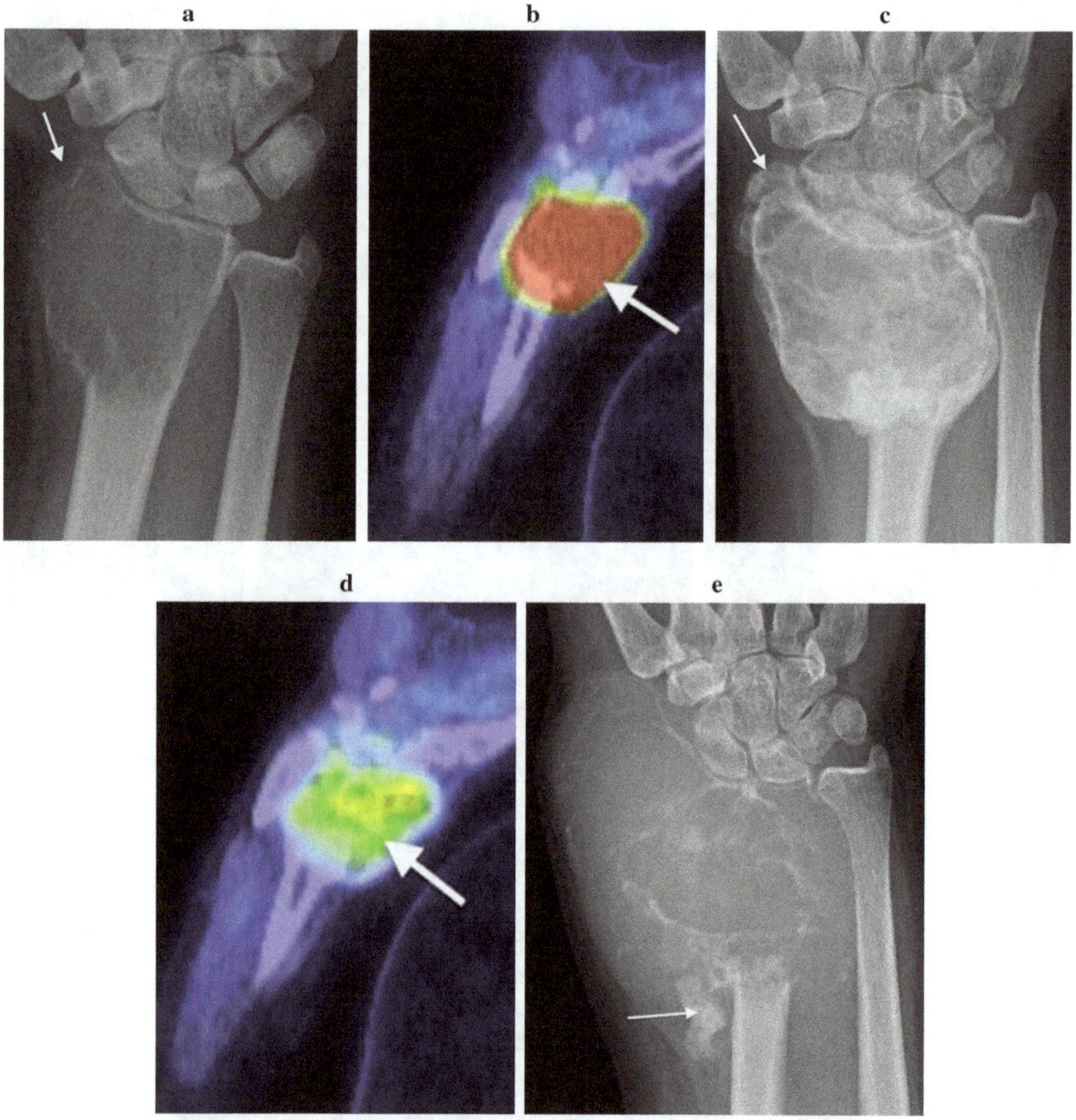

Fig. 5 Patient 5: pre denosumab, **a** frontal plain radiograph illustrates a distal radial GCTB with moderate expansion and cortical thinning. A breach of the radial styloid articular surface (arrow) with soft tissue extending into the carpal joint was confirmed on MR imaging and this lesion was graded as Campanacci grade 3. **b** Fused PET/CT image confirms marked metabolic activity with an increased SUV of 19.5 (arrow). Post denosumab at 2 months, **c** frontal plain radiograph demonstrates an increase in size of the lesion despite marginal sclerosis with reconstitution of the radial articular surface (arrow) and quite marked intralesional matrix consolidation. **d** Fused PET/CT image confirms reduced activity of the lesion with a significant decrease in the SUV to 4.5 (arrow). Post surgical, **e** frontal plain radiograph 2 months post surgery shows tumour recurrence with rapid growth, progressive bone destruction and extrusion of cement (arrow)

Improved wrist mobility and function was also noted in all patients within 8 weeks of denosumab therapy as seen in prior studies [6, 28].

Radiological features indicative of a positive response to denosumab are marginal sclerosis of the tumour and cortical thickening which was clearly seen all patients after 2 months of denosumab treatment. Similar radiological findings have been described in other studies where denosumab treatment ranged from 2 months to 2 years [27, 29–33]. One of our cases demonstrated reconstitution of cortical bone with repair of a focal defect in the articular surface. Intralesional consolidation was more variable with mild to more marked matrix osteosclerosis. In our cases, marginal and intralesional osteosclerosis was best appreciated on plain radiographs and the CT component of the PET/CT. PET/CT also revealed a decrease in

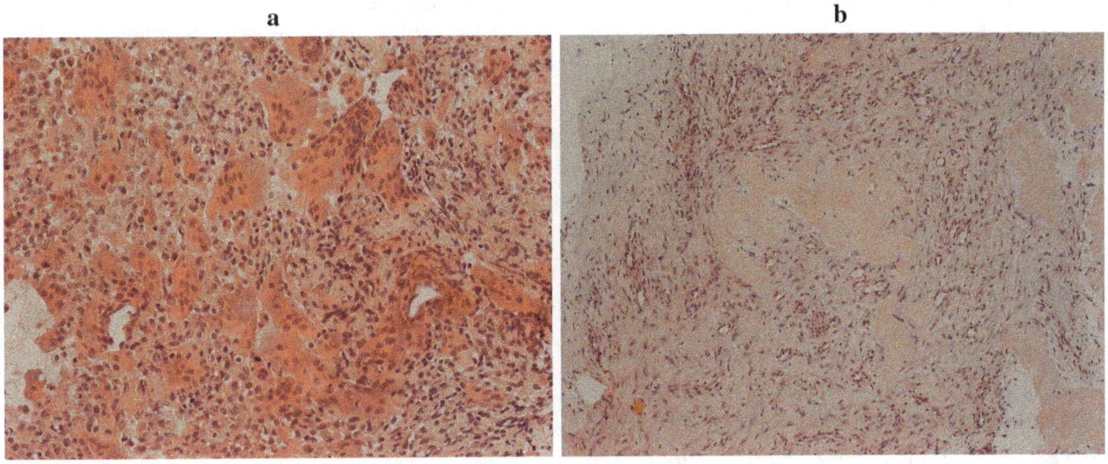

Fig. 6 Histology: pre denosumab, **a** numerous osteoclast-like giant cells, some of which have a very large number of nuclei, and surrounding mononuclear cells. Post denosumab, **b** well-vascularised fibrous tissue in which there is focal osteoid/woven bone formation and absence of osteoclasts

average SUV from 14.8 pre-treatment to 4.7 at 2 months, indicating that PET/CT may be a sensitive monitor for the response to denosumab. MRI did not aid in evaluating the efficacy of denosumab therapy, although increased tumour heterogeneity on T2-weighted images with areas of decreased gadolinium uptake were observed. MRI findings of increased intralesional heterogeneity, cortical thickening and irregularity and linear perilesional fluid like signal following short term denosumab therapy have previously been described and misinterpreted as disease progression [33]. These MR features were present in our cases and represent an appropriate response to denosumab treatment. It has been suggested that increased MRI tumour heterogeneity and T2 low signal may reflect central necrosis and osteosclerosis in the tumour [29, 30]. Histopathological findings in our denosumab treated cases did not show evidence of necrosis but did show prominent intralesional ossification and fibrosis, disappearance of osteoclastic giant cells and a reduction in the number of mononuclear stromal cells, as previously described [6, 29, 30, 34, 35].

In one of our cases, ongoing post operative infilling and sclerosis was noted around the cement on plain radiographs despite no post-operative denosumab treatment. This case continues to have an excellent clinical and radiological response with no evidence of recurrent symptoms or tumour 3 years and 9 months post surgery. The findings in this case suggest that there may be some continued response to short term denosumab therapy.

An overall reduction in GCTB size has been noted following denosumab treatment for an average duration of 15.3 (12.1–23.6) months [17]. In our series none of the lesions decreased in size when imaged after 2 months of denosumab treatment and the Campanacci grade 3 lesion was larger than on presentation radiographs.

Local recurrence occurred in one case, the Campanacci grade 3 lesion that had aggressive radiological features pre-denosumab with involvement of the cortex, breach of the radial styloid articular surface and a small soft tissue mass evident on MRI. In this case, after 2 months of denosumab treatment, despite an overall increase in tumour size, disappearance of the soft tissue component and reconstitution of the articular cortex, was noted, as well as matrix osteosclerosis and reduced metabolic activity on PET (SUV 19.5–4.5). This allowed the patient the opportunity of initial surgical curettage with the chance for an improved functional outcome.

Previous studies have shown that denosumab results in a decrease in tumour progression, with surgical down-staging to a less morbid surgical salvage procedure than originally planned in 38% (n = 84/222; average duration of denosumab treatment 15.3 months) and 61% (n = 16/26; average duration of denosumab treatment 6 months) of patients [17, 18]. In our experience of treating GCTBs with neoadjuvant denosumab, we found that treatment for more than 3 months often resulted in marked intralesional sclerosis and extensive perilesional new bone formation. This makes curettage of some GCTBs more difficult, and, as noted by some observers [36], can create uncertainty with regard to the adequacy of tumour excision. In this study we show that a short course of denosumab results in reconstitution of cortical and subarticular bone and sufficient marginal sclerosis to define the tumour margin whilst not causing marked intralesional sclerosis. The sarcoma surgeon who treated all cases, was of the opinion that this treatment regime facilitated curettage of the lesion with preservation of the native joint, local functional anatomy and wrist function.

It has been suggested that, although the newly formed bone at the tumour periphery allows for a sufficient mechanical scaffold for curettage to be done without fear of the bone collapsing, this rim of sclerotic bone may contain neoplastic stromal cells that may become active and express RANKL after denosumab treatment is stopped [36]. Another advantage of performing curettage earlier following a short course of denosumab is prevention of too thick a rim of peripheral bone from being formed; this decreases the chances of neoplastic tissue being left behind post-curettage in the thickened rim of perilesional new bone thus facilitating complete tumour removal. A recent study of 35 patients with locally advanced Campanacci grade 3 GCTB supports a short course (3 months) of denosumab treatment prior to surgical curettage; however, postulates that a longer duration of denosumab therapy should be administered for en bloc tumour resection, which may be facilitated by more marked tumour sclerosis with a lower risk of recurrence [35].

Conclusion

Our results indicate that GCTB of the distal forearm responds clinically, radiologically and histologically within 3 months of denosumab treatment. Short term denosumab was well tolerated and thought to facilitate surgical curettage in all cases, with preservation of the native joint and a good surgical outcome apart from one case of recurrence in a Campanacci grade 3 lesion. Limitations of this study include its retrospective nature, and clearly small sample size. However, the rarity of GCTB, especially with regard to a particular anatomic site makes the reporting of larger numbers challenging in a single institution. Co-ordinated, multi-institutional studies are likely to be needed in order to fully assess this treatment regime and whether a short course of neoadjuvant denosumab would be similarly effective for GCTBs in other bones.

Abbreviations

GCTB: giant cell tumour of bone; RANKL: receptor activator of nuclear factor kappa-B ligand; PMMA: polymethylmethacrylate; MMWS: modified Mayo Wrist Score (MMWS); MRI: magnetic resonance imaging; PET/CT: positron emission tomography with fluorodeoxyglucose integrated with computed tomography; STIR: short tau inversion recovery; SUV: standardized uptake value; VFFG: vascularized free fibular graft.

Authors' contributions

CM collected, analysed and interpreted the data, plain radiographs and magnetic resonance imaging, and was a major contributor in writing the manuscript. MG performed surgical curettage and cementoplasty, analyzed and interpreted patient data, and contributed to the writing the manuscript. KB analyzed and interpreted the PET/CT scans. BH administered the denosumab and acquired clinical data. HG performed the vascularised free fibular graft and joint reconstruction in the tumour recurrence. NA performed the biopsy and surgical curettage histological examinations, and was a major contributor in writing the manuscript. All authors read and approved the final manuscript.

Acknowledgements

The authors thank Sarah Turton for typing the manuscript. This study was supported by the European Union as part of EuroSarc (FP7-27842) and EuroBoNeT (FP6-18814) consortiums.

Competing interests

The authors declare that they have no competing interests.

Funding

No funding was received.

References

1. Thomas DM, Skubitz KM. Giant cell tumour of bone. Curr Opin Oncol. 2009;21:338–44.
2. Athanasou NA, Bansal M, Forsyth R, Reid RP, Sapi Z. Giant cell tumour of bone. In: Fletcher CDM, Bridge JA, Hogendoorn PCW, Mertens F, editors. WHO classification of tumours of soft tissue and bone. 4th ed. Lyon: International Agency for Research on Cancer; 2013. p. 321–4.
3. Unni KK. Dahlin's bone tumours: general aspects and data on 11,087 cases. New York: Lippincott-Raven; 1996.
4. Roux S, Amazit L, Meduri G, Guiochon-Mantel A, Milgrom E, Mariette X. RANK (receptor activator of nuclear factor kappa B) and RANK ligand are expressed in giant cell tumors of bone. Am J Clin Pathol. 2002;117:210–6.
5. Lau YS, Sabokbar A, Gibbons CL, Giele H, Athanasou N. Phenotypic and molecular studies of giant-cell tumours of bone and soft tissue. Hum Pathol. 2005;36:945–54.
6. Thomas D, Henshaw R, Skubitz K, Chawla S, Staddon A, Blay JY, Roudier M, Smith J, Ye Z, Sohn W, Dansey R, Jun S. Denosumab in patients with giant-cell tumour of bone: an open-label, phase 2 study. Lancet Oncol. 2010;11:275–80.
7. Thomas DM. RANKL, denosumab, and giant cell tumor of bone. Curr Opin Oncol. 2012;24:397–403.
8. Skubitz KM. Giant cell tumor of bone: current treatment options. Curr Treat Options Oncol. 2014;15(3):507–18.
9. Campanacci M, Baldini N, Boriani S, Sudanese A. Giant-cell tumour of bone. J Bone Jt Surg Am. 1987;69:106–14.
10. Balke M, Schremper L, Gerbert C, et al. Giant cell tumours of bone: treatment and outcome of 214 cases. J Cancer Res Clin Oncol. 2008;134(9):969–78.
11. Kivioja AH, Blomqvist C, Hietaniemi K, et al. Cement is recommended in intralesional surgery of giant cell tumours; a Scandinavian sarcoma group study of 294 patients followed for a median time of 5 years. Acta Orthop. 2008;79:86–93.
12. Van der Heijden L, Dijkstra PD, van de Sande MA, et al. The clinical approach toward giant cell tumor of bone. Oncologist. 2014;19:550–61.
13. Klenke FM, Wenger DE, Inwards CY, Rose PS, Sim FH. Giant cell tumor of bone: risk factors for recurrence. Clin Orthop Relat Res. 2011;469:591–9.
14. Becker WT, Dohle J, Bernd L, et al. Local recurrence of giant cell tumor of bone after intralesional treatment with and without adjuvant therapy. J Bone Jt Surg Am. 2008;90:1060–7.
15. Van der Griend RA, Funderburk CH. The treatment of giant-cell tumours in the distal part of the radius. J Bone Jt Surg Am. 1993;75:899–908.
16. Harness NG, Mankin HJ. Giant-cell tumour of the distal forearm. J Hand Surg Am. 2004;29:188–93.
17. Rutkowski P, Ferrari S, Grimer RJ, et al. Surgical downstaging in an open label phase II trial of denosumab in patients with giant cell tumour of bone. Ann Surg Oncol. 2015;22:2860–8.
18. Chawla S, Henshaw R, Seeger L, Choy E, Blay JY, Ferrari S, et al. Safety and efficacy of denosumab for adults and skeletally mature adolescents with giant cell tumour of bone: interim analysis of an open-label, parallel-group, phase 2 study. Lancet Oncol. 2013;14:901–8.
19. Sheth DS, Healey H, Sobel M, Lane JM, Marcove RC. Giant cell tumour of the distal radius. J Hand Surg. 1995;20A:432–40.
20. Lui YP, Li KH, Sun BH. Which treatment is best for giant cell tumours of the distal radius? A meta-analysis. Clin Orthop Relat Res. 2012;470:2886–94.
21. Blackley HR, Wunder JS, Davis AM, White LM, Kandel R, Bell RS. Treatment of giant-cell tumors of long bones with curettage and bone-grafting. J Bone Jt Surg Am. 1999;81:811–20.
22. Klenke FM, Wenger DE, Inwards CY, Rose PS, Sim FH. Recurrent giant cell tumor of long bones: analysis of surgical management. Clin Orthop Relat Res. 2011;469:1181–7.

23. Humail SM, Ghulam MK, Zaidi IH. Reconstruction of the distal radius with non-vascularised fibular graft after resection of giant cell tumour of bone. J Orthop Surg (Hong Kong). 2014;22:356–9.
24. Park MJ, Ganjoo KN, Ladd AL. Denosumab, a potential alternative to the surgical treatment of distal radius giant cell tumour of bone: case report. J Hand Surg Am. 2015;40:1620–4.
25. Pauli C, Fuchs B, Pfirrmann C, Bridge JA, Hofer S, Bode B. Response of an aggressive periosteal aneurysmal bone cyst of the radius to denosumab therapy. World J Surg Oncol. 2014;12:17.
26. Taylor RM, Kashima TG, Hemingway FK, Dongre A, Knowles HJ, Athanasou NA. CD14-mononuclear stromal cells support (CD14+) monocyte-osteoclast differentiation in aneurysmal bone cyst. Lab Invest. 2012;92:600–5.
27. Matcuk GR, Patel DB, Schein AJ, White EA, Menendez LR. Giant cell tumour: rapid recurrence after cessation of long term denosumab therapy. Skelet Radiol. 2015;44:1027–31.
28. Martin-Broto J, Cleeland CS, Glare PA, et al. Effects of denosumab on pain and analgesic use in giant cell tumor of bone: interim results from a phase II study. Acta Oncol. 2014;53(9):1173–9.
29. Hakozaki M, Tajino T, Yamada H, et al. Radiological and pathological characteristics of giant cell tumour of bone treated with denosumab. Diagn Pathol. 2014;9:111.
30. Branstetter DG, Nelson SD, Manivel JC, Blay JY, Chawla S, Thomas DM, Jun S, Jacobs I. Denosumab induces tumor reduction and bone formation in patients with giant-cell tumor of bone. Clin Cancer Res. 2012;18:4415–24.
31. Chakarun CJ, Forrester DM, Gottsegen CJ, Patel DB, White EA, Matcuk GR Jr. Giant cell tumor of bone: review, mimics, and new developments in treatment. Radiographics. 2013;33:197–211.
32. Akaike K, Suehara Y, Takagi T, et al. An eggshell-like mineralized recurrent lesion in the popliteal region after treatment of giant cell tumor of the bone with denosumab. Skelet Radiol. 2014;43:1767–72.
33. Von Borstel DO, Taguibao RA, Strle NA, Burns JE. Giant cell tumour of the bone: aggressive case initially treated with denosumab and intralesional surgery. Skelet Radiol. 2017;46:571–8.
34. Girolami I, Mancini I, Simoni A, et al. Denosumab treated giant cell tumour of bone: a morphological, immunohistochemical and molecular analysis of a series. J Clin Pathol. 2016;69:240–7.
35. Borkowska A, Goryn T, Pienkowski A, et al. Denosumab treatment of inoperable or locally advanced giant cell tumour of bone. Oncol Lett. 2016;12:4312–8.
36. Gaston CL, Grimer RJ, Parry M, Stacchiotti S, Dei Tos AP, Gelderblom H, et al. Current status and unanswered questions on the use of denosumab in giant cell tumour of bone. Clin Sarcoma Res. 2016;6:15.

23

Aggressive fibromatosis response to tamoxifen: lack of correlation between MRI and symptomatic response

M. Libertini[1], I. Mitra[1,2], W. T. A. van der Graaf[1,3], A. B. Miah[1,3], I. Judson[1,3], R. L. Jones[1,3], K. Thomas[2], E. Moskovic[1,3], Z. Szucs[1], C. Benson[1] and C. Messiou[1,2,3*]

Abstract

Background: One of the commonly used systemic agents for the treatment of aggressive fibromatosis is the anti-oestrogen drug tamoxifen. However, data on efficacy and optimum methods of response assessment are limited, consisting mainly of small case series and reports.

Methods: A retrospective database was used to identify consecutive patients diagnosed with aggressive fibromatosis (AF) and treated with tamoxifen plus/minus non-steroidal anti-inflammatory drugs at our tertiary referral centre between 2007 and 2014. MRI and symptom changes were recorded.

Results: Thirty-two patients (13 male 19 female, median age 41 years) were included. Median duration of treatment with tamoxifen was 316 days. Of 9 patients with progressive disease by RECIST 1.1 (28%): 4 patients experienced worsening symptoms; 3 patients had improved symptoms and 2 had no change in symptoms. Of 22 patients with stable disease (69%): 11 had no change in symptoms; 6 had improved symptoms and 5 patients had worsening symptoms. One patient achieved a partial response with improved symptoms.

Conclusions: No relationship was identified between symptomatic benefit and response by RECIST 1.1 on MRI. Prospective studies in AF should incorporate endpoints focusing on patient symptoms.

Keywords: Aggressive fibromatosis, Anti-oestrogen therapy, Symptoms, MRI features, T2 weighted signal

Background

Aggressive fibromatosis (AF), also named desmoid-type fibromatosis, is characterised by monoclonal myofibroblastic proliferation in soft tissues. It is a rare disease accounting for 3% of all soft tissue neoplasms, with an incidence of 2–5 people per million per year [1]. It has a female predominance and a peak incidence in the third to fourth decades [2]. AF is often sporadic, however, there is a reported increased incidence of 3.5–32% in patients with familial adenomatous polyposis (FAP) or Gardner's variant [3, 4]. AF is usually solitary but multifocal tumours have been reported [5]. It may arise from any anatomical site, commonly the extremities, abdominal and chest wall and paravertebral tissues [6, 7]. Although AF is slow growing without metastatic potential, its unpredictable behaviour, propensity for progressive infiltration and local invasion makes treatment challenging. Currently there is no established evidence-based approach to treatment [8], although a consensus approach based on wide consultation with physicians and patient groups has been published [9]. Active surveillance is now often used in asymptomatic cases [10]. High local recurrence rates of 15–50% [11–14] up to 87% [15] in younger patients, despite apparently complete resection, have reduced the popularity of surgical resection as initial management. Radiotherapy can help improve local control [16] however, side effects, including radiation-induced malignancies have to be considered especially in young patients [17].

*Correspondence: Christina.Messiou@rmh.nhs.uk
[2] Department of Radiology, The Royal Marsden NHS Foundation Trust, 203 Fulham Road, London SW3 6JJ, UK

Drugs used in the treatment of AF, include hormonal therapy (e.g. tamoxifen and toremifene) [18], Non steroidal antinflammatory drugs (NSAIDs) and cytotoxic chemotherapeutic agents, such as anthracycline-based regimens [19] (including pegylated liposomal doxorubicin [20]) and vinblastine plus methotrexate [21]. Tyrosine kinase inhibitors, including imatinib [22], sorafenib [23] and pazopanib [24] can also play a role in the treatment of AF. A recent phase I study demonstrated demonstrated promising efficacy of a γ-secretase inhibitor in desmoid tumours [25].

For many centres, first line systemic treatment of non-resectable or symptomatic desmoid-type fibromatosis consists of hormonal manipulation, with or without a NSAID. Particularly in centres within the United Kingdom, this is heavily influenced by lack of reimbursed alternatives, availability and the low side effect profile. Immunohistochemical studies have demonstrated the presence of oestrogen receptor-beta in 90% of desmoid-type tumours [26]. This is supported by the tendency of fibromatosis to occur more often in women, particularly during pregnancy/within 1 year post partum [27], or on oral contraception, and there are reports of spontaneous regression during menopause and post-partum [2, 28]. Several publications have documented the effectiveness of hormonal manipulation in AF treatment [29–32]. Despite the lack of randomised prospective data, it has been reported that antioestrogen therapy can be effective in about half of patients [18]. Tamoxifen is a non-steroidal triphenylethylene derivative that binds to oestrogen receptors. One suggested mechanism for the anti-proliferative action of tamoxifen is regulation of the synthesis of the cytokine transforming growth factor-β (TGF-β) [32] and its receptors, which are also involved in AF pathogenesis.

There are several means of monitoring treatment response, including clinical evaluation of tumour size and symptoms as well as radiological. The Response Evaluation Criteria in Solid Tumours (RECIST 1.1) [33] are currently employed within clinical trials. Magnetic resonance imaging (MRI) has become the imaging modality of choice for soft tissue lesions, due to better evaluation of the tumour and its relationship with surrounding structures such as nerves and vessels. Given the chronic nature of the disease, the lack of radiation exposure makes MRI ideal for follow up studies. Furthermore, in lesions undergoing radiation or drug therapy, MR surveillance has been used to assess response to treatment with a decrease in T2-weighted signal and lesion size being suggested as indicators of treatment response [34].

The variable content of spindle cells, collagen and myxoid tissue of AF correlates with the observation that these lesions often show heterogeneous signals on MRI [35]. In particular, the highly cellular, actively growing lesions tend to be of high signal on T2-weighted MR images [6, 36, 37]. Interspersed low signal bands correspond with the collagen bundles. As the lesion matures, the increase in collagen deposition and decreased cellularity result in a decrease in T2 signal [38, 39]. However to date it has not been possible to predict behaviour based on MRI signal [40, 41].

The main aims of this study were to assess MRI response and symptom control in patients with AF treated with tamoxifen with or without NSAIDs.

Methods

Patient selection

The prospectively collected Royal Marsden Hospital sarcoma database was used to identify consecutive patients diagnosed with AF and treated with tamoxifen at our tertiary referral centre between 2007 and 2014. Institutional approval was obtained. Inclusion criteria were patients aged 18 years and over, treated with tamoxifen, with a baseline and at least one follow-up MRI scan. Demographic data, disease characteristics, previous treatments, date of starting and stopping tamoxifen, toxicity and clinical symptoms were collected from clinical notes. Descriptive statistical analysis was applied: progression-free survival (PFS) was calculated using the Kaplan–Meier method.

Imaging data

Baseline MRI images, defined as the last MRI performed prior to tamoxifen treatment, and subsequent follow up MRI images were identified for each patient. Where available a pre-baseline MRI was also collected. On average 3 (range 2–6) follow up MRIs were assessed for each patient. The minimum MRI protocol for inclusion in the study was axial T1W, T2W, STIR and coronal T2W and STIR images. All images were re-reviewed by a specialist soft tissue radiologist (CM). Tumour size, RECIST 1.1 assessment and T2-weighted signal changes were documented at each time point.

Results

Between 2007 and 2014 a total of 35 patients were treated with tamoxifen at the Royal Marsden Hospital. Baseline imaging was not available for 3 patients, and they were therefore not eligible for this study. Of the remaining 32 cases, the median age at the time of commencing tamoxifen was 41 years (range 19–68 years). There was a 3:2 female to male ratio [19 (60%): 13 (40%)]. One patient (3%) had a diagnosis of FAP. The most common site of origin was limb and limb girdle (18; 56%), followed by chest wall (5; 15%), pelvis (3; 10%), abdominal wall (3; 10%), paravertebral tissues (1; 3%) and head/neck (2; 6%).

Fourteen patients (44%) received tamoxifen as first-line treatment. Eighteen of 32 patients (56%) had been treated previously, with surgery, radiotherapy, steroid injections, NSAIDs or doxorubicin chemotherapy. Patient and disease characteristics are summarised in Table 1.

Tamoxifen treatment was started due to tumour growth and worsening symptoms, mostly characterised by pain, including neuropathic and somatic pain, and decreased range of movement. Four patients (12%) were asymptomatic at the time of starting tamoxifen.

The average length of time on tamoxifen was 316 days, ranging from 1 month to 3 years (33–997 days). Tamoxifen dosages used were 40 mg (15 patients), 20 mg (15 patients), 10 mg (1 patient) and unknown (1 patient). Twenty-four patients (75%) received tamoxifen in association with a NSAID (naproxen or diclofenac). Thirteen of the 32 patients (41%) suffered from tamoxifen-related side effects, most commonly hot flushes and mood swings. Two patients had their 40 mg dose reduced to 20 mg due to side effects. One of those was a 40-year old male who experienced increased tiredness and the other a 27-year old male who suffered from mood swings, fatigue and hot flushes.

The most common reasons for stopping tamoxifen were tumour progression (10, 31%), and grade 2–3 side effects (8, 25%), such as hot flushes, mood swings and fatigue. Four patients (13%) stopped due to lack of any perceived benefit and 3 (9%) due to worsening symptoms. One patient with stable disease stopped tamoxifen as she was planning on starting a family and she was aware of possible associated birth defects [42]. One patient stopped

Table 1 Patient and disease characteristics

	#	(%)	[range]
Number of patients	32		
Male	14	(40%)	
Female	19	(60%)	
Median age on starting tamoxifen	41		[19–68]
Site of origin			
Extremities (including girdle)	18	(56%)	
Chest wall	5	(15%)	
Pelvis	3	(10%)	
Abdominal wall	3	(10%)	
Paravertebral	1	(3%)	
Head and neck	2	(6%)	
Sporadic disease	31	(97%)	
FAP-associated	1	(3%)	
Previous treatments	18	(56%)	
Local treatment			
Surgery	10	(31%)	
Surgery and RT	7	(21%)	
RT alone	0		
Systemic treatment	4	(12%)	
No previous treatment	14	(44%)	

tamoxifen because of pregnancy. Two patients died for reasons unrelated to AF. One patient stopped tamoxifen due to side effects, and subsequently received an anti-tumour necrosis factor (anti-TNF)-α agent, adalimumab [43], for his rheumatoid arthritis and the AF decreased in size. Two patients continue on tamoxifen.

Tamoxifen with or without a NSAID, resulted in symptom improvement in 10 patients (31%)—5 patients on 40 mg tamoxifen, 4 patients on 20 mg tamoxifen and 1 patient on 10 mg tamoxifen (8 of these 10 patients were also taking NSAIDs). Worsening symptoms were experienced by 9 patients (28%)—2 patients on 40 mg tamoxifen, 6 patients on 20 mg tamoxifen and 1 unknown (6 of these 9 patients were also taking NSAIDs). Thirteen patients did not experience any change in symptoms (41%)—9 patients on 40 mg tamoxifen, 4 patients on 20 mg tamoxifen (10 of these 13 patients were also taking NSAIDs). The majority of patients with symptomatic benefit did not have significant changes in size or signal on MRI (Fig. 1a, b).

The median tumour size on starting tamoxifen was 60 mm (range 23–165 mm). There was a varied response in tumour size. Eighteen patients (56%) had increase in tumour size, 6 patients (19%) had a reduction in tumour size and 8 patients (25%) had no change in tumour size. By RECIST 1.1, 9 patients (28%) had progressive disease—6 patients on 40 mg tamoxifen, 2 patients on 20 mg tamoxifen and 1 unknown; 22 patients (69%) had stable disease—8 patients on 40 mg tamoxifen, 13 patients on 20 mg tamoxifen, 1 patient on 10 mg tamoxifen and 1 patient (3%) had a partial response—40 mg tamoxifen. Median progression-free survival (PFS) per RECIST 1.1 was 10 months with (95% CI 6.4–24.6); PFS at 1 and 2 years was 50% (95% CI 32–66) and 34% (95% CI 19–51), respectively (Fig. 2), with a median follow-up of 45.5 months (range 14–105).

We divided our series into three RECIST 1.1 criteria-based groups: progressive disease, stable disease and partial response. Of 9 patients with progressive disease (28%): 4 patients experienced worsening symptoms with increased pain; 3 patients had an improvement in pain and increase in range of movement and no change in symptoms was observed in the remaining 2 patients. T2 signal increase was observed in 1 case, which correlated with clinical deterioration; in 8 of 9 cases there was no change in T2 signal. Of 22 patients with stable disease (69%): 11 had no change in symptoms with T2 signal reduction in 3 cases and increase in 1; 6 experienced symptom improvement: 1 of 6 had a correlating T2 signal reduction. Five patients complained of worsening symptoms without any change in T2 signal.

One patient achieved a partial response (3%). This patient was a 35-year old male affected by AF involving

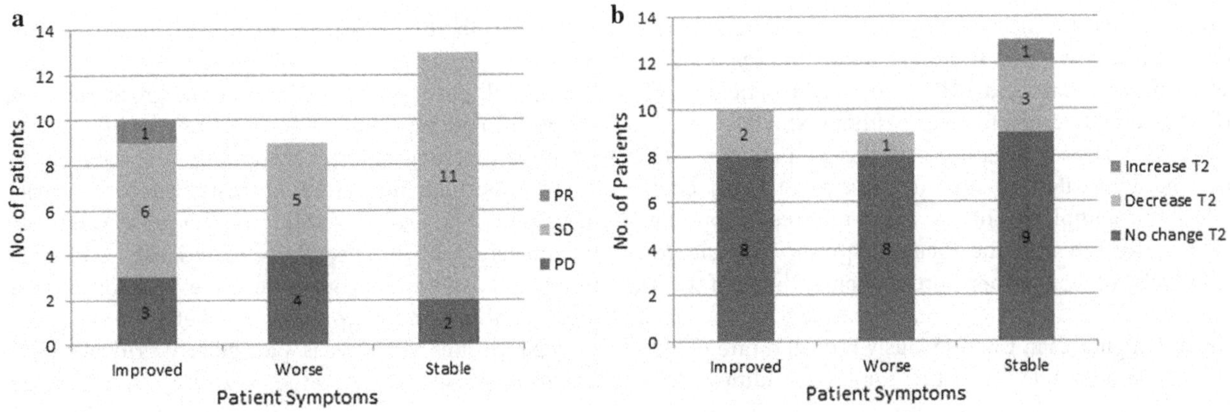

Fig. 1 Barcharts of patient symptoms and corresponding RECIST 1.1 status (**a**) and T2W MRI signal changes (**b**)

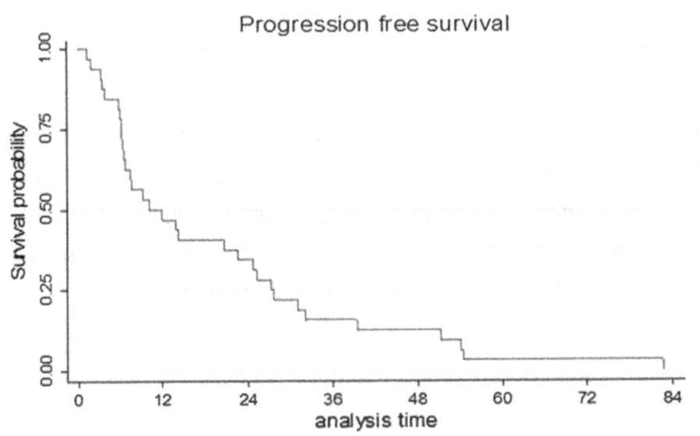

Fig. 2 Kaplan–Meier progression free survival analysis after treatment with tamoxifen. Median PFS was 10 months (95% CI 6.4–24.6)

the right anterior abdominal wall with abdominal pain at baseline. This patient is still on treatment, and has completed 476 days of therapy at the time of analysis. After 18 months of treatment, he experienced an improvement in symptoms with a reduction in pain. The symptomatic improvement corresponded with a decrease in size and T2 signal on MRI (Fig. 3).

Additional pre-baseline MRI scans were available for 14 patients. Thirteen out of 14 patients' tumours were increasing in size prior to starting tamoxifen. Six continued to increase following tamoxifen; 5 showed some decrease in size; 2 became stable having demonstrated growth prior to starting tamoxifen.

Discussion

Aggressive fibromatosis is a challenging disease with an unpredictable behaviour. The unsatisfactory outcomes of surgery and the fact that growth arrest and regression can occur spontaneously have led to the increased adoption of active surveillance as the initial approach to management [44]. However hormonal manipulation has been commonly used particularly in the United Kingdom as first-line systemic therapy in AF [10].

Our study of 32 patients is limited by the retrospective design and the collection of symptomatic changes by

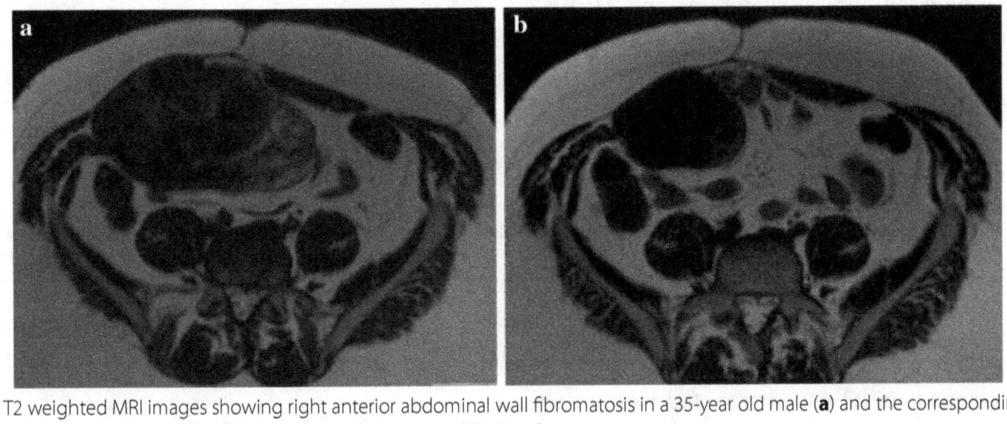

Fig. 3 Axial T2 weighted MRI images showing right anterior abdominal wall fibromatosis in a 35-year old male (**a**) and the corresponding MRI after 7 months of treatment with tamoxifen (**b**) show decrease in size and T2 signal

retrospective case note review rather than prospective dedicated questionnaires. However, to our knowledge, this is the largest single series evaluating the relationship between symptoms and MRI response in patients with AF treated with tamoxifen with/without NSAIDs.

Within this case series, 14 of the 32 patients (44%) received tamoxifen as first-line treatment. This could reflect the complexity of the cases referred to our tertiary centre but also the focus on preserving function and quality of life. Furthermore, we found that 8 of the 32 patients (25%) had to stop tamoxifen due to side effects, which is higher than the previously reported rate of 10% [45] and remarkable given the, for this condition, relatively low dose of tamoxifen prescribed in our patients [29, 46].

In our series 18 of the 32 patients (56%) had an increase in tumour size and among these, 28% were defined as disease progression by RECIST 1.1. This is in keeping with the rates of disease progression stated in a systematic review [18]. However, our stable disease and partial response rates of 69 and 3% respectively, do not correlate with the 18 and 58% rates previously quoted, raising the possibility of an overestimation in the reported efficacy of tamoxifen in AF. Importantly, 31% of patients did report symptomatic benefit, although the positive contribution of NSAIDs cannot be excluded. Seventy-five percent of cases in this series were treated with concomitant NSAIDs, which may have influenced the results, since prostaglandin blockage has been shown to provide some benefit in the treatment of AF [47].

Interestingly, one patient treated with a fully human monoclonal antibody tumor necrosis factor inhibitor (TNFi), adalimumab, used for rheumatoid arthritis showed a response after tamoxifen discontinuation, suggesting either a possible late tamoxifen effect or a role of immunomodulation in AF pathogenesis and treatment.

Among the population of patients with stable disease, representing the most heterogeneous group, we found a discordance between clinical symptoms and MRI T2 changes. This could be explained by the fact that cases with a slight increase/decrease in size are included within the category of RECIST 1.1 stable disease.

Although MRI is accepted to be the best imaging modality for visualising AF [38] this study suggests that it is less useful in demonstrating therapeutic benefit on tamoxifen ± NSAIDs. This study has not demonstrated a clear relationship between MRI features (size/signal) and reported symptoms. This limitation may not be restricted to assessment of tamoxifen effects as Sheth et al. also reported that RECIST were not sensitive to clinically determined response in 23 patients treated with a variety of local and systemic therapies [48]. Although there is thought provoking evidence that FDG PET/CT gives some early indication of response in patients treated with imatinib, the risk:benefit ratio of the radiation doses involved must be given careful consideration particularly where multiple assessments for non malignant pathology are performed, especially in young patients [49].

Our study suggests that symptoms are arguably the most important indicators of response to tamoxifen in patients with AF. According to this observation, the incorporation of prospective validated pain scores and functional assessment tools into the evaluation of treatment in this disease would give a better indication of therapeutic benefit. This is particularly critical for the design of prospective AF studies where we suggest that endpoints should focus on patient symptoms. However, some experience with MRI in patients treated on pazopanib indicate that MRI may be more useful in assessing response to other agents [25].

For those patients with previous pre-baseline images available for comparison, a few cases showed a decrease in the rate of tumour growth. However, it is difficult to extrapolate definitive conclusions from these data because the number of patients with pre-baseline images was low and AF is known to have such a varied natural history with prolonged periods of stabilisation and eventual regression in nearly 28% of cases in one reported series [50].

Conclusions

We showed for the first time that symptomatic benefit, MRI T2 signal changes and tumour size correlate poorly. Therefore, MRI is of limited value in assessing therapeutic benefit in patients treated with tamoxifen ± NSAIDs. This highlights the importance of robust systems to collect data on patients' symptoms and quality of life.

Authors' contributions

Concept and design (CM, IM, ML, CB, KT, IJ, AM, RJ, EM, ZS, WG); Data collection (CM, IM, ML); Data Analysis (ML, KT). Writing and interpretation (All authors). All authors read and approved the final manuscript.

Author details

[1] Sarcoma Unit, Royal Marsden NHS Foundation Trust, London, UK. [2] Department of Radiology, The Royal Marsden NHS Foundation Trust, 203 Fulham Road, London SW3 6JJ, UK. [3] Institute of Cancer Research, Sutton, UK.

Acknowledgements

We acknowledge National Health Service funding to the National Institute for Health Research Biomedical Research Centre, Clinical Research Facility in Imaging and the Cancer Research Network. The views expressed in this publication are those of the author(s) and not necessarily those of the National Health Service, the National Institute for Health Research or the Department of Health.

Presented at 21th Connective Tissue Oncology Society Annual Meeting, 2016, Lisbon, Paper 033.

Competing interests

The authors declare that they have no competing interests.

Funding
Michela Libertini received support from European School of Oncology (ESO) within the ESO training programme 2016. All authors were supported by NHS funding to the NIHR Biomedical Research Centre at the Royal Marsden Hospital.

References

1. Van Broekhoven DL, Verhoef C, Grünhagen DJ, et al. Prognostic value of CTNNB1 gene mutation in primary sporadic aggressive fibromatosis. Ann Surg Oncol. 2015;5:1464–70.
2. Shields CJ, Winter DC, Kirwan WO, Redmond HP. Desmoid tumours. Eur J Surg Oncol. 2001;27:701–6.
3. Clark SK, Philips RK. Desmoids in familial adenomatous polyposis. Br J Surg. 1996;83:1494–504.
4. Bertario L, Russo A, Sala P, Varesco L, Giarola M, Mondini P, et al. Hereditary colorectal tumour registry. Multiple approach to the exploration of genotype-phenotype correlations in familial adenomatous polyposis. J Clin Oncol. 2003;21:1698–707.
5. Sundaram M, Duffrin H, McGuire MH, Vas W. Synchronous multicenteric desmoids tumors (aggressive fibromatosis) of the extremities. Skeletal Radiol. 1988;17:16–9.
6. Shingare AB, Ramaiya NH, Jagannathan JP, Krajewski KM, Giardino AA, Butrynski JE, Raut CP. A to Z of desmoid tumours. AJR. 2011;197:W1008–14.
7. Goldblum JR, Fletcher JA. Desmoid-type fibromatosis. In:Fletcher CDM, Bridge JA, Hogendoorn PCW, Mertens F, editors. World Health Organization classification of tumours of softtissue and bone. Lyon: IARC Press; 2013. p. 72–3.
8. Kasper B. Systemic treatment approaches for sporadic desmoids-type fibromatosis: scarce evidence and recommendations. Oncol Res Treat. 2015;38:244–8.
9. Kasper B, Baumgarten C, Garcia J, et al. An update on the managment of sporadic desmoid-type fibromatosis:a European Consensus Initiative between Sarcoma PAtients EuroNet (SPAEN) and European Organisation for Research and Treatment of Cancer (EORTC)/Soft Tissue and Bone Sarcoma Group (STBSG). Ann Oncol. 2017;28:2399–408.
10. Gronchi A, Colombo C, Le Péchoux C, et al. Sporadic desmoid-type fibromatosis: a stepwise approach to a non-metastasising neoplasm-A position paper from the Italian and the French Sarcoma Group. Ann Oncol. 2014;25:578–83.
11. Reitamo JJ, Sheinin TM, Pekka H. The desmoid syndrome. New aspects in the cause, pathogenesis and treatment of the desmoid tumor. Am J Surg. 1986;15:230–7.
12. Alman BA, Pajerski ME, Diaz-Cano S, Corboy K, Wolfe HJ. Aggressive fibromatosis (desmoid tumor) is a monoclonal disorder. Diagn Mol Pathol. 1997;6:98–101.
13. Merchant NB, Lewis JJ, Woodruff JM, Leung DH, Brennan MF. Extremity and trunk desmoid tumors: a multifactorial analysis of outcome. Cancer. 1999;86:2045–52.
14. Lev D, Kotilingam D, Wei C, et al. Optimizing treatment of desmoid tumors. J Clin Oncol. 2007;25:1785–91.
15. Romero JA, Kim EE, Kim CG, Chung WK, Isiklar I. Different biologic features of desmoids tumours in adult and juvenile patients: MR demonstration. J Comput Assist Tomogr. 1995;19:782–7.
16. Keus R, Nout RA, Blay JY, et al. Results of a phase II pilot study of moderate dose radiotherapy for inoperable desmoid-type fibromatosis—an EORTC STBSG and ROG study (EORTC 62991–22998). Ann Oncol. 2013;24:2672–6.
17. Guadagnolo BA, Zagars GK, Ballo MT. Long-term outcomes for desmoid tumors treated with radiation therapy. Int J Radiat Oncol Biol Phys. 2008;71:441–7.
18. Bocale D, Rotelli MT, Cavallini A, Altomare F. Anti-oestrogen therapy in the treatment of desmoids tumours: a systematic review. Colorectal Dis. 2011;13:e388–95.
19. Garbay D, Le Cesne A, Penel N, et al. Chemotherapy in patients with desmoid tumors: a study from the French Sarcoma Group (FSG). Ann Oncol. 2012;23:182–6.
20. Constantinidou A, Jones RL, Scurr M, Al-Muderis O, Judson I. Pegylated liposomal doxorubicin, an effective, well-tolerated treatment for refractory aggressive fibromatosis. Eur J Cancer. 2009;45:2930–4.
21. Park K-H, Choi YJ, Kim KW, Ro KH, Kang CH, Song SH, Park JH. Combination chemotherapy with methotrexate and vinblastine for surgically unresectable, aggressive fibromatosis. Jpn J Clin Oncol. 2016;46:845–9.
22. Penel N, Le Cesne A, Bui BN, et al. Chemotherapy in patients with desmoid tumors: a study from the French Sarcoma Group (FSG). Ann Oncol. 2012;23:182–6.
23. Gounder MM, Lefkowitz RA, Keohan ML, et al. Activity of sorafenib against desmoid tumor/deep fibromatosis. Clin Cancer Res. 2011;17:4082–90.
24. Szucs Z, Messiou C, Wong HH, et al. Pazopanib, a promising option for the treatment of aggressive fibromatosis. Anticancer Drugs. 2017. https://doi.org/10.1097/cad.0000000000000474.
25. Hughes DP, Kummar S, Lazar AJ. New, tolerable γ-secretase inhibitor takes desmoid down a notch. Clin Cancer Res. 2015;21:7–9.
26. Deyrup AT, Tretiakova M, Montag AG. Estrogen receptor-beta expression in extraabdominal fibromatoses: an analysis of 40 cases. Cancer. 2006;106:208–13.
27. Fiore M, Coppola S, Cannell AJ, et al. Desmoid-type fibromatosis and pregnancy: a multi-institutional analysis of recurrence and obstetric risk. Ann Surg. 2014;259:973–8.
28. Lotfi AM, Dozois RR, Gordon H, Hruska LS, Weiland LH, Carryer PW, Hurt RD. Mesenteric fibromatosis complicating familial adenomatous polyposis: predisposing factors and results of treatment. Int J Colorectal Dis. 1989;4:30–6.
29. Hansmann A, Vogel CAT, Unger A, Moeslein G. High dose tamoxifen and sulindac as first line treatment for desmoids tumors. Cancer. 2004;100:612–20.
30. Skapek SX, Anderson JR, Da Hill, et al. Safety and efficacy of high dose tamoxifen and sulindac for desmoids tumor in children: results of a Children's Oncology Group (COG) Phase II study. Paediatr Blood Cancer. 2013;60:1108–12.
31. Fiore M, Colombo C, Radaelli S, Callegaro D, et al. Hormonal manipulation with toremifene in sporadic desmoids-type fibromatosis. Eur J Cancer. 2015;51:2800–7.
32. Carthy JM, Sundqvist A, Heldin A, van Dam H, Kletsas D, Heldin CH, Moustakas A. Tamoxifen inhibits TGF-β-mediated activation of myofibroblasts by blocking non-smad signaling through ERK1/2. J Cell Physiol. 2015;230:3084–92.
33. Eisenhauer EA, Therasse P, Bogaerts J, et al. New response evaluation criteria in solid tumors: re-vised RECIST guideline (version 1.1). Eur J Cancer. 2009;45:228–47.
34. Murphey MD, Ruble CM, Tyszko SM, Zbojniewicz AM, Potter BK, Miettinem M. From the archives of the AFIP: musculoskeletal fibromatoses-radiologic-pathologic correlation. RadioGraphics. 2009;29:2143–73.
35. Walker EA, Petscavage JM, Brian PL, et al. Imaging features of superficial and deep fibromatoses in the adult population. Sarcoma. 2012;2012:215810.
36. Lee JC, Thomas JM, Phillips S, Fisher C, Moskovic E. Aggressive fibromatosis: MRI features with pathologic correlation. AJR. 2006;186:247–54.
37. Dinauer PA, Brixey CJ, Moncur JT, Fanburg-Smith JC, Murphey MD. Pathologic and MR imaging features of benign fibrous soft-tissue tumours in adults. Radiographics. 2007;27:173–87.
38. Sundaram M, McGuire MH, Schajowicz F. Soft tissue masses: histologic basis for decreased signal (short T2) on T2-weighted MR images. AJR. 1987;148:1247–50.
39. Otero S, Moskovic EC, Strauss DC, Benson C, Miah AB, Thway K. Desmoid-type fibromatosis. Clin. Radiology. 2015;70:1038–45.
40. Castellazzi G, Vanel D, Le Cesne A, et al. Can the MRI signal of aggressive fibromatosis be used to predict its behavior? Eur J Radiol. 2009;69:222–9.
41. Kamali F, Wang W-L, Guadagnolo BA, et al. MRI may be used as a prognostic indicator in patients with extra-abdominal desmoid tumours. Br J Radiol. 2016;89:20150308.
42. Rodriguez-Wallberg KA, Oktay K. Fertility preservation in women with breast cancer. Clin Obstet Gynecol. 2010;53:753–62.
43. Weinblatt ME, Keystone EC, Furst DE, et al. Adalimumab, a fully human anti-tumor necrosis factor α monoclonal antibody, for the treatment of rheumatoid arthritis in patients taking concomitant methotrexate. Arthritis Rheum. 2003;48:35–42.
44. Fiore M, Rimareix F, Mariani L, et al. Desmoid type fibromatosis: a front line conservative approach to select patients for surgical treatment. Ann Surg Oncol. 2009;16:2587–93.
45. Brooks MD, Ebbs SR, Colletta AA, Baum M. Desmoid tumors treated with triphenylethylenes. Eur J Cancer. 1992;28A:1014–8.

46. Quast DR, Schneider R, Burdzik E, Hoppe S, Molsein G. Long-term outcome of sporadic and FAP-associated desmoid tumors treated with high-dose selective estrogen receptor modulators and sulindac: a single-center long-term observational study in 134 patients. Fam Cancer. 2016;15:31–40.
47. Hial V, Horakova Z, Shaff FE, Beaven MA. Alteration of tumor growth by aspirin and indomethacin: studies with two transplantable tumors in mouse. Eur J Pharmacol. 1976;37:367–76.
48. Sheth PJ, Del Moral S, Wilky BA, et al. Desmoid fibromatosis: MRI features of response to systemic therapy. Skeletal Radiol. 2016;45:1365–73.
49. Kasper B, Dimitrakopoulou-Strauss A, Pilz LR, Strauss LG, Sachpekidis C, Hohenberger P. Positron emission tomography as a surrogate marker for evaluation of treatment response in patients with desmoid tumors under therapy with imatinib. Biomed Res Int. 2013;2013:389672.
50. Bonvalot S, Ternès N, Fiore M, et al. Spontaneous regression of primary abdominal wall desmoid tumors: more common than previously thought. Ann Surg Oncol. 2013;20:4096–102.

Treatment patterns and survival among older adults in the United States with advanced soft-tissue sarcomas

Rohan C. Parikh[1*], Maria Lorenzo[2], Lisa M. Hess[3], Sean D. Candrilli[1], Steven Nicol[3] and James A. Kaye[4]

Abstract

Background: To describe patient and tumor characteristics, treatments, and survival among older adults in the United States with advanced soft-tissue sarcoma (STS), across and by categories of specifically defined histologic subtypes.

Methods: We conducted a retrospective cohort analysis using the SEER. The study population comprised patients ≥ 65 years old with advanced STS (excluding osteosarcoma, Kaposi sarcoma, and gastrointestinal stromal tumors) diagnosed from January 1, 2001 to December 31, 2011.

Results: Of 4274 study patients, 2103 (49.2%) were male. Mean age was 77.8 years, and 1539 (36.0%) had distant disease at initial diagnosis. The most common histologic categories were leiomyosarcoma (922[21.6%]), undifferentiated pleomorphic sarcoma (652[15.3%]), and liposarcoma (554[13.0%]). Overall, 1227 (28.7%) patients received first-line systemic therapy. Among these patients, 325 (26.5%) received docetaxel plus gemcitabine and 231 (18.8%) received doxorubicin alone. Only 476 patients received second-line therapy (11.1%), most commonly doxorubicin alone (n = 101). Median overall survival (95% confidence interval) from advanced STS diagnosis was 8.9 (8.3, 9.7) months.

Conclusions: Although previous studies of younger populations reported anthracycline-based therapy predominated in first line, our study of older advanced STS patients found that docetaxel plus gemcitabine was most commonly used. Despite variation by histologic category, prognosis remains poor for older adult patients with advanced STS.

Keywords: Soft-tissue sarcoma, Chemotherapy, Observational study

Background

Soft-tissue sarcoma (STS) refers to a rare and heterogeneous group of malignant tumors comprising more than 50 histologic subtypes derived from connective tissues and other cells of mesenchymal origin. Soft-tissue sarcoma accounts for approximately 1% of all incident malignancies [1] and an estimated 13,040 new cases will be diagnosed in the United States (US) in 2018, with 7370 dying from the disease [2]. In 2014, the age-adjusted incidence rate, for STS for patients 65 years of age and older was 11.3 per 100,000, compared to 2.3 per 100,000 for patients younger than 65 years of age [3].

Among all patients diagnosed with STS, the 5-year overall survival is approximately 50% [4]. Tumor histology, stage, and primary site are prognostic factors [4, 5]; 5-year overall survival is 83% in patients with localized disease and 16% in patients with distant metastases at initial diagnosis [6]. Eventually, either at initial diagnosis or after recurrence from a more limited extent of disease, 40–50% of patients with STS will have metastatic or unresectable locally-advanced disease (collectively referred to as "advanced STS") [7].

Treatment options for patients with advanced STS have historically been limited; cytotoxic chemotherapy has been the mainstay of therapy for decades. Active drugs

*Correspondence: rparikh@rti.org
[1] RTI Health Solutions, 200 Park Offices Drive, Research Triangle Park, NC 27560, USA

include doxorubicin, ifosfamide, gemcitabine, taxanes, and several others; these may be administered either as single agents or in combination regimens [4, 8]. The intent of these treatments is palliative for the majority of patients [4, 8, 9]. Until recently, clinical trials—including those demonstrating superiority of combination chemotherapy over monotherapy and those leading to the regulatory approval of newer agents such as olaratumab, trabectedin, and pazopanib—have found improvements in response rates and progression-free survival [4, 10–14]. However, olaratumab is the only newer agent to date that has also demonstrated a statistically significant improvement in overall survival [11].

Few studies have examined utilization of systemic treatments for STS in the general population of the US, especially in older patients with advanced disease. Furthermore, there is little published information on variation in outcomes according to tumor histology, especially among older adults. Thus, the objectives of this study were to describe real-world, population-based treatment patterns and survival among older adult patients with advanced STS, overall and by groupings of specific histologic subtypes (hereafter "histologic categories").

Methods

Data source

The Surveillance, Epidemiology, and End Results (SEER), which contains administrative claims data for Medicare enrollees, was used for the study. The SEER cancer registry comprises nine state population-based and seven metropolitan or regional population-based registries that routinely collect information on 98% of newly diagnosed (incident) cancer cases, in persons residing in SEER areas [15]. SEER areas have been shown to be nationally representative [16] and capture approximately one-quarter of the total US population [15].

Along with detailed information on incident cancer, the database provides comprehensive longitudinal health care utilization data from Medicare. The Medicare claims database provides information on all services covered under Medicare Part A benefits, including inpatient, skilled nursing facility, home health care, and hospice care. In addition, the database provides information on approximately 95% of services covered under Medicare Part B, including physician visits, outpatient care, durable medical equipment, and home health care. This study was deemed exempt from Institutional Review Board review in accordance with the US Code of Federal Regulations [45CFR46.101(b)] as these data do not contain any variables that could identify an individual subject either directly or indirectly.

Study population

Patients with a new diagnosis of STS between January 1, 2001 and December 31, 2011 were eligible for this study. Medicare claims data were available through 2013. Patients with STS (except osteosarcoma, Kaposi sarcoma, and gastrointestinal stromal tumors) were identified in the SEER database using International Classification of Diseases for Oncology, 3rd Edition (ICD-O-3), morphology codes as listed in Appendix 1: Table 6 [17]. In order to reduce the number of strata analyzed specific histologic subtypes (i.e., individual ICD-O-3 codes) were grouped into broader categories for analysis based on the 2013 World Health Organization's (WHO) Classification of Tumours of Soft Tissue and Bone [18]: (1) leiomyosarcoma (smooth muscle tumors), (2) undifferentiated pleomorphic sarcoma (UPS; previously known as malignant fibrous histiocytoma), (3) liposarcoma (adipocytic tumors), (4) vascular sarcomas, (5) fibroblastic/myofibroblastic sarcoma, (6) nerve sheath sarcoma, (7) rhabdomyosarcoma (skeletal muscle tumors), (8) synovial sarcoma, and (9) others or not otherwise specified (NOS). The term "histologic category" was used in this study to distinguish these categories from the individual "histologic subtypes" they contain.

Advanced disease was defined as metastatic disease or as the presence of nodal metastases and no surgery (assuming patients who did not receive surgery were not suitable for surgical resection). Metastatic disease and nodal metastases were identified using the American Joint Commission on Cancer's Cancer Staging Manual [19] or the National Cancer Institute's (NCI's) SEER Summary Staging Manual [20]. Patients were also considered to have advanced STS if they had an initial diagnosis of localized disease with later progression to advanced STS as identified by either a medical claim with an International Classification of Diseases, 9th Revision, Clinical Modification (ICD-9-CM) diagnosis code for a secondary neoplasm (ICD-9-CM 196.0-198.89) or initiation of systemic therapy more than 6 months after surgery. The 6-month lag period was chosen to avoid interpreting adjuvant therapy as treatment for advanced disease.

Additionally, eligible patients were 65 years or older at the time of advanced STS diagnosis and were enrolled in both Medicare parts A and B without any health maintenance organization (HMO) enrollment from 6 months before initial STS diagnosis to death or end of study. Patients with HMO coverage (provided outside of the Medicare system) were excluded because claims data for these patients would not be complete, as the linked data for this study were limited to Medicare. Of the patients initially diagnosed with localized or regional disease according to SEER data, only those with evidence of advanced STS in Medicare claims that occurred at a date later than the initial STS diagnosis were included in the study (i.e., patients were excluded if there were contradictory initial diagnosis codes [i.e., localized or regional STS diagnosis and secondary neoplasm claims] on the same date, or if patients had no surgery after initial STS diagnosis and no secondary neoplasm claim). Study index date for each patient (start of follow-up) was defined as the date of the first observed evidence of advanced STS.

Demographic and clinical characteristics

Demographic characteristics including age, sex, race, SEER registry location, and urban or rural residency were tabulated. Clinical characteristics that were assessed at initial STS diagnosis included cancer stage, tumor location, and histologic subtype (with subsequent categorization described previously). We also computed a modified Charlson Comorbidity Index (CCI) score to obtain a measure of each patient's overall comorbidity burden at the time of the index diagnosis [21–23]. CCI scores were calculated for each patient based on evidence of the relevant diagnoses from 6-months prior to advanced STS diagnosis to advanced STS diagnosis (i.e., during 6-month pre-index date period). ICD-9-CM diagnosis codes for cancer were excluded from the CCI calculation for this study so as to not overestimate the baseline comorbidity burden, as all patients in this study had cancer.

Treatment patterns

Treatments were identified using evidence of relevant Healthcare Common Procedure Coding System (HCPCS) codes, ICD-9-CM procedure codes, and certain ICD-9-CM diagnostic codes and administrative revenue codes. In addition to HCPCS and ICD-9-CM codes, Medicare Part D prescription data were used to identify chemotherapy use for a subset of the cohort with this data (2007–2012). Among patients who received systemic treatment, up to five lines of treatment were identified. Specific therapies were examined based upon options included in the National Comprehensive Cancer Network (NCCN) Guidelines [24]. First-line treatment was examined among all patients, with at least one claim for an HCPCS-identifiable chemotherapeutic, biologic, or targeted therapy agent after their index date. The first observed date of treatment after the index date signaled the start of first-line treatment. First-line treatment was defined as the combination of all agents observed within 21 days after (and inclusive of) treatment initiation. After the end of this 21-day period, the use of any new agent signaled the start of the next line of treatment. Discontinuation of one or more of the agents without the addition of another agent was not considered a new line of treatment. In addition, patients with at least 6 months between apparent cessation of their previous line of treatment and reuptake of an identical regimen were defined as having initiated a next line of treatment. End of a line of treatment was defined as: (1) a 6-month gap in treatment regimen, (2) interruption by next line of treatment, or (3) treatment continuation until the end of study or death. Cancer-directed therapy was defined as receipt of any of broad treatment categories of surgery, radiation, chemotherapy, biologic therapy, or targeted therapy, while supportive care was defined as no receipt of treatment from any of the broad cancer-directed therapies.

Statistical analyses

Descriptive statistics [i.e., means, medians, ranges, and standard deviations (SDs) of continuous variables and frequency counts and percentages for categorical variables] were computed. Overall survival from advanced STS diagnosis was measured using the death information available from SEER and Medicare data, and survival time end points were analyzed using the Kaplan–Meier estimates with median survival time and 95% confidence intervals (CIs) reported in months. Patients alive at the end of study period were censored for this analysis. Treatment patterns and survival were assessed in the overall advanced STS population and by histologic category. Additionally, survival was estimated separately for patients who received cancer-directed treatment and those who received supportive care only. All analyses were conducted using SAS Version 9.4 (Cary, NC: SAS Institute, Inc.; 2011). The SEER-Medicare data use agreement required that no cell sizes less than 11 be reported for any demographic or other characteristic, or combination of characteristics; thus, if sufficient sample size was not available, data were not reported and indicated with "–".

Results

A total of 4274 patients with advanced STS met the inclusion criteria for this study (Table 1). Patients were on average 77.8 years of age (SD, 7.3; range 65–104 years) at the time of advanced STS diagnosis and 49.2% were male (Table 2). The mean (SD) CCI score was 2.8 (2.33), and 69.2, 18.3, and 6.5% of patients had a history of hypertension, congestive heart failure, and myocardial infarction, respectively.

At initial diagnosis, 36.0% of patients had metastatic (distant) disease; the remaining majority (64.0%) were diagnosed at earlier stages of disease and had claims based indicators of progression to advanced STS (Table 2) with a mean (SD) interval of 16.6 (23.0) months from initial diagnosis. Nodal disease (without any distant metastases) was observed only among 1.6% of patients at

Table 1 Study population selection process

	Number of patients
Initial sample included in the SEER database	142,689
Initial diagnosis date on or after January 1, 2001	135,608
Patients whose first diagnosis recorded in the SEER database was STS	21,167
Patients with evidence (i.e., claim in Medicare data or diagnosis in SEER database) of metastatic disease	8537
Initially diagnosed at metastatic stage[a]	3391
Initially diagnosed at non-metastatic stage[a]	5146
Patients 65 years or older at time of metastatic STS diagnosis	6712
Patients who were alive at initial diagnosis of STS (i.e., reporting source other than autopsy or death certificate)	6705
Patients who were not enrolled in an HMO for at least 6 months prior to initial diagnosis of STS to end of follow-up period	5166
Patients who have continuous enrollment in Medicare Part A and B (non-HMO) for at least 6 months prior to initial diagnosis of STS until end of follow-up period	4353
Patients who are not lost to follow-up prior to the assigned advanced STS diagnosis date[b]	4324
Patients with a date of advanced STS diagnosis different than initial STS diagnosis (patients excluded if no surgery after initial STS diagnosis and no secondary neoplasm claim)	4298
Patients with a date of advanced STS diagnosis different than initial STS diagnosis (patients excluded if initial STS diagnosis and secondary neoplasm claim on the same date)	4274
Final study population	*4274*

HMO health maintenance organization, *SEER* Survey, Epidemiology, and End Results, *STS* soft-tissue sarcoma

[a] Only for descriptive purposes and no exclusion was made based on this criterion

[b] Day of diagnosis, which is reported as month and years, was assigned as 15th of each month and hence some patients who either die or are lost to follow-up before the 15th of the month have a negative length of follow-up

initial diagnosis. The most common histologic category was leiomyosarcoma (n=922; 21.6%), followed by UPS (n=652; 15.3%), liposarcoma (n=554; 13.0%), vascular sarcoma (n=357; 8.4%), fibroblastic/myofibroblastic sarcoma (n=227; 5.3%), nerve sheath sarcoma (n=106; 2.5%), rhabdomyosarcoma (n=98; 2.3%), and synovial sarcoma (n=49; 1.1%); the remaining 30.6% (n=1309) had other or NOS histologic categories. A few variations in patient and tumor characteristics by tumor histology were evident: 66.7% of patients with leiomyosarcoma were female; patients with synovial sarcoma had a mean age of 74.1 years, and 54.1, 40.8, 48.7% of patients with rhabdomyosarcoma, synovial sarcoma, and other/NOS histology, respectively, had distant stage of disease at initial STS diagnosis (Table 2). Overall, the most common specified anatomic tumor site was lower limb (21.9%) (Appendix 2: Table 7), and the most common known tumor grade was undifferentiated (30.7%) (Table 2). The average observed follow-up time from advanced STS diagnosis was 1.7 years (SD, 2.36) (Table 2).

Cancer-directed treatment was received by 62.1% of patients. Radiation was received by 40.0% of patients and surgery was received by 10.3% of patients. The mean (SD) age of patients who received cancer-directed treatment was 76.5 (6.9) years and the mean (SD) CCI score was 2.5 (2.1), with hypertension, diabetes (without complications), chronic pulmonary disease, peripheral vascular disease, and congestive heart failure observed among 68.9, 28.4, 24.4, 18.1, and 14.6% of patients, respectively (Additional file 1: Table S1). Chemotherapy, biologic therapy, and targeted therapy were received by 27.5, 1.9, and 1.3% of patients, respectively. Among the 28.7% of all patients with advanced STS who received chemotherapy, biologic therapy, or targeted therapy (n=1227), the mean duration of first-line therapy was 4.1 months (SD, 4.1) (Table 3). Second-line therapy was received by 11.1% (n=476) of all patients; the mean duration of second-line treatment was 4.6 months (SD, 5.3). Among the 4.4% of all patients with advanced STS who received at least third-line therapy (n=189), the mean duration of third-line therapy was 4 months (SD, 3.4). The proportion of patients receiving up to three lines of treatment and duration of each line of treatment by histologic category is shown in Table 3. First-line chemotherapy was most commonly received by patients with synovial sarcoma (42.9%), leiomyosarcoma (37.0%), and vascular sarcoma (36.4%).

Overall, the most common regimen during first-line therapy was docetaxel plus gemcitabine (26.5%), followed by doxorubicin monotherapy (18.8%), gemcitabine monotherapy (9.1%), paclitaxel monotherapy (5.5%), and bevacizumab monotherapy (3.3%). Docetaxel plus gemcitabine was the most common first-line therapy for patients with all histologic categories except liposarcoma

Table 2 Patient and tumor characteristics, overall and by histologic categories

	All patients	Leiomyo-sarcomas	Undifferentiated pleomorphic sarcoma	Liposarcomas	Vascular sarcomas	Fibroblastic/ myofibroblastic sarcomas	Nerve sheath sarcomas	Rhabdomyo-sarcomas	Synovial sarcomas	Others/NOS
N	4274	922	652	554	357	227	106	98	49	1309
Sex (n, %)										
Male	2103 (49.2)	307 (33.3)	390 (59.8)	329 (59.4)	195 (54.6)	122 (53.7)	64 (60.4)	43 (43.9)	28 (57.1)	625 (47.8)
Female	2171 (50.8)	615 (66.7)	262 (40.2)	225 (40.6)	162 (45.4)	105 (46.3)	42 (39.6)	55 (56.1)	21 (42.9)	684 (52.2)
Race										
White	3729 (87.3)	783 (84.9)	576 (88.3)	499 (90.1)	309 (86.6)	203 (89.4)	96 (90.6)	82 (83.7)	43 (87.8)	1138 (86.9)
Black	337 (7.9)	106 (11.5)	46 (7.1)	23 (4.2)	21 (5.9)	–	–	–	–	106 (8.1)
Other	197 (4.6)	31 (3.4)	26 (4.0)	32 (5.8)	25 (7.0)	–	–	–	–	63 (4.8)
Age at *advanced* diagnosis										
Mean (SD)	77.8 (7.3)	76.8 (7.2)	79.4 (7.2)	77.5 (7.1)	78.2 (7.5)	77.8 (7.1)	77.7 (7.6)	76.8 (7.3)	74.1 (6.5)	78.0 (7.4)
Median	77.4	76.1	79.7	76.6	77.9	77.8	77.3	76.6	73.5	77.5
Min, Max	65.0, 104.1	65.0, 102.9	65.1, 99.3	65.1, 96.8	65.6, 101.8	65.7, 97.4	65.5, 95.9	65.3, 95.3	65.7, 91.0	65.1, 104.1
Pre-index date Charlson Comorbidity Index (CCI) score[a]										
Mean (SD)	2.8 (2.3)	2.5 (2.2)	2.8 (2.4)	2.8 (2.3)	2.9 (2.7)	2.8 (2.2)	2.8 (2.3)	2.6 (2.1)	3.0 (2.3)	2.8 (2.4)
Median	2.0	2.0	2.0	2.0	2.0	2.0	2.0	2.0	2.0	2.0
Min, Max	0.0, 15.0	0.0, 14.0	0.0, 15.0	0.0, 12.0	0.0, 12.0	0.0, 11.0	0.0, 10.0	0.0, 9.0	0.0, 8.0	0.0, 15.0
Stage of disease at initial diagnosis of STS (n, %)										
Localized	1731 (40.5)	345 (37.4)	379 (58.1)	260 (46.9)	150 (42.0)	121 (53.3)	36 (34.0)	25 (25.5)	18 (36.7)	397 (30.3)
Regional—direct extension only	938 (22.0)	200 (21.7)	135 (20.7)	177 (32.0)	62 (17.4)	59 (26.0)	32 (30.2)	14 (14.3)	11 (22.5)	248 (19.0)
Regional—lymph nodes involved only	29 (0.7)	–	–	–	–	–	–	–	0 (0.0)	–
Regional—direct extension and lymph nodes	37 (0.9)	–	–	–	–	–	–	–	0 (0.0)	–
Distant	1539 (36.0)	363 (39.4)	133 (20.4)	114 (20.6)	138 (38.7)	45 (19.8)	36 (34.0)	53 (54.1)	20 (40.8)	637 (48.7)
Grade of cancer at time of initial diagnosis of STS (n, %)										
Well or moderately differentiated (grade 1 or 2)	646 (15.1)	152 (16.5)	36 (5.5)	239 (43.1)	40 (11.2)	50 (22.0)	–	–	–	116 (8.9)
Poorly differentiated (grade 3)	908 (21.2)	192 (20.8)	151 (23.2)	101 (18.2)	81 (22.7)	35 (15.4)	–	–	16 (32.7)	294 (22.5)
Undifferentiated (grade 4)	1310 (30.7)	250 (27.1)	228 (35.0)	129 (23.3)	61 (17.1)	63 (27.8)	28 (26.4)	34 (34.7)	–	510 (39.0)
Unknown	1410 (33.0)	328 (35.6)	237 (36.4)	85 (15.3)	175 (49.0)	79 (34.8)	54 (50.9)	39 (39.8)	24 (49.0)	389 (29.7)

Table 2 (continued)

	All patients	Leiomyo-sarcomas	Undifferentiated pleomorphic sarcoma	Liposarcomas	Vascular sarcomas	Fibroblastic/ myofibroblastic sarcomas	Nerve sheath sarcomas	Rhabdomyo-sarcomas	Synovial sarcomas	Others/NOS
Total follow-up time (years)[b]										
Mean (SD)	1.7 (2.4)	1.8 (2.2)	2.0 (2.8)	2.6 (2.8)	1.1 (1.7)	2.5 (2.7)	1.4 (2.1)	0.8 (1.5)	1.4 (1.8)	1.3 (2.0)
Median	0.7	1.0	0.8	1.5	0.5	1.6	0.5	0.3	0.6	0.5
Min, Max	0.0, 12.8	0.0, 12.2	0.0, 12.3	0.0, 12.3	0.0, 12.5	0.0, 12.5	0.0, 9.9	0.0, 9.8	0.0, 8.8	0.0, 12.8

ICD-9-CM International Classification of Diseases, 9th Revision, Clinical Modification, *Max* maximum, *Min* minimum, *NOS* not otherwise specified, *SD* standard deviation, *STS* soft-tissue sarcoma

[a] Because the objective of the CCI score was to evaluate underlying comorbidity burden independent of STS, ICD-9-CM diagnosis codes for cancer were excluded from the CCI calculation for this study

[b] Follow-up time calculated as the number of months between the study index date (first diagnosis of advanced STS) and the earliest of death, loss of eligibility, or end of the Medicare database (December 31, 2013)

Table 3 Treatment line progression, overall and by histologic categories

	Histologic categories									
	All patients	Leiomyosarcomas	Undifferentiated pleomorphic Sarcoma	Liposarcomas	Vascular sarcomas	Fibroblastic/myofibroblastic sarcomas	Nerve sheath sarcomas	Rhabdomyosarcomas	Synovial sarcomas	Others/NOS
	n (%)	n (%)	n (%)	n (%)	n (%)	n (%)	n (%)	n (%)	n (%)	n (%)
All patients	4274	922	652	554	357	227	106	98	49	1309
Receiving first-line systemic[a] treatment	1227 (28.7)	341 (37.0)	158 (24.2)	140 (25.3)	130 (36.4)	58 (25.6)	24 (22.6)	28 (28.6)	21 (42.9)	327 (25.0)
Duration, mean (SD)	4.1 (4.1)	4.1 (4.2)	4.4 (5.7)	4.3 (4.7)	4.4 (3.4)	4.2 (3.8)	3.3 (2.5)	4.5 (2.9)	3.9 (3.3)	3.8 (3.2)
Median	3.0	3.1	2.6	3.0	3.5	3.6	3.1	3.7	3.0	2.8
Receiving second-line systemic[a] treatment	476 (11.1)	148 (16.1)	64 (9.8)	45 (8.1)	60 (16.8)	19 (8.4)	–	15 (15.3)	–	109 (8.3)
Duration, mean (SD)	4.6 (5.3)	4.5 (4.0)	5.1 (8.6)	5.5 (5.4)	4.6 (5.2)	4.7 (3.6)	–	3.2 (2.2)	–	4.3 (4.7)
Median	3.0	3.3	2.9	4.0	3.4	4.8	–	2.6	–	2.9
Receiving third-line systemic[a] treatment	189 (4.4)	66 (7.2)	24 (3.7)	15 (2.7)	21 (5.9)	–	–	–	–	46 (3.5)
Duration, mean (SD)	4.0 (3.4)	4.6 (3.6)	3.3 (3.8)	2.8 (2.2)	5.1 (3.6)	–	–	–	–	3.4 (2.8)
Median	3.0	3.7	2.3	2.1	5.1	–	–	–	–	2.6

Oral chemotherapy was not covered by Medicare until 2007

SD standard deviation

[a] Systemic therapy includes chemotherapy, biologic therapy, or targeted therapy

(for whom it was doxorubicin monotherapy [24.3%]) and vascular sarcoma (for whom it was paclitaxel monotherapy [40.0%]) (Table 4). During first-line therapy, doxorubicin plus ifosfamide was received by 3.0% and ifosfamide monotherapy was received by 2.7% of patients. Among all patients who received doxorubicin alone or a doxorubicin-based first-line therapy (n = 371), 29.7% received liposomal doxorubicin, and 5.9% received the cardioprotective agent dexrazoxane.

Among patients who received second-line (n = 476) and third-line (n = 189) therapy, doxorubicin monotherapy (second line, 21.2%; third line, 14.8%), docetaxel plus gemcitabine (second line, 17.4%; third line, 11.1%), and gemcitabine monotherapy (second line, 8.6%; third line, 11.1%) were most common (Table 4). Among the 476 patients who received second-line therapy, the most common treatment sequence was first-line docetaxel plus gemcitabine followed by second-line doxorubicin monotherapy (n = 56, 11.8%). Among the 189 patients who received third-line therapy, the most common sequence was first-line doxorubicin followed by second-line gemcitabine and then third-line docetaxel plus gemcitabine (n ≤ 11). Among patients who received second- or third-line therapy, ≤ 11 received dexrazoxane.

Among patients who received supportive care only (n = 1618, 37.86%), the mean (SD) age was 80.0 (7.5) years (Additional file 1: Table S1). Hypertension (69.6%), diabetes without complications (28.7%), chronic pulmonary disease (28.1%), congestive heart failure (24.5%), and peripheral vascular disease (22.6%) were the most common baseline comorbidities and the mean (SD) CCI score was 3.1 (2.6).

The majority of patients (n = 3565; 83.4%) died during study follow-up, with a median survival (95% CI) of 8.9 months (8.3, 9.7) from the time of advanced STS diagnosis. Median survival (95% CI) from advanced STS diagnosis among patients who received cancer-directed therapy was 13.6 months (12.9, 14.6), and among those who received supportive care it was 2.8 months (2.6, 3.4) (Table 5 and Fig. 1). Survival estimates for each histologic category is shown in Table 5. Estimated survival from advanced STS diagnosis varied by histologic category with median survival ranging from 21.4 months (15.6, 26.8) for patients with fibroblastic/myofibroblastic sarcoma to 3.0 months (1.8, 5.7) for patients with rhabdomyosarcoma.

Discussion

This study assessed recent real-world treatment patterns and estimated survival of a population-based cohort of older adults diagnosed with advanced STS in the US. More than 60% of patients were initially diagnosed at an earlier stage of disease and progressed to advanced STS with mean time to progression of 16.6 months. Consistent with previous studies [25–27], leiomyosarcoma, UPS and liposarcoma were the most common histological categories of STS in this study population.

Among patients initiating first-line systemic therapy, the most common regimen was docetaxel plus gemcitabine combination therapy (26.5%); the next most common first-line regimen (18.8%) was doxorubicin only. Both a recent medical record review study in the US [25] and the Sarcoma Treatment and Burden of Illness in North America and Europe chart review study [26] found that anthracyclines were used most commonly among first-line therapies (either alone or in combination) in younger patient populations. In this study of older adults, docetaxel plus gemcitabine was the most commonly used first-line therapy for most histologic categories except for vascular sarcomas (for which paclitaxel was most commonly used) and liposarcoma (for which doxorubicin was most commonly used). The use of paclitaxel for vascular sarcomas is consistent with evidence suggesting that vascular sarcomas may be relatively more responsive to taxanes and as such are recommended by NCCN guidelines [24, 28–30]. A relatively lower use of doxorubicin or related drugs was observed in this study, plausibly because the older age of the study population (mean age, 77.8 years) may increase concerns about adverse events, particularly doxorubicin-associated cardiotoxicity [27]. In the current study, 18.3% of the patients had a history of congestive heart failure and 25.8% of patients had a history of chronic pulmonary disease. Additionally, 69.2% of the patients in this study had hypertension that, along with age, is known to increase the risk of doxorubicin-associated cardiotoxicity [31, 32]. Prior research has addressed the issues of doxorubicin-based therapies and cardiovascular risk factors in the older adult population [33–35]. It is possible that the low use of doxorubicin observed in this study cohort is related to these issues, but the study design and available data do not allow for a thorough investigation of this potential relationship. Further understanding of physician preferences with regard to administration of doxorubicin-based therapy among older adult patients is needed to adequately comprehend observed treatment patterns. Knowledge about the appropriate care of the older patient remains limited, but data from this study begin to fill this gap and suggest directions for future research related to toxicity risk, disease progression, recurrence and survival outcomes, and their relationship with patient age in the setting of advanced STS.

As observed in other studies, gemcitabine was used most commonly during second-line therapy (either alone or in combination) [25, 26]. We also noted that

Table 4 Top 5 most frequent regimens during first-, second-, and third-line therapy

First-line therapy All patients (N = 1227)	n (%)	Second-line therapy All patients (N = 476)	n (%)	Third-line therapy All patients (N = 189)	n (%)
Docetaxel–gemcitabine	325 (26.5)	Doxorubicin	101 (21.2)	Doxorubicin	28 (14.8)
Doxorubicin	231 (18.8)	Docetaxel–gemcitabine	83 (17.4)	Docetaxel–gemcitabine	21 (11.1)
Gemcitabine	112 (9.1)	Gemcitabine	41 (8.6)	Gemcitabine	21 (11.1)
Paclitaxel	68 (5.5)	Paclitaxel	21 (4.4)	Ifosfamide	15 (7.9)
Bevacizumab	41 (3.3)	Ifosfamide	20 (4.2)	Dacarbazine	–
Leiomyosarcomas (N = 341)		**Leiomyosarcomas (N = 148)**		**Leiomyosarcomas (N = 66)**	
Docetaxel–gemcitabine	136 (39.9)	Doxorubicin	41 (27.7)	Doxorubicin	12 (18.2)
Doxorubicin	64 (18.8)	Docetaxel–gemcitabine	35 (23.7)	Docetaxel–gemcitabine	–
Gemcitabine	43 (12.6)	Gemcitabine	–	Gemcitabine	–
Carboplatin-paclitaxel	–	Docetaxel	–	Carboplatin-paclitaxel	–
Dacarbazine-doxorubicin	–	Dacarbazine	–	Ifosfamide	–
Doxorubicin–ifosfamide	–				
Temozolomide	–				
Undifferentiated pleomorphic sarcoma (N = 158)		**Undifferentiated pleomorphic sarcoma (N = 64)**		**Undifferentiated pleomorphic sarcoma (N = 24)**	
Docetaxel–gemcitabine	36 (22.8)	Docetaxel–gemcitabine	1 3 (20.3)	Doxorubicin	–
Doxorubicin	32 (20.3)	Doxorubicin	–	Docetaxel–gemcitabine	–
Gemcitabine	13 (8.2)	Ifosfamide	–	Dacarbazine	–
Ifosfamide	11 (7.0)	Gemcitabine	–	Ifosfamide	–
Doxorubicin–ifosfamide	–	Paclitaxel	–		
		Temozolomide	–		
Liposarcomas (N = 140)		**Liposarcomas (N = 45)**		**Liposarcomas (N = 15)**	
Doxorubicin	34 (24.3)	Docetaxel–gemcitabine	11 (24.4)	Ifosfamide	–
Docetaxel–gemcitabine	31 (22.1)	Doxorubicin	–	Gemcitabine	–
Bevacizumab	13 (9.3)	Gemcitabine	–		
Gemcitabine	12 (8.6)	Docetaxel-doxorubicin-gemcitabine	–		
Doxorubicin–ifosfamide	–	Ifosfamide	–		
Ifosfamide	–				
Vascular sarcomas (N = 130)		**Vascular sarcomas (N = 60)**		**Vascular sarcomas (N = 21)**	
Paclitaxel	52 (40.0)	Doxorubicin	18 (30.0)	Doxorubicin	–
Doxorubicin	22 (16.9)	Paclitaxel	–	Doxorubicin–ifosfamide	–
Docetaxel–gemcitabine	–	Docetaxel–gemcitabine	–	Docetaxel	–
Doxorubicin–ifosfamide	–	Gemcitabine	–	Docetaxel–gemcitabine	–
Docetaxel	–	Docetaxel	–	Paclitaxel	–
Fibroblastic/Myofibroblastic sarcomas (N = 58)		**Fibroblastic/Myofibroblastic sarcomas (N = 19)**		**Fibroblastic/Myofibroblastic sarcomas (N = -)**	
Docetaxel–gemcitabine	16 (27.6)	Bevacizumab	–	Docetaxel–gemcitabine	–
Doxorubicin	–	Docetaxel–gemcitabine	–	Gemcitabine	–
Bevacizumab	–	Bevacizumab-temozolomide	–		
Gemcitabine	–	Gemcitabine	–		
Cisplatin	–	Temozolomide	–		
Doxorubicin–ifosfamide	–				

Table 4 (continued)

Nerve sheath sarcomas (N = 24)		**Nerve sheath sarcomas (N = -)**		**Nerve sheath sarcomas (N = -)**	
Doxorubicin	–	Doxorubicin	–		
Docetaxel–gemcitabine	–				
Gemcitabine	–				
Doxorubicin–ifosfamide	–				
Ifosfamide	–				
Rhabdomyosarcomas (N = 28)		**Rhabdomyosarcomas (N = 15)**		**Rhabdomyosarcomas (N = -)**	
Docetaxel–gemcitabine	–	Doxorubicin	–		
Carboplatin-paclitaxel	–	Cyclophosphamide-doxorubicin-vincristine	–		
Cyclophosphamide-dactinomycin-vincristine	–				
Cyclophosphamide-doxorubicin	–				
Cyclophosphamide-doxorubicin-vincristine	–				
Doxorubicin	–				
Synovial sarcomas (N = 21)		**Synovial sarcomas (N = -)**		**Synovial sarcomas (N = -)**	
Docetaxel–gemcitabine	–	Dacarbazine	–		
Doxorubicin	–	Doxorubicin	–		
Temozolomide	–	Ifosfamide	–		
Others/NOS (N = 327)		**Others/NOS (N = 109)**		**Others/NOS (N = 46)**	
Docetaxel–gemcitabine	81 (24.8)	Docetaxel–gemcitabine	14 (12.8)	Gemcitabine	–
Doxorubicin	61 (18.7)	Doxorubicin	14 (12.8)	Ifosfamide	–
Gemcitabine	30 (9.2)	Gemcitabine	12 (11.0)	Dacarbazine	–
Carboplatin-paclitaxel	16 (4.9)	Carboplatin-paclitaxel	–	Docetaxel–gemcitabine	–
Paclitaxel	12 (3.7)	Docetaxel	–	Doxorubicin	–
		Doxorubicin–ifosfamide	–		
		Ifosfamide	–		

Only showing treatment regimens received by more than 1 patient

NOS not otherwise specified

dexrazoxane was not at all commonly used in this population among those who were treated with doxorubicin.

Approximately 62% of the study population received cancer-directed therapy. As compared to patients receiving cancer-directed therapy, patients receiving supportive care only had a mean age of 80.0 years (cancer-directed therapy: 76.5 years) at the time of being diagnosed with advanced disease and had a baseline comorbidity burden (mean CCI score) of 3.1 (cancer-directed therapy: 2.5), and 24.5% (cancer-directed therapy: 14.6%) had a history of congestive heart failure. Therefore, it seems likely that many of these patients may have been considered to not be candidates for chemotherapy, particularly with a cardiotoxic agent. The mean non-cancer CCI scores observed in this study for the overall population, patients receiving cancer-directed treatment, and patients receiving supportive care only are in line with those reported by Davis et al. among metastatic lung cancer patients [36].

Median overall survival in the entire study population was estimated to be less than 9 months. Patients who received supportive care lived only less than 3 months. The shorter survival of the group that received only supportive care, in addition to being related to not receiving anticancer treatment per se, is likely to be confounded by selection of patients for treatment who had a more favorable prognosis or better ability to tolerate treatment.

A study by Italiano et al. [7] (median age range 53–59 years), which included patients from the time frame of this study (i.e., 2002–2006), found that patients with synchronous or metachronous metastatic STS had an overall survival of 18 months from the time of metastatic diagnosis. Patients in the study by Italiano et al. [7] had relatively longer survival than those in this study, plausibly because patients in this study were considerably

Table 5 Overall survival by treatment status and histologic categories

Overall	Survival from initial diagnosis of advanced STS					
	Total	Died	Censored	Median length of survival (in months)	95% CI	
All advanced STS patients	4274	3565	709	8.9	8.3	9.7
Treatment status						
Received cancer-directed treatment	2656	2185	471	13.6	12.9	14.6
Received supportive care only	1618	1380	238	2.8	2.6	3.4
Histologic categories						
Fibroblastic/myofibroblastic sarcomas	227	160	67	21.4	15.6	26.8
Leiomyosarcomas	922	781	141	12.9	10.9	14.6
Liposarcomas	554	395	159	21.1	17.4	27.1
Nerve sheath sarcomas	106	88	18	6.2	3.6	9.3
Rhabdomyosarcomas	98	–	–	3.0	1.8	5.7
Synovial sarcomas	49	–	–	8.6	5.3	13.8
Undifferentiated pleomorphic sarcomas	652	539	113	9.6	8.2	11.4
Vascular sarcomas	357	327	30	6.0	4.8	7.3
Others/NOS	1309	1139	170	5.4	4.8	6.1

CI confidence interval, *NOS* not otherwise specified, *STS* soft-tissue sarcoma

older. Similar to this study, survival did vary by histologic category in the study by Italiano et al. [7]. For example, patients with leiomyosarcoma, UPS, and nerve sheath sarcoma had a median survival of 12.9, 9.6, and 6.2 months, respectively, in this study and 19.4, 11.2, and 8.6 months, respectively, in the Italiano et al. [7] study.

An array of treatments (e.g. eribulin, olaratumab, pazopanib, trabectedin) became available for this population in the last decade [11, 13, 14, 37]; however, effectiveness of these treatments specifically among older adult patients with advanced STS is yet to established. Other treatments like oral cyclophosphamide plus prednisone [34] may also be feasible for older adult patients for whom treatment with doxorubicin may not be an option. Overall survival, progression-free survival, and response rates of patients with advanced STS may improve as these treatments will become part of routine care provided to this population.

This study is subject to several limitations inherent in analyses of Medicare claims data and the use of such data in studies of advanced cancer, in particular. For patients who were not initially diagnosed at the metastatic stage of the disease, ICD-9-CM diagnosis codes were used to identify evidence of metastatic disease during the follow-up period. However, the use of ICD-9-CM codes to identify metastatic disease has been shown to have sensitivity, specificity, and positive predictive value of less than 80%, and thus the use of ICD-9-CM diagnosis codes in the Medicare claims data may have resulted in inaccurate or under-identification of an advanced STS population [38, 39]. As described in the study methods, one of the criteria used to identify progression to metastatic disease was the initiation of systemic therapy at least 6 months after surgery. This criterion may have resulted in selection bias because patients who had disease progression but did not receive systemic therapy would have been omitted from the supportive care-only group. Although, the 6-month lag period after surgery was used to avoid interpreting adjuvant therapy as treatment for advanced disease, patients who progressed and received systemic therapy for advanced disease would have been omitted from the cancer-directed therapy group. Lines of therapy are not reported in claims data; therefore, an algorithm had to be defined to estimate the lines of therapy. This may have misclassified treatments by line of therapy, as the reasons for treatment changes were not available in the data. The Medicare Part D database was available for only a subset of the cohort (32.4%); however, only a small proportion of all chemotherapy (2%) claims were identified from the Medicare Part D database, so the risk of missing important treatment data is relatively low despite this limitation. An array of treatments (i.e., eribulin, olaratumab, pazopanib, trabectedin) became available for this population in the last decade, although these agents are not fully represented in the study dataset. Future research should evaluate the use and outcomes of these novel treatments in the older adult population. Finally, this study included only patients aged 65 years or older, and although SEER-Medicare data is representative of the US population 65 years and older for age and gender, participating SEER sites may not be representative with regard to distribution of race, income, urban residence,

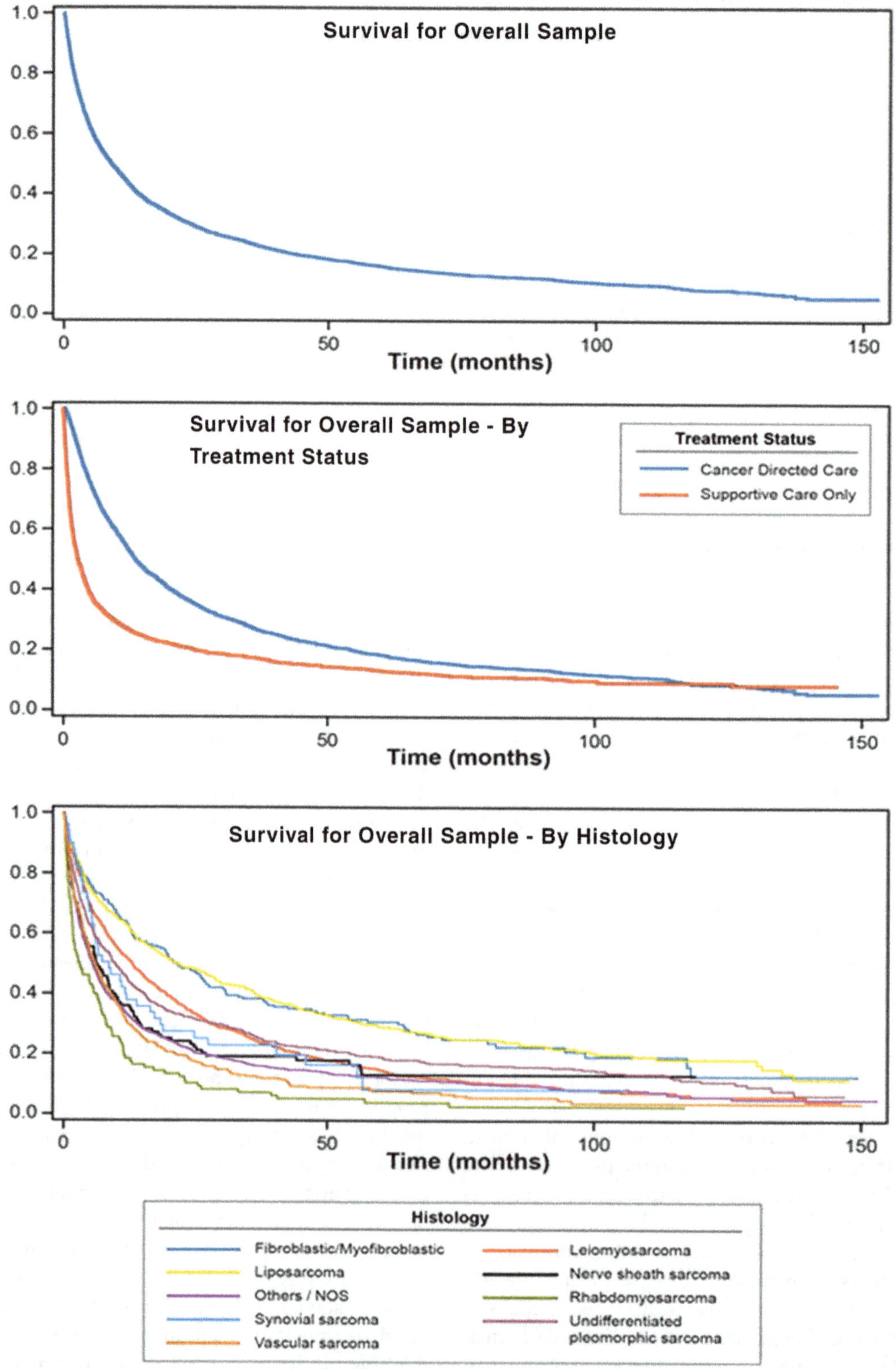

Fig. 1 Survival estimates from diagnosis of advanced soft-tissue sarcoma

HMO enrollment as well as cancer mortality [15] and thus the results should not be generalized to the entire population of older adult patients with advanced STS.

Despite these limitations, this study documents real-world treatment patterns that may help inform providers, researchers, and policymakers about the care of older patients with STS in the US. As real-world data including new therapeutic options become available, our results provide a basis for analyzing changes in treatment patterns and outcomes over time. This study demonstrates that the prognosis is poor for older adult patients with advanced STS, highlighting the unmet medical need in this population.

Conclusion

Although previous studies of younger populations reported anthracycline-based therapy predominated in first line, our study of older adults with advanced STS found that doxorubicin was not commonly used. Despite variation by histologic category, prognosis was observed to be poor for older adult patients with advanced STS in this study.

Abbreviations

CCI: Charlson Comorbidity Index; CI: confidence interval; HCPCS: Healthcare Common Procedure Coding System; ICD-9-CM: International Classification of Diseases, 9th Revision, Clinical Modification; ICD-O-3: International Classification of Diseases for Oncology, 3rd Edition; NCCN: National Comprehensive Cancer Network; NCI: National Cancer Institute; NOS: not otherwise specified; SD: standard deviation; SEER: The Surveillance, Epidemiology, and End Results; STS: soft-tissue sarcoma; UPS: undifferentiated pleomorphic sarcoma; US: United States.

Authors' contributions

All authors have participated in the content of the manuscript from initial study design, protocol development and interpretation of the data. RP drafted the manuscript and conducted the study analyses. All other authors contributed significant scientific/intellectual content and provided critical revisions to the draft manuscript. All authors meet the criteria for authorship in accordance with the authorship standards of the International Committee of Medical Journal Editors (ICMJE) *Recommendations for the Conduct, Reporting, Editing and Publication of Scholarly Work in Medical Journals* (http://www.ICMJE.org). All authors read and approved the final manuscript.

Author details

[1] RTI Health Solutions, 200 Park Offices Drive, Research Triangle Park, NC 27560, USA. [2] Eli Lilly and Company Limited, Lilly Research Centre, Erl Wood Manor, Sunninghill Road, Windlesham, Surrey GU20 6PH, UK. [3] Eli Lilly and Company, Lilly Corporate Center, Indianapolis, IN 46285, USA. [4] RTI Health Solutions, 307 Waverley Oaks Road, Suite 101, Waltham, MA 02452, USA.

Acknowledgements

The authors acknowledge Eleanor Sibal (RTI Health Solutions) for medical writing support.

Competing interests

This study was performed under a research contract between RTI Health Solutions and Eli Lilly and Company and was funded by Eli Lilly and Company. RCP, SDC, and JAK are salaried employees of RTI Health Solutions. ML, LMH, and SN are salaried employees of Eli Lilly and Company.

Funding

This work was funded by Eli Lilly and Company, Indianapolis, IN, United States.

Appendix 1

See Table 6.

Table 6 Advanced soft-tissue sarcoma histologic categories and subtypes. Source: World Health Organization [17]

Histologic subtype (ICD-O-3)	Description[a]
Fibroblastic/myofibroblastic sarcomas	
8810/3	Fibrosarcoma, NOS
8811/3	Fibromyxosarcoma
8814/3	Infantile fibrosarcoma
8815/3	Solitary fibrous tumor, malignant
8825/3	Myofibroblastic sarcoma
8832/3	Dermatofibrosarcoma, NOS
Leiomyosarcomas	
8890/3	Leiomyosarcoma, NOS
8891/3	Epithelioid leiomyosarcoma
8896/3	Myxoid leiomyosarcoma
Liposarcomas	
8850/3	Liposarcoma, NOS
8851/3	Liposarcoma, well differentiated
8852/3	Myxoid liposarcoma
8853/3	Round cell liposarcoma
8854/3	Pleomorphic liposarcoma
8855/3	Mixed liposarcoma
8857/3	Fibroblastic liposarcoma
8858/3	Dedifferentiated liposarcoma
Nerve sheath sarcomas	
9540/3	Malignant peripheral nerve sheath tumor
9560/3	Malignant neurilemoma
9561/3	Malignant triton tumor
9571/3	Malignant Perineurioma
9580/3	Malignant granular cell tumor
Others/NOS	
8800/3	Sarcoma, NOS
8801/3	Undifferentiated spindle cell sarcoma
8802/3	Undifferentiated pleomorphic sarcoma
8803/3	Undifferentiated round cell sarcoma
8804/3	Undifferentiated epithelioid sarcoma
8805/3	Undifferentiated sarcoma
8806/3	Desmoplastic small round cell tumor
8840/3	Myxosarcoma
8842/3	Ossifying fibromyxoid tumor, atypical
8860/3	Angiomyolipoma
8894/3	Angiomyosarcoma
8895/3	Myosarcoma
8940/3	Mixed tumor, malignant, NOS
8963/3	Malignant rhabdoid tumor
8982/3	Myoepithelial carcinoma
8990/3	Mesenchymoma, malignant
9020/3	Phyllodes tumor, malignant
9044/3	Clear cell sarcoma, NOS (except of kidney)
9133/3	Epithelioid hemangioendothelioma, malignant
9231/3	Myxoid chondrosarcoma
9251/3	Malignant giant cell tumor of soft parts
9364/3	Peripheral neuroectodermal tumor
Rhabdomyosarcomas	
8900/3	Rhabdomyosarcoma, NOS
8901/3	Pleomorphic rhabdomyosarcoma, adult type
8902/3	Mixed type rhabdomyosarcoma
8910/3	Embryonal rhabdomyosarcoma, NOS
8912/3	Spindle cell rhabdomyosarcoma
8920/3	Alveolar rhabdomyosarcoma
Synovial sarcomas	
9040/3	Synovial sarcoma, NOS
9041/3	Synovial sarcoma, spindle cell
9042/3	Synovial sarcoma, epithelioid cell
9043/3	Synovial sarcoma, biphasic
Undifferentiated pleomorphic sarcoma (previously known as malignant fibrous histiocytoma or MFH)	
8830/3	Malignant fibrous histiocytoma
Vascular sarcomas	
9120/3	Hemangiosarcoma
9130/3	Hemangioendothelioma, malignant
9150/3	Hemangiopericytoma, malignant
9161/3	Hemangioblastoma; angioblastoma
9170/3	Lymphangiosarcoma

NOS not otherwise specified

Appendix 2

See Table 7.

Table 7 Patient and tumor characteristics, overall and by histologic categories

	All patients	Leiomyo-sarcomas	Undifferentiated pleomorphic sarcoma	Liposarcomas	Vascular sarcomas	Fibroblastic/ myofibroblastic sarcomas	Nerve sheath sarcomas	Rhabdomyo-sarcomas	Synovial sarcomas	Others/NOS
N	4274	922	652	554	357	227	106	98	49	1309
Location of residence (n, %)										
Big metro	2358 (55.2)	507 (55.0)	362 (55.5)	294 (53.1)	198 (55.5)	133 (58.6)	55 (51.9)	54 (55.1)	25 (51.0)	730 (55.8)
Less urban	1269 (29.7)	267 (29.0)	187 (28.7)	172 (31.1)	111 (31.1)	65 (28.6)	40 (37.7)	29 (29.6)	16 (32.7)	382 (29.2)
Metro	255 (6.0)	55 (6.0)	39 (6.0)	35 (6.3)	21 (5.9)	–	–	–	–	83 (6.3)
Rural	320 (7.5)	78 (8.5)	60 (9.2)	41 (7.4)	–	17 (7.5)	–	–	–	87 (6.7)
Urban	71 (1.7)	15 (1.6)	–	12 (2.2)	–	–	0 (0.0)	–	0 (0.0)	27 (2.1)
SEER region (n, %)										
Northeast	981 (23.0)	197 (21.4)	147 (22.6)	143 (25.8)	75 (21.0)	59 (26.0)	29 (27.4)	24 (24.5)	13 (26.5)	294 (22.5)
Midwest	472 (11.0)	124 (13.5)	57 (8.7)	47 (8.5)	35 (9.8)	29 (12.8)	12 (11.3)	13 (13.3)	–	149 (11.4)
South	971 (22.7)	238 (25.8)	170 (26.1)	106 (19.1)	94 (26.3)	27 (11.9)	16 (15.1)	18 (18.4)	–	292 (22.3)
West	1850 (43.3)	363 (39.4)	278 (42.6)	258 (46.6)	153 (42.9)	112 (49.3)	49 (46.2)	43 (43.9)	20 (40.8)	574 (43.9)
Anatomic location of primary tumor at the time of initial diagnosis of STS (n, %)										
Axilla	526 (12.3)	110 (11.9)	65 (10.0)	105 (19.0)	41 (11.5)	37 (16.3)	13 (12.3)	–	–	140 (10.7)
Breast	123 (2.9)	12 (1.3)	–	–	28 (7.8)	–	–	–	0 (0.0)	67 (5.1)
Genitourinary	106 (2.5)	34 (3.7)	–	–	12 (3.4)	–	–	–	–	38 (2.9)
Head or neck	354 (8.3)	31 (3.4)	104 (16.0)	13 (2.4)	108 (30.3)	13 (5.7)	17 (16.0)	–	–	61 (4.7)
Lower limb	937 (21.9)	125 (13.6)	236 (36.2)	122 (22.0)	41 (11.5)	58 (25.6)	22 (20.8)	19 (19.4)	16 (32.7)	298 (22.8)
Mediastinum, lung, or pleura	221 (5.2)	29 (3.2)	12 (1.8)	–	16 (4.5)	28 (12.3)	–	–	–	110 (8.4)
Pelvis	416 (9.7)	83 (9.0)	66 (10.1)	49 (8.8)	30 (8.4)	23 (10.1)	11 (10.4)	–	–	144 (11.0)
Retroperitoneal	396 (9.3)	118 (12.8)	19 (2.9)	174 (31.4)	–	–	–	–	0 (0.0)	70 (5.4)
Trunk	283 (6.6)	59 (6.4)	39 (6.0)	26 (4.7)	25 (7.0)	16 (7.1)	–	–	–	99 (7.6)
Upper limb	309 (7.2)	36 (3.9)	89 (13.7)	32 (5.8)	11 (3.1)	30 (13.2)	–	–	–	87 (6.7)
Uterus	366 (8.6)	228 (24.7)	–	15 (2.7)	0 (0.0)	–	–	21 (21.4)	0 (0.0)	92 (7.0)
Other	237 (5.6)	57 (6.2)	–	–	41 (11.5)	–	–	–	–	103 (7.9)

References

1. Wibmer C, Leithner A, Zielonke N, Sperl M, Windhager R. Increasing incidence rates of soft tissue sarcomas? A population-based epidemiologic study and literature review. Ann Oncol. 2010;21(5):1106–11.
2. Siegel RL, Miller KD, Jemal A. Cancer statistics, 2018. CA Cancer J Clin. 2018;68:7–30.
3. National Cancer Institute (NCI). Age-adjusted SEER incidence rates. https://seer.cancer.gov/faststats/selections.php?series=age. Accessed 10 Jan 2018.
4. Schöffski P, Cornillie J, Wozniak A, Li H, Hompes D. Soft tissue sarcoma: an update on systemic treatment options for patients with advanced disease. Oncol Res Treat. 2014;37(6):355–62.
5. National Cancer Institute (NCI). Adult soft tissue sarcoma treatment (PDQ); 2017. https://www.cancer.gov/types/soft-tissue-sarcoma/patient/adult-soft-tissue-treatment-pdq. Accessed 30 March 2017.
6. American Cancer Society (ACS). Survival by Stage of Soft Tissue Sarcoma; 2016. https://www.cancer.org/cancer/soft-tissue-sarcoma/detection-diagnosis-staging/survival-rates.html. Accessed 21 Sept 2017.
7. Italiano A, Mathoulin-Pelissier S, Cesne AL, Terrier P, Bonvalot S, Collin F, et al. Trends in survival for patients with metastatic soft-tissue sarcoma. Cancer. 2011;117(5):1049–54.
8. Spira AI, Ettinger DS. The use of chemotherapy in soft-tissue sarcomas. Oncologist. 2002;7(4):348–59.
9. Karavasilis V, Seddon BM, Ashley S, Al-Muderis O, Fisher C, Judson I. Significant clinical benefit of first-line palliative chemotherapy in advanced soft-tissue sarcoma: retrospective analysis and identification of prognostic factors in 488 patients. Cancer. 2008;112(7):1585–91.
10. Judson I, Verweij J, Gelderblom H, Hartmann JT, Schöffski P, Blay JY, et al. Doxorubicin alone versus intensified doxorubicin plus ifosfamide for first-line treatment of advanced soft-tissue sarcoma: a randomised controlled phase 3 trial. Lancet Oncol. 2014;15(4):415–23.
11. Tap WD, Jones RL, Van Tine BA, Chmielowski B, Elias AD, Adkins D, et al. Olaratumab and doxorubicin versus doxorubicin alone for treatment of soft-tissue sarcoma: an open-label phase 1b and randomised phase 2 trial. Lancet. 2016;388(10043):488–97.
12. United States Food and Drug Administration (FDA). FDA grants accelerated approval to new treatment for advanced soft tissue sarcoma [press release]; 2016. https://www.fda.gov/newsevents/newsroom/pressannouncements/ucm525878.htm. Accessed 7 July 2017.
13. Demetri GD, Von Mehren M, Jones RL, Hensley ML, Schuetze SM, Staddon A, Milhem M, Elias A, Ganjoo K, Tawbi H, Van Tine BA. Efficacy and safety of trabectedin or dacarbazine for metastatic liposarcoma or leiomyosarcoma after failure of conventional chemotherapy: results of a phase III randomized multicenter clinical trial. J Clin Oncol. 2015;34(8):786–93.
14. van der Graaf WT, Blay JY, Chawla SP, Kim DW, Bui-Nguyen B, Casali PG, Schöffski P, Aglietta M, Staddon AP, Beppu Y, Le Cesne A. Pazopanib for metastatic soft-tissue sarcoma (PALETTE): a randomised, double-blind, placebo-controlled phase 3 trial. Lancet. 2012;379(9829):1879–86.
15. Warren JL, Klabunde CN, Schrag D, Bach PB, Riley GF. Overview of the SEER-Medicare data: content, research applications, and generalizability to the United States elderly population. Med Care. 2002;40(Suppl 8):IV-3-18.
16. Nattinger AB, McAuliffe TL, Schapira MM. Generalizability of the Surveillance, Epidemiology, and End Results registry population: factors relevant to epidemiologic and health care research. J Clin Epidemiol. 1997;50(8):939–45.
17. World Health Organization (WHO). International classification of diseases for oncology (ICD-O), 3rd edition, 1st revision; 2013. http://apps.who.int/iris/bitstream/10665/96612/1/9789241548496_eng.pdf. Accessed June 2017.
18. Christopher DM, Fletcher JA, Bridge PC, editors. WHO classification of tumours of soft tissue and bone. 4th ed. Lyon: World Health Organization; 2013. p. 110–1.
19. American Joint Committee on Cancer. Cancer staging manual. 6th edition; 2002. https://cancerstaging.org/references-tools/deskreferences/Pages/default.aspx. Accessed 26 June 2017.
20. National Cancer Institute (NCI). SEER summary staging manual—2000: codes and coding instructions; 2000. https://seer.cancer.gov/tools/ssm/. Accessed 9 June 2017.
21. Charlson ME, Pompei P, Ales KL, MacKenzie CR. A new method of classifying prognostic comorbidity in longitudinal studies: development and validation. J Chronic Dis. 1987;40(5):373–83.
22. Charlson ME, Charlson RE, Peterson JC, Marinopoulos SS, Briggs WM, Hollenberg JP. The Charlson Comorbidity Index is adapted to predict costs of chronic disease in primary care patients. J Clin Epidemiol. 2008;61(12):1234–40.
23. Deyo RA, Cherkin DC, Ciol MA. Adapting a clinical comorbidity index for use with ICD-9-CM administrative databases. J Clin Epidemiol. 1992;45(6):613–9.
24. National Comprehensive Cancer Network (NCCN). Soft tissue sarcoma. NCCN Clinical Practice Guidelines in Oncology; 2017 https://www.nccn.org/professionals/physician_gls/pdf/sarcoma.pdf. Accessed June 2017.
25. Wagner MJ, Amodu LI, Duh MS, Korves C, Solleza F, Manson SC, et al. A retrospective chart review of drug treatment patterns and clinical outcomes among patients with metastatic or recurrent soft tissue sarcoma refractory to one or more prior chemotherapy treatments. BMC Cancer. 2015;15:175.
26. Leahy M, Garcia Del Muro X, Reichardt P, Judson I, Staddon A, Verweij J, et al. Chemotherapy treatment patterns and clinical outcomes in patients with metastatic soft tissue sarcoma. The Sarcoma treatment and Burden of Illness in North America and Europe (SABINE) study. Ann Oncol. 2012;23(10):2763–70.
27. Matushansky I, Dela Cruz F, Insel BJ, Hershman DL, Neugut AI. Chemotherapy use in elderly patients with soft tissue sarcoma: a population-based study. Cancer Invest. 2013;31(2):83–91.
28. Skubitz KM, Haddad PA. Paclitaxel and pegylated-liposomal doxorubicin are both active in angiosarcoma. Cancer. 2005;104(2):361–6.
29. Penel N, Bui BN, Bay JO, Cupissol D, Ray-Coquard I, Piperno-Neumann S, et al. Phase II trial of weekly paclitaxel for unresectable angiosarcoma: the ANGIOTAX Study. J Clin Oncol. 2008;26(32):5269–74.
30. Schlemmer M, Reichardt P, Verweij J, Hartmann JT, Judson I, Thyss A, et al. Paclitaxel in patients with advanced angiosarcomas of soft tissue: a retrospective study of the EORTC soft tissue and bone sarcoma group. Eur J Cancer. 2008;44(16):2433–6.
31. Chatterjee K, Zhang J, Honbo N, Karliner JS. Doxorubicin cardiomyopathy. Cardiology. 2010;115(2):155–62.
32. Volkova M, Russell R 3rd. Anthracycline cardiotoxicity: prevalence, pathogenesis and treatment. Curr Cardiol Rev. 2011;7(4):214–20.
33. Hershman DL, McBride RB, Eisenberger A, Tsai WY, Grann VR, Jacobson JS. Doxorubicin, cardiac risk factors, and cardiac toxicity in elderly patients with diffuse B-cell non-Hodgkin's lymphoma. J Clin Oncol. 2008;26(19):3159–65.
34. Mir O, Domont J, Cioffi A, Bonvalot S, Boulet B, Le Pechoux C, Terrier P, Spielmann M, Le Cesne A. Feasibility of metronomic oral cyclophosphamide plus prednisolone in elderly patients with inoperable or metastatic soft tissue sarcoma. Eur J Cancer. 2011;47(4):515–9.
35. Ferreira AL, Matsubara LS, Matsubara BB. Anthracycline-induced cardiotoxicity. Cardiovasc Hematol Agents Med Chem (Former Curr Med ChemistryCardiovasc Hematol Agents). 2008;6(4):278–81.
36. Davis KL, Goyal RK, Able SL, Brown J, Li L, Kaye JA. Real-world treatment patterns and costs in a US Medicare population with metastatic squamous non-small cell lung cancer. Lung Cancer. 2015;87(2):176–85.
37. Schöffski P, Chawla S, Maki RG, Italiano A, Gelderblom H, Choy E, et al. Eribulin versus dacarbazine in previously treated patients with advanced liposarcoma or leiomyosarcoma: a randomised, open-label, multicentre, phase 3 trial. Lancet. 2016;387(10028):1629–37.
38. National Cancer Institute (NCI). Measures that are limited or not available in the data; 2015. https://healthcaredelivery.cancer.gov/seermedicare/considerations/measures.html. Accessed 21 Sept 2017.
39. Chawla N, Yabroff KR, Mariotto A, McNeel TS, Schrag D, Warren JL. Limited validity of diagnosis codes in Medicare claims for identifying cancer metastases and inferring stage. Ann Epidemiol. 2014;24(9):666–72.

PDGF/PDGFR effects in osteosarcoma and the "add-on" strategy

Jie Xu, Lu Xie and Wei Guo*

Abstract

New treatment options for advanced osteosarcoma have remained limited. The platelet-derived growth factor (PDGF)/platelet-derived growth factor receptor (PDGFR) pathway plays an important role in the development and metastasis of osteosarcoma, via either direct autocrine stimulation of tumor cells, or paracrine stimulation on tumor stromal cells. It promotes angiogenesis to overcome hypoxia in the tumor microenvironment, and modulates tumor interstitial fluid pressure to control the influx and efflux of other agents. Targeting the PDGF/PDGFR pathway is a promising therapeutic method to overcome drug resistance and improve patients' outcome in osteosarcoma. Further evidence is needed to define the detailed mechanism. Results from clinical trials using PDGF/PDGFR inhibitor as a single agent were disappointing, both in osteosarcoma and soft tissue sarcoma. However, when combined with other agents, named as "add-on" strategy, a synergistic antitumor effect has been confirmed in soft tissue sarcoma, and should be attempted in osteosarcoma.

Keywords: PDGF, PDGFR, Osteosarcoma, Add-on therapy

Background

Osteosarcoma is the most common primary bone malignancy in adolescents and young adults, with an incidence rate of 4.4 cases per 1 million each year in people aged 0–24 years [1]. Current multidisciplinary treatments have led to a dramatic improvement in prognosis for patients with localized osteosarcoma; long-term survival rates of less than 20% improved to 65–70% [2]. Unfortunately, with metastatic disease, the rate of long-term survival is greatly reduced to 20–30% [3, 4]. Although several clinical trials have been conducted, and new drugs such as sorafenib and everolimus have been tested in metastatic osteosarcoma, the overall outcome has not significantly improved over the past few decades [5–7]. The event-free survival for refractory or relapsed osteosarcoma is as low as 12% at 4 months [7].

Platelet-derived growth factors (PDGFs) and their receptors (PDGFRs) are major players in oncogenesis and drug resistance, and are attractive oncologic targets in cancer [8]. PDGFs/PDGFRs are frequently expressed in various tumors, and their expression levels correlate with tumor growth, invasiveness, drug resistance, and poor clinical outcomes [9]. The PDGF pathway is also a key signal for tumor stromal cells recruitment such as cancer-associated fibroblasts [10], which play an important role in the maintenance of tumor microenvironment. The exact mechanism leading to the development and metastasis of osteosarcoma is not fully understood. The PDGF receptor does not appear to be as central to proliferation for osteosarcoma cultures as Bcr/Abl is for chronic myelogenous leukemia. Although PDGF is known to stimulate proliferation and differentiation of osteoblasts and osteoclasts [11], its role in osteosarcoma, specifically PDGF ligands and their receptors, is poorly understood. Whether treatment with PDGF/PDGF receptor antagonists will be beneficial for osteosarcoma is the subject of ongoing studies. In this article, we summarize the preclinical and clinical studies of the PDGF pathway in osteosarcoma, and discuss the mechanism and future directions.

Overview of PDGF signaling

Activation and function of PDGF/PDGFR pathway

The platelet-derived growth factor (PDGF) signaling network consists of four ligands, PDGF-A, PDGF-B,

*Correspondence: bonetumor@163.com
Peking University People's Hospital, Beijing 100044, China

PDGF-C, and PDGF-D, and two receptors, PDGFR-α and PDGFR-β. All PDGFs function as disulfide-linked homodimers, but only PDGF-A and -B can form functional heterodimers. Before binding to the protein tyrosine kinase receptors PDGFR-α and PDGFR-β, the four PDGF ligands are inactive in their monomeric forms. The receptor isoforms dimerize upon binding, leading to three possible receptor combinations, namely -AA, -BB, and -AB, causing the subsequent activation of kinase. Kinase activation is visualized as tyrosine phosphorylation of the receptor molecules, which occurs between the dimerized receptor molecules (transphosphorylation). The receptor molecules then undergo conformational changes that allow a basal kinase activity to phosphorylate a critical tyrosine residue, thereby "unlocking" the kinase, leading to full enzymatic activity directed toward other tyrosine residues in the receptor molecules, as well as other substrates for the kinase [12, 13].

More than 10 different molecules bind selectively to phosphorylated residues in the PDGF receptors, including the Src family, SHP-2 tyrosine phosphatase, phospholipase C-γ (PLC-γ), and the GTPase activating protein (GAP) for Ras. Furthermore, the receptors bind and activate signal transducers and activators of transcription (STATs). Finally, some of the receptors binding molecules lack intrinsic enzymatic activities, but can form complexes with other signaling molecules. For example, the regulatory subunit p85 of the PI3K forms a complex with the p110 catalytic subunit, and Grb2 activates Ras and the Erk MAP-kinase pathway by binding with SOS1. In addition, the PDGF receptors bind other adaptors (e.g., Shc, Nck, Crk, and GAB) and mediate interactions with numerous different downstream signaling molecules [14, 15]. The activation of these signaling pathways leads to cell survival, proliferation, angiogenesis, and cell migration.

PDGFs and PDGFRs are expressed by a large variety of normal human tissues and organs. PDGFs are major mitogens for many cell types of mesenchymal or neuroectodermal in origin. PDGFs have chemo-attractant properties and are involved in erythropoiesis, wound healing, bone formation, and angiogenesis. Much evidence suggests involvement in the normal development of important organs such as kidney, brain, and cardiovascular and respiratory systems [16]. During normal development, cell proliferation significantly increases as a consequence of PDGF overexpression and decreases in PDGF null mutants.

PDGF/PDGFR pathway in tumor development and metastasis

A complex interplay between cancer cells, endothelial cells, and other stromal cells occurs in tumor angiogenesis. The PDGF/PDGFR pathway plays an important role in the development and metastasis of tumors in at least three different ways: (1) direct autocrine stimulation of tumor cells [17]; (2) paracrine stimulation of tumor stromal cells [12] and promotion of angiogenesis to overcome hypoxia in the tumor microenvironment [18]; (3) modulation of tumor interstitial fluid pressure (IFP) to control the influx and efflux of agents [19].

The mode of action of PDGF and PDGFR involvement in tumor development and progression is mainly through direct autocrine stimulation of tumor cell growth and cell autonomy, whereas in normal tissues paracrine stimulation is predominant [20]. Direct blockade of autocrine stimulation using inhibitors of PDGFR in cell lines and xenograft models show positive results in tumors such as lung cancer [21], hepatic cancer [22], gastrointestinal stromal tumor (GIST) [23], dermatofibrosarcoma protuberans [24], and osteosarcoma, which expressed PDGFR-α on the cell surface [25]. The levels of phosphorylation of both PDGFRs and the downstream signaling proteins such as protein kinase B (AKT) and extracellular regulated kinase (ERK) are downregulated by PDGFR antibodies or small molecular tyrosine kinase inhibitors (TKIs) [25].

In addition to direct autocrine stimulation, the PDGF/PDGFR pathway exerts paracrine stimulation on tumor stromal cells. PDGF promotes the formation of a rich stromal compartment, characterized by deposition of extracellular matrix components and blood vessel formation [26]. Experimental models showed that VEGF-null cells require PDGFR to recruit fibroblasts in tumor stroma [27]. Cancer-associated fibroblasts (CAFs), which secrete several active factors to stimulate angiogenesis and tumor invasion, constitute a functionally important component of tumor stroma in many types of cancer [28].

Clinical data indicate that carcinomas with desmoplastic stroma, consisting of fibroblast cells and extracellular matrix, are associated with a poor prognosis [29]. An experimental model of glioma revealed that PDGF-B enhances angiogenesis by stimulating VEGF expression in tumor-associated endothelial cells and by recruiting pericytes [30]. Several other preclinical models demonstrated that using antibodies or TKIs to disrupt the paracrine signaling with PDGFR can significantly reduce tumor growth by inhibiting tumor cell growth, recruitment of fibroblasts, and angiogenesis in xenograft tumor models or genetic mouse models of cancer [31], such as melanoma [26], cervical cancer [32], and colon cancer [33].

Targeting the PDGF/PDGFR pathway can regulate the influx and efflux of agents and thus modify the uptake of drugs. Previous data showed that connective tissue cells control interstitial fluid pressure (IFP) by exerting tension on the collagen/microfibrillar network via collagen binding integrin a_2b_1 [34, 35]. Experiments using transgenic mice carrying PDGFR-β receptor mutations suggest a function for PDGF signaling through PI3K in IFP homeostasis by modulating the tension between cells and extracellular matrix structures [35]. Previous studies reported that the inhibition of PDGFR reduced interstitial hypertension and increased transcapillary transport in tumors. An increased tumor uptake of the tracer compound ^{51}Cr-EDTA and paclitaxel, after inhibition of PDGF receptor using TKIs in tumor stroma, was previously demonstrated [18, 19, 36].

An increased tumor uptake of cytotoxic drugs has therefore been proposed as the mechanism and further promotes combination treatment with PDGF antagonists and chemotherapy, which is called an "add-on" strategy. "Add-on" strategy has been used in a variety of tumors with different partners, such as fludarabine phosphate (F-AMP) in GIST [37], doxorubicin in breast cancer [38], and fucoxanthin in chronic myeloid leukemia [39]. Because of the mild adverse effect of PDGF antagonists, most combinations are safe and well-tolerated.

PDGF/PDGFR pathway in osteosarcoma

Expression of PDGFs/PDGFRs in osteosarcoma

The expression of PDGF/PDGF receptors in osteosarcoma has been tested in immunohistochemical (IHC) studies of specimens and various cell lines. A significant heterogeneity has been found in this pathway because the proportion of positive staining varies widely from study to study (4–90%). However, the association of higher expression of PDGF with higher proliferation and poorer prognosis seems universally accepted. One of the early immunohistochemical studies demonstrated that of 37 cases of osteosarcoma, 38% showed PDGF and PDGFR expression, with 11 (30%) cases having expression of both, and correlation of PDGF-positive tumors with higher proliferation (MIB-1 index) compared with PDGF-negative tumors [40]. Another immunohistochemical study also demonstrated that 23 osteosarcoma specimens each expressed both PDGF-A and PDGF-a receptor with 52 and 43% staining strongly positive (>25% of the cells stained), respectively [41]. A study with 57 osteosarcoma samples showed that high levels of PDGF-AA expression were associated with a significantly lower 5-year disease-free survival compared with low-level expression of PDGF-AA (21.22% vs. 42.72%). PDGF-a receptor expression, although exhibiting a similar trend, failed to achieve significance [42]. A flow cytometry study of patient-derived osteosarcoma cell lines showed high expression of PDGFR-β in the co-expression with insulin receptors [43].

In a clinical trial for imatinib and osteosarcoma, a frequent expression of PDGF-AA (80.4%) and PDGF-a receptor (79.6%) and their correlation with inferior event-free survival ($P<0.05$) was reported. PDGF-BB and PDGF-b-receptor expressions were also frequent (75.4 and 86%, respectively); however, statistically significant inferior event-free survival was not demonstrated ($P=0.15$) [44]. On the contrary, in a larger study of 100 patients, 96 showed PDGFRA expression ranging from 4 to 90%. Overall and disease-free survival analysis did not reveal any differences between osteosarcoma patients, according to the level of PDGFRA expression [45]. Another study showed more than 50% positive expression of PDGFs/PDGFRs but no relationship with patients' outcome [46].

Targeting PDGF/PDGFR pathway in osteosarcoma

By definition, autocrine growth is suggested to occur in cells expressing both ligand and its cognate receptor, and osteosarcomas meet these criteria [17]. Co-expression of PDGF and PDGFRs has been confirmed in osteosarcoma cell lines, as well as in human osteosarcoma samples, as mentioned above. Recently, antagonists specific for PDGF/PDGFR have been developed and used to investigate the role of PDGFR stimulation in various diseases [14, 15, 47]. Typically, there are two kinds of inhibitors, (1) the antibody or other binders can target the receptors and prevent their activation or promote their degradation specifically [48, 49], and (2) several tyrosine kinase inhibitors of PDGF receptor kinases (TKIs), including imatinib, sunitinib, sorafenib, and pazopanib, which are not specific and are multi-targeted [47, 50–52] (Table 1). For most TKIs studied in osteosarcoma clinical trials, anti-angiogenesis was considered a more dominant mechanism compared with anti-PDGF effect. The only exception was imatinib.

Imatinib

Imatinib mesylate (Gleevec, STI571, Novartis Pharmaceuticals) was the first TKI developed as an ATP competitive inhibitor of ABL tyrosine kinase that has been highly effective in chronic myelomonocytic leukemia [53, 54]. Imatinib also inhibits other tyrosine kinase receptors except for ABL, including PDGFR and c-kit,

Table 1 The IC_{50} values and targets of the approved kinase inhibitors against PDGFRs

Kinase name	Imatinib	Dasatinib	Nilotinib	Sorafenib	Sunitinib	Pazopanib
IC_{50} values						
PDGFR-α [49]	2.5	2.6	2.4	1.0	13	20
PDGFR-α [T674I] [50]	8500		4100	100	19	170
PDGFR-α [V561D] [50]	9.1	2.9	15	5.6	14	21
PDGFR-β [53]	68	1.1	60	34	5.7	42
Primary targets [53, 54]	Abl, PDGFR, Kit	Abl, Src	Kit, Abl, PDGFR	Raf, VEGFR, PDGFR, Kit, Flt3	PDGFR, VEGFR, Kit, Flt3	VEGFR, PDGFR, Kit
Secondary targets [53, 54]	Raf	PDGFR, Kit				FGFR

Primary targets: The targets that are inhibited at the lowest concentrations (regardless of absolute concentrations)

Secondary targets: The targets that are inhibited by about tenfold higher inhibitor concentrations

and was approved for treatment of c-kit positive gastrointestinal stromal tumors (GIST) and dermatofibrosarcoma protuberans [24]. Given the activation of PDGF/PDGFR pathway, several in vitro and in vivo experiments have been performed with osteosarcomas.

Because PDGF acts as a potent mitogen in several osteosarcoma cell lines [55, 56] and patient-derived cell cultures [44], the inhibition of the PDGF pathway results in a reduction of cell proliferation due to caspase-dependent apoptosis [44, 56, 57], an arrest of the cell cycle, and an inhibition of cell migration. Imatinib exhibits a dose-dependent anti-proliferative effect in all cell lines studied [56]. To further define the inhibition effect of PDGF pathway, the expression of downstream signaling protein has been tested. Greater than 50% inhibition of PDGFR phosphorylation and its downstream signaling molecules such as AKT and ERK is observed after treatment with imatinib. An in vivo study shows a redundancy in growth factor loops in osteosarcoma. Implantation of TE-85 and MG-63 cells into the tibia of nude mice revealed that lower levels of PDGF were sufficient to satisfy the PDGFRs [17]. However, unlike the promising results from in vitro studies, the effect of imatinib alone in animal models was limited [17], which disallows use of a PDGF inhibitor as a single drug.

Less efficacy as a single drug was also demonstrated in two open labeled, single arm phase 2 clinical trials, namely NCT00031915 and NCT0003066. In the NCT00031915 trial, imatinib was used in patients with one of 10 different subtypes of advanced sarcoma. Patients were treated with imatinib 300 mg bid. In 27 patients with osteosarcoma, no complete response (CR) or partial response (PR) but only 5 stable disease (SDs) were recorded [58]. In another phase 2 trial by the Children's Oncology Group (COG), NCT0003066, imatinib was administered daily for 28 day courses at a dose of 440 mg/m^2/day. In 70 eligible patients, only one PR was seen among 24 patients with Ewing sarcoma. No objective responses were confirmed in osteosarcomas [59]. The failure of these clinical trials suggests that use of imatinib alone in advanced osteosarcoma is not appropriate.

Although imatinib alone had no antitumor effect in mice harboring OS tumors or in clinical trials, using imatinib as an add-on therapy is more promising. Synergistic antiproliferative effects of imatinib and doxorubicin has been noticed in PDGFR-expressing osteosarcoma cells both in vitro and in vivo [60]. Combined antiproliferative activity with cisplatin has also been demonstrated in experimental Ewing sarcoma [61]. The synergistic effect can be partly explained by the reversion of multidrug-resistance (MDR) related transporters [62]. The on-going clinical trials using imatinib as add-on therapy could give us more information (Table 2).

As a target of multiple TKIs, the activity of imatinib can also be explained by other mechanisms, such as the inhibition of transforming growth factor(TGF) and its cross-talk with c-Myc, which was upregulated in MG63 cell lines. Imatinib can also inhibit cell proliferation by blocking TGF and c-Myc [63].

Olaratumab

Olaratumab is a human immunoglobulin G subclass 1 mAb with selective, high affinity binding to the extracellular domain of PDGFR-α, disrupting receptor ligand interactions with resulting downregulation of downstream signal transduction [64]. Preclinical studies of olaratumab alone [65] or in combination with doxorubicin have demonstrated antitumor activity in human sarcoma xenograft models, and several other kinds of cancers [66, 67].

A recent evaluation of the effect of olaratumab in osteosarcoma [25] concluded that in vitro olaratumab treatment of osteosarcoma and rhabdoid tumor cell lines reduced proliferation and inhibited invasion driven by

Table 2 Ongoing study using "add-on" strategy with PDGF/PDGFR inhibitors in solid tumors

Regimen	Mechanism of partner	Diagnosis	Phase	Study design	Start date	Recruitment	ClinicalTrials.gov Identifier
Imatinib+							
Pemetrexed	Cytotoxic drugs	Pleural mesothelioma	2	Single group, open label	11/2014	Active, not recruiting	NCT02303899
Temzolomide	Cytotoxic drugs	Melanoma	1/2	Single group, open label	01/2003	Active, not recruiting	NCT00667953
Regoragenib	Multi-targeted TKI	GIST	2	Randomized, open label	02/2015	Recruiting	NCT02365441
BYL719	PI3K inhibitor	GIST	1	Single group, open label	02/2013	Active, not recruiting	NCT01735968
Pembrolizumab	Check point inhibitor	Melanoma	1/2	Single group, open label	11/2016	Recruiting	NCT02812693
Letrozole	Antihormonal drug	Breast cancer	2	Single group, open label	10/2003	Active, not recruiting	NCT00338728
Binimetinib	MEK inhibitor	GIST	1b/2	Single group, open label	11/2013	Recruiting	NCT01991379
BGJ398	FGFR inhibitor	GIST	1b/2	Single group, open label	10/2014	Active, not recruiting	NCT02257541
Ipilimumab	Check point inhibitor	Cancer	1	Single group, open label	02/2013	Recruiting	NCT01738139
Olaratumab+							
Paclitaxel/carboplatin	Cytotoxic drugs	NSCLC	2	Randomized, open label	01/2010	Active, not recruiting	NCT00918203
Nab-paclitaxel/gemcitabine	Cytotoxic drugs	Pancreatic cancer	1b/2	Randomized, double-blind	01/2017	Recruiting	NCT03086369
ADM	Cytotoxic drugs	STS	3	Randomized, double-blind	09/2015	Active, not recruiting	NCT02451943
Standard chemos	Cytotoxic drugs	Pediatric cancer	1	Non-randomized, open label	08/2016	Recruiting	NCT02677116
ADM	Cytotoxic drugs	STS	2	Non-randomized, open label	02/2016	Recruiting	NCT02584309
Gemcitabine/ADM	Cytotoxic drugs	STS	1b/2	Randomized, double-blind	03/2016	Recruiting	NCT02659020
Trabectedin/ADM	Cytotoxic drugs	Leiomyosarcoma	1	Non-randomized, open label	Not yet	Not yet recruiting	NCT03437070
ADM	Cytotoxic drugs	STS	1	Single group, open label	10/2016	Active, not recruiting	NCT02783599
ADM	Cytotoxic drugs	Cancer	1	Non-randomized, open label	03/2016	Active, not recruiting	NCT02377752
ADM/ifosfamide	Cytotoxic drugs	STS	1	Single group, open label	10/2017	Recruiting	NCT03283696
Pembrolizumab	Check point inhibitor	STS	1	Non-randomized, open label	07/2017	Recruiting	NCT03126591

PI3K phosphatidylinositol 3-kinase, *STS* soft tissue sarcoma, *ADM* adriamycin

individual platelet-derived growth factors (PDGFs) or serum. Furthermore, olaratumab delayed primary tumor growth in mouse models of pediatric osteosarcoma and malignant rhabdoid tumor, and this activity was enhanced by combination with either doxorubicin or cisplatin [25].

Similar to imatinib, the use of olaratumab alone is unsatisfactory in clinical trials, whereas its combination with other drugs seems more promising. Two phase 1 studies evaluated the effect of olaratumab as a single agent in patients with advanced sarcomas [68, 69]. In both studies, olaratumab was well tolerated and without dose-limiting toxicities. However, no objective radiological response was recorded in either study. The best response of SD was shown in 12 (63%) and 7 (44%) patients, respectively. When combined with doxorubicin, a recent phase 2 study (JGDG) on soft tissue sarcoma showed a surprising effect of olaratumab as an "add-on" agent [70]. In the pivotal trial, the combination of olaratumab with doxorubicin reduced the risk of death by 48% compared with doxorubicin alone (HR, 0.52; 95% CI 0.34–0.79, $P < 0.05$). Median overall survival in the intent-to-treat population ($n = 129$) was improved by 11.8 months. The median overall survival was 26.5 months with the combination versus 14.7 months with doxorubicin alone. Olaratumab has been also tested in other malignancies, such as GIST [23] and lung cancer [23]. Unlike the success of add-on therapy in soft tissue sarcoma, a 131-patient phase 2 trial in treatment-naïve adult patients with advanced non-small cell lung cancer (NSCLC) failed to show any advantage when olaratumab was added to the classical carboplatin/paclitaxel regimen, with an increasing risk of neutropenia, thrombocytopenia, and fatigue in the experimental arm [21] (Table 3).

Development and possible mechanisms for add-on strategy

Promising strategy in add-on therapy

Given the unsatisfactory result of clinical trials using imatinib as a single drug, it is clear that targeting PDGF/PDGFR alone would not be sufficient to control the growth of osteosarcoma, even in tumor cells that express PDGF/PDGFR highly. The PDGF signaling pathway does not appear to be the main driver of osteosarcoma cells, especially in the presence of other growth-promoting factors such as VEGF. Osteosarcomas have rich vascularity and many growth signals, which may also influence the unfavorable results obtained in clinical trials. The application of PDGF/PDGFR pathway targeted therapy would therefore be expected to be effective only if added to other therapy.

Data from phase I and phase 2 trials showed that the adverse effect of most PDGF/PDGFR inhibitors was mild, which allow the opportunity of delivering "add-on" therapy. Adding olaratumab to ADM, the first-line chemo agent in soft tissue sarcoma, has achieved great success [70]. The strategy of "add-on" therapy is used in many ongoing studies in different types of solid tumors (Table 3). The addition of PDGF/PDGFR inhibitors to standard chemotherapy of osteosarcoma should be attempted in the future to overcome drug-resistance and to improve patients' outcome.

Possible mechanisms for add-on strategy

Two possible mechanisms can explain the results of combination drug therapy using PDGF/PDGFR inhibitors.

The first hypothesis is overcoming tissue hypoxia in tumor microenvironment, a common phenomenon in sarcomas. Tissue hypoxia occurs where there is an imbalance between oxygen supply and consumption. Hypoxia occurs in solid tumors as a result of an inadequate supply of oxygen, due to exponential cellular proliferation and an inefficient vascular supply. It is an adverse prognostic indicator in cancer as it is associated with resistance to therapy [71, 72]. The crosstalk between hypoxia inducible factor (HIF-11α) and PDGF has been investigated in several cell lines [73, 74]. The use of PDGF inhibitors could improve hypoxia in tumor tissue, therefore leaving them more sensitive to other drugs [8].

The second hypothesis is based on a regulation of tumor interstitial fluid pressure (IFP) brought by PDGF inhibition, which could eventually increase tumor uptake of other agents [19, 75]. Lowering of tumor interstitial hypertension, which acts as a barrier for tumor transvascular transport, has been proposed as a general strategy to enhance tumor uptake and therapeutic effects of anticancer drugs. As mentioned above, the effects of PDGF antagonists on chemo responses as a mediator of tumor hypertension have been tested in various types of malignancies [18, 19, 34–36]. Although treatment with only PDG Fantagonists had no effect on tumor growth, uptake

Table 3 Published phase 1/2 studies of olaratumab

Author	Phase	N	Diagnosis	ORR	CBR	PFS	OS
Chiorean [69]	1	19	Solid tumors	0	NA	NA	NA
Doi [68]	1	16	Solid tumors	0	NA	NA	NA
Tap [70]	1b	15	Soft tissue sarcoma	NA	NA	NA	NA
Tap [70]	2	129	Soft tissue sarcoma	Olaratumab+ ADM 18.2% ADM alone 11.9%	NA	6.6 months 4.1 months	26.5 14.7
Wagner [25]	2	21	GIST	PDGFR-a mutation(+) PDGFR-a mutation(−)	50.0 14.3	32.1 weeks 6.1 weeks	NR 24.9 weeks
Gerber [23]	2	131	NSCLC	olaratumab+ P/C P/C	NA	4.4 months 4.4 months	11.8 months 11.5 months

N number; *ORR* objective response rate, =CR+PR; *CBR* clinical benefit rate, =CR+PR+SD at 12 weeks; *PFS* progression free survival; *OS* overall survival; *NA* not available; *ADM* adriamycin; *NR* not reached; *P/C* paclitaxel/carboplatin of classical cytotoxic drugs in tumors was increased by treatment with PDGF antagonists.

Future research in PDGF/PDGFR pathway

PDGF/PDGFR pathway in stromal cells

The development and progression of cancer depend on the microenvironment. Cancer cells themselves cannot explain growth and formation of the primary or metastasis, and a combination of proliferating tumor cells and their partners, including cancer stem cells, immune cells, mesenchymal stromal cells, and/or CAFs all contribute to the tumor bulk [76–78]. Studies of other types of malignant tumors strongly suggest that PDGF isoforms secreted by cancer cells affect the stromal microenvironment by inducing fibroblast proliferation, migration, infiltration, myofibroblastic conversion, and overproduction of ECM components, and finally promoting tumorigenesis indirectly in a paracrine manner [14, 26].

Compared to tumor cells, stromal cells show a higher expression of PDGFRs [79, 80]. According to the conclusion of the JGDG study, no difference was found in objective response rate or survival considering the expression level of PDGFR, indicating that the indirect manner of targeting tumor microenvironment may be more important in therapy with PDGF/PDGFR inhibitors. More studies of PDGF/PDGFR pathways in stromal cells of osteosarcoma are needed to explore further the mechanism and activity, including but not limited to the associations between the PDGFR status of stromal cells and the extent of malignancy, the ability of metastasis, response to treatment, and survival conditions.

PDGF/PDGFR inhibitors in drug-resistant cells

Although synergistic antiproliferative effects of PDGF/PDGFR inhibitors, such as imatinib and olaratumab, and classical cytotoxic agents (i.e., AMD, cisplatin) were observed in both in vitro and in vivo experiments, the effects of these inhibitors on drug-resistant cells have not been explored. Intratumoral and intertumoral heterogeneity was found in drug-resistant osteosarcoma cell lines [81] and in samples from refractory patients [82, 83]. Relapsed osteosarcoma is characterized by complex signaling and drug resistance pathways. However, the abnormal efflux of cytotoxic agents demonstrated a common mechanism of multiple drug resistance [84, 85]. The effect of PDGF inhibitors to upregulate drug uptake in tumor cells and to overcome tissue hypoxia has been described above, but the mechanism of reversal of drug is not well understood. More research is needed with drug-resistant cells to confirm this action.

Conclusion

New treatment options for advanced osteosarcoma remain limited. The PDGF/PDGFR pathway plays an important role in the development and metastasis of osteosarcoma, via both tumor cells and stromal cells. Targeting the PDGF/PDGFR pathway is a promising therapeutic method to overcome drug-resistance and to improve patients' outcome. The "add-on" strategy, adding PDGF/PDGFR inhibitors to other existing agents, should be attempted in the future.

Authors' contributions

LX and JX did literature search and made all the tables. WG designed this review. LX, JX, and WG analyzed and interpreted the data. JX wrote the manuscript. All the authors reviewed the article for intellectual content, provided comments, and gave their final approval. All authors read and approved the final manuscript.

Acknowledgements

None.

Competing interests

The authors declare that they have no competing interests.

Funding

None.

References

1. Mirabello L, Troisi RJ, Savage SA. Osteosarcoma incidence and survival rates from 1973 to 2004: data from the surveillance, epidemiology, and end results program. Cancer. 2009;115(7):1531–43.
2. Bacci G, et al. Neoadjuvant chemotherapy for osteosarcoma of the extremities in preadolescent patients: the Rizzoli Institute experience. J Pediatr Hematol Oncol. 2008;30(12):908–12.
3. Pratt CB. Treatment of osteosarcoma 1972–1997: an American perspective. Pediatr Hematol Oncol. 1998;15(3):207–10.
4. Isakoff MS, et al. Osteosarcoma: current treatment and a collaborative pathway to success. J Clin Oncol. 2015;33(27):3029–35.
5. Grignani G, et al. Sorafenib and everolimus for patients with unresectable high-grade osteosarcoma progressing after standard treatment: a non-randomised phase 2 clinical trial. Lancet Oncol. 2015;16(1):98–107.
6. Grignani G, et al. A phase II trial of sorafenib in relapsed and unresectable high-grade osteosarcoma after failure of standard multimodal therapy: an Italian Sarcoma Group study. Ann Oncol. 2012;23(2):508–16.
7. Lagmay JP, et al. Outcome of patients with recurrent osteosarcoma enrolled in seven phase II trials through children's cancer group, pediatric oncology group, and children's oncology group: learning from the past to move forward. J Clin Oncol. 2016;34(25):3031–8.
8. Wang Y, et al. The platelet-derived growth factors (PDGFs) and their receptors (PDGFRs) are major players in oncogenesis, drug resistance, and attractive oncologic targets in cancer. Growth Factors. 2016;34(1–2):64–71.
9. Paulsson J, Ehnman M, Ostman A. PDGF receptors in tumor biology: prognostic and predictive potential. Future Oncol. 2014;10(9):1695–708.
10. Tejada ML, et al. Tumor-driven paracrine platelet-derived growth factor receptor alpha signaling is a key determinant of stromal cell recruitment in a model of human lung carcinoma. Clin Cancer Res. 2006;12(9):2676–88.
11. Zhang L, et al. Human osteoblasts synthesize and respond to platelet-derived growth factor. Am J Physiol. 1991;261(2 Pt 1):C348–54.
12. Heldin CH, Westermark B. Mechanism of action and in vivo role of platelet-derived growth factor. Physiol Rev. 1999;79(4):1283–316.

13. Baxter RM, et al. Full activation of the platelet-derived growth factor beta-receptor kinase involves multiple events. J Biol Chem. 1998;273(27):17050–5.
14. Heldin CH. Targeting the PDGF signaling pathway in tumor treatment. Cell Commun Signal. 2013;11:97.
15. Papadopoulos N, Lennartsson J. The PDGF/PDGFR pathway as a drug target. Mol Aspects Med. 2017. https://doi.org/10.1016/j.mam.2017.11.007.
16. Andrae J, Gallini R, Betsholtz C. Role of platelet-derived growth factors in physiology and medicine. Genes Dev. 2008;22(10):1276–312.
17. Benini S, et al. Redundancy of autocrine loops in human osteosarcoma cells. Int J Cancer. 1999;80(4):581–8.
18. Pietras K, et al. Inhibition of PDGF receptor signaling in tumor stroma enhances antitumor effect of chemotherapy. Cancer Res. 2002;62(19):5476–84.
19. Pietras K, et al. Inhibition of platelet-derived growth factor receptors reduces interstitial hypertension and increases transcapillary transport in tumors. Cancer Res. 2001;61(7):2929–34.
20. Betsholtz C. Biology of platelet-derived growth factors in development. Birth Defects Res C Embryo Today. 2003;69(4):272–85.
21. Gerber DE, et al. Phase II study of olaratumab with paclitaxel/carboplatin (P/C) or P/C alone in previously untreated advanced NSCLC. Lung Cancer. 2017;111:108–15.
22. Kikuchi A, et al. Platelet-derived growth factor receptor alpha contributes to human hepatic stellate cell proliferation and migration. Am J Pathol. 2017;187(10):2273–87.
23. Wagner AJ, et al. A phase II study of a human anti-PDGFRalpha monoclonal antibody (olaratumab, IMC-3G3) in previously treated patients with metastatic gastrointestinal stromal tumors. Ann Oncol. 2017;28(3):541–6.
24. Kosela-Paterczyk H, Rutkowski P. Dermatofibrosarcoma protuberans and gastrointestinal stromal tumor as models for targeted therapy in soft tissue sarcomas. Expert Rev Anticancer Ther. 2017;17(12):1107–16.
25. Lowery CD, et al. Olaratumab exerts antitumor activity in preclinical models of pediatric bone and soft tissue tumors through inhibition of platelet-derived growth factor receptor alpha. Clin Cancer Res. 2018;24(4):847–57.
26. Forsberg K, et al. Platelet-derived growth factor (PDGF) in oncogenesis: development of a vascular connective tissue stroma in xenotransplanted human melanoma producing PDGF-BB. Proc Natl Acad Sci USA. 1993;90(2):393–7.
27. Dong J, et al. VEGF-null cells require PDGFR alpha signaling-mediated stromal fibroblast recruitment for tumorigenesis. EMBO J. 2004;23(14):2800–10.
28. Kalluri R, Zeisberg M. Fibroblasts in cancer. Nat Rev Cancer. 2006;6(5):392–401.
29. Ostman A, Augsten M. Cancer-associated fibroblasts and tumor growth–bystanders turning into key players. Curr Opin Genet Dev. 2009;19(1):67–73.
30. Guo P, et al. Platelet-derived growth factor-B enhances glioma angiogenesis by stimulating vascular endothelial growth factor expression in tumor endothelia and by promoting pericyte recruitment. Am J Pathol. 2003;162(4):1083–93.
31. Skobe M, Fusenig NE. Tumorigenic conversion of immortal human keratinocytes through stromal cell activation. Proc Natl Acad Sci USA. 1998;95(3):1050–5.
32. Pietras K, et al. Functions of paracrine PDGF signaling in the proangio genic tumor stroma revealed by pharmacological targeting. PLoS Med. 2008;5(1):e19.
33. Kitadai Y, et al. Targeting the expression of platelet-derived growth factor receptor by reactive stroma inhibits growth and metastasis of human colon carcinoma. Am J Pathol. 2006;169(6):2054–65.
34. Reed RK, et al. Control of interstitial fluid pressure: role of beta1-integ rins. Semin Nephrol. 2001;21(3):222–30.
35. Rodt SA, et al. A novel physiological function for platelet-derived growth factor-BB in rat dermis. J Physiol. 1996;495(Pt 1):193–200.
36. Pietras K, et al. STI571 enhances the therapeutic index of epothilone B by a tumor-selective increase of drug uptake. Clin Cancer Res. 2003;9(10 Pt 1):3779–87.
37. Pessetto ZY, et al. Drug repurposing identifies a synergistic combina tion therapy with imatinib mesylate for gastrointestinal stromal tumor. Mol Cancer Ther. 2014;13(10):2276–87.
38. Chen Y, et al. Co-delivery of doxorubicin and imatinib by pH sensitive cleavable PEGylated nanoliposomes with folate-mediated targeting to overcome multidrug resistance. Int J Pharm. 2018;542(1–2):266–79.
39. Almeida TP, et al. Cytotoxic activity of fucoxanthin, alone and in combination with the cancer drugs imatinib and doxorubicin, in CML cell lines. Environ Toxicol Pharmacol. 2018;59:24–33.
40. Oda Y, et al. Expression of growth factors and their receptors in human osteosarcomas. Immunohistochemical detection of epidermal growth factor, platelet-derived growth factor and their receptors: its correlation with proliferating activities and p53 expression. Gen Diagn Pathol. 1995;141(2):97–103.
41. Sulzbacher I, et al. Platelet-derived growth factor-AA and -alpha receptor expression suggests an autocrine and/or paracrine loop in osteosarcoma. Mod Pathol. 2000;13(6):632–7.
42. Sulzbacher I, et al. Expression of platelet-derived growth factor-AA is associated with tumor progression in osteosarcoma. Mod Pathol. 2003;16(1):66–71.
43. Hassan SE, et al. Cell surface receptor expression patterns in osteosarcoma. Cancer. 2012;118(3):740–9.
44. Kubo T, et al. Platelet-derived growth factor receptor as a prognostic marker and a therapeutic target for imatinib mesylate therapy in osteosarcoma. Cancer. 2008;112(10):2119–29.
45. Sulzbacher I, et al. Expression of platelet-derived growth factor-alpha receptor in human osteosarcoma is not a predictor of outcome. Pathology. 2010;42(7):664–8.
46. Abdeen A, et al. Correlation between clinical outcome and growth factor pathway expression in osteogenic sarcoma. Cancer. 2009;115(22):5243–50.
47. Heldin CH. Targeting the PDGF signaling pathway in the treatment of non-malignant diseases. J Neuroimmune Pharmacol. 2014;9(2):69–79.
48. Shen J, et al. Development of a fully human anti-PDGFRbeta antibody that suppresses growth of human tumor xenografts and enhances antitumor activity of an anti-VEGFR2 antibody. Neoplasia. 2009;11(6):594–604.
49. Jayson GC, et al. Blockade of platelet-derived growth factor receptor-beta by CDP860, a humanized, PEGylated di-Fab', leads to fluid accumulation and is associated with increased tumor vascularized volume. J Clin Oncol. 2005;23(5):973–81.
50. Kaminski WE, et al. Basis of hematopoietic defects in platelet-derived growth factor (PDGF)-B and PDGF beta-receptor null mice. Blood. 2001;97(7):1990–8.
51. Kitagawa D, et al. Activity-based kinase profiling of approved tyrosine kinase inhibitors. Genes Cells. 2013;18(2):110–22.
52. Socinski MA. Multitargeted receptor tyrosine kinase inhibition: an antiangiogenic strategy in non-small cell lung cancer. Cancer Treat Rev. 2011;37(8):611–7.
53. Druker BJ, et al. Effects of a selective inhibitor of the Abl tyrosine kinase on the growth of Bcr-Abl positive cells. Nat Med. 1996;2(5):561–6.
54. Carroll M, et al. CGP 57148, a tyrosine kinase inhibitor, inhibits the growth of cells expressing BCR-ABL, TEL-ABL, and TEL-PDGFR fusion proteins. Blood. 1997;90(12):4947–52.
55. McGary EC, et al. Inhibition of platelet-derived growth factor-mediated proliferation of osteosarcoma cells by the novel tyrosine kinase inhibitor STI571. Clin Cancer Res. 2002;8(11):3584–91.
56. Gobin B, et al. Imatinib mesylate exerts anti-proliferative effects on osteosarcoma cells and inhibits the tumour growth in immunocompetent murine models. PLoS ONE. 2014;9(3):e90795.
57. Yoshitani K, et al. Growth inhibition of rat osteosarcoma and malignant fibrous histiocytoma cells by tyrosine kinase inhibitor STI571. Vivo. 2003;17(3):255–8.
58. Chugh R, et al. Phase II multicenter trial of imatinib in 10 histologic subtypes of sarcoma using a bayesian hierarchical statistical model. J Clin Oncol. 2009;27(19):3148–53.
59. Bond M, et al. A phase II study of imatinib mesylate in children with refractory or relapsed solid tumors: a Children's Oncology Group study. Pediatr Blood Cancer. 2008;50(2):254–8.
60. Yamaguchi SI, et al. Synergistic antiproliferative effect of imatinib and adriamycin in platelet-derived growth factor receptor-expressing osteosarcoma cells. Cancer Sci. 2015;106(7):875–82.
61. Yerushalmi R, et al. Combined antiproliferative activity of imatinib mesylate (STI 571) with radiation or cisplatin in vitro. Exp Oncol. 2007;29(2):126–31.

62. Gomes CM, et al. Multidrug resistance mediated by ABC transporters in osteosarcoma cell lines: mRNA analysis and functional radiotracer studies. Nucl Med Biol. 2006;33(7):831–40.
63. Matsuyama S, et al. SB-431542 and Gleevec inhibit transforming growth factor-beta-induced proliferation of human osteosarcoma cells. Cancer Res. 2003;63(22):7791–8.
64. Pender A, Jones RL. Olaratumab: a platelet-derived growth factor receptor-alpha-blocking antibody for the treatment of soft tissue sarcoma. Clin Pharmacol. 2017;9:159–64.
65. Loizos N, et al. Targeting the platelet-derived growth factor receptor alpha with a neutralizing human monoclonal antibody inhibits the growth of tumor xenografts: implications as a potential therapeutic target. Mol Cancer Ther. 2005;4(3):369–79.
66. Wang YX, et al. Inhibiting platelet-derived growth factor beta reduces Ewing's sarcoma growth and metastasis in a novel orthotopic human xenograft model. Vivo. 2009;23(6):903–9.
67. Stock P, et al. Platelet-derived growth factor receptor-alpha: a novel therapeutic target in human hepatocellular cancer. Mol Cancer Ther. 2007;6(7):1932–41.
68. Doi T, et al. Phase I study of olaratumab in Japanese patients with advanced solid tumors. Cancer Sci. 2014;105(7):862–9.
69. Chiorean EG, et al. A phase I study of olaratumab, an anti-platelet-derived growth factor receptor alpha (PDGFRalpha) monoclonal antibody, in patients with advanced solid tumors. Cancer Chemother Pharmacol. 2014;73(3):595–604.
70. Tap WD, et al. Olaratumab and doxorubicin versus doxorubicin alone for treatment of soft-tissue sarcoma: an open-label phase 1b and randomised phase 2 trial. Lancet. 2016;388(10043):488–97.
71. Cosse JP, Michiels C. Tumour hypoxia affects the responsiveness of cancer cells to chemotherapy and promotes cancer progression. Anticancer Agents Med Chem. 2008;8(7):790–7.
72. Shannon AM, et al. Tumour hypoxia, chemotherapeutic resistance and hypoxia-related therapies. Cancer Treat Rev. 2003;29(4):297–307.
73. Karakiulakis G, et al. Cell type-specific effect of hypoxia and platelet-derived growth factor-BB on extracellular matrix turnover and its consequences for lung remodeling. J Biol Chem. 2007;282(2):908–15.
74. Yoshida D, et al. Hypoxia inducible factor 1-alpha regulates of platelet derived growth factor-B in human glioblastoma cells. J Neurooncol. 2006;76(1):13–21.
75. Wu Q, et al. Chemoresistance to gemcitabine in hepatoma cells induces epithelial-mesenchymal transition and involves activation of PDGF-D pathway. Oncotarget. 2013;4(11):1999–2009.
76. Gialeli C, et al. PDGF/PDGFR signaling and targeting in cancer growth and progression: focus on tumor microenvironment and cancer-associated fibroblasts. Curr Pharm Des. 2014;20(17):2843–8.
77. Cortini M, Avnet S, Baldini N. Mesenchymal stroma: role in osteosarcoma progression. Cancer Lett. 2017;405:90–9.
78. Bonuccelli G, et al. Role of mesenchymal stem cells in osteosarcoma and metabolic reprogramming of tumor cells. Oncotarget. 2014;5(17):7575–88.
79. Roskoski R Jr. The role of small molecule platelet-derived growth factor receptor (PDGFR) inhibitors in the treatment of neoplastic disorders. Pharmacol Res. 2018;129:65–83.
80. Ostman A. PDGF receptors in tumor stroma: biological effects and associations with prognosis and response to treatment. Adv Drug Deliv Rev. 2017;121:117–23.
81. Collier CD, et al. Micrometastatic drug screening platform shows heterogeneous response to map chemotherapy in osteosarcoma cell lines. Clin Orthop Relat Res. 2018. https://doi.org/10.1007/s11999.0000000000000059.
82. Egas-Bejar D, et al. Theranostic profiling for actionable aberrations in advanced high risk osteosarcoma with aggressive biology reveals high molecular diversity: the human fingerprint hypothesis. Oncoscience. 2014;1(2):167–79.
83. Subbiah V, et al. Personalized comprehensive molecular profiling of high risk osteosarcoma: implications and limitations for precision medicine. Oncotarget. 2015;6(38):40642–54.
84. Ma Q, et al. Hypoxia promotes chemotherapy resistance by down-regulating SKA1 gene expression in human osteosarcoma. Cancer Biol Ther. 2017;18(3):177–85.
85. Liu T, et al. Targeting ABCB1 (MDR1) in multi-drug resistant osteosarcoma cells using the CRISPR-Cas9 system to reverse drug resistance. Oncotarget. 2016;7(50):83502–13.

26

Smoking is predictive of poorer distant metastasis-free and progression free-survival in soft tissue sarcoma patients treated with pre-operative radiotherapy or chemoradiotherapy

Nicholas P. Gannon[1], David M. King[1] and Manpreet Bedi[2*]

Abstract

Background: Soft tissue sarcomas (STS) are often treated with pre-operative radiation (RT), with or without chemotherapy, followed by wide local excision. Prognosis for these patients involves an interplay of tumor and patient characteristics. Known prognostic determinants include tumor size, grade, response to therapy, and patient characteristics such as age. While smoking is negatively correlated with outcomes in various malignancies, the impact on STS is unknown. We aimed to assess if smoking impacts overall (OS), distant metastasis-free (DMFS), and progression-free (PFS) survival in patients with STS treated with pre-operative RT.

Methods: Between 2000 and 2015, 166 patients with STS were identified from our prospective database. Patient variables were retrospectively reviewed. Smoking was defined as a ≥ 10 pack year history of current and former smokers. Survival was evaluated using the fisher exact test for univariate (UVA) and logistic regression for multivariate (MVA) analysis.

Results: Fifty-seven (34.3%) patients had smoking histories of ≥ 10 pack years. On UVA, smoking was associated with decreased DMFS ($p = 0.0009$) and PFS ($p = 0.0036$), but not OS ($p = 0.05$). Smoking held significance on MVA for both DMFS and PFS. Current smokers and patients with ≥ 24-month follow-up demonstrated decreased DMFS and PFS on UVA and MVA.

Conclusions: Current smokers and patients with a significant smoking history demonstrated decreased DMFS and PFS in STS patients treated with pre-operative RT. Smoking may cause immunologic compromise and therefore lead to higher rates of progression and distant metastasis.

Keywords: Cancer, Smoking, Nicotine, Metastatic survival, Prognosis

Background

Soft tissue sarcomas (STS) are rare, heterogeneous solid tumors of mesenchymal origin. Approximately 12,000 new cases of STS are diagnosed per year in the United States with a mortality rate of 40% [1]. Historical standard-of-care treatment has included extremity amputation in an effort to reduce recurrence rates and improve survival. However, there has been an evolution towards limb-salvage therapy with wide local excision and radiation (RT) with or without chemotherapy. Pre-operative RT followed by wide local excision has been widely accepted as appropriate management and leads to excellent rates of local control and survival [2–10].

Despite excellent local control rates, many patients with STS develop metastases and succumb to their

*Correspondence: mbedi@mcw.edu
[2] Department of Radiation Oncology, Medical College of Wisconsin, 9200 West Wisconsin Ave, Milwaukee, WI 53226, USA
Full list of author information is available at the end of the article

disease. Factors associated with survival in STS include inherent tumor biology, response to therapy, and patient characteristics. Similar findings have been shown when assessing overall survival (OS), local recurrence, distant recurrence, or post-metastasis survival [11–14]. While the previous investigations included large cohorts and reported consistently reproducible results, many did not analyze patient lifestyle behaviors with survival outcomes.

Smoking has been strongly correlated with the pathogenesis of many malignancies including, but not limited to, head and neck, lung, and bladder cancer [15], and smoking has been shown to impact disease outcomes in these cancers. Studies have also demonstrated increased cancer mortality risks amongst both men and women, current and former smokers [16, 17]. Shopland et al. projected that smoking leads to 21.5% of cancer related deaths in women and 45% of cancer related deaths in men [17].

Contrary to other malignancies, there has been no direct link demonstrated between smoking and the incidence of STS. Similarly, sparse information exists on the significance of smoking associated survival in STS. The investigations that have gathered/reported smoking history and correlated it with various measures of survival conclude no significance [18–20].

In the present study, we retrospectively analyzed a cohort of STS patients treated with pre-operative RT or chemoradiotherapy (CRT) followed by limb-sparing surgery. The primary objective of this investigation was to assess if smoking correlates with OS, distant metastasis-free survival (DMFS), and progression-free survival (PFS).

Methods

This research was reviewed and approved by the Medical College of Wisconsin Institutional Review Board (IRB) and all investigators completed training in both human research and patient privacy.

Patient population

All patients with primary STS of the extremity and trunk who received pre-operative RT with or without pre-operative chemotherapy followed by surgical resection between November 2000 and August 2015 were reviewed from a prospectively collected database. Patients were staged according to the 2010 American Joint Committee on Cancer (AJCC) system seventh edition. Exclusion criteria included metastatic disease on initial presentation, age < 18 years old, STS of locations other than the extremity or trunk, post-operative RT, recurrent sarcomas, and histopathologic types demonstrating rhabdomyosarcoma, extraosseous primitive neuroectodermal tumor, Ewing's sarcoma, osteosarcoma, Kaposi's sarcoma, angiosarcoma, aggressive fibromatosis, or dermatofibrosarcoma protuberans. Patients who did not have complete medical records including treatment information and a pathology report, and follow-up of less than 6 months were also excluded. Patient demographic, clinical, and pathological information were recorded.

Treatment

All patients with STS were discussed at a multi-disciplinary sarcoma board consisting of surgical and musculoskeletal oncologists, medical and radiation oncologists, musculoskeletal radiologists, and pathologists with specialty training in bone and soft tissue pathology. Tumor board treatment recommendations were presented and discussed with the patient.

Radiation and chemotherapy

All patients were administered pre-operative RT. Patients received a median dose of 50 gray (Gy) using 3D-conformal radiation or intensity-modulated RT (IMRT).

Chemotherapy was discussed and offered to patients who were aged < 70 years, with large (> 5 cm), deep, and high-grade lesions. Chemotherapy was delivered prior to initiation of radiation therapy, using combination doxorubicin–ifosfamide for 1–3 cycles, dependent on patient tolerance and clinical efficacy.

Surgery

Limb-salvage resection was performed 4–6 weeks following RT. Surgery was grossly approached through normal tissue planes and included sacrifice of tumor-violated arteries and veins. Neurovascular structures were preserved whenever possible. Surgical goals were to achieve negative margins (R0). Vascular and reconstructive plastic surgeons were consulted and involved in cases with difficult wound closures, specifically those requiring free or rotational tissue transfer.

Statistical analyses

Following exclusion criteria, the sample size for this analysis included 166 patients with available smoking history, defined as a binary variable. Patients who had at least a 10 pack year (20 cigarettes/day/year × 10 years) history of smoking were deemed as smokers, a routinely employed threshold by the oncologic community and former literature. OS, DMFS, PFS rates were estimated using the Kaplan–Meier estimate of the survival function. The log-rank test was used to compare two survival curves. The Fisher exact test was used for univariate (UVA) and a logistic regression analysis was used for multivariate analysis (MVA). For all analyses, type I error was maintained at 0.05 and all tests were two-sided. All statistical analyses were performed using MedCalc (Version 15.6, MedCalc Software bvba, Ostend, Belgium).

Results

Patient characteristics

A total of 166 patients received pre-operative RT with or without chemotherapy followed by surgical resection at our institution and were eligible for study inclusion. Of the 57 patients with smoking history, 23 patients were current smokers. Management of patients with positive smoking history is included in Table 1. The median age at diagnosis for the smoking and non-smoking groups were 60 and 55, respectively. The median follow-up was 3.8 years. Subset analysis was performed on 119 patients having a follow-up of ≥ 24 months, 14 patients being smokers. Patient, tumor, and treatment information is summarized in Table 2.

Outcomes

We first looked at all patients following exclusion criteria (≥ 6 month follow up). Smoking trended towards significance for OS on UVA ($p = 0.05$) and MVA ($p = 0.06$). Patients with at least a 10 pack year history of smoking had worse DMFS on UVA ($p = 0.0009$) and MVA ($p = 0.0038$, 95% CI 1.51–5.14) as well as worse PFS on UVA ($p = 0.0036$) and MVA ($p = 0.0151$, 95% CI 1.37–4.49). The median DMFS for non-smokers was not met versus 44.75 months for patients who were smokers (Fig. 1). The median PFS for non-smokers was not met versus 49 months for smokers (Fig. 2).

Analysis of a subset group of patients with ≥ 24-month follow-up revealed that smoking impacted DMFS ($p < 0.0001$) and PFS ($p = 0.0004$) on UVA, and DMFS ($p = 0.0001$, 95% CI 2.14–9.61) and PFS ($p = 0.005$, 95% CI 1.45–8.21) on MVA.

We further analyzed a second subset of patients who were current smokers at the time of treatment. Current smoking impacted DMFS on UVA ($p = 0.0005$) and MVA ($p = 0.0009$, 95% CI 1.62–6.50), and PFS on UVA ($p = 0.0014$) and MVA ($p = 0.0109$, 95% CI 1.24–5.09).

In addition to smoking, variables significant for the entire group for DMFS on MVA were age at diagnosis ($p = 0.0218$, 95% CI 1.01–1.04), tumor size ≥ 10 cm ($p = 0.0088$, 95% CI 1.56–5.18), low to intermediate grade disease ($p = 0.04$, 95% CI 0.16–0.99), and a synovial sarcoma histology ($p = 0.02$, 95% CI 1.04–12.6). Tumor size ≥ 10 cm ($p = 0.0012$, 95% CI 1.49–5.12) and tumor location of lower extremity ($p = 0.0116$, 95% CI 1.11–4.87) were the only other significant variables for PFS on MVA in addition to smoking. Variables significant on UVA for OS, PFS and DMFS are located in Table 3.

Table 1 Management of positive smoking history

	OS	DMFS	PFS	Total
Chemotherapy alone	0	0	0	0
Radiotherapy alone	8	16	15	39
Chemoradiotherapy	11	9	9	29

Table 2 Patient, tumor, and treatment characteristics

	Number of patients (%) 166
Median age	Smoking: 60 Non-smoking: 55
Smoking	No: 109 (65.6) Yes: 57 (34.4)
Current smoker	No: 143 (86.1) Yes: 23 (13.9)
Cardiovascular disease	No: 143 (86.1) Yes: 23 (13.9)
Lung disease	No: 147 (88.6) COPD: 18 (10.8) Primary malignancy: 1 (0.6)
Diabetes mellitus	No: 145 (87.3) Yes: 21 (12.7)
Grade	Low: 16 (9.6) Intermediate: 50 (30.1) High: 100 (60.2)
Histology	Undifferentiated/MFH: 45 (27.1) Liposarcoma: 33 (19.9) Synovial cell: 33 (19.9) Myxofibrosarcoma: 23 (13.9) Leiomyosarcoma: 15 (9.0) MPNST: 6 (3.6) Extraskeletal myxoid chondrosarcoma: 4 (2.4) Fibrosarcoma: 3 (1.8) Solitary fibrous: 3 (1.8) Clear cell: 1 (0.6)
Stage	I: 24 (14.4) II: 25 (15.1) III: 117 (70.5)
Karnofsky performance status	80–100: 141 (84.9) ≤ 70: 25 (15.1)
Tumor location	Upper extremity: 39 (23.5) Lower extremity: 127 (76.5)
Distant lung metastasis	42 (25.3)
Tumor size	< 10 cm: 94 (56.6) ≥ 10 cm: 72 (43.4)
Chemotherapy	No: 107 (64.5) Yes: 59 (35.5)

Discussion

Many variables are associated with outcomes in STS treated with pre-operative RT with or without chemotherapy followed by limb-salvage surgery. Factors demonstrated in previous reports include response to treatment, primary tumor biology (grade), tumor size, and individual patient characteristics, such as age. Previous studies have demonstrated that smoking does not

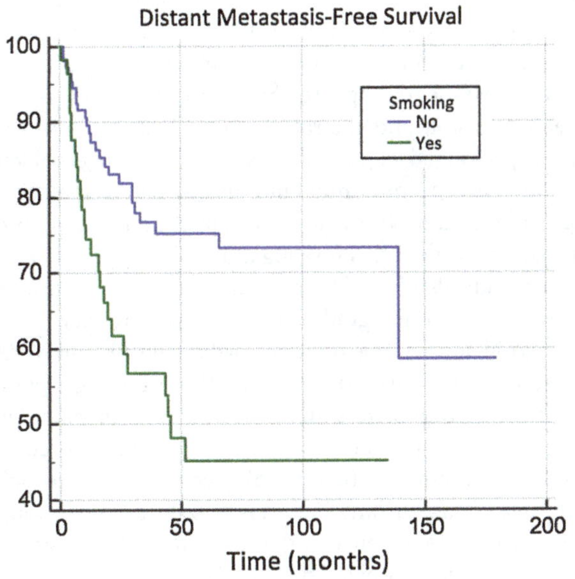

Fig. 1 Distant metastasis-free survival and smoking

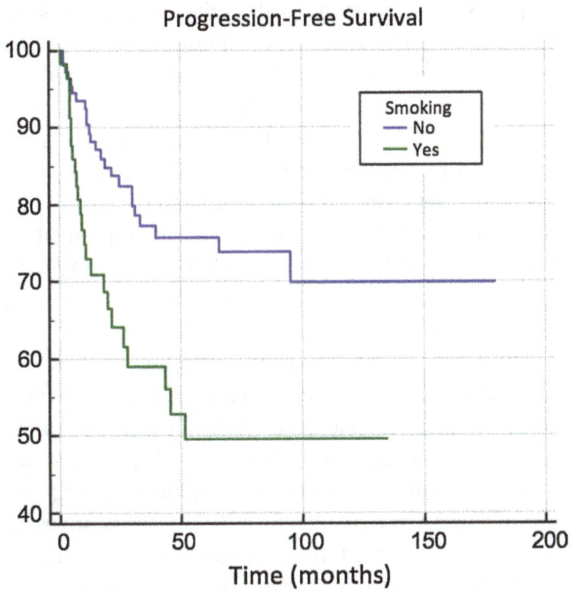

Fig. 2 Progression-free survival and smoking

seem to be a significant risk factor in the development of STS. Our data, however, indicates that a significant smoking history may increase the risk of patients with STS developing metastatic disease.

Consistent with previous findings, the current study found smoking does not appear to influence OS despite a trend towards significance, perhaps a product of our modest cohort size, lessened statistical power, or short follow-up time. Contrary to other studies, we show cigarette use of at least 10 years was associated with

Table 3 UVA for overall, distant-metastasis free, and progression-free survival

Variable	p-value		
	OS	DMFS	PFS
Age	0.0005	0.0218	NS
Smoking	0.05	0.0038	0.0151
Cardiovascular disease	NS	NS	NS
Diabetes	NS	NS	NS
High-grade	0.04	0.04	NS
Histology	NS	0.02	NS
Karnofsky performance status	NS	NS	NS
Tumor location	0.03	NS	0.0116
Tumor size	0.008	0.0088	0.0012
Chemotherapy	NS	NS	NS

NS not-significant

decreased DMFS and PFS on UVA and MVA. Alamanda et al. conducted a 5-year retrospective cohort study using 397 patients with extremity STS and found smoking non-predictive of sarcoma-specific death ($p = 0.59$), distant metastasis ($p = 0.9323$), or local recurrence ($p = 0.5451$) [18]. The authors also noted obese patients had a higher prevalence of smoking than non-obese patients, having no adverse effect on survival [18]. The risk of developing metastatic disease at 6 months in STS is much lower than at 2–3 years [21]. Here we show DMFS and PFS is similar for those patients with ≥ 6- and ≥ 24-month follow-up, as well as current smokers. Behnke et al. demonstrated that smoking status does not contribute to malignant course of disease nor is it correlated with postoperative infection after STS resection [19]. Similarly, smoking history of seventy-seven patients with STS of the thigh provided little prognostic value for local recurrence or distant metastasis, but was associated with an increased risk of death in patients aged less than 50 years, leading authors to conclude smoking prematurely ages STS patients prognostically [20]. This investigation also found increasing age is an independent prognostic indicator for STS patients.

Our cohort selectively included those patients having received only pre-operative RT or CRT, possibly producing conflicting results with those investigations that have concluded smoking has no correlation with all measures of survival [18–20]. Survival differences may contrast from those previous studies which included all patients regardless of treatment course (pre-operative, post-operative RT). The use of neoadjuvant chemotherapy has been shown to increase DMFS in patients < 70 years old with clinical stage III disease of the trunk and extremity [22], although the multimodality synergy of combination RT and chemotherapy remains unknown. At our institution, neoadjuvant chemotherapy is recommended in deep STS that are high grade and ≥ 5 cm in size. In addition, chemotherapy is recommended to select histologies including synovial sarcoma, leiomyosarcoma, myxoid and dedifferentiated liposarcoma, and poorly differentiated sarcoma. No single factor should determine the decision to administer neoadjuvant chemotherapy, and all patients should be discussed at a multidisciplinary sarcoma tumor board. The authors recommend several factors be considered prior to chemotherapy administration including depth, grade, size, and histology. Other factors such as patient preference, significant medical comorbidities, performance status, and positive smoking history should also be evaluated. Additional explanations for discrepancies between our study and those aforementioned are the specific differences in smoking habits/histories, genetic predisposition, and socioeconomic status between the populations examined, or how smoking status was experimentally defined (≥ 10 pack years in the current study).

Although the connection between smoking and disease progression is suggested in our data, the exact mechanism by which smoking increases the risk of disease progression is poorly understood. The present investigation suggests the potential influence of smoking on the immunologic cascade in STS. Previous studies have suggested cigarette exposure affects a wide range of host defense mechanisms, including decreased cytotoxic T cell activity and increased inflammatory response [23–26]. Inflammation from smoking increases mutations and silences tumor suppressor genes through various stress mechanisms. Smoking also promotes angio- and lymphangiogenesis, thereby increasing potential for tumor spread [23].

Lu et al. showed that cigarette smoke exposure increased the incidence of lung metastases following a B16-MO5 melanoma tumor challenge [27]. This study also showed that the carcinogens from cigarette smoke alter the immunity associated with increased tumor load by impairment of NK cell-dependent tumor immune surveillance [27]. Moreover, smokers have been shown to have decreased number and proportion of circulating NK cells, an effect seen in current smokers and those who report smoking cessation for more than 20 years [28]. This evidence suggests the complete restoration of NK cell levels following cessation appears to be profoundly suppressed or irreversible. Due to the myriad effects of cigarette smoke, it is conceivable NK cells are only one of many contributory factors of disease evolution.

Inflammatory mediators such as direct carcinogens, toxins, and oxidative compounds found in cigarette smoke are well established to activate nuclear factor-kappa B (NFκB), inducing expression of several growth factors that can increase tumor cell proliferation, survival, and migration through the phosphoinositide 3 kinase (PI3K)-Akt pathway [29]. Inflammatory macrophages, neutrophils, and mast cells produce extracellular matrix-degrading proteases and other factors that enable invasion and migration [30]. Thus, patients who had a prolonged exposure to smoke carcinogens likely had decreased immunity and dysregulated molecular signaling, leading to distant metastasis and disease progression as seen in this investigation.

This study also found that larger tumors (≥ 10 cm), age at diagnosis, tumor grade, and synovial sarcoma histology significantly impacted OS, DMFS, and PFS on MVA. Several studies have corroborated these findings, possibly having prognostic significance for STS independent of cohort subtype composition and patient differences. Increased tumor size (per 1 cm) predicted sarcoma-specific death and distant metastasis, but was not significant for local recurrence [18]. Others have demonstrated increasing size as a prognostic indicator for survival and distant metastasis [19, 31]. Age > 50 is associated with decreased postmetastatic survival [31] and sarcoma-specific death, but not distant metastasis or local recurrence [18, 32]. Another survival predictor, tumor grade, is well known to influence oncologic outcomes, as patients with high grade disease and a metastatic presentation have a poorer prognosis [31, 33]. Coindre et al. found patients with grade 3 tumors had poorer OS, along with an increased rate of local recurrence and distant metastasis [32]. Others have shown similar findings as higher tumor grade contributes to increased likelihood of distant metastasis and mortality [34–37]. Interestingly, histological diagnosis of synovial sarcoma was associated with a 13-fold increased risk of death when compared with other sarcomas after prognostic factors had been accounted for [13]. Tumor size (> 5 cm), non-extremity location, metastatic disease on initial presentation, and monophasic subtype was associated with poorer overall survival in synovial sarcoma; monophasic subtype was also associated with poorer PFS [38]. Further investigations have documented synovial sarcoma to represent a poor prognosis compared with other STS histologies [39, 40].

Limitations to this study include a modest cohort size and the heterogeneous sarcoma profile contained herein. While follow-up time was limited, several confounding variables can alter the OS of STS patients. Therefore, any effect of smoking on OS may take years to determine. Another limitation was the retrospective nature of our study which inherently introduced biases as a byproduct of this design. Smoking history was also represented as a dichotomous term, narrowing our intra-study variables. Other limitations include potential bias of selecting only pre-operative RT and chemotherapy/

RT patients, although this is the general recommendation from our center. Additionally, history was gathered under the assumption that the self-reporting of smoking history was accurate. Future investigations should consider gathering a comprehensive smoking history including: pack years, use of other tobacco products, use of nicotine replacement therapy, and length of abstinence (if applicable).

Conclusion

Current and former smoking is associated with DMFS and PFS in STS patients treated with pre-operative RT. Smoking may lead to immunologic compromise, likely increasing the potential for tumor spread. A complete smoking history may allow physicians to better predict survival rates, and as such, should be gathered in future cohort studies as a potential correlative variable and prognostic indicator. Additional information regarding the extent of smoking may further delineate the role smoking has on the prognosis of STS patients.

Abbreviations

CI: confidence interval; CRT: chemoradiotherapy; DMFS: distant metastasis-free survival; Gy: gray; IMRT: intensity-modulated RT; KPS: Karnofsky performance status; MVA: multivariate analysis; NFκB: nuclear factor-kappa B; OS: overall survival; PFS: progression-free survival; PI3K: phosphoinositide 3 kinase; RT: radiation; STS: soft tissue sarcoma; UVA: univariate analysis.

Authors' contributions

NPG: conducted a literature search, analysis, and drafted the manuscript. DK: formulated project design, assisted with manuscript construction and editing, and supervised the study. MB: assisted with the literature search, formulated project design, performed data analysis, and assisted in manuscript construction and editing. All authors read and approved the final manuscript.

Author details

[1] Department of Orthopaedic Surgery, Medical College of Wisconsin, Milwaukee, WI 53226, USA. [2] Department of Radiation Oncology, Medical College of Wisconsin, 9200 West Wisconsin Ave, Milwaukee, WI 53226, USA.

Acknowledgements

We would like to thank the Department of Radiation Oncology for their support of this work.

Competing interests

The authors declare that they have no competing interests.

Funding

No funding was received for this work.

References

1. Siegel RL, Miller KD, Jemal A. Cancer statistics. CA Cancer J Clin. 2016;66(1):7–30.
2. Suit HD, Spiro I. Role of radiation in the management of adult patients with sarcoma of soft tissue. Semin Surg Oncol. 1994;10(5):347–56.
3. Rosenberg SA, Tepper J, Glatstein E, Costa J, Baker A, Brennan M, DeMoss EV, Seipp C, Sindelar WF, Sugarbaker P, Wesley R. The treatment of soft-tissue sarcomas of the extremities: prospective randomized evaluations of (1) limb-sparing surgery plus radiation therapy compared with amputation and (2) the role of adjuvant chemotherapy. Ann Surg. 1982;196(3):305–15.
4. Suit HD, Mankin HJ, Wood WC, Proppe KH. Preoperative, intraoperative, and postoperative radiation in the treatment of primary soft tissue sarcoma. Cancer. 1985;55(11):2659–67.
5. Mundt AJ, Awan A, Sibley GS, Simon M, Rubin SJ, Samuels B, Wong W, Beckett M, Vijayakumar S, Weichselbaum RR. Conservative surgery and adjuvant radiation therapy in the management of adult soft tissue sarcoma of the extremities: clinical and radiobiological results. Int J Radiat Oncol Biol Phys. 1995;32(4):977–85.
6. Yang JC, Chang AE, Baker AR, Sindelar WF, Danforth DN, Topalian SL, DeLaney T, Glatstein E, Steinberg SM, Merino MJ, Rosenberg SA. Randomized prospective study of the benefit of adjuvant radiation therapy in the treatment of soft tissue sarcomas of the extremity. J Clin Oncol. 1998;16(1):197–203.
7. Sarcoma Meta-analysis Collaboration. Adjuvant chemotherapy for localised resectable soft-tissue sarcoma of adults: meta-analysis of individual data. Lancet. 1997;350(9092):1647–54.
8. DeLaney TF, Spiro IJ, Suit HD, Gebhardt MC, Hornicek FJ, Mankin HJ, Rosenberg AL, Rosenthal DI, Miryousefi F, Ancukiewicz M, Harmon DC. Neoadjuvant chemotherapy and radiotherapy for large extremity soft-tissue sarcomas. Int J Radiat Oncol Biol Phys. 2003;56(4):1117–27.
9. Schuetze SM, Rubin BP, Vernon C, Hawkins DS, Bruckner JD, Conrad EU 3rd, Eary JF. Use of positron emission tomography in localized extremity soft tissue sarcoma treated with neoadjuvant chemotherapy. Cancer. 2005;103(2):339–48.
10. MacDermed DM, Miller LL, Peabody TD, Simon MA, Luu HH, Haydon RC, Montag AG, Undevia SD, Connell PP. Primary tumor necrosis predicts distant control in locally advanced soft-tissue sarcomas after preoperative concurrent chemoradiotherapy. Int J Radiat Oncol Biol Phys. 2010;76(4):1147–53.
11. Stefanovski PD, Bidoli E, De Paoli A, Buonadonna A, Boz G, Libra M, Morassut S, Rossi C, Carbone A, Frustaci S. Prognostic factors in soft tissue sarcomas: a study of 395 patients. Eur J Surg Oncol. 2002;28(2):153–64.
12. Pisters PW, Leung DH, Woodruff J, Shi W, Brennan MF. Analysis of prognostic factors in 1,041 patients with localized soft tissue sarcomas of the extremities. J Clin Oncol. 1996;14(5):1679–89.
13. Singer S, Corson JM, Bonin R, Labow B, Eberlein TJ. Prognostic factors predictive of survival and local recurrence for extremity soft tissue sarcoma. Ann Surg. 1994;219(2):165–73.
14. Stojadinovic A, Leung DH, Allen P, Lewis JJ, Jaques DP, Brennan MF. Primary adult soft tissue sarcoma: time-dependent influence of prognostic variables. J Clin Oncol. 2002;20(21):4344–52.
15. Sasco AJ, Secretan MB, Straif K. Tobacco smoking and cancer: a brief review of recent epidemiological evidence. Lung Cancer. 2004;45(Suppl 2):S3–9.
16. CDC. The surgeon general's 1989 report on reducing the health consequences of smoking: 25 years of progress. MMWR. 1989;38(2):1–32.
17. Shopland DR, Eyre HJ, Pechacek TF. Smoking-attributable cancer mortality in 1991: is lung cancer now the leading cause of death among smokers in the United States? J Natl Cancer Inst. 1991;83(16):1142–8.
18. Alamanda VK, Moore DC, Song Y, Schwartz HS, Holt GE. Obesity does not affect survival outcomes in extremity soft tissue sarcoma. Clin Orthop Relat Res. 2014;472(9):2799–806.
19. Behnke NK, Alamanda VK, Song Y, Archer KR, Halpern JL, Schwartz HS, Holt GE. Does postoperative infection after soft tissue sarcoma resection affect oncologic outcomes? J Surg Oncol. 2014;109(5):415–20.
20. Newcomer AE, Dylinski D, Rubin BP, Joyce MJ, Hoeltge G, Bershadsky B, Lietman SA. Prognosticators in thigh soft tissue sarcomas. J Surg Oncol. 2011;103(1):85–91.
21. Bedi M, King DM, Charlson J, Whitfield R, Hackbarth DA, Zambrano EV, Wang D. Multimodality management of metastatic patients with soft tissue sarcomas may prolong survival. Am J Clin Oncol. 2014;37(3):272–7.
22. Bedi M, King DM, Shivakoti M, Wang T, Zambrano EV, Charlson J, Hackbarth D, Neilson J, Whitfield R, Wang D. Prognostic variables in patients with primary soft tissue sarcoma of the extremity and trunk treated with neoadjuvant radiotherapy or neoadjuvant sequential chemoradiotherapy. Radiat Oncol. 2013;8:60.
23. Stämpfli MR, Anderson GP. How cigarette smoke skews immune responses to promote infection, lung disease and cancer. Nat Rev Immunol. 2009;9(5):377–84.
24. Sopori M. Effects of cigarette smoke on the immune system. Nat Rev Immunol. 2002;2(5):372–7.
25. Holt PG. Immune and inflammatory function in cigarette smokers. Thorax. 1987;42(4):241–9.

26. Ng SP, Silverstone AE, Lai ZW, Zelikoff JT. Effects of prenatal exposure to cigarette smoke on offspring tumor susceptibility and associated immune mechanisms. Toxicol Sci. 2006;89(1):135–44.
27. Lu LM, Zavitz CC, Chen B, Kianpour S, Wan Y, Stämpfli MR. Cigarette smoke impairs NK cell-dependent tumor immune surveillance. J Immunol. 2007;178(2):936–43.
28. Tollerud DJ, Clark JW, Brown LM, Meuland CY, Mann DL, Pankiw-Trost LK, Blattner WA, Hoover RN. Association of cigarette smoking with decreased numbers of circulating natural killer cells. Am Rev Respir Dis. 1989;139(1):194–8.
29. Vivanco I, Sawyers CL. The phosphatidylinositol 3-Kinase AKT pathway in human cancer. Nat Rev Cancer. 2002;2(7):489–501.
30. Hanahan D, Weinberg RA. Hallmarks of cancer: the next generation. Cell. 2011;144(5):646–74.
31. Billingsley KG, Lewis JJ, Leung DH, Casper ES, Woodruff JM, Brennan MF. Multifactorial analysis of the survival of patients with distant metastasis arising from primary extremity sarcoma. Cancer. 1999;85(2):389–95.
32. Coindre JM, Terrier P, Bui NB, Bonichon F, Collin F, Le Doussal V, Mandard AM, Vilain MO, Jacquemier J, Duplay H, Sastre X, Barlier C, Henry-Amar M, Macé-Lesech J, Contesso G. Prognostic factors in adult patients with locally controlled soft tissue sarcoma. A study of 546 patients from the French Federation of Cancer Centers Sarcoma Group. J Clin Oncol. 1996;14(3):869–77.
33. Mendenhall WM, Indelicato DJ, Scarborough MT, Zlotecki RA, Gibbs CP, Mendenhall NP, Mendenhall CM, Enneking WF. The management of adult soft tissue sarcomas. Am J Clin Oncol. 2009;32(4):436–42.
34. Markhede G, Angervall L, Stener B. A multivariate analysis of the prognosis after surgical treatment of malignant soft-tissue tumors. Cancer. 1982;49(8):1721–33.
35. Gaynor JJ, Tan CC, Casper ES, Collin CF, Friedrich C, Shiu M, Hajdu SI, Brennan MF. Refinement of clinicopathologic staging for localized soft tissue sarcoma of the extremity: a study of 423 adults. J Clin Oncol. 1992;10(8):1317–29.
36. Saddegh MK, Lindholm J, Lundberg A, Nilsonne U, Kreicbergs A. Staging of soft-tissue sarcomas. Prognostic analysis of clinical and pathological features. J Bone Joint Surg Br. 1992;74(4):495–500.
37. Ravaud A, Bui NB, Coindre JM, Lagarde P, Tramond P, Bonichon F, Stöckle E, Kantor G, Trojani M, Chauvergne J, Marée D. Prognostic variables for the selection of patients with operable soft tissue sarcomas to be considered in adjuvant chemotherapy trials. Br J Cancer. 1992;66(5):961–9.
38. Koh KH, Cho EY, Kim DW, Seo SW. Multivariate analysis of prognostic factors in synovial sarcoma. Orthopedics. 2009;32(11):824.
39. Spillane AJ, A'Hern R, Judson IR, Fisher C, Thomas JM. Synovial sarcoma: a clinicopathologic, staging, and prognostic assessment. J Clin Oncol. 2000;18(22):3794–803.
40. Trassard M, Le Doussal V, Hacène K, Terrier P, Ranchère D, Guillou L, Fiche M, Collin F, Vilain MO, Bertand G, Jacquemire J, Sastre-Garau X, Bui NB, Bonichon F, Coindre JM. Prognostic factors in localized primary synovial sarcoma: a multicenter study of 128 adult patients. J Clin Oncol. 2001;19(2):525–34.

27

Utility of VS38c in the diagnostic and prognostic assessment of osteosarcoma and other bone tumours/tumour-like lesions

E. S. Hookway[1], Z. Orosz[1], Y. Uchihara[1], A. Grigoriadis[2], A. B. Hassan[1], U. Oppermann[1] and N. A. Athanasou[1*]

Abstract

Background: VS38c is a monoclonal antibody that recognises a rough endoplasmic reticulum (rER) intracellular antigen termed cytoskeleton-linking membrane protein 63. rER is typically found in viable tumour cells and is abundant in osteosarcoma cells. The aim of this study was to determine the diagnostic and prognostic utility of VS38c in the histological assessment of osteosarcoma and other bone tumours/tumour-like leisons.

Methods: Immunohistochemical staining with VS38c was carried out on formalin-fixed specimens of osteosarcoma (pre/post-chemotherapy) and a wide range of benign and malignant bone lesions. In addition, VS38c staining of cultures of MG63 and Sa0S2 osteosarcoma cell cultures. (±cisplatin and actinomycin D-treatment) was analysed.

Results: VS38c strongly stained tumour cells in all low-grade and high-grade osteosarcomas and in undifferentiated sarcomas and high-grade chondrosarcomas. There was little or no VS38c staining of low-grade chondrosarcomas or chordomas and variable staining of Ewing sarcomas. Osteoblasts in benign bone-forming tumours and mononuclear stromal cells in chondroblastomas, giant cell tumours and non-ossifying fibromas strongly stained for VS38c. VS38c staining was absent in cisplatin and actinomycin D treated Sa0S2 and MG63 cells. In specimens of osteosarcoma post-neoadjuvant therapy, VS38c staining was absent in most morphologically necrotic areas of tumor although some cells with pyknotic nuclei stained for VS38c in these areas. Most tumour cells exhibiting atypical nuclear forms were not stained by VS38c.

Conclusions: Our findings show that VS38c is a sensitive but not specific diagnostic marker of osteosarcoma. Staining with VS38c identifies viable osteosarcoma cells, a feature which may be useful in the assessment of percentage tumour necrosis post-neoadjuvant chemotherapy.

Keywords: Osteosarcoma, VS38c, Rough endoplasmic reticulum, Bone tumour, Therapy

Background

VS38c is a monoclonal antibody that recognises an intracellular antigen identified as the rough endoplasmic reticulum (rER) cytoskeleton-linking membrane protein P63 (CLIMP 63) which has also been termed P63 and cytoskeletal-associated protein 4 [1]. CLIMP-63 is a stable, abundant rER protein that plays a role in protein transport. The VS38c monoclonal antibody strongly stains immunoglobulin-producing plasma cells and facilitates the immunohistochemical diagnosis of myeloma [2, 3]. VS38c staining of tumour cells in neuroendocrine carcinoma, melanoma and osteosarcoma has also been reported [4–7]. A common feature of all tumour cells that stain with VS38c is that they ultrastructurally contain numerous cytoplasmic ribosomes and abundant rER.

Regular protein production is a functional characteristic of viable cells, and loss or inactivation of ribosomes and rER has been noted in necrotic tumour cells [8, 9]. Several types of cell death involve changes in ER [10, 11], and ER stress has been shown to play a role in the necrosis of osteosarcoma cells [12–14]. Osteosarcomas are

*Correspondence: nick.athanasou@ndorms.ox.ac.uk
[1] Nuffield Department of Orthopaedics, Rheumatology and Musculoskeletal and Sciences, University of Oxford, Nuffield Orthopaedic Centre, Oxford OX3 7HE, UK

usually treated pre-operatively by a course of neoadjuvant chemotherapy with assessment of the response evaluated by determining histologically the extent of necrosis in the resected tumour specimen [15–19]; this percentage measure of tumour necrosis provides important prognostic information and gives a guide to as to whether adjuvant chemotherapy is required. Osteosarcoma cells can exhibit nuclear abnormalities post-chemotherapy and it is not certain whether such cells are viable or apoptotic in this context [20–26]. There are no formal morphological criteria that can be used to determine whether an osteosarcoma cell is viable or not and it can be difficult to assess accurately the extent of necrosis in an osteosarcoma specimen.

In this study, we have sought to determine the diagnostic and prognostic utility of VS38c in the assessment of osteosarcoma and other primary bone tumours. We have examined VS38c staining in a wide range of benign and malignant bone tumours, including osteosarcoma subtypes, in order to assess the sensitivity and specificity of this marker for the diagnosis of osteosarcoma. In addition, as ER changes have been noted in necrotic tumour cells, and active protein production is a feature of cell viability, we have examined VS38c staining in osteosarcomas that have received neoadjuvant chemotherapy in order to determine if expression of this marker can be used to identify viable tumour cells and to facilitate the evaluation of percentage tumour necrosis in osteosarcoma specimens.

Methods

Specimens analysed

Paraffin-embedded tissue from 178 specimens of bone tumours as well as specimens of normal compact and cancellous bone, femoral articular surface and growth plate, were retrieved from the files of the Nuffield Orthopedic Centre Histopathology Department, Oxford (Table 1). 61 cases of high-grade osteosarcoma were analysed including 25 cases that had histology pre/post-neoadjuvant chemotherapy. Criteria for the histological diagnosis of the bone tumours were those of the 2013 WHO Classification of Tumours of Soft Tissue and Bone [27]. Samples were derived from biopsies and resection specimens fixed in 10% buffered formalin and decalcified in 5% nitric acid. Histology was assessed using a Nikon Eclipse 80i microscope.

Immunohistochemistry

5 μm sections of formalin-fixed paraffin-embedded tissue were cut and then stained by an indirect immunoperoxidase technique using chemMate Envision (Dako, UK). After blocking endogenous peroxidase, sections were incubated with the monoclonal antibody VS38C (Dako, UK) with antigen unmasking pretreatment. Antigens were detected by incubation with labelled polymer and diaminobenzidine. Sections of myeloma were employed as a positive control. Negative controls consisted of sections which were incubated with normal mouse IgG1 (10 or 20 μg/mL, Sigma-Aldrich, Dorset, UK) substituted for the monoclonal antibody. The VS38c staining was scored as strong or weak relative to the positive control. Where the majority of lesional cells were not stained with VS38c, an assessment of the percentage of VS38-positive cells relative to the total number of (lesional) cells was noted.

Table 1 VS38c staining of benign and malignant bone tumours/tumour-like lesions

Osteoid osteoma	(4)
Osteoblastoma	(4)
Osteosarcoma—high-grade	
Osteoblastic	(46)
Chondroblastic	(6)
Telangiectatic	(6)
Giant-cell rich	(1)
Small cell	(2)
Osteosarcoma—low grade	
Intramedullary	(2)
Parosteal	(4)
Fibrous dysplasia[a]	(8)
Osteochondroma[a]	(3)
Enchondroma[a]	(6)
Chondroblastoma	(4)
Chondromyxoid fibroma[a]	(3)
Atypical cartilaginous tumour/Chondrosarcoma, Grade I	(12)
Chondrosarcoma, Grade II/III	(8)
Ewing sarcoma[a]	(16)
Giant cell tumour of bone	(12)
Aneurysmal bone cyst	(4)
Simple bone cyst	(2)
Osteofibrous dysplasia	(4)
Adamantinoma	(3)
Chordoma[a]	(6)
Undifferentiated sarcoma	(4)
Langerhans cell histiocytosis[a]	(4)
Fracture	(2)
Myositis ossificans	(2)

(), number of cases

[a] Tumours where fewer than 10% lesional stained cells with VS38c

Expression of VS38c in MG63 and Sa0S2 cells

MG63 and SAOS2 human osteosarcoma cells were cultured in Iscove's Modified Dulbecco's Medium (Sigma-Aldrich, Dorset, UK) supplemented with 10% fetal calf serum [28]. To determine expression of VSC38c, cells were plated at either low (10^5 cells) or high (10^6 cells) density in a 6 well plate and allowed to adhere overnight. Cells were then treated for 24 h in the presence of either cisplatin (1 μg/mL), actinomycin D (10 μg/mL) or vehicle control. Cultures were fixed in formalin and stained as above by immunohistochemistry with the antibody VS38c.

Results

VS38c staining of normal bone and cartilage

Strong cytoplasmic staining of osteoblasts with VS38c was noted in compact and cancellous woven and lamellar bone in areas of bone remodelling (Fig. 1). A few osteocytes in woven bone and a few marrow stromal cells and flattened bone lining cells were also weakly VS38c positive. Osteoclasts and fat cells in bone, fibroblasts in periosteal dense connective tissue, and endothelial cells/ smooth muscle cells in blood vessels were negative for VS38c. Chondrocytes in hyaline articular cartilage and in the reserve and proliferating zones of growth plate cartilage were unstained; hypertrophic and mineralizing cartilage cells in the growth plate stained with VS38c.

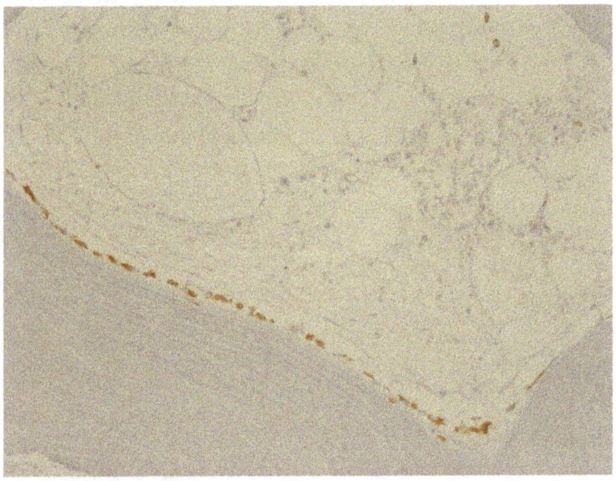

Fig. 1 Immunohistochemistry with monoclonal antibody VS38c showing strong staining of osteoblasts in remodelling cancellous bone. (original magnification ×200)

VS38c staining of osteosarcoma and other bone-forming tumours and tumour-like lesions

Tumour cells in all high-grade osteoblastic osteosarcomas (Fig. 2a), as well as small cell and telangiectatic (Fig. 2b) sub-types strongly stained for VS38c; tumour cells in chondroblastic and fibroblastic areas of high-grade osteosarcoma were also strongly stained by VS38c. VS38c also strongly stained osteogenic tumour cells in intramedullary low-grade osteosarcoma and parosteal osteosarcoma. In other primary bone-forming tumours, osteoid osteoma and osteoblastoma, there was also strong VS38c staining of osteoblasts lining the surface of woven bone; some newly formed woven bone trabeculae in these lesions also showed VS38c staining of osteocytes. In four cases of fibrous dysplasia, there was strong VS38c staining of mononuclear stromal cells in the intertrabecular fibrous tissue, the remaining cases showing little (<10%) or no staining. In osteofibrous dysplasia, VS38c strongly stained plump osteoblasts rimming woven bone and stromal cells in the fibrous stroma. Osteoblasts in reactive woven bone in fracture callus and myositis ossificans were also strongly VS38c positive.

VS38c staining of other primary bone tumours

No staining or weak staining of a few (<10%) cartilage cells was noted with VS38c in benign cartilage tumours including enchondroma, osteochondroma and chondromyxoid fibroma; some cellular enchondromas of

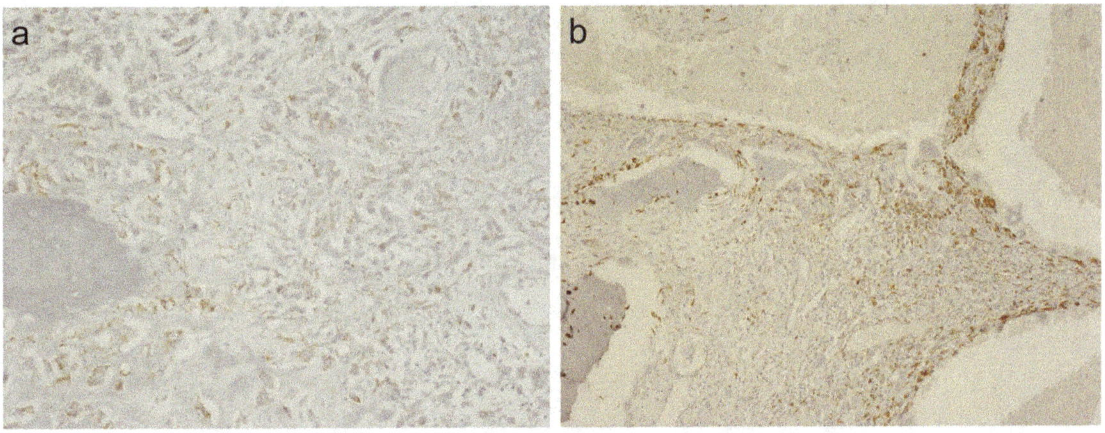

Fig. 2 Immunohistochemistry with monoclonal antibody VS38c showing strong staining of osteoid-forming tumour cells in: (**a**) high-grade osteoblastic osteosarcoma and (**b**) telangiectatic osteosarcoma. (original magnification: **a** ×200; **b** ×100)

the hand, however, showed more prominent staining of cartilage cells. In contrast, VS38c strongly stained chondroblasts in chondroblastoma. Atypical cartilaginous tumour/chondrosarcoma grade 1 showed a similar pattern of VS38c staining to that seen in most enchondromas, but malignant cells in high-grade chondrosarcomas strongly and diffusely stained with VS38c (Fig. 3a, b). In dedifferentiated chondrosarcoma, the low-grade chondrosarcoma component showed little staining with VS38c whereas the high-grade sarcoma component was strongly stained (Fig. 3c).

In giant cell tumour of bone, mononuclear cells strongly stained with VS38c but osteoclast-like giant cells were negative (Fig. 4a). A similar pattern of staining was noted in non-ossifying fibroma and aneurysmal bone cyst where reactive woven bone and scattered fibroblastic cells in the cyst wall were also stained by VS38c.

All tumor cells in primary high-grade undifferentiated spindle cell/pleomorphic sarcoma of bone stained strongly with VS38c. Ten of 16 cases of Ewing sarcoma were also strongly and diffusely stained with VS38c, (Fig. 4b), but six cases showed staining of a few (<10%) cells. Most chordomas were VS38c-negative but two cases showed weak staining of a few (<10%) cells. VS38c strongly stained adamantinomas in both epithelial and mesenchymal components.

VS38c staining of osteosarcomas receiving neoadjuvant chemotherapy

Strong VS38c staining of osteosarcoma cells was noted in all pre-treatment biopsies of the 25 cases of osteosarcoma that had received pre-operative neoadjuvant therapy. VS38c strongly stained areas containing residual viable tumour in resection specimens of these treated osteosarcomas (Fig. 5). Absence of VS38c staining was noted in areas of tumour necrosis where there was only amorphous cellular debris or ghost cells i.e. where nucleated tumour cells could not be identified morphologically (Figs. 5, 6a). In morphologically necrotic areas of tumour, a variable number of cells with pyknotic nuclei stained with VS38c (Fig. 6b). In some tumours, there were scattered atypical cells with vacuolated cytoplasm

Fig. 3 Immunohistochemistry with monoclonal antibody VS38c showing: **a** strong staining of cartilage tumour cells in high-grade chondrosarcoma; **b** absence of staining of cartilage tumour cells in low-grade chondrosarcoma; **c** in dedifferentiated chondrosarcoma absence of staining in the low-grade chondrosarcoma component and strong staining in the dedifferentiated pleomorphic sarcoma component. (original magnification: **a** ×400; **b** ×400; **c** ×100)

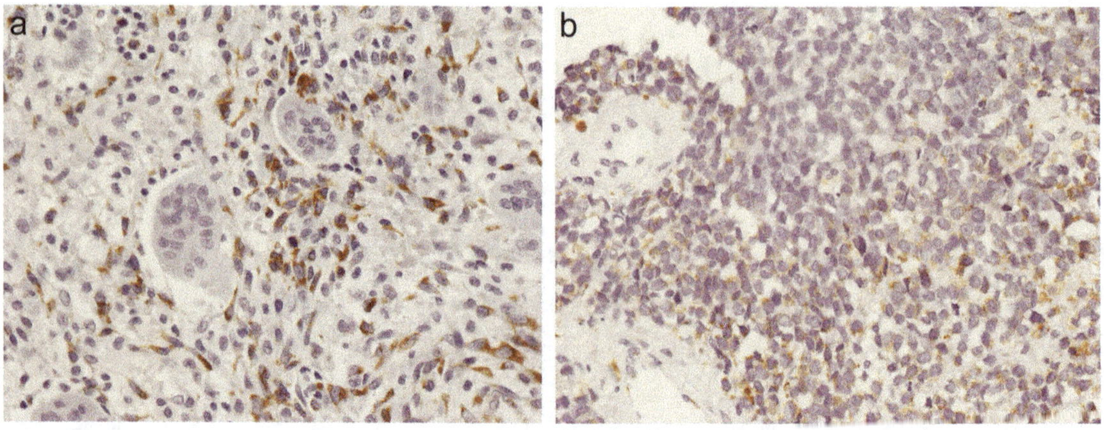

Fig. 4 Immunohistochemistry with monoclonal antibody VS38c showing: **a** staining of mononuclear cells but not giant cells in giant cell tumour of bone; and **b** staining of tumour cells in Ewing sarcoma. (original magnification: **a** ×400; **b** ×400)

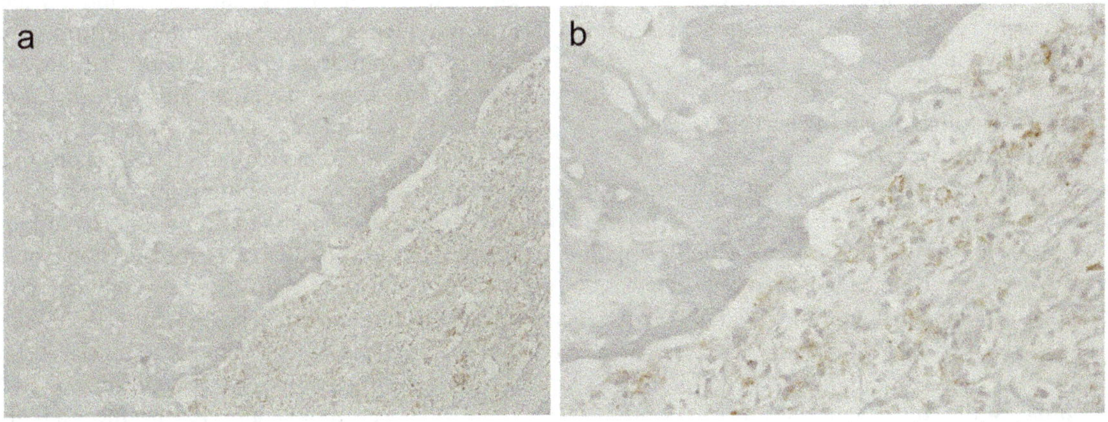

Fig. 5 Immunohistochemistry with monoclonal antibody VS38c of an osteosarcoma that had received neoadjuvant therapy showing: **a** low and **b** high-power views of VS38c staining of residual viable tumour (right) and absence of staining in necrotic areas of tumour (left) (original magnification: **a** ×100; **b** ×400)

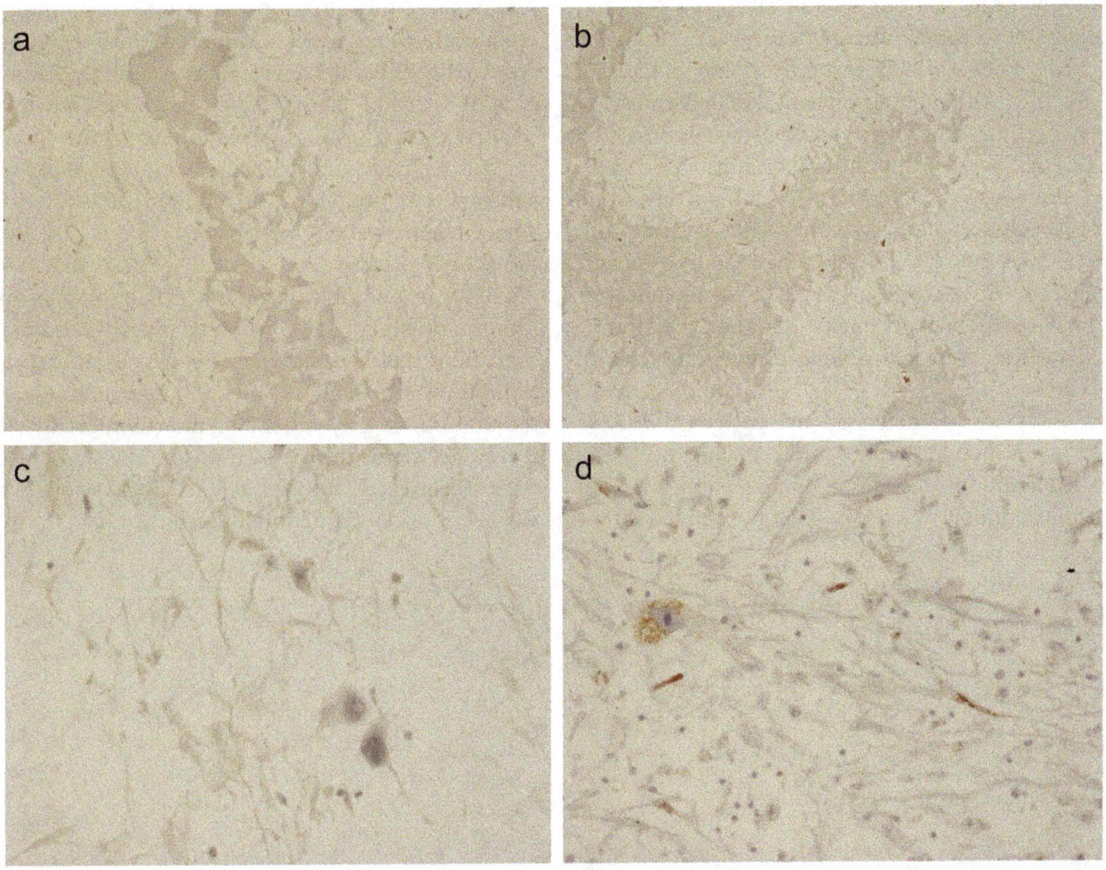

Fig. 6 Immunohistochemistry with monoclonal antibody VS38c of an osteosarcoma that had received neoadjuvant therapy showing in necrotic areas of the tumour: **a** absence and **b** variable VS38c staining of cells with pyknotic nuclei and **c** absence and **d** variable staining with VS38c of atypical cells with vacuolated cytoplasm (original magnification: **a** ×200; **b** ×200; **c** ×400; **d** ×400)

and bizarre homogenization of nuclear chromatin; most of these cells were negative for VS38c (Fig. 6c) but a few were noted to be VS38c positive (Fig. 6d).

VS38c staining of cultured osteosarcoma cells treated by cisplatin and actinomycin D

Control cultures of MG63 and Sa0S2 osteosarcoma cells contained viable tumour cells that strongly expressed VS38c (Fig. 7a). In parallel cultures to which cisplatin and actinomycin D had been added, there was necrosis of tumour cells which did not stain for VS38c (Fig. 7b).

Discussion

Osteosarcoma is the most common primary malignant tumour of bone. Histological diagnosis of osteosarcoma is based on the identification of cytologically malignant tumour cells that form osteoid/bone. These matrix protein-producing malignant cells ultrastructurally contain numerous ribosomes and rER. In this study, we have shown that tumour cells in all high-grade and low-grade osteosarcomas are stained by the monoclonal antibody VS38c which recognises the CLIMP-63 protein on rER. Although absence of VS38c expression effectively excludes the diagnosis of osteosarcoma, the diagnostic specificity of this antibody is limited because, as noted previously [5], VS38c also stains other bone tumours. Absence of staining with VS38c was noted in cultures of actinomycin D/cisplatin-treated osteosarcoma cells and in necrotic areas of (post-neoadjuvant therapy) osteosarcoma specimens, a finding which may be useful in evaluating percentage tumour necrosis in osteosarcoma.

In this study we characterised the pattern of VS38c staining in primary benign and malignant bone tumours. In addition to osteosarcoma and other benign bone-forming tumours, VS38c strongly stained other high-grade primary malignant bone tumours, including undifferentiated spindle-cell/pleomorphic sarcoma and Grade II/III chondrosarcoma. VS38c staining was also noted in most Ewing sarcomas, although the number of stained cells was highly variable. Atypical cartilaginous tumour/chondrosarcoma grade 1 and chordoma were either negative or showed little staining with VS38c. In a number of giant-cell rich lesions of bone, including giant-cell tumour, non-ossifying fibroma, chondroblastoma and aneurysmal bone cyst, VS38c strongly stained mononuclear cells but not osteoclastic giant cells. VS38c staining of such a wide range of bone tumours clearly limits its diagnostic specificity but, given its strong and consistent staining of osteosarcoma, it may be useful as a highly sensitive if not specific positive marker of this tumour.

Although a number of factors, (e.g. tumour site, size and histological subtype) influence disease survival in osteosarcoma, the extent of chemotherapy-induced necrosis has been shown to correlate most strongly with prognosis. Multi-drug neoadjuvant chemotherapy for high-grade osteosarcoma is now routinely employed and systematic pathological evaluation of the resection specimen of a treated osteosarcoma has been shown to yield important prognostic information about the chemotherapeutic response and to provide a guide as to whether adjuvant chemotherapy is required [16–19]. In cases where chemotherapy-induced necrosis is 90% or more, the 5 year disease free survival is more than 80% [27, 29–36]. Loss of ribosomes and rER is seen in necrotic tumour cells [10, 11]. We noted that, in osteosarcoma specimens that had received neoadjuvant therapy, VS38c staining was strongly positive in areas of residual viable tumour but largely absent in morphologically necrotic areas of tumour; this pattern of staining was reflected in osteosarcoma cell cultures, where VS38c strongly stained viable but not necrotic tumour cells.

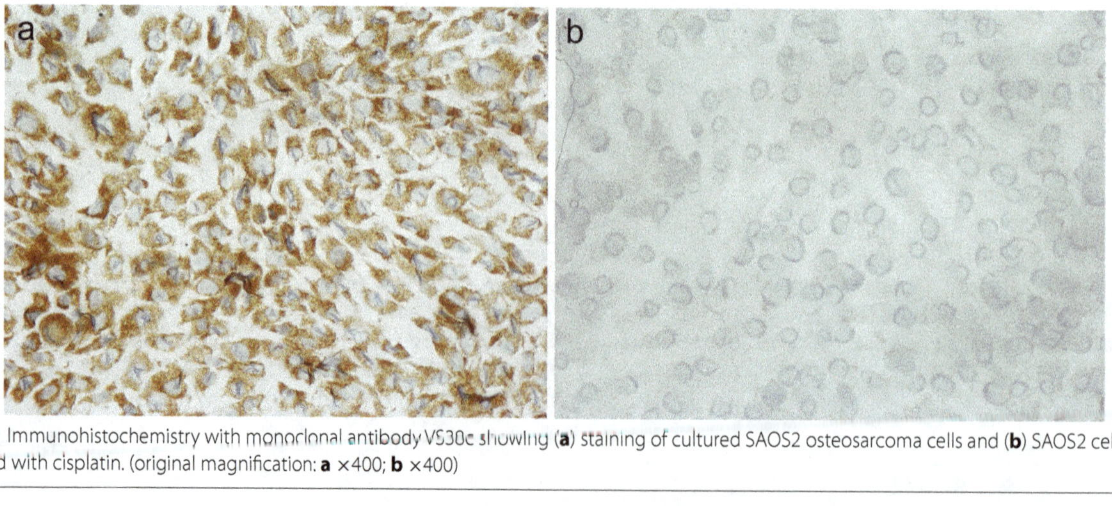

Fig. 7 Immunohistochemistry with monoclonal antibody VS38c showing (**a**) staining of cultured SAOS2 osteosarcoma cells and (**b**) SAOS2 cells treated with cisplatin. (original magnification: **a** ×400; **b** ×400)

Qualitative assessment of the percentage area of tumour necrosis in pathological specimens of osteosarcoma is believed to correlate well with quantitative morphometric analysis [15–19]. However, there are no studies, to our knowledge, which have proved that morphological assessment of tumour necrosis in osteosarcoma is accurate. Most histopathologists rely on the identification of cytoplasmic and nuclear alterations indicative of cell death, such as pyknosis, karyorrhexis and karyolysis, to determine tumour necrosis in chemotherapy-treated osteosarcomas. Necrotic areas of tumour often contain ghost cells which show a variable degree of loss of nuclear and cytoplasmic detail. However, irreversible cell death or necrosis is difficult to distinguish morphologically from reversible degenerative change or apoptosis affecting individual cells or small groups of cells. Preoperative neo-adjuvant chemotherapy of osteosarcomas not only results in necrosis, but also changes in the tumour stroma which maybe partly calcified, contain hypermineralised bone or areas of reparative fibrosis, neovascularisation and inflammation [22–24, 26]. A major challenge to the surgical pathologist is the interpretation of atypical cells containing vacuolated cytoplasm and hyperchromatic nuclei with smudged or clumped chromatin found in some post-treatment osteosarcoma specimens. These atypical cells are often found in areas where there is not only necrosis but also fibrosis and it can be difficult to determine morphologically whether such cells are apoptotic/necrotic or viable. We found that most of these cells were VS38c negative, indicating that they did not contain rER. However, a few of these cells were VS38c positive. Cells with pyknotic nuclei are not uncommonly seen in areas of tumour necrosis in post-chemotherapy osteosarcoma specimens. Pyknosis is a nuclear feature seen in both apoptotic and necrotic cells and we noted that some tumour cells with pyknotic nuclei were VS38c positive; this indicates that such cells contain rER and that they are thus potentially capable of protein production, a feature characteristic of viable tumour cells.

In conclusion, our findings indicate that VS38c is a highly sensitive but not specific diagnostic marker for osteosarcoma. VS38c staining was seen in other primary benign and malignant bone tumours but it was not prominent in some low-grade tumours such as atypical cartilaginous tumour. VS38c staining outlined areas of residual viable tumour in post-chemotherapy osteosarcoma specimens and aided assessment of percentage tumor necrosis. However, although there was little or no VS38c staining in most areas of tumour necrosis in osteosarcoma specimens, there was variable staining of atypical cells with clumped chromatin and vacuolated cytoplasm and cells with pyknotic nuclei. The status of these VS38c positive cells in these necrotic areas is uncertain and more studies are needed to determine whether the morphological assessment of percentage tumour necrosis truly reflects the extent of viable and necrotic tumour in osteosarcoma specimens.

Authors' contributions

EH collected and analysed the data and contributed to writing the manuscript. ZO and YU collected data. AG, AH, and UO interpreted the data and contributed to the writing of the manuscript. NA conceived the experiments, analysed the data and wrote the manuscript. All authors read and approved the final manuscript.

Author details

[1] Nuffield Department of Orthopaedics, Rheumatology and Musculoskeletal and Sciences, University of Oxford, Nuffield Orthopaedic Centre, Oxford OX3 7HE, UK. [2] Department of Craniofacial Development and Stem Cell Biology, Guy's Hospital, King's College, London, UK.

Acknowledgements

We would like to thank Sarah Turton for typing the manuscript.

Competing interests

The authors declare that they have no competing interests.

Funding

This study was supported by the European Union through funding of the EuroBoNet and Eurosarc consortiums. The funders played no role in the design of experiments, collection of data, interpretation of results or writing the manuscript.

References

1. Sandoz PA. Gisou van der Gout. How many lives does CLIMP 63 have? Biochem Soc Trans. 2015;43:222–8.
2. Turley H, Jones M, Erber W, Mayne K, de Waele M, Gatter K. VS38: a new monoclonal antibody for detecting plasma cell differentiation in routine sections. J Clin Pathol. 1994;47:418–22.
3. Banham AH, Turley H, Pulford K, Gatter K, Mason DY. The plasma cell associated antigen detectable by antibody VS38 is the p63 rough endoplasmic reticulum protein. J Clin Pathol. 1997;50:485–9.
4. Banerjee SS, Shanks JH, Hasleton PS. VS38 immunostaining in neuroendocrine tumours. Histopathology. 1997;30:256–9.
5. Sulzbacher I, Fuchs M, Chott A, Lang S. Expression of VS38 in osteoblasts and stroma cells of bone tumors. Pathol Res Pract. 1997;193:613–6.
6. Al-Janabi K, Cassidy M. Specificity of plasma cell antibody VS38. J Clin Pathol. 1996;49:694.
7. Shanks JH, Banerjee SS. VS38 immunostaining in melanocytic lesions. J Clin Pathol. 1996;49:205–7.
8. Orvoine RH, Messier PE, Cantin M, Seidman JM. Light and electron microscope study of osmotically induced tumor necrosis. Cancer Res. 1978;38:1960–6.
9. Pelletier N, Casamayor-Pallejà M, De Luca K, Mondière P, Saltel F, Jurdic P, et al. The endoplasmic reticulum is a key component of the plasma cell death pathway. J Immunol. 2006;176:1340–7.
10. Galluzzi L, Maiuri MC, Vitale I, Zischka H, Castedo M, Zitvogel L, et al. Cell death modalities: classification and pathophysiological implications. Cell Death Differ. 2007;14:1237–43.
11. Kroemer G, Galluzzi L, Vandenabeele P, Abrams J, Alnemri ES, Baehrecke EH, et al. Classification of cell death: recommendations of the Nomenclature Committee on cell death. Cell Death Differ. 2009;16:3–11.
12. Chiu H-W, Tseng Y-C, Hsu Y-H, Lin Y-F, Foo N-P, Guo H-R, et al. Arsenic trioxide induces programmed cell death through stimulation of ER stress and inhibition of the ubiquitin–proteasome system in human sarcoma cells. Cancer Lett. 2015;356:762–72.

13. Kamiński M, Masaoka M, Karbowski M, Kedzior J, Nishizawa Y, Usukura J, et al. Ultrastructural basis for the transition of cell death mode from apoptosis to necrosis in menadione-treated osteosarcoma 143B cells. J Electron Microsc (Tokyo). 2003;52:313–25.
14. Tao H, Tao L, Shen C, Liu B, Yang Z, Tao H. Silencing of Barkor/ATG14 sensitizes osteosarcoma cells to cisplatin-induced apoptosis. Int J Mol Med. 2013;33:271–6.
15. Rosen G, Caparros B, Huvos AG, Kosloff C, Nirenberg A, Cacavio A, et al. Preoperative chemotherapy for osteogenic sarcoma: selection of post-operative adjuvant chemotherapy based on the response of the primary tumor to preoperative chemotherapy. Cancer. 1982;49:1221–30.
16. Raymond AK, Chawla SP, Carrasco CH, Ayala AG, Fanning CV, Grice B, et al. Osteosarcoma chemotherapy effect: a prognostic factor. Semin Diagn Pathol. 1987;4:212–36.
17. Bramwell VH, Burgers M, Sneath R, Souhami R, van Oosterom AT, Voûte PA, et al. A comparison of two short intensive adjuvant chemotherapy regimens in operable osteosarcoma of limbs in children and young adults: the first study of the European Osteosarcoma Intergroup. J Clin Oncol. 1992;10:1579–91.
18. Davis AM, Bell RS, Goodwin PJ. Prognostic factors in osteosarcoma: a critical review. J Clin Oncol. 1994;12:423–31.
19. Saeter G, Elomaa I, Wahlqvist Y, Alvegård TA, Wiebe T, Monge O, et al. Prognostic factors in bone sarcomas. Acta Orthop Scand. 1997;68(Suppl 273):156–60.
20. Patterson K. The pathologic handling of skeletal tumors. Am J Clin Pathol. 1998;109(4 Suppl 1):S53–66.
21. Wold LE. Practical approach to processing osteosarcomas in the surgical pathology laboratory. Pediatr Dev Pathol. 1998;1:449–54.
22. Huvos AG, Rosen G, Marcove RC. Primary osteogenic sarcoma: pathologic aspects in 20 patients after treatment with chemotherapy en bloc resection, and prosthetic bone replacement. Arch Pathol Lab Med. 1977;101:14–8.
23. Picci P, Bacci G, Campanacci M, Gasparini M, Pilotti S, Cerasoli S, et al. Histologic evaluation of necrosis in osteosarcoma induced by chemotherapy. Regional mapping of viable and nonviable tumor. Cancer. 1985;56:1515–21.
24. Ayala AG, Raymond AK, Jaffe N. The pathologist's role in the diagnosis and treatment of osteosarcoma in children. Hum Pathol. 1984;15:258–66.
25. Weatherby RP, Unni KK. Practical aspects of handling orthopedic specimens in the surgical pathology laboratory. Pathol Annu. 1982;17(Pt 2):1–31.
26. Coffin CM, Lowichik A, Zhou H. Treatment effects in pediatric soft tissue and bone tumors. Am J Clin Pathol. 2005;123:75–90.
27. Fletcher CDM, Bridge JA, Hogendoorn PCW, Mertens F. editors. WHO classification of tumours of soft tissue and bone, 4th edn. Lyon: IARC; 2013.
28. Athanasou NA. Cell and organ culture in the understanding of the bone and its neoplasms. In: Helliwell TR, editors. Pathology of bone and joint neoplasms. Saunders: Philadelphia; 1999. p. 34–58.
29. Dahlin DC. Osteosarcoma of bone and a consideration of prognostic variables. Cancer Treat Rep. 1978;62:189–92.
30. Goidanich IF, Battaglia L, Lenzi L, Silva E. Osteogenic sarcoma analysis of factors influencing prognosis in 100 cases. Clin Orthop Relat Res. 1966;48:209–22.
31. Hauben EI, Weeden S, Pringle J, Van Marck EA, Hogendoorn PCW. Does the histological subtype of high-grade central osteosarcoma influence the response to treatment with chemotherapy and does it affect overall survival? A study on 570 patients of two consecutive trials of the European Osteosarcoma Intergroup. Eur J Cancer. 2002;38:1218–25.
32. Bacci G, Bertoni F, Longhi A, Ferrari S, Forni C, Biagini R, et al. Neoadjuvant chemotherapy for high-grade central osteosarcoma of the extremity. Cancer. 2003;97:3068–75.
33. Glasser DB, Lane JM, Huvos AG, Marcove RC, Rosen G. Survival, prognosis, and therapeutic response in osteogenic sarcoma. The Memorial Hospital experience. Cancer. 1992;69:698–708.
34. Rosen G, Marcove RC, Caparros B, Nirenberg A, Kosloff C, Huvos AG. Primary osteogenic sarcoma: the rationale for preoperative chemotherapy and delayed surgery. Cancer. 1979;43:2163–77.
35. Benjamin RS, Chawla SP, Carrasco CH, Raymond AK, Murray JA, Armen T, et al. Preoperative chemotherapy for osteosarcoma with intravenous adriamycin and intra-arterial cis-platinum. Ann Oncol. 1992;3(suppl_2):S3–6.
36. Willén H. Tumor necrosis and prognosis in osteosarcoma. Acta Orthop Scand. 1997;68(Suppl 273):126–9.

Permissions

All chapters in this book were first published in CSR, by BioMed Central; hereby published with permission under the Creative Commons Attribution License or equivalent. Every chapter published in this book has been scrutinized by our experts. Their significance has been extensively debated. The topics covered herein carry significant findings which will fuel the growth of the discipline. They may even be implemented as practical applications or may be referred to as a beginning point for another development.

The contributors of this book come from diverse backgrounds, making this book a truly international effort. This book will bring forth new frontiers with its revolutionizing research information and detailed analysis of the nascent developments around the world.

We would like to thank all the contributing authors for lending their expertise to make the book truly unique. They have played a crucial role in the development of this book. Without their invaluable contributions this book wouldn't have been possible. They have made vital efforts to compile up to date information on the varied aspects of this subject to make this book a valuable addition to the collection of many professionals and students.

This book was conceptualized with the vision of imparting up-to-date information and advanced data in this field. To ensure the same, a matchless editorial board was set up. Every individual on the board went through rigorous rounds of assessment to prove their worth. After which they invested a large part of their time researching and compiling the most relevant data for our readers.

The editorial board has been involved in producing this book since its inception. They have spent rigorous hours researching and exploring the diverse topics which have resulted in the successful publishing of this book. They have passed on their knowledge of decades through this book. To expedite this challenging task, the publisher supported the team at every step. A small team of assistant editors was also appointed to further simplify the editing procedure and attain best results for the readers.

Apart from the editorial board, the designing team has also invested a significant amount of their time in understanding the subject and creating the most relevant covers. They scrutinized every image to scout for the most suitable representation of the subject and create an appropriate cover for the book.

The publishing team has been an ardent support to the editorial, designing and production team. Their endless efforts to recruit the best for this project, has resulted in the accomplishment of this book. They are a veteran in the field of academics and their pool of knowledge is as vast as their experience in printing. Their expertise and guidance has proved useful at every step. Their uncompromising quality standards have made this book an exceptional effort. Their encouragement from time to time has been an inspiration for everyone.

The publisher and the editorial board hope that this book will prove to be a valuable piece of knowledge for researchers, students, practitioners and scholars across the globe.

List of Contributors

Emilie P Buddingh, S Eriaty N Ruslan, R Maarten Egeler and Arjan C Lankester
Department of Pediatrics, J6-S, Leiden University Medical Center, 2300 RC Leiden, The Netherlands

Christianne M A Reijnders, Marieke L Kuijjer, Pancras C W Hogendoorn and Anne-Marie Cleton-Jansen
Department of Pathology, Leiden University Medical Center, Leiden, The Netherlands

Karoly Szuhai
Department of Molecular Cell Biology, Leiden University Medical Center, Leiden, The Netherlands

Helene Roelofs
Department of Immunohematology and Blood Transfusion, Leiden University Medical Center, Leiden, The Netherlands

L. Gatto, M. Nannini and M. Saponara
Department of Specialized, Experimental, and Diagnostic Medicine, S.Orsola-Malpighi Hospital, University of Bologna, Bologna, Italy

G. Brandi, G. Biasco and M. A. Pantaleo
Department of Specialized, Experimental, and Diagnostic Medicine, S.Orsola-Malpighi Hospital, University of Bologna, Bologna, Italy
Interdepartmental Centre of Cancer Research "G. Prodi", University of Bologna, Bologna, Italy

V. Di Scioscio
Department of Radiology, S.Orsola Malpighi Hospital, Bologna University, Bologna, Italy

G. Beltramo
Centro Diagnostico Italiano, Reparto Cyberknife, Milan, Italy

G. P. Frezza
Radiation Oncology Unit, Bellaria Hospital, Bologna, Italy

G. Ercolani and A. D. Pinna
Department of General and Emergency Surgery and Organ Transplantation, S. Orsola-Malpighi Hospital, University of Bologna, Bologna, Italy

A. Astoli and M. Urbini
Interdepartmental Centre of Cancer Research "G. Prodi", University of Bologna, Bologna, Italy

Kirsten Sundby Hall
Department of Oncology, Oslo University Hospital, The Norwegian Radium Hospital, Ullernchausseen 70, 0379 Oslo, Norway

Oyvind Bruland
Department of Oncology, Oslo University Hospital, The Norwegian Radium Hospital, Ullernchausseen 70, 0379 Oslo, Norway
Institute for Clinical Medicine, Faculty of Medicine, University of Oslo, Blindern, 0450 Oslo, Norway

Mercy Varghese
Department of Oncology, Oslo University Hospital, The Norwegian Radium Hospital, Ullernchausseen 70, 0379 Oslo, Norway
Department of Surgery, Nordland Hospital, 8092 Bodoe, Norway

Anne Marit Wiedswang
Department of Radiology, Oslo University Hospital, The Norwegian Radium Hospital, Ullernchausseen 70, 0379 Oslo, Norway

Ingvild Lobmaier
Department of Pathology, Oslo University Hospital, The Norwegian Radium Hospital, Ullernchausseen 70, 0379 Oslo, Norway

Bård Røsok
Gastrointestinal and pediatric surgery, Section for Hepatopancreatobiliary Surgery, Oslo University Hospital Rikshospitalet, Sognsvannsveien 20, 0424 Oslo, Norway

Robert S. Benjamin
Department of Sarcoma Medical Oncology, The University of Texas M. D. Anderson Cancer Center, Texas, Houston 77030, USA

Rohan Gupta, Neda Heshami and Chouhan Jay
The University of Texas at Houston Internal Medicine Residency Program, Houston, TX, USA

Naveen Ramesh
The University of Texas Graduate School of Biomedical Sciences at Houston, Houston, TX, USA

Juhee Song and Xiudong Lei
Division of Quantitative Sciences, The University of Texas MD Anderson Cancer Center, Houston, TX, USA

Erfe Jean Rose and Joseph L. Nates
Department of Critical Care, The University of Texas MD Anderson Cancer Center, Houston, TX, USA

Kristen Carter, Dejka M. Araujo, Robert S. Benjamin, Shreyaskumar Patel and Vinod Ravi
Department of Sarcoma Medical Oncology, The University of Texas MD Anderson Cancer Center, 1515 Holcombe Blvd # 450, Houston, TX 77030, USA

Bernadette Brennan
Department of Paediatric Oncology, Royal Manchester Children's Hospital, Oxford Road, Manchester M13 9WL, UK

Nicola Dennis and Matthew Francis
Knowledge and Intelligence Service West Midlands, Public Health England, Birmingham, UK

Charles Stiller and John Broggio
National Cancer Registration and Analysis Service, Public Health England, Birmingham, UK

Robert Grimer
Department of Orthopaedic Oncology, Royal Orthopaedic Hospital, Birmingham, UK

Rahul Rajeev, Mohit Patel, Thejus T. Jayakrishnan, Fabian M. Johnston and Kiran K. Turaga
Division of Surgical Oncology, Department of Surgery, Medical College of Wisconsin, 9200 West Wisconsin Avenue, Milwaukee, WI 53226, USA

Meena Bedi
Department of Radiation Oncology, Medical College of Wisconsin, 8701 Watertown Plank Rd., Milwaukee, WI 53226, USA

John Charlson
Section of Hematology and Oncology, Medical College of Wisconsin, 9200 West Wisconsin Avenue, Milwaukee, WI 53226, USA

Emanuela Marchesi and Irene Quattrini
Italian Sarcoma Group, Istituto Ortopedico Rizzoli, Via Pupilli 1, 40136 Bologna, Italy

Celeste Cagnazzo, Giovanni Grignani and Lorenzo D'Ambrosio
Division of Medical Oncology, Candiolo Cancer Institute-FPO, IRCCS, Candiolo, Italy

Martina Piccinni Leopardi
Chemotherapy Unit, Orthopedic Rizzoli Institute, Bologna, Italy

Chiara Villa, Silvia Stacchiotti and Paolo Giovanni Casali
Adult Mesenchymal Tumour and Rare Cancer Medical Oncology Unit, Fondazione IRCCS Istituto Nazionale Tumori, Milan, Italy

Piero Picci
Laboratory of Experimental Oncology, Orthopedic Rizzoli Institute, Bologna, Italy

Susie Bae and Jayesh Desai
Department of Medical Oncology, Peter MacCallum Cancer Centre, St Andrews Place, East Melbourne, VIC 3002, Australia

Philip Crowe
Department of Surgery, Prince of Wales Hospital, Barker St, Randwick, NSW 2031, Australia

Raghu Gowda
Department of Radiation Oncology, Royal Adelaide Hospital, North Terrace, Adelaide, SA 5000, Australia

Warren Joubert
Department of Medical Oncology, Princess Alexandra Hospital, 199 Ipswich Rd, Woolloongabba, QLD 4102, Australia

Richard Carey-Smith
Department of Orthopaedic Surgery, Sir Charles Gardner Hospital, Hospital Ave, Nedlands, WA 6009, Australia

Paul Stalley
Department of Orthopaedic Surgery, Royal Prince Alfred Hospital, Missenden Rd, Camperdown, NSW 2050, Australia

Ian Judson
The Institute of Cancer Research, Royal Marsden NHS Foundation Trust, Fulham Road, London SW3 6JJ, UK

Ramesh Bulusu
Addenbrooke's Hospital, Cambridge University Hospitals, Cambridge, UK

Beatrice Seddon
University College Hospital, University College London Hospitals NHS Foundation Trust, London, UK

Adam Dangoor
Bristol Cancer Institute, University Hospitals, Bristol NHS Trust, Bristol, UK

Newton Wong
Southmead Hospital, North Bristol NHS Trust, Bristol, UK

Satvinder Mudan
Royal Marsden NHS Foundation Trust London, London, UK

Robert M. Conry
Division of Hematology Oncology, University of Alabama at Birmingham, 2145 Bonner Way, Birmingham, AL 35243, USA

Michael G. Rodriguez
Department of Radiology, University of Alabama at Birmingham, 619 19th St South, Birmingham, AL 35249, USA

Joseph G. Pressey
Department of Pediatrics, University of Alabama at Birmingham, 1600 7th Avenue South, Birmingham, AL 35233, USA
Cancer & Blood Disorders Institute, Cincinnati Children's Hospital Medical Center, Cincinnati, OH, USA

G M O'Kane, E M Walsh, R Emerson and D N Carney
Department of Medical Oncology, Mater Misericordiae University Hospital, Eccles Street, Dublin 7, Ireland

K A Cadoo
Gynaecologic Medical Oncology Service, Memorial Sloan-Kettering Cancer Centre, 300 East 66th Street, New York, NY 10065, USA

P Dervan and C O'Keane
Department of Histopathology, Mater Misericordiae University Hospital, Eccles Street, Dublin 7, Ireland

B Hurson, G O'Toole and S Dudeney
Department of Orthopaedic Surgery, Cappagh National Orthopaedic Hospital, Finglas, Dublin 11, Ireland

E Kavanagh and S Eustace
5 Department of Radiology, Mater Misericordiae University Hospital, Eccles Street,Dublin 7, Ireland

Lars Tharun
Institute of Pathology, University Hospital Cologne, Cologne, Germany

Eva Roth
Department of Pediatric Oncology, Hematology and Immunology, University Hospital Heidelberg, Heidelberg, Germany

Dominik Sturm
Department of Pediatric Oncology, Hematology and Immunology, University Hospital Heidelberg, Heidelberg, Germany
Division of Pediatric Neurooncology, German Cancer Consortium (DKTK), German Cancer Research Center (DKFZ), Heidelberg, Germany

Christoph Plass
Division of Epigenomics and Cancer Risk Factors, German Cancer Research Center (DKFZ), Heidelberg, Germany

Iver Petersen
Institute of Pathology, University Hospital, Jena, Germany

Uta Flucke
Department of Pathology, Radboud University Hospital, Nijmegen, The Netherlands

Craig Gerrand
Newcastle upon Tyne Hospitals NHS Foundation Trust, Freeman Hospital, Newcastle upon Tyne NE7 7DN, UK

Nick Athanasou
Nuffield Orthopaedic Centre, Oxford OX3 7LD, UK

Bernadette Brennan
Royal Manchester Children's Hospital, Manchester M13 9WL, UK

Robert Grimer
Royal Orthopaedic Hospital, Birmingham B31 2AP, UK

Ian Judson
The Royal Marsden, Sutton SM2 5PT, UK

Bruce Morland
Birmingham Children's Hospital, Birmingham B4 6NH, UK

David Peake
Queen Elizabeth Hospital, Birmingham B15 2TH, UK

Beatrice Seddon and Jeremy Whelan
University College Hospital, London NW1 2PG, UK

Jason Joseph, Naveen Ramesh, Robert Benjamin, Shreyaskumar Patel and Vinod Ravi
Department of Sarcoma Medical Oncology, Unit 0450, The University of Texas MD Anderson Cancer Center, 1515 Holcombe Blvd., Houston, TX 77030, USA

Wei-lien Wang
Department of Pathology, The University of Texas MD Anderson Cancer Center, Houston, TX, USA

Madhavi Patnana
Department of Diagnostic Radiology, The University of Texas MD Anderson Cancer Center, Houston, TX, USA

Catherine McCarthy
Department of Radiology, Nuffield Orthopaedic Centre, Windmill Road, Oxford OX3 7HE, UK

Monika Hofer and Olaf Ansorge
Department of Neuropathology, Oxford University Hospitals Oxford, Oxford OX3 9DU, UK

Marianna Vlychou and Nick A. Athanasou
Nuffield Department of Orthopaedics, Rheumatology and Musculoskeletal Sciences, Nuffield Orthopaedic Centre, University of Oxford, Windmill Road, Oxford OX3 7HE, UK

Robar Khundkar and Paul Critchley
Sarcoma Service, Nuffield Orthopedic Centre, Windmill Road, Oxford OX3 7HE, UK

Simon Cudlip
Department of Neurosurgery, Oxford University Hospitals, Oxford OX3 9DU, UK

Michael Ziegele and David M. King
Department of Orthopaedic Surgery, Medical College of Wisconsin, 9200 West Wisconsin Ave, Milwaukee, WI 53226, USA

Manpreet Bedi
Department of Radiation Oncology, Medical College of Wisconsin, 9200 West Wisconsin Ave, Milwaukee, WI 53226, USA

Sarah Bétrian and Christine Chevreau
Departments of Oncology and Clinical Research, Institut Claudius Regaud, Institut Universitaire du Cancer, Toulouse Oncopole, 1 avenue Irène Joliot-Curie, 31059 Toulouse Cedex, France

Christophe Bergeron and Perrine Marec-Berard
Departments of Oncology and Clinical Research, Centre Léon Berard and Institut d'Hématologie et d'Oncologie Pédiatrique, Lyon, France

Jean-Yves Blay, Philippe A. Cassier, Jérome Fayette and Isabelle Ray-Coquard
Departments of Oncology and Clinical Research, Centre Léon Berard, Lyon, France

Emmanuelle Bompas
Departments of Oncology and Clinical Research, Institut de Cancérologie de l'Ouest, Rene Gauducheau, St Herblain, France

Laure Chevallier and Magali Girodet
Clinical Research Department, CRA, Centre Léon Berard, Lyon, France

Cécile Guillemet
Departments of Oncology and Clinical Research, Centre Henri Becquerel, Rouen, France

Axel Le Cesne
Departments of Oncology and Clinical Research, Institut Gustave Roussy, Paris, France

Jens Jakob
Department of Surgery, Division of Surgical Oncology, University Hospital Mannheim, University of Heidelberg, Mannheim, Germany

Henry G. Smith, Michelle J. Wilkinson, Tim Pencavel, Aisha B. Miah, Joseph M. Thomas, Dirk C. Strauss and Andrew J. Hayes
Sarcoma Unit, Department of Academic Surgery, Royal Marsden Hospital NHS Foundation Trust, Fulham Road, London SW3 6JJ, UK

Per-Ulf Tunn
Department of Orthopedic Oncology,Helios Klinikum Berlin-Buch, Sarcoma Center Berlin-Brandenburg, Berlin, Germany

Lothar R. Pilz
Medical Faculty Mannheim, University of Heidelberg, Mannheim, Germany.

Peter Hohenberger
Department of Surgery, Division of Surgical Oncology and Thoracic Surgery, University Hospital Mannheim, University of Heidelberg, Mannheim, Germany

Marco Gambarotti, Piero Picci and Daniel Vanel
Department of Pathology, Rizzoli Institute, Bologna, Italy

Angelo Paolo Dei Tos
Department of Pathology, Rizzoli Institute, Bologna, Italy
Department of Pathology, Treviso Regional Hospital, Treviso, Italy
University of Padua School of Medicine, Padua, Italy

Alberto Righi
Department of Pathology, Rizzoli Institute, Bologna, Italy
Istituto Ortopedico Rizzoli, Via di Barbiano 1/10, 40136 Bologna, Italy

Marta Sbaraglia
Department of Pathology, Treviso Regional Hospital, Treviso, Italy

Giuseppe Bianchi
Orthopaedic Oncology Department, Rizzoli Institute, Bologna, Italy

Nicholas Calvert, Richard Carey-Smith and David Wood
Department of Orthopaedic Surgery, Sir Charles Gairdner Hospital, Nedlands, WA 6009, Australia

Evan Ingley
Murdoch University, Murdoch, WA 6150, Australia
Harry Perkins Institute of Medical Research, The University of Western Australia, 6 Verdun Street, Nedlands, WA 6009, Australia

Jiansha Wu and Sophie Sneddon
Harry Perkins Institute of Medical Research, The University of Western Australia, 6 Verdun Street, Nedlands, WA 6009, Australia

Jennifer Woodhouse
Hollywood Functional Rehabilitation Centre, 117 Stirling Hwy, Nedlands, WA 6009, Australia

Kristin Teiken, Mark Kuehnel, Hans Kreipe, Florian Laenger, Kais Hussein and Danny Jonigk
Institute of Pathology, Hannover Medical School (MHH), Carl-Neuberg-Str. 1, 30625 Hannover, Germany

Jan Rehkaemper
Institute of Pathology, University of Muenster, Domagkstraße 17, 48149 Muenster, Germany

Catherine L. McCarthy, Christopher L. M. H. Gibbons, Kevin M. Bradley, A. Bass Hassan, Henk Giele and Nicholas A. Athanasou
Nuffield Orthopaedic Centre, Windmill Road, Headington, Oxford OX3 7HE, UK

M. Libertini, Z. Szucs and C. Benson
Sarcoma Unit, Royal Marsden NHS Foundation Trust, London, UK

I. Mitra
Sarcoma Unit, Royal Marsden NHS Foundation Trust, London, UK
Department of Radiology, The Royal Marsden NHS Foundation Trust, 203 Fulham Road, London SW3 6JJ, UK

C. Messiou
Sarcoma Unit, Royal Marsden NHS Foundation Trust, London, UK
Department of Radiology, The Royal Marsden NHS Foundation Trust, 203 Fulham Road, London SW3 6JJ, UK
Institute of Cancer Research, Sutton, UK

W. T. A. van der Graaf, A. B. Miah, I. Judson, R. L. Jones and E. Moskovic
Sarcoma Unit, Royal Marsden NHS Foundation Trust, London, UK
Institute of Cancer Research, Sutton, UK

K. Thomas
Department of Radiology, The Royal Marsden NHS Foundation Trust, 203 Fulham Road, London SW3 6JJ, UK

Rohan C. Parikh and Sean D. Candrilli
RTI Health Solutions, 200 Park Offices Drive, Research Triangle Park, NC 27560, USA

Maria Lorenzo
Eli Lilly and Company Limited, Lilly Research Centre, Erl Wood Manor, Sunninghill Road, Windlesham, Surrey GU20 6PH, UK

Lisa M. Hess and Steven Nicol
Eli Lilly and Company, Lilly Corporate Center, Indianapolis, IN 46285, USA

James A. Kaye
RTI Health Solutions, 307 Waverley Oaks Road, Suite 101, Waltham, MA 02452, USA

Jie Xu, Lu Xie and Wei Guo
Peking University People's Hospital, Beijing 100044, China

Nicholas P. Gannon and David M. King
Department of Orthopaedic Surgery, Medical College of Wisconsin, Milwaukee, WI 53226, USA

Manpreet Bedi
Department of Radiation Oncology, Medical College of Wisconsin, 9200 West Wisconsin Ave, Milwaukee, WI 53226, USA

E. S. Hookway, Z. Orosz, Y. Uchihara, A. B. Hassan, U. Oppermann and N. A. Athanasou
Nuffield Department of Orthopaedics, Rheumatology and Musculoskeletal and Sciences, University of Oxford, Nuffield Orthopaedic Centre, Oxford OX3 7HE, UK

A. Grigoriadis
Department of Craniofacial Development and Stem Cell Biology, Guy's Hospital, King's College, London, UK

Index

www.ingramcontent.com/pod-product-compliance
Lightning Source LLC
LaVergne TN
LVHW080918210926
848485LV00004B/681